Pain Relief in Advanced Cancer

This book is dedicated to Andy and Vicki as representatives of the many patients with whom I have been privileged to share in professional partnership, and to my wife, Deirdre, my children and my colleagues at Sir Michael Sobell House.

For Churchill Livingstone

Copy editor: Susan Brown
Production controller: Mark Sanderson
Design: Design Resources Unit and Charles Simpson
Sales promotion executive: Maria O'Connor

Pain Relief in Advanced Cancer

Robert Twycross MA DM FRCP

Macmillan Clinical Reader in Palliative Medicine, University of Oxford
Consultant Physician, Sir Michael Sobell House, Churchill Hospital, Oxford
Senior Research Fellow, St Peter's College, Oxford
Director, WHO Collaborating Centre for Palliative Cancer Care
Chairman, International School for Cancer Care

Churchill Livingstone
EDINBURGH
LONDON
MADRID
MELBOURNE
NEW YORK
AND
TOKYO
1994

CHURCHILL LIVINGSTONE
Medical Division of Longman Group Ltd

Distributed in the United States of America by Churchill
Livingstone Inc., 650 Avenue of the Americas, New York,
N. Y. 10011, and by associated companies, branches and
representatives throughout the world.

First published 1994

ISBN 0–443–04119–9

British Library Cataloguing in Publication Data
A catalogue record for this book is available from the British
Library.

Library of Congress Cataloguing in Publication Data
A catalog record for this book is available from the library of
congress.

Produced by Longman Singapore Publishers (Pte) Ltd.
Printed in Singapore

Contents

Preface

It is over 10 years since 'Symptom control in far advanced cancer: pain relief', the forerunner to this book, was published. Since then there has been a dramatic increase in knowledge about pain mechanisms, analgesics and pain relief. This is reflected in the expansion from 17 to 27 chapters. The book has been written primarily with the Senior Registrar in Palliative Medicine in mind — to provide a sound basis for future specialist medical practice. It will also be of value to doctors already established in palliative care, particularly those who teach.

The original book was co-authored by Sylvia Lack, who works in the USA. This gave it a transatlantic flavour. It has not been possible to continue this partnership, and the transatlantic dimension has inevitably decreased. On the other hand, my involvement with several other countries has resulted in a broader international dimension. Thus, drugs not currently available in the UK (or the USA) such as dipyrone and tramadol are included. Likewise, the Edmonton injector is discussed alongside the syringe driver.

The amount of data and information currently being brought into the public domain is staggering. It makes the attempt to provide a relatively comprehensive and relatively cheap textbook on the relief of cancer pain an impossible task. A secondary aim of the book, however, is to enable the reader to participate more fully in conferences on pain. If this aim is achieved, the effort of preparation will be adequately rewarded.

There are inevitably still areas of controversy including, in some instances, definition of terms. I have, however, tried to indicate where terms are those of the International Association for the Study of Pain and where not. The emerging consensus concerning neuropathic pain is, I think, fairly represented.

Some readers will, of course, wish to pursue their personal study of cancer pain beyond the contents of this book. The range of available textbooks is daunting. However, the third edition of the *Textbook of Pain* (Wall PD,

Melzack R (eds) Churchill Livingstone, Edinburgh 1993) and the *Proceedings of the VIIth World Congress* are recommended as sources for further reading, together with the new *Pain Reviews* journal.

My debt to colleagues both local and distant is considerable. Some have provided references and articles; others have answered innumerable questions on specific topics; others have commented on the early drafts of some chapters. Ray Hill and Jennifer Laird were particularly helpful in relation to basic pain mechanisms. Chris Fenn gave much advice about gastric injury and nonsteroidal anti-inflammatory drugs. Stephen Golding provided the imaging examples featured in Chapter 5. Carol Davis and Tim Lovel were most helpful in relation to nebulized morphine, and John Thompson and Ruben Bild in relation to TENS and psychological methods respectively. I am grateful also to Keith Budd for the 'working definitions' of primary and secondary analgesics. A number of illustrations were prepared by Sylvia Barker at Oxford Medical Illustration.

Finally, I am particularly grateful to Michael Minton for shouldering more than the lion's share of the clinical supervision at Sobell House for an extended period. Karen Allen undertook the mammoth task of typing and retyping the ever-changing script.

Robert Twycross
1994

Drug names

Generic drug names are generally the same regardless of the country of use. Important exceptions are:

UK	USA
activated dimethicone	simethicone
adrenaline	epinephrine
dextropropoxyphene	propoxyphene
diamorphine (di-acetylmorphine)	heroin
frusemide	furosemide
hyoscine	scopolamine
lignocaine	lidocaine
paracetamol	acetaminophen
pethidine	meperidine

In addition readers should note that prednisolone and its inactive prodrug, prednisone, are identical in potency and efficacy.

Not all the drugs referred to are universally available. The reader is advised to check with his own National Formulary or drug compendium if he is in doubt.

Abbreviations

General

BNF	British National Formulary
BP	British Pharmacopoeia
IASP	International Association for the Study of Pain
UK	United Kingdom
USA	United States of America
USP	United States Pharmacopoeia
WHO	World Health Organization

Medical

CNS	central nervous system
COAD	chronic obstructive airways disease
CSF	cerebrospinal fluid
CT	computed tomography
H_1, H_2	histamine type 1, type 2 receptors
MAOI (s)	mono-amine oxidase inhibitor(s)
MRI	magnetic resonance imaging
NSAID(s)	nonsteroidal anti-inflammatory drug(s)
PCA	patient controlled analgesia
PG(s)	prostaglandin(s)
5HT	5-hydroxytryptamine (serotonin)

Drug administration

b.i.d.	twice daily; alternative, b.d.
daily	once a day
ED	epidural
IM	intramuscular
IT	intrathecal
IV	intravenous
m/r	modified release; alternative, slow release

nocte	at bedtime
PO	per os, by mouth
PR	per rectum, by rectum
q4h, q6h	every 4 hours, every 6 hours etc.
q.i.d.	four times a day (per 24 hours); alternative, q.d.s.
SC	subcutaneous
SL	sublingual
stat	immediately
t.i.d.	three times a day (per 24 hours); alternative, t.d.s.

Units

CI	confidence intervals
cm	centimetre(s)
g	gram(s)
Gy	Gray(s), a measure of irradiation
h	hour(s)
Hg	mercury
IU	international unit(s)
kg	kilogram(s)
L	litre(s)
mEq	milliequivalent(s)
mg	milligram(s)
ml	millilitre(s)
mm	millimetre(s)
mmol	millimole(s)
min	minute(s)
µg	microgram
SD	standard deviation
SE	standard error

The extent of the problem

INCIDENCE AND PREVALENCE OF PAIN IN CANCER

Pain is experienced by 20–50% of cancer patients at diagnosis and varies according to the primary site; and by up to 75% of patients with advanced cancer (Kane et al 1984, Bonica 1990). Data for the common primary sites or conditions are listed in Table 1.1. Pain is:

- moderate or severe in 40–50%
- very severe or excruciating in 25–30% (Bonica 1990).

Table 1.1 Prevalence of pain in advanced or terminal cancer

Primary site of cancer	Patients with pain	
	Mean[a]	Range
Oesophagus	87	80–93
Sarcoma	85	75–89
Bone (metastasis)	83	55–96
Pancreas	81	72–100
Bone (primary)	80	70–85
Liver/biliary	79	65–100
Stomach	78	67–93
Cervix uteri	75	40–100
Breast	74	56–100
Bronchus	73	57–88
Ovary	72	49–100
Prostate	72	55–100
CNS	70	55–83
Colon–rectum	70	47–95
Urinary organs	69	62–100
Oral–pharynx	66	54–80
Soft tissue	60	50–82
Lymphomas	58	20–69
Leukaemia	54	5–76

[a] Derived from 3–6 reports.
From Bonica 1990

Table 1.2 Evaluation of WHO Method for Relief of Cancer Pain

Study	Year	Country	Number of patients	Pain control (%)
Rappaz et al	1985	Switzerland	63	90
Ventafridda et al	1987	Italy	1229	71
Walker et al	1988	UK	20	100
Takeda	1989	Japan	205	86
Vijayaram et al	1989	India	88	86
Schug et al	1990	W Germany	174	92
Zech	1990	W Germany	1070	70
WHO Collaborating		25 countries	261[a]	75
Centre in Milan			110[b]	50

[a] Centres familiar with WHO method.
[b] Centres not familiar with WHO method.
From Stjernsward 1991

When translated into global terms, the problem is one of massive proportions (WHO 1990):

- in developed countries, 25% of the population dies from cancer
- *everyday*, at least 4 million people globally are suffering from cancer pain
- many of these do not obtain adequate relief.

Reports of the use of the World Health Organization (WHO) Method for Relief of Cancer Pain indicate, however, that pain can be completely relieved in 80–90% of patients and that 'acceptable relief' is possible in most of the remainder (Table 1.2).

STUDIES OF PALLIATIVE CARE

There are now innumerable studies of different aspects of palliative care, particularly in the United Kingdom (UK) and the United States of America (USA). Reference here is limited to a few which are of historical interest.

St. Christopher's Hospice study

A review of over 3000 case notes at St. Christopher's Hospice, London, indicated that pain was 'difficult to relieve' in 34 patients (1%) (Saunders 1981). The Home Care Service at St. Joseph's Hospice, London, adopting a similar approach, recorded unsatisfactory relief in about 10% of patients (Lamerton 1978). The higher percentage possibly relates to the reluctance of some patients to take tablets or medicine. Other patients decline the offer of admission to hospitals for further treatment and prefer to 'soldier on' at home.

Spouse's memory of pain

Data are also available from two studies of widows and widowers conducted 10 years apart in the vicinity of St. Christopher's Hospice, London (Parkes 1985). All the patients had been under 65 and died about one year before

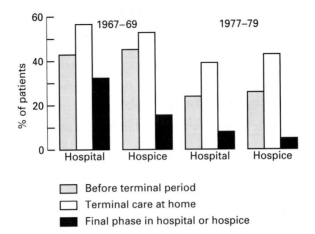

Fig. 1.1   Percentage of patients whose mean pain was rated as severe or greater by the surviving spouse 13 months after bereavement. (Reproduced with permission from Parkes 1985.)

an interview with the surviving spouse. The data therefore reflect the spouses' *memory* of the patient's pain, and possibly the spouse's own distress at the time. Although helpful in comparing different modes of care, they cannot be compared with records made at the time of the patient's illness, or with the patient's own report of pain.

In 1967–69 patients at St. Christopher's Hospice suffered significantly less pain than those dying in other hospitals in the area (Fig. 1.1). In 1977–79 pain relief was even better at St. Christopher's, but so too at other hospitals in the area. Thus, by 1977–79 there was no longer any significant difference between St. Christopher's Hospice and other hospitals in the area in terms of the severity of reported pain.

National hospice study

The National Hospice Study in the USA in the early 1980s showed an increase in the percentage of patients with unrelieved pain before death in those cared for in hospital or by a home care hospice programme (Table 1.3). At the time of the final evaluation, however, only one third of patients were able to respond to the question about pain intensity. In the other two thirds the answer was supplied by the 'primary care person' (i.e. key carer)

Table 1.3   National Hospice Study USA: terminal cancer patients with persistent pain (%)

Care setting	Number of patients	Evaluation	
		Penultimate	Final
Hospital	297	14	22
Home care hospice	833	7	13
Inpatient hospice	624	3	5

From Morris et al 1986

who tended to record pain more readily than the patients. Thus, when first interviewed, 31% of patients said they had no pain, whereas only 19% of primary care persons put the patient in the 'no pain' category. The increased percentage of patients in pain may, therefore, have been spurious.

Veterans Administration Hospital study

A second study in the USA compared traditional care with specialist palliative care at a Veterans Administration (VA) Hospital in a randomized controlled trial of over 200 patients. The mean pain scores at several points in time did not show any statistically significant differences (Kane et al 1984). The 11 bed palliative care unit was, however, in the VA hospital and some of the palliative care patients were cared for on the general wards by palliative care staff before being transferred to the palliative care unit. The general wards, therefore, would have been influenced by the staff of the palliative care unit. In addition, before the trial, the general wards would have benefited from the educational impact of ward consultations. To use the results to claim that 'specialist palliative care is no better' is not legitimate. Rather, the results suggest that the principles of pain management as practised in specialist palliative care units are transferable to other settings. Significant differences in favour of palliative care were, in fact, noted in relation to satisfaction with 'interpersonal care' and involvement in decision making.

REASONS FOR UNRELIEVED PAIN

Reasons for the gap between what is possible and what is achieved include (WHO 1986, Cleeland et al 1986, Dorrepaal et al 1989, Hill 1990):

- a lack of awareness that established methods already exist for cancer pain management
- a lack of systematic teaching of medical students, doctors, nurses and other health care workers about cancer pain management
- fears about addiction in both cancer patients and the wider public if strong opioids are more readily available for medical purposes
- nonavailability of necessary pain relief drugs in many parts of the world (Kanner & Portenoy 1986)
- use of special 'triplicate prescription' forms for Controlled Drugs which, in practice, discourage the use of strong opioids (Jage 1991, Kimbel 1991, Tunca & Yelken 1991, Zenz & Sorge 1991, Kimbel 1992)
- a lack of concern by national governments.

A more detailed list is given in Box 1.A.

OPIOPHOBIA

It has been suggested that 'opiophobia' is a major reason for poor cancer pain management, and that this stems from measures designed to control the abuse of drugs by addicts (Zenz & Willweber-Strumpf 1993). 'Opiophobia'

BOX 1.A
COMMON REASONS FOR UNRELIEVED PAIN

Associated with patient or family:
- belief that pain in cancer is inevitable and untreatable
- failure to contact doctor
- patient misleads doctor by 'putting on a brave face'
- patient fails to take prescribed medication as does not 'believe' in tablets
- belief that one should take analgesics only 'if absolutely necessary'
- noncompliance because of fears of 'addiction'
- noncompliance because of a belief that tolerance will rapidly develop, leaving nothing 'for when things get really bad'
- patient stops medication because of adverse effects and does not notify doctor.

Associated with doctor or nurse:
- doctor ignores the patient's pain, believing it to be inevitable and untreatable
- unawareness of the intensity of the patient's pain
- failure to get behind the 'brave face'
- doctor prescribes an analgesic which is too weak to relieve the pain
- prescription of an analgesic to be taken 'as needed'
- failure to appreciate that standard doses derived from postoperative studies are not relevant for cancer pain
- failure to give a patient adequate instructions about the use of analgesics
- because of lack of knowledge about analgesic potency, doctor either reduces or fails to increase the relative analgesic dose when transferring from one opioid to another
- fear that patient will become 'addicted' if a strong opioid is prescribed
- doctor believes that morphine should be reserved until patient is 'really terminal' (moribund), and continues to prescribe inadequate doses of less effective drugs
- failure to monitor the patient's progress
- lack of knowledge about other pain relieving drugs for use when opioids are ineffective
- failure to use nondrug measures when appropriate
- failure to give psychological support to the patient and family.

may be the explanation for the wide variation in morphine use in Western Europe (Fig. 1.2). The Danish figure, however, includes morphine used in maintenance programmes for addicts.

Most Western European countries are very restrictive about opioid use. Except in Belgium, Ireland, the Netherlands and the UK, special prescription forms or books are required. In Italy, Spain and Portugal, doctors have to apply to the authorities in person to obtain the special prescription forms. Doctors in Spain and Portugal also have to pay for them. In Spain and Italy, the patient needs a special identity card before the doctor is allowed to prescribe a strong opioid. In Spain, the card is valid for only 3 months. Further, if the dose is changed within 1 month, the patient must obtain a new card. The period for which a prescription remains valid varies (Table 1.4). A short period may prevent a patient from taking an extended holiday (Zenz & Willweber-Strumpf 1993).

National legislation in this area often dates back to before the Second World War when the main concern was to prevent drug trafficking and abuse, and cancer was not as common. In addition, the value of oral opioids

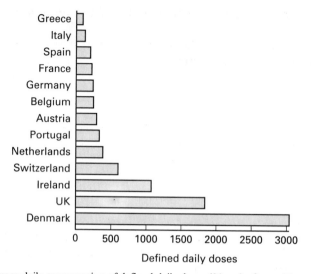

Fig. 1.2 Average daily consumption of defined daily doses (30 mg) of morphine per million inhabitants 1986–90 in Western Europe. UK figure = morphine + diamorphine. (Based on Zenz & Willweber-Strumpf 1993.)

Table 1.4 Prescribing regulations in Western Europe in 1992 for morphine tablets

Country	Maximum amount prescribable (days)	Prescription validity
Austria	–	7 days (initial) 4 weeks (continuing)
Belgium	–	12 weeks
Denmark	–	2 years
France	14	14 days
Germany	7	7 days
Greece	5	5 days
Ireland	–	Unlimited
Italy	8	10 days
Netherlands	–	Unlimited
Portugal	–	10 days
Spain	–	Unlimited
Switzerland	–	12 weeks
United Kingdom	–	13 weeks

Source: Zenz & Willweber-Strumpf 1993

for cancer pain was not so well recognized. These regulations, however, now commonly obstruct the provision of strong opioids to cancer patients.

At a meeting in 1992 in Brussels, attended by palliative care and pain specialists and by government representatives from 10 European countries, there was agreement that the dose and duration of opioid treatment should be determined only by the needs of the patient. The following statement was issued:

● our first goal must be adequate care of cancer patients and to give relief by all available means

- cancer pain relief programmes are not in conflict with control of drug abuse
- governments and clinicians should work together closely to guarantee *both* cancer pain relief for all patients *and* control of drug abuse
- future common European narcotic laws should be based on scientific data concerning both effectiveness of cancer pain relief and prevention of drug abuse
- the WHO Method for Relief of Cancer Pain provides an excellent basis for improving standards of cancer pain management
- no patient should live with unrelieved cancer pain, where relief is possible.

IMPACT OF UNRELIEVED PAIN

In one study (Twycross & Fairfield 1982), 73% of patients had had pain for more than 8 weeks when first admitted to a palliative care unit, and 57% for more than 16 weeks (Fig. 1.3). A similar percentage stated that it was severe, very severe or excruciating.

The impact of unrelieved pain varies according to its cause. In cancer, the pain is usually continuous and tends to get worse, which leads to mental and physical exhaustion. The patient becomes demoralized and increasingly fearful as yet another day of pain is anticipated. Severe anxiety, depression and delirium are all more common in cancer patients with pain (Massie & Holland 1992, Heim & Oei 1993).

The National Committee on the Treatment of Intractable Pain in the USA has many letters on file from relatives, friends and doctors describing

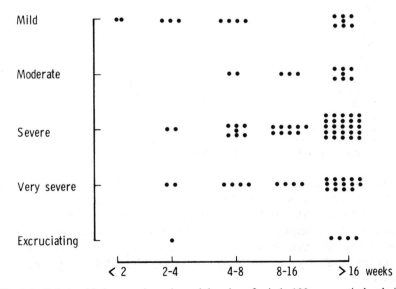

Fig. 1.3 Relationship between intensity and duration of pain in 100 consecutively admitted cancer patients with pain. ● represents 1 patient. (Reproduced with permission from Twycross & Fairfield 1982.)

BOX 1.B
EXTRACTS FROM LETTERS FROM RELATIVES

"I have lost my mother with incurable uterine cancer. Her pain was so horrid that she lost her mind and ate her bottom lip completely off from clenching her top teeth so tightly. My 13 year-old sister and I watched this for 6 weeks. We would enter the small hospital and hear her screams as soon as we closed the door. The nurses had no way to quieten her. She was immune to conventional pain killers."

"This July we lost our dad with cancer of the kidney. He was a beautiful 65 year-old retired contractor in January. The pain that man went through in May and June is undescribable. They would inject morphine into his buttocks and it would run out through his constantly injected flesh and onto the bedsheet."

"My brother just died of terminal cancer. He had a painful death. It deeply hurt us in the immediate family to sit alongside his bed last week and see him in great pain and have his request for relief, either a shot or pill, turned down because it wasn't time for another shot."

---

patients who spent their last months in severe pain (Box 1.B). An article tells of a family doctor in the USA who did not have the triplicate forms required by state law to prescribe strong opioids:

■ CASE HISTORY

When Mary developed oesophageal cancer, she was referred to a cancer centre in another city where she was treated with surgery and irradiation. She continued to have persistent mediastinal pain which caused insomnia, anorexia and weight loss. She was always tired and irritable. Her family doctor prescribed a weak opioid but this did not help. On the next visit to the cancer centre a strong opioid was prescribed which provided relief. Mary slept and ate better, and enjoyed life again. When she asked for a repeat prescription from her family doctor, he refused. He said that he did not have any triplicate forms, nor did he intend to obtain any. He believed that none of his patients needed drugs with an addictive potential. When she again lost weight and sleep because of pain, Mary's husband drove 360 k to the cancer centre for the effective medication (Hill 1987).

And from a country without readily available medicinal morphine:

"To see your son (24 years old with osteogenic sarcoma) cry out with pain running down the hospital corridor, to beg the resident doctor for an injection so he could have a period of 1–2 hours, or maybe 3 hours, of less pain, that is a crime committed here by the Health Authorities in the name of crime prevention.

Just think of how many people in our city, in our state, in the whole country who are having the same problem. I urge the Health Authorities and the Federal Police to examine this issue more carefully. Please, please, for the love of God, find a way for these medications to be freed for doctors to prescribe them more easily" (Schisler E 1988 Personal Communication).

'GOOD ENOUGH' PAIN RELIEF

At St. Christopher's Hospice, London, when evaluating pain relief, patients are divided into two broad categories (Haram 1978):

- those in whom there is 'good relief from pain'
- those in whom 'pain is difficult to relieve'.

Considering the many factors that can influence pain relief, either for good or ill, this is in fact a sensible way of summarizing the relief obtained. When considering pain management, one has to bear in mind that:

- pain relief is not an 'all or none' phenomenon
- all pains are not equally responsive to analgesics
- some pains continue to be brought on by activity and/or weightbearing
- relief is not generally a 'once only' exercise; old pains may re-emerge as the disease progresses or new pains develop.

When these factors are taken into account, one can restate the primary goal of pain management as seeking to help a patient move from a position in which he is mastered by the pain to one in which he establishes mastery over the pain. When a patient is mastered by pain, the pain becomes overwhelming and all-embracing. When sufficiently improved, a patient may say:

> 'I still have the pain, but it doesn't worry me now.'
> 'It's still there, but it's not what you'd call pain.'
> 'I can get on with things and forget it now.'

Of course, the ultimate goal remains complete relief. But, in practice, partial relief is acceptable provided the patient is significantly more comfortable, physically and mentally rested, and both patient and family are showing their mastery of the situation. Then there is little need to pursue relentlessly the ultimate goal using invasive techniques which do not guarantee success and may well be complicated by weakness, numbness or incontinence.

The concept of 'mastery over pain' has been validated by the Wisconsin Brief Pain Inventory (Daut & Cleeland 1982). When using this inventory, patients score both pain intensity and activity interference (Fig. 1.4). Parameters are scored on a scale of 0–10. Patients with pain rated 1–3 record little impact by the pain on either activity or enjoyment of life (Table 1.5). In other words, despite residual pain, the patient is enjoying a good quality of life.

■ CASE HISTORY

A 66 year-old man with intrapelvic spread of a bladder cancer was referred for outpatient evaluation at Sobell House. He was exhausted and in great distress because of insomnia caused by 'round the clock' frequency of micturition and by pain in the lower abdomen and legs. The frequency of micturition and insomnia were both corrected by drug therapy. On the other hand, he continued to experience 'a golf ball' sensation in the perineum, 'but it's not really painful', and intermittent pain in the right L5 dermatome. This

Circle the one number that describes how, during the past week, pain has interfered with your:

A. General Activity

0	1	2	3	4	5	6	7	8	9	10
Does not interfere										Completely interferes

B. Mood

0	1	2	3	4	5	6	7	8	9	10
Does not interfere										Completely interferes

C. Walking ability

0	1	2	3	4	5	6	7	8	9	10
Does not interfere										Completely interferes

D. Normal work (includes both work outside the home and housework)

0	1	2	3	4	5	6	7	8	9	10
Does not interfere										Completely interferes

E. Relations with other people

0	1	2	3	4	5	6	7	8	9	10
Does not interfere										Completely interferes

F. Sleep

0	1	2	3	4	5	6	7	8	9	10
Does not interfere										Completely interferes

G. Enjoyment of life

0	1	2	3	4	5	6	7	8	9	10
Does not interfere										Completely interferes

Fig. 1.4 Wisconsin Brief Pain Inventory: interference factors.

Table 1.5 Relationship between worst pain rating and interference ratings of cancer patients

Worst pain rating	Number of patients	Activity interference (mean)	Enjoyment interference (mean)
1	13	0.2	0.8
2	16	1.5	1.9
3	33	1.4	1.6
4	41	2.6	2.8
5	100	4.4	4.4
6	45	5.4	5.0
7	54	6.2	5.7
8	39	6.2	5.8
9	17	7.5	6.3
10	49	7.1	6.8

From Daut & Cleeland 1982

was usually mild but, occasionally, could be more troublesome. As lowering the dose of morphine did not make the pain worse, it was concluded that this particular pain was probably at best only partly opioid responsive. The residual pain had only minimal impact on the patient's activity and enjoyment of life. It was decided therefore not to recommend a nerve block or other invasive procedure at this stage.

The contrast between the man's condition at his initial evaluation and subsequent reviews continued to be considerable, despite occasional trouble with constipation or frayed emotions. So, was his pain relieved or was it not? In absolute terms, no: but, in his estimation, yes.

REALISTIC EXPECTATIONS

Many cancer patients with persistent pain have expectations of relief which are unnecessarily low. Thus, when first seen, all patients should be assured that the situation can be improved and that it is possible to relieve most, if not all, of their pain. It is always possible to achieve *at least* some improvement within 48 h. It is often wise, however, to aim at 'graded relief'. Because some pains respond more readily to treatment than others, improvement must be evaluated in relation to each pain.

The initial target is a painfree, sleepful night. Some patients have not had a good night's rest for weeks or months and are exhausted and demoralized. To sleep through the night painfree and wake refreshed is a boost to both the patient's and the doctor's morale. Next, one aims for relief at rest in bed or chair during the day; finally, for freedom from pain on movement. The former is always eventually possible; the latter sometimes not. Relief at night and when resting during the day, however, gives the patient new hope and incentive, and enables him to begin to live again despite limited mobility. Freed from the nightmare of constant pain, his last weeks or months take on a new look.

The doctor must be determined to succeed and be prepared to spend time evaluating and re-evaluating the patient's pain and other distressing symptoms. In addition, a balance is needed between marking time therapeutically (while capitalizing on the impact of improved sleep and morale) and pressing on decisively with further initiatives. If this skill is not developed, the doctor and patient become trapped in the 'one step behind' syndrome. Most of the right things will be done, but always several days or weeks too late (Fenton 1992). The 'one step behind' syndrome is graphically illustrated in the account of a 90 year-old man admitted to a London teaching hospital with bone pain and who died still in pain 3 months later (Hunt et al 1977).

CANCER PAIN RELIEF PROGRAMME

A global problem demands a global response. Cancer pain relief is an integral component of the WHO Comprehensive Cancer Control Programme begun in 1980. This has three main goals (Stjernsward et al 1985):

- primary prevention

- early diagnosis and curative treatment
- pain relief and palliative care.

In most parts of the world the majority of cancer patients present with advanced disease. For them, the only realistic option is pain relief and palliative care. In consequence, the WHO prepared a Method for Relief of Cancer Pain (WHO 1986).

The monograph incorporating the Method is the second most translated WHO publication ever. In addition to English, it is available in 19 other languages: Arabic, Brazilian, Bulgarian, Chinese, Croatian, Czech, French, German, Gujarati, Hindi, Hungarian, Italian, Japanese, Portuguese, Russian, Spanish, Thai, Turkish and Vietnamese. This publication, with over a quarter of a million copies sold, reflects the growing awareness of the problem of cancer pain. The WHO Method emphasizes that a small number of relatively

Table 1.6 National policies on cancer pain relief and palliative care

Country	Title of document	Issued by	Year
Canada	Douleurs cancereuses (Cancer pain)	Ministry of Health & Welfare, Canada	1984
France	Soigner et accompagner jusqu'au bout. Soulager la souffrance (Caring and accompanying until the end. Alleviate the suffering)	Ministry of Social Affairs & Employment, Ministry of Health and the Family, France	1986
Australia	Management of severe pain	National Health and Medical Research Council, Australia	1988
Japan	Manual care for terminally ill cancer patients	Ministry of Health and Japanese Medical Association, Japan	1889
Sweden	The management of pain in the terminal stage of life	National Board of Health and Welfare, Sweden	1989
Finland	Syopapotilaan kivun hoito (Treatment of pain in cancer patients)	National Board of Health, Finland Laakintohallituksven Oppassarja Nro 5	1989
Italy	Decreta Art. I Gazzetta Ufficiale della Repubblica Italiana (Decree on prescription of opioid drugs)	Ministry of Health, Italy	1989
Mexico	Health policy for cancer pain relief	Ministry of Health, Mexico	1990
Netherlands	Pijn en pijnbehandeling bij de patient met kanker (Pain and pain treatment for patients with cancer)	Dutch chapter of IASP subsidised by the Ministry of Health, Welfare and Cultural Affairs, The Netherlands	1990
Vietnam	Cancer pain policy statement	Ministry of Health, Socialist Republic of Vietnam	1990
Philippines	Guidelines on cancer pain relief	Philippines Cancer Control Programme, Department of Health, Republic of the Philippines	1991

From Stjernsward et al 1992

inexpensive drugs, including morphine, are the mainstay of cancer pain management. Field testing has demonstrated the efficacy of the guidelines in most cancer patients (see Table 1.2).

Governments are being encouraged by the WHO to set up statutory cancer control programmes. Cameroon, Chile, Cuba, India, Indonesia, Pakistan, Singapore and Zimbabwe have done so, and have specifically incorporated cancer pain relief and/or palliative care as key priorities. Several other countries have established national policies on cancer pain relief and palliative care (Table 1.6).

In the USA, the state of Wisconsin established an initiative for improving cancer pain management which has been replicated in many other states (Joranson et al 1987, Champlin 1992, Spross 1992). Other initiatives which should have a major impact include:

- a Committee on Cancer Pain set up by the American Society of Clinical Oncology
- a Task Force on Cancer Pain set up by the International Association for the Study of Pain (IASP).

Cancer pain management will remain an ongoing challenge. Even so:

'Quality of life and comfort before death could be considerably improved by a relatively small reshuffling of resources. It only requires the will to do so' (Stjernsward 1988).

This then is the challenge to Ministries of Health, the medical profession, major cancer centres and national Cancer Societies. Are we prepared to face the facts and demand a redistribution of the massive resources available for research into curative treatments so as to enable the majority of cancer patients to receive satisfactory pain relief and palliative care during the end stage of their disease?

REFERENCES

Bonica J J 1990 Cancer pain: current status and future needs. In: Bonica J J (ed) The management of pain, 2 edn. Lea & Febiger, Philadelphia, pp 400–445
Champlin L 1992 Inadequate analgesia: patients endure pain, fear addiction. Geriatrics 47 (8): 71–74
Cleeland C S, Cleeland L M, Dar R, Rinehardt L C 1986 Factors influencing physician management of cancer pain. Cancer 58: 796–800
Daut R L, Cleeland C S 1982 The prevalence and severity of pain in cancer. Cancer 50: 1913–1918
Dorrepaal L K, Aaronson N K, van Dam F S A M 1989 Pain experience and pain management among hospitalized cancer patients. A clinical study. Cancer 63: 593–598
Dutch chapter of IASP (Nederlandse Vereniging ter Bestudering van Pijn) 1990. Pijn en pijnbehandeling bij de patient met kanker. Oostersingel 59, 9700 R B Groningen, Academisch Ziekenhuis, Groningen
Fenton A 1992 The ultimate failure. British Medical Journal 305: 1027
Haram B J 1978 Facts and figures. In: Saunders C M (ed) The management of terminal disease. Edward Arnold, London, pp 12–18
Heim H M, Oei T P S 1993 Comparison of prostate cancer patients with and without pain. Pain 53: 159–162

Hill C S 1987 Painful prescriptions. Journal of the American Medical Association 257: 2081
Hill C S 1990 Relationship among cultural, educational, and regulatory agency influences on optimum cancer pain treatment. Journal of Pain and Symptom Management 5: S37–S45
Hunt J M, Stollar T D, Littlejohns D W, Twycross R G, Vere D W 1977 Patients with protracted pain: a survey conducted at the London Hospital. Journal of Medical Ethics 3: 61–73
Garattini S 1993 Pain relief: narcotic drug use for severe pain. Lancet 341: 1061–1062
Jage J 1991 Opioids and the fear of addiction in Germany. Cancer Pain Release 5(2): 1
Joranson D E, Dahl J L, Engber D 1987 Wisconsin initiative for improving cancer pain management. Journal of Pain and Symptom Management 2: 111–113
Kane R L, Wales J, Bernstein L, Leibowitz A, Kaplan S 1984 A randomized controlled trial of hospice care. Lancet i: 890–894
Kanner R M, Portenoy R K 1986 Unavailability of narcotic analgesics for ambulatory cancer patients in New York city. Journal of Pain and Symptom Management 1: 87–89
Kimbel K H 1991 Germany: bureaucracy versus analgesia. Lancet 337: 905
Kimbel K H 1992 Germany: changes in analgesics law. Lancet 339: 1044
Lamerton R 1978 Annual Report of Macmillan Home Care Service. St. Joseph's Hospice, London
Massie M J, Holland J C 1992 The cancer patient with pain: psychiatric complications and their management. Journal of Pain and Symptom Management 7: 99–109
Ministry of Health (Italy) 1989 Decreta Art: 1 gazzetta Ufficiale della Repubblica Italiana. Ministry of Health, Rome
Ministry of Health (Japan) and Japanese Medical Association 1989 Manual of care for terminally ill cancer patients. Ministry of Health and Japanese Medical Association, Tokyo
Ministry of Health (Mexico) 1990 Health policy for cancer pain relief. Secretaria de Salud, Estados Unidos Mexicanos. (Book no. 2 of laws, decrees, agreements and various documents that regulate the administrative activities of the Health Secretariat and the Health Sector.)
Ministry of Health (Vietnam) 1990 Cancer pain policy statement. Ministry of Health, Socialist Republic of Vietnam
Ministry of Health and Welfare (Canada) 1984 Cancer pain: a monograph on the management of pain. Department of Supply and Services, Ottawa
Ministry of Social Affairs and Employment, Ministry of Health and the Family (France) 1986 Soigner et accompagner jusqu'au bout: Soulager la souffrance. Ministry of Social Affairs and Employment, Ministry of Health and the Family, Paris
Morris J N, Mor V, Goldberg R J, Sherwood S, Greer D S, Hiris J 1986 The effect of treatment setting and patient characteristics on pain in terminal cancer patients: A report from the National Hospice Study. Journal of Chronic Diseases 39: 27–35
National Board of Health (Finland) 1989 Vainio A (ed) Syopapotilaan kivun hoito, Laakintohallituksven Oppassarja Nro 5. National Board of Health, Helsinki
National Board of Health and Welfare (Sweden) 1989 The management of pain in the terminal stage of life. National Board of Health and Welfare, Stockholm
National Health and Medical Research Council 1988 Management of severe pain. Australian Government Publishing Service, Canberra
Parkes C M 1985 Terminal care: Home, hospital, or hospice? Lancet i: 155–157
Philippines Cancer Control Program 1991 Guidelines on cancer pain relief. Department of Health, Republic of the Philippines
Rappaz O, Tripiana J, Rapin C-H, Stjernsward J, Junod J O 1985 Soins palliatifs et traitement de la douleur cancereuse en geriatrie. Revue Therapeutique/Therapeutische Umschau 42: 843–848
Saunders C M 1981 Current views of pain relief and terminal care. In: Swerdlow M (ed) The therapy of pain. MTP Press, Lancaster, pp 215–241
Schug S A, Zech K, Dorr U 1990 Cancer pain management according to WHO analgesic guidelines. Journal of Pain and Symptom Management 5: 27–32
Spross J A 1992 Cancer pain relief: an international perspective. Oncology Nursing Forum 19 (7) suppl: 5–11
Stjernsward J 1988 WHO cancer pain relief programme. In: Hanks G W (ed) Pain and cancer (Cancer Survey Series) Vol 7. Oxford University Press, Oxford, pp 195–208
Stjernsward J 1991 WHO cancer pain relief programme and future challenges. In: Takeda F (ed) Cancer pain relief and quality of life. WHO Collaborating Center for Cancer Pain Relief and Quality of Life Saitama, Japan, pp 5–9
Stjernsward J, Koroltchouk V, Teoh N 1992 National policies for cancer pain relief and palliative care. Palliative Medicine 6: 273–276

Stjernsward J, Stanley K, Eddy D, Tsechkovski M, Sobin L, Koza I, Notaney K H 1985 Cancer control: strategies and priorities. World Health Forum 6: 160–164

Takeda F 1989 The management of cancer pain in Japan. In: Twycross R G (ed) The Edinburgh symposium on pain control and medical education. Royal Society of Medicine, London, pp 17–21

Tunca M, Yelken J 1991 Undertreatment of cancer pain. Lancet 337: 1294

Twycross R G, Fairfield S 1982 Pain in far-advanced cancer. Pain 14: 303–310

Ventafridda V, Tamburini M, Caraceni A, De Conno F, Naldi F 1987 A validation study of the W.H.O. method for cancer pain relief. Cancer 59: 851–856

Vijayaram S, Bhargava M K, Ramamani P V, Chadrasekhar N S, Sudharshan R, Heranjal R, Lobo B 1989 Experience with oral morphine for cancer pain relief. Journal of Pain and Symptom Management 4: 130–134

Walker V A, Hoskin P J, Hanks G W, White I D 1988 Evaluation of WHO analgesic guidelines for cancer pain in a hospital-based palliative care unit. Journal of Pain and Symptom Management 3: 145–149

World Health Organization 1986 Cancer pain relief. World Health Organization, Geneva

WHO Expert Committee Report 1990 Cancer pain relief and palliative care. Technical report series No. 804. World Health Organization, Geneva

Zech D 1990 Pain control according to WHO guidelines in 1140 cancer patients. Presented at the First Congress of the European Association for Palliative Care, Paris

Zenz M, Sorge J 1991 Is the therapeutic use of opioids adversely affected by prejudice and law? Recent Results in Cancer Research 121: 43–50

Zenz M, Willweber-Strumpf A 1993 Opiophobia and cancer pain in Europe. Lancet 341: 1075–1076

CHAPTER	
2	# Pain and suffering

ACUTE VERSUS CHRONIC PAIN

Acute pain and its associated responses are provoked by noxious stimulation produced by injury or disease, or by extreme function of muscle or viscera without actual tissue damage (Box 2.A). Severe acute pain is accompanied by a 'fight or flight' response, like acute anxiety, whereas chronic pain is often associated with vegetative features similar to those seen in depression (Table 2.1). This means that a patient may have severe chronic pain but not look distressed. It is easy for the doctor without personal experience of chronic pain to forget this.

Most people's understanding of pain is usually taken from personal experience of acute pain — toothache, headache, bruise or sprain — all of which pass relatively quickly. In contrast, chronic pain is a situation rather than an event and it:

- is impossible to predict when it will end
- often gets worse rather than better

BOX 2.A
USEFUL DEFINITIONS

Acute pain (Bonica 1990)
A complex constellation of unpleasant sensory, perceptual, and emotional experiences with associated autonomic, psychological and behavioural reponses.

Chronic pain (Bonica 1990)
Pain which persists a month beyond the usual course of an acute disease or a reasonable time for an injury to heal, or is associated with a chronic pathological process which causes continuous pain or pain which recurs at intervals for months or years.

Table 2.1   Acute versus chronic pain

	Acute	Chronic	
Time course	Transient	Persistent	

Meaning to patient	Positive:
	    draws attention to
	    injury or illness
		Negative:
		  serves no useful
		  purpose
			Positive:
			    as patient obtains
			    secondary gain

Accompanying features	Fight or flight:
	    pupillary dilatation
	    increased sweating
	    increased respiratory rate
	    increased heart rate
	    shunting of blood from
	      viscera to muscles
		Vegetative:
		  sleep disturbance
		  anorexia
		  decreased libido
		  anhedonia
		  constipation
		  somatic pre-occupation
		  personality change
		  lethargy	

- often conveys a negative message
- frequently expands to occupy the patient's whole attention and isolates him from the world around.

There is, in fact, no standard definition of chronic pain. It is commonly defined as pain of more than 6 months duration (Sternbach 1974). While of benefit in limiting referrals, such a definition does not make pathophysiological sense. Most acute conditions heal in 2–3 weeks. If pain is still present after cure, it should be considered chronic (Box 2.A). For example, a fracture of the wrist usually becomes painfree within 2 weeks. If the pain is still present after 2 months, something is wrong. It is possible that the patient is developing a sympathetically maintained pain ('reflex sympathetic dystrophy'). If left for 6 months before being considered chronic pain, it may well have become resistant to treatment (Bonica 1990).

'CHRONIC BENIGN PAIN'

'Chronic benign pain' is a term which was introduced in the 1970s to distinguish chronic pain of nonmalignant origin from chronic cancer pain (Sternbach et al 1976). It was almost immediately pointed out that benign denotes 'a state of gentleness, kindness, mild or favourable outcome' and, therefore, is not an appropriate description for any form of chronic pain (Boas 1976). To quote John Bonica:

> 'As one who has observed thousands of patients suffering chronic pain and also has personally suffered persistent pain since 1974, I have a deep conviction that chronic pain is never 'benign' but is rather a malefic force that is deleterious to the patient, the family, and society' (Bonica 1990).

The term 'chronic benign pain', therefore, should not be used. The term 'chronic pain of nonmalignant origin' or 'chronic noncancer pain' should be used instead.

CHRONIC PAIN SYNDROME

About 20 years ago, it was suggested that the term 'chronic pain syndrome' (CPS) could be used for patients who complain of persistent, intractable pain in the absence of an identifiable pathological condition which would account for the level of distress (Black 1975). In addition, there are features of depression, insomnia, irritability or anxiety, fatigue, psychosocial mal-adjustment, marital problems, somatizing, hypochondriasis, and functional symptoms (Tunks 1990). There will also be:

- a history of multiple medical consultations
- a history of many nonproductive diagnostic procedures
- an excessive pre-occupation with the pain on the part of the patient, the family and friends.

It was emphasized that CPS must be differentiated from chronic nociception in, for example, patients with arthritis. It is clearly equally important to differentiate CPS from chronic neuropathic pain. In other words, CPS refers to a 'ragbag' of patients whose chronic pain is determined primarily by psychological factors and secondarily by physical inactivity (Tunks 1990).

CPS patients have become dependent on their pain as a way of avoiding the challenges of life. They obtain considerable 'secondary gain' from their suffering and have a vested interest in maintaining ill health (Freud 1963, Aronoff & Wilson 1978). They exhibit 'pain behaviours' which have the perpetuation of the sick role as their goal. Additional roles may also be adopted, such as the 'medication dependent role', the 'rehabilitation role', and the 'diagnosis confounding role' (Bergman & Werblun 1978).

Treatment of CPS is a combination of specific psychological and physical therapies. Several types of treatment are available, including:

- operant-conditioning (Fordyce 1973)
- cognitive-behavioural (Turk & Meichenbaum 1989).

Such approaches are concerned with enabling the patient to understand his condition better and to re-inforce mental and physical coping strategies. Cognitive-behavioural therapy provides a greater opportunity for the patient to question, re-appraise and acquire self-control over maladaptive thoughts, feelings, behaviours and physiological responses. There is no reason, however, why operant-conditioning techniques should not be incorporated into a programme of cognitive-behavioural therapy (see p. 544).

The overriding message of cognitive-behavioural approaches is that:

- patients are not helpless
- pain need not be the overriding determinant of their lives.

Rather, various resources are available for confronting pain. Treatment, therefore, encourages patients to develop a problem solving orientation and a sense of resourcefulness, instead of a sense of helplessness and withdrawal revolving around bed, doctors and pharmacists.

Specific psychological therapies are of value in selected cancer patients, particularly those with evidence of gross somatization (Turk & Fernandez 1990). In advanced cancer, however, some patients may well not live long enough to complete the course of therapy.

CANCER PAIN

Cancer pain is as distinct from chronic pain of nonmalignant origin as the latter is from acute pain. Cancer patients in pain exhibit a mixture of both 'fight and flight' and vegetative reactions. The former is particularly manifest when pain is associated with symptoms of deterioration, such as anorexia, weight loss, decreasing exercise tolerance, and increasing physical dependence. For the patient, this constellation of signs and symptoms has inescapable significance. The message from his body states clearly: 'Unless a miracle happens, I will not survive for long.' The patient realizes that he is on a collision course with death. Such a realization, even if partly subconscious, evokes an instinctive autonomic response.

OVERWHELMING CANCER PAIN

After several weeks or months of pain, particularly if associated with insomnia, many cancer patients become overwhelmed by pain. Pain envelops their whole mental outlook. Such patients often find it difficult to describe the location or the nature of the pain precisely:

'But I'm all pain, doctor.'

'The pain is in my chest and my back and my arm and my head — it's really all over.'

'I feel as if my body is enclosed in a pressure balloon and the balloon is slowly collapsing, squeezing every bone and every joint in my body as it closes around me.'

The last statement was made by a woman with breast cancer with pain in the lumbar spine. She had earlier described her pain as a knife sticking into her back. By the time she was admitted to her local palliative care unit, she had developed paraparesis and a bedsore, and her entire life had become one all-embracing pain.

In the majority of patients the response to the continuing pain is vegetative; the patient withdraws mentally and physically, and looks depressed. In some, anxiety predominates (Box 2.B), or a mixture of agitated and depressive features co-exist.

In all cases of overwhelming pain, the key to success is breaking the vicious circle of insomnia $\longrightarrow$ fatigue $\longrightarrow$ pain $\longrightarrow$ insomnia. Because the patient is exhausted and demoralized, it may take 3–4 weeks to achieve maximum relief. Unless this is understood, patient and staff morale can drop irretrievably after a few days of inpatient treatment if the pain persists. On the other hand, the doctor can and should promise some early improvement, particularly in relation to rest and comfort at night.

BOX 2.B
OVERWHELMING PAIN

Severe pain compounded by:

- insomnia
- fatigue
- mental exhaustion
- loss of morale
- distrust of caregivers.

Type 1
Physical reluctance
Depression
Dependence on present
   unsatisfactory medication

Type 2
Fear of movement or being moved
Marked anxiety/agitation
No faith in any medication

These patients look distressed.

It takes several weeks to achieve maximum benefit.

The initial key to success is painfree sleepful nights.

Type 2 is a medical emergency: treat with combination of analgesic and an anxiolytic, and review within hours.

With overwhelming pain it is advisable, if possible, to review the first day's treatment before deciding on the medication for the first night. Some patients will seem dependent on their former inadequate medication. Presumably this is because it is the best they have had so far. They may be determined that no one, not even the palliative care doctor, is going to deprive them of it. Generally, in this circumstance, patients should be allowed to keep their old medication and to use it as necessary in addition to the new medication. Patients can be provided with a chart to record when and how much of the old medication is used.

When anxiety is prominent, treatment comprises both an analgesic and an anxiolytic, together with psychological evaluation and initial psychological support. The choice and dose of each drug will depend to a large extent on what the patient had previously been taking. Overwhelming pain accompanied by marked anxiety is best regarded as an emergency, and a considerable amount of time needs to be allocated to its treatment. Ideally, one experienced doctor should be responsible for all medical aspects of care over the first few days in order to establish a good working relationship with both the patient and the family.

It is, of course, possible to have both marked anxiety and pain without the pain being overwhelming. Moderate anxiety will usually lessen when pain is relieved and the patient's fears and concerns addressed. Extreme anxiety is not always immediately apparent but may be manifested in one or more of the following ways:

- attention seeking behaviour

- fear of being left alone
- overactivity
- misperceptions — usually unpleasant
- nightmares
- continued insomnia despite pain relief.

Insomnia may also be a feature of depression. Screening with the Hospital Anxiety and Depression (HAD) Scale, for example, may help identify those who are depressed and who will need an antidepressant instead of an anxiolytic (Massie 1990).

SOMATIZATION

Mood and morale have an impact on the intensity of all symptoms. Some patients, however, express negative emotions through physical symptoms. The following case histories illustrate this:

■ CASE HISTORY

A 55 year-old man with recently diagnosed cancer of the oesophagus was still in pain despite receiving m/r morphine tablets, *6000 mg* (100 mg × 60) b.i.d. Following inpatient admission to a palliative care unit, he became painfree on 30 mg b.i.d. and diazepam 10 mg nocte. He returned home, converted the spare bedroom into a workshop, and was able to spend many happy hours there. The key to success was *evaluation, explaining and setting positive rehabilitation goals*.

■ CASE HISTORY

A 34 year-old woman was admitted to a palliative care unit suffering from disseminated breast cancer. In the past she had two stillbirths and now had a much treasured 3 year-old son. When relatively well she had coped with her situation on an intellectual level, and made all the necessary arrangements for her approaching death. As she weakened it became clear that she had not come to terms with her illness emotionally. Now she was asking, 'Why all this? Why me?'. She grieved over losses already sustained. For example, she wanted to be able to meet her son after playschool and to cuddle him but could no longer do so. She missed her home but, because of her condition, could make only brief visits. She lamented her increasing dependence and was overwhelmed by the thought that she might lose control over physical functions. Her grief was manifested in crushing, intractable pain. She said, 'I am resigned to the fact that this is my lot. It is the pain I cannot accept. Dying is all right, but there is no reason for this pain, no purpose in it. I am no longer angry with God for my fate, but why this pain?'

Oral morphine in daily doses of up to 1500 mg was ineffective. Complaints of shattering pain continued and she was miserable and often withdrawn. The slightest movement caused her to cringe in pain. Care to pressure areas was no longer permitted. For relief, large and frequent doses of IV diazepam were required. Epidural morphine was commenced and was continued for 5 weeks.

In time she came to terms with her situation. As this occurred, her need for analgesia became less and eventually she was painfree on oral morphine 10 mg q4h. She improved to the point where she was able to be wheeled down the road on an ambulance trolley to buy a present for her son, and to visit the local art gallery the day before she died (Lichter 1991).

■ CASE HISTORY

A 79 year-old woman, previously exceptionally fit, developed epigastric pain. When investigated she was found to have cancer of the pancreas. The pain was initially readily controlled by m/r morphine 30 mg b.i.d.. She then began to experience intense central abdominal colic for several hours every few days. Between attacks she was her normal vivacious self. When the pain was present she would moan and groan and express feelings such as 'I can't go on', 'I'd rather die than have this pain', 'If I were a dog you'd put me down'. She was virtually inconsolable.

The pain was clearly functional and radiological investigations demonstrated no cause for it except morphine induced constipation. It was not possible to reduce the dose of morphine because a reduction was followed within 1–2 days by another severe episode of pain — which needed more morphine to control it. Eventually it seemed to the palliative care doctor that the patient had accepted that the pain was functional and not caused by the cancer. Within a few days, however, she began to experience intermittent attacks of cramp in the left quadratus lumborum muscle related to a myofascial trigger point. This was explained to her and she was treated with local massage whenever she had an attack. Because the attacks continued, she was treated by local injection of bupivacaine into the trigger point. Then, after a day or so, she began to experience functional intestinal pains again.

Although visited regularly by a psychologist, it was not possible to enable her to vocalize her fears and her anger.

In the first example, management was relatively straightforward. In the second, it was necessary to stay alongside for many weeks, sharing the woman's anguish until it eventually resolved. In the third example, there was no such ending. The woman remained locked in her recurring anguish and most of her final months were spent in bed in a palliative care unit.

The last case history is, in fact, a typical example of a common problem in patients with unresolved fears, unexpressed anger and emotional conflicts. Functional abdominal pain (irritable bowel syndrome) probably had been her way of expressing negative emotions throughout her life. Not surprisingly, it proved impossible to change a long established pattern of behaviour. The situation progressed into a vicious spiral of more morphine, more laxatives and more sedatives until the patient finally succumbed to a combination of inactivity and medication.

Such situations are extremely demanding for the nurses, doctors and others involved. They engender feelings of failure and of guilt. Good communication between team members is essential to clarify goals (which may change) and to provide mutual, ongoing support.

SUFFERING

Few patients contemplate their approaching death without distress. Most use their psychological resources to contain their anguish, rage, or fear about what is happening to them. For many people a palliative care unit is 'a safe place to suffer', i.e. a place where they feel safe enough to explore their feelings more openly (Stedeford 1987).

Pain and suffering are not identical (Fishman 1990). Suffering, therefore, must be distinguished from pain and other symptoms with which it may be associated. Patients may tolerate severe pain without considering themselves to be suffering if they know that:

- the pain has an identified cause
- it can be dealt with
- it will be relatively short lived.

On the other hand, even relatively minor symptoms may cause suffering if they are believed or known to:

- have a life threatening cause
- be intractable
- reflect a hopeless prognosis.

Indeed, suffering may occur in the absence of any symptoms, for example when witnessing the physical deterioration of a loved one (Gates 1993). Suffering is experienced by persons, not by bodies (Cassell 1991). It stems from a threat to the integrity of the person as a complex social and psychological entity. Helplessness is a potent source of suffering (Cassell 1991).

■ CASE HISTORY

A 35 year-old sculptress with widespread breast cancer was treated by doctors using the most advanced knowledge and technology, and acting with kindness and true concern. But, at every stage, the treatment as well as the disease was a source of suffering to her. For example, she had not anticipated that the irradiated breast would be disfiguring. After the removal of her ovaries and the prescription of hormones, she became hirsute, obese, and devoid of libido. When the cancer spread to her neck, the hand she used for sculpting became weak. The loss of creative potential resulted in severe depression. She then sustained a pathological fracture of the femur, and treatment was delayed while her doctors openly disagreed about the advisability of pinning it. She was uncertain and frightened about her future.

Each time there was a response to treatment and hope rekindled, there would be a subsequent new manifestation of disease. Thus, when a new course of chemotherapy was started, she was torn between a desire to live and the fear that, if she allowed hope to rekindle, she would once again be devastated when the treatment failed.

She feared the future. Each day was seen as heralding increased sickness, pain, or disability, never as the beginning of better times. She felt isolated because she was no longer like other people and could not do what others did; and she feared that her friends would stop visiting her (Cassell 1991).

This account is a reminder that:

- cancer is usually devastating in its impact on the patient
- suffering may be caused both by the disease and its treatment
- suffering is not limited to physical symptoms
- in order to identify sources of suffering, it is necessary to evaluate the patient psychologically and to ask open questions.

This woman's suffering extended to threats to the social and private dimensions of her life. She suffered from the effects of both the disease and the treatment on her appearance and abilities, and from her perception of the future.

TOTAL PAIN

The phrase 'total pain' was coined by Dame Cicely Saunders to emphasize the multidimensional ramifications of pain in advanced cancer (Saunders 1967):

- physical
- psychological
- social
- spiritual.

In some respects, the concepts of suffering and somatization constitute a better working model. However, because many people still use 'total pain' as a means of emphasizing that pain is a somatopsychic experience, a description is included here.

Patients with cancer sometimes describe their whole life as painful. Those caring for them must, therefore, address all aspects of discomfort and distress if the pain is to be relieved. Although the doctor may be able to discriminate between separate areas of 'life pain', the patient often cannot — for him the pain is total and all embracing.

■ CASE HISTORY

A 54 year-old woman with a past history of sarcoma of the stomach was referred for psychiatric consultation when admitted for biopsy of an enlarged submandibular gland and for assessment of chronic pain in her left side (Table 2.2).

When seen, she appeared to be in considerable discomfort and was preoccupied with what she described as a severe and sharp pain. Signs of depression were noted (psychomotor retardation, poor eye contact, low pitched monotonous voice, and expressions of fatigue and despair). She was aware of her diagnosis and the possibility of recurrence and death.

However, she talked almost exclusively about her pain, which had been the only reason for her seeking help. The pain had been constant and severe for 3 months, and it significantly impeded both domestic and social activities. The pain concerned her much more than did the enlarged node, which she dismissed by stating that the surgeons would cut it out as they had 2 years earlier.

Table 2.2 Past history of 54 year-old woman

Number of years ago	Event
5	Second marriage ended in divorce
4	Partial gastrectomy for sarcoma
3	Inpatient treatment for depression; 7 year-old son temporarily entrusted to alcoholic ex-husband
2	Excision biopsy of submandibular gland is positive for sarcoma; no evidence of other recurrence
1	Outpatient treatment for depression
¼	Pain in left flank

The pain in her side was a different story altogether. It was new and she was afraid that it represented a new direction of tumour spread. Exploration of this notion revealed concern that this would mean death was imminent. The woman confessed that in recent months she had been spending more and more of her time preoccupied with thoughts about her death.

She was encouraged to elaborate some of her thoughts and the rest of the interview was focused on this. Among her greatest fears was leaving behind her 11 year-old son in the care of his untrustworthy father. She also expressed the fear that death would be painful and that in the end her doctors would abandon her. She cried spontaneously during this part of the discussion. At the end of the interview, the woman's mood had improved dramatically. She was more animated, and eye contact with the interviewer had increased.

Next day, the woman enthusiastically summoned the psychiatrist to her bedside and reported that the pain in her side had disappeared immediately after their meeting and had not returned. It was the first time in 3 months that she had been without pain. Because of complications with the subsequent biopsy, however, she remained in hospital for several more weeks but without a recurrence of pain (Kuhn & Bradnan 1979).

If the pain conveys a negative message, the intensity of the pain increases. Thus, a pain which was 'just a backache' and which responded to codeine required morphine when the cause was found to be metastatic cancer (Cassell 1982). Further, patients whose pain has lasted many months are anxious as they look into the future and anticipate only continuing and increasing pain. A new or worsening pain implies further deterioration — a step closer to death.

■ CASE HISTORY

A 56 year-old man with cancer of the prostate and spinal metastases became paraplegic. He lay in a general hospital bed for 11 weeks with no knowledge of why he had become paraplegic, or that it had anything to do with his cancer which he thought was cured. Because he was considered terminal, he received no physiotherapy and few visits from a doctor. He was turned every 2 hours, and had a large sacral bedsore. Thus, he spent 2 hours out of every 4 facing the wall instead of the door. This increased his depression which in turn increased his pain. Transfer to a palliative care unit, physiotherapy, honesty about his disease, and explanation about future expectations enabled him to become wheelchair independent, and return home for 3 months. His pain eased even though drug doses were unchanged. He was re-admitted to the palliative care unit only the day before he died.

Social pain

Social pain means the suffering associated with anticipated or actual separation or loss. Patients realize that they are going to be separated from their family by death. Often the hospital hastens that separation by restrictions on visiting. It is important, therefore, that steps are taken to avoid anything which separates terminally ill patients from their family and friends. A patient's pain may be relieved better by allowing grandchildren to visit than by increasing opioid dosage. Social isolation at home can also contribute to social pain.

Pain may also be exacerbated by interpersonal or financial problems, as shown in the following accounts:

■ CASE HISTORY

A 45 year-old man with advanced pancreatic cancer became so angry and depressed by his deterioration that he disrupted his whole household. He had always been a domineering father but, when suffering from persistent pain, this tendency took on an angry and vicious aspect. Two of his teenage sons ran away from home and his wife attempted suicide. At this point he was admitted to a palliative care unit. His pain was greatly exacerbated by the family problems the illness had caused. With the help of the social worker, the runaways were found and, in time, brought back into the family. These aspects of care, together with analgesics, relieved his pain and he in turn was then able to re-establish normal family relationships.

■ CASE HISTORY

A 38 year-old Italian immigrant came to the USA with his wife and three small children in the hope of making his fortune. He had set up a small business in horticulture and had minimal medical insurance. He was then found to have advanced cancer of the rectum. He was referred to a home palliative care unit programme because of intractable rectal and abdominal pain. When the pain had been reduced by analgesics, he was more able to talk about his problems. An outstanding hospital bill for $12 000 was a major anxiety. He knew he was leaving his wife and three young children with a hospital bill to pay off at the rate of $50 per week.

Spiritual pain

■ CASE HISTORY

An active member of a Christian church was in hospital dying of cancer.

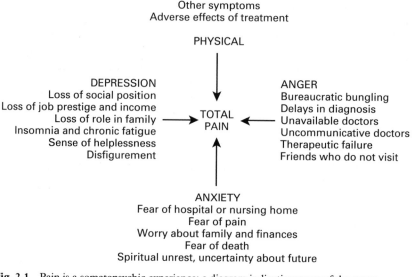

Fig. 2.1 Pain is a somatopsychic experience: a diagram indicating some of the many nonphysical influences which modify perception of pain.

She was in constant pain. This and the prospect of death created tremendous anxiety. Several relatives spent much of the day with the woman but this appeared not to help. A church visitor invited the family members present to pray with her and the patient. Although initially self-conscious, their discomfort gave way to a sense of serenity as they prayed together. The patient's pain completely subsided and, a few days later, she died peacefully in her sleep. Her sister subsequently phoned the church visitor to thank her for her help. 'We were all praying for Betty individually, but none of us had realized the importance of praying together with her. The experience has deepened our relationship with God and with one another' (Shlemon et al 1978).

In palliative care, the contribution of any one person or treatment is not generally as dramatic as this. The story is included, in part, to help redress the tendency nowadays to undervalue the role of the clergy and their helpers.

Others have modified the description of total pain (Fig. 2.1). The essential message however remains unchanged, namely, that pain is a somatopsychic experience, and nonphysical aspects must be addressed.

REFERENCES

Aronoff G M, Wilson R R 1978 How to teach your patients to control chronic pain. Behavioural Medicine 5: 29–35
Bergman J I, Werblun M N 1978 Chronic pain. A review for the family physician. Journal of Family Practice 7: 685–693
Black R G 1975 The chronic pain syndrome. Surgical Clinics of North America 55: 999–1011
Boas R A 1976 Chronic benign pain. Pain 2: 359
Bonica J J 1990 Definitions and taxonomy of pain. In: Bonica J J (ed). The management of pain, 2 edn. Lea & Febiger, Philadelphia, pp 18–27

Cassell E J 1982 The nature of suffering and the goals of medicine. New England Journal of Medicine 306: 639–645

Cassell E J 1991 The nature of suffering and the goals of medicine. Oxford University Press, Oxford

Fishman B 1990 The treatment of suffering in patients with cancer pain: cognitive-behavioral approaches. In: Foley K M, Bonica J J, Ventafridda V (eds) Advances in pain research and therapy vol 16. Raven Press, New York pp 301–316

Fordyce W 1973 An operant conditioning method for managing chronic pain. Postgraduate Medicine 53: 123–128

Freud S 1963 The standard edition of the complete psychological works of Sigmund Freud. Hogarth Press, London

Gates R P 1993 A different kind of cancer pain: the issue of family pain. American Journal of Hospice and Palliative Care 10: 11–12

Kuhn C C, Bradnan W A 1979 Pain as a substitute for the fear of death. Psychosomatics 20: 494–495

Lichter I 1991 Some psychological causes of distress in the terminally ill. Palliative Medicine 5: 138–146

Massie M J 1990 Depression. In: Holland J C, Rowland J H (eds) Handbook of Psychooncology. Oxford University Press, Oxford, pp 283–290

Saunders C M 1967 The management of terminal illness. Hospital Medicine Publications, London

Shlemon B L, Linn D, Linn M 1978. To heal as Jesus healed. Ave Maria Press, Notre Dame, Indiana, p 49

Stedeford A 1987 Hospice: a safe place to suffer? Palliative Medicine 1: 73–74

Sternbach R A 1974 Pain patients: traits and treatments. New York, Academic Press

Sternbach R A, Ignelzi R J, Deems L M, Timmermans G 1976 Transcutaneous electrical analgesia: a follow-up analysis. Pain 2: 35–41

Tunks E 1990 Is there a chronic pain syndrome? In: Lipton S, Tunks E, Zoppi M (eds) Advances in pain research and therapy. Raven Press, New York, pp 257–266

Turk D C, Fernandez E 1990 On the putative uniqueness of cancer pain: do psychological principles apply? Behaviour Research and Therapy 28: 1–13

Turk D C, Meichenbaum D H 1989 A cognitive-behavioural approach to pain management. In: Wall P D, Melzack R (eds) Textbook of pain. Churchill Livingstone, Edinburgh, pp 1001–1009

Basic science

DEFINITION OF PAIN

More than 2000 years ago, Aristotle described pain, along with pleasure, as a 'passion of the soul'. He further emphasized that pain is not just a physical sensation by omitting it from his list of the five senses (sight, hearing, smell, taste, touch). This fundamental truth about pain has been incorporated in the definition of pain proposed by the International Association for the Study of Pain (IASP):

> 'Pain is an unpleasant sensory and emotional experience associated with actual or potential tissue damage, or described in terms of such damage' (IASP 1986).

The definition is followed by a long explanatory note (Box 3.A) which further stresses that pain is a somatopsychic experience (Fig. 3.1).

It is this dualistic model of pain which gives rise to one of the more popular definitions of pain, namely, pain is what the patient says hurts. The following equation, therefore, does *not* exist:

x units of noxious stimulus = y units of pain experienced.

A classical description of the *falsehood* of this equation can be found in an article 'Pain in men wounded in battle' (Beecher 1946). In the Second World War, over 200 seriously injured soldiers were asked about pain and their need of analgesia shortly after entry into a Forward Hospital. Only 24% said they had severe pain and only a similar number (27%) requested medication (Table 3.1).

Pain threshold varies both between and within ethnic groups even under controlled conditions in the laboratory (Box 3.B). What some people describe merely as warmth is reported as painful by others (Hardy et al 1952). In one study, normal subjects from a single ethnic group could be separated into (Keele 1967):

- hypersensitives (22%)

BOX 3.A
DEFINITION OF PAIN PROPOSED BY THE INTERNATIONAL ASSOCIATION FOR THE STUDY OF PAIN (IASP 1986)

An unpleasant sensory and emotional experience associated with actual or potential tissue damage, or described in terms of such damage.

Note: Pain is always subjective. Each individual learns the application of the word through experiences related to injury in early life. Biologists recognize that those stimuli which cause pain are liable to damage tissue. Accordingly, pain is that experience which we associate with actual or potential tissue damage. It is unquestionably a sensation in a part or parts of the body, but it is also always unpleasant and therefore also an emotional experience. Experiences which resemble pain, e.g. pricking, but are not unpleasant should not be called pain. Unpleasant abnormal experiences (dysaesthesiae) may also be pain but are not necessarily so because, subjectively, they may not have the usual sensory qualities of pain.

Many people report pain in the absence of tissue damage or any likely pathophysiological cause; usually this happens for psychological reasons. There is no way to distinguish their experience from that due to tissue damage if we take the subjective report. If they regard their experience as pain and if they report it in the same ways as pain caused by tissue damage, it should be accepted as pain. This definition avoids tying pain to the stimulus. Activity induced in the nociceptor and nociceptive pathways by a noxious stimulus is not pain, which is always a psychological state, even though we may well appreciate that pain most often has a proximate physical cause.

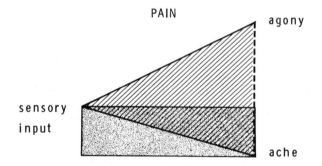

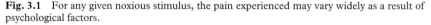

Fig. 3.1 For any given noxious stimulus, the pain experienced may vary widely as a result of psychological factors.

Table 3.1 Pain experienced by 215 severely injured soldiers

Pain intensity	Percentage[a]
No pain	32
Slight	26
Moderate	19
Severe	24

[a] Figures rounded to nearest whole number.
From Beecher 1946

- normosensitives (61%)
- hyposensitives (17%).

Hyposensitive subjects experience less pain even, for example, after myocardial infarction. Differences in pain sensitivity relate partly to differences in endogenous opioid production (Buchsbaum et al 1977). Ethnic and cultural factors (attitudes, beliefs, emotions, psychological states) are also important (Bates et al 1993).

TERMINOLOGY

Strictly speaking it is wrong to speak of a 'painful stimulus' which is converted to 'pain signals' in 'pain fibres' and then conducted to the brain where the information is registered as 'pain' (Woolf 1991). 'Noxious stimulus' is a preferable term (Box 3.B), with 'nociception' as the activity produced in the nervous system by potential or actual tissue damaging stimuli. Pain is the perception of nociception and, as already emphasized, its intensity is determined by an interaction between sensorineural activity and other factors (Portenoy 1992).

NEURO-ANATOMY

Peripheral nerve

Research papers use two different classifications based on fibre diameter to describe nerve fibres. One classification uses Roman numbers I–IV (Lloyd & Chang 1948), whereas the other uses a mixture of Roman and Greek letters (Gasser & Grundfest 1939). A–alpha, A–gamma and B are motor

---

BOX 3.B
USEFUL DEFINITIONS

Sensation threshold
The least stimulus at which a person perceives a sensation.
Note: this is uniform for all ethnic groups under laboratory conditions. Elsewhere, attention and suggestion radically modify the sensation threshold.

Pain threshold (IASP 1986)
The least experience of pain which a subject can recognize.

Pain tolerance level (IASP 1986)
The greatest level of pain which a subject is prepared to tolerate.

Noxious stimulus (IASP 1986)
A noxious stimulus is one which is damaging to normal tissues.

Nociceptor (IASP 1986)
A receptor preferentially sensitive to a noxious stimulus or to a stimulus which would become noxious if prolonged.

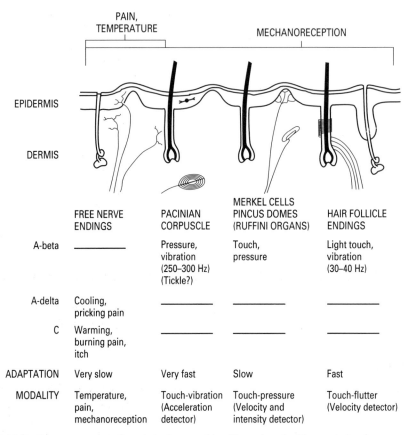

Fig. 3.2 Sensory neurones from hairy human skin. (Reproduced with permission from Shepherd 1988.)

fibres; A–beta, A–delta and C are sensory fibres (Fig. 3.2). Fibres which subserve pain are A–delta (III) and C (IV).

There are morphologically distinct nerve endings in almost all tissues which, when activated, give rise to pain. These nerve endings are called nociceptors (Box 3.B). Nociceptors are normally inactive but are excited by mechanical, thermal and chemical stimuli (Table 3.2). Unless sensitized they respond only to noxious, or potentially noxious stimuli.

A–delta nociceptors respond particularly well to pinching or squeezing the skin, or to a pinprick. C nociceptors respond to noxious mechanical, thermal and chemical stimuli. They are also sensitive to many pain producing substances such as *acetylcholine, bradykinin, histamine, potassium, capsaicin* and *strong acids*. Because of their responses to several types of noxious stimuli, C nociceptors are known as 'polymodal nociceptors'. A common property of both A–delta and C nociceptors is sensitization when exposed to repeated noxious stimuli (see p. 43).

The 'first' or 'fast' sharp pain which one experiences when stubbing a toe is mediated by A–delta fibres. The 'second' or 'slow' diffuse, throbbing,

Table 3.2   Contrasting characteristics of nociceptive fibres

	A-delta	C
Description	A-mechanoheat nociceptors[a]	C-polymodal nociceptors
Size	Larger (myelinated)	Smaller (unmyelinated)
Number	Fewer	Many more
Conduction	Faster	Slower
Content	Neuropeptides +/–	Neuropeptides +++
Functions	'First' pain (sharp)	'Second' pain (diffuse, throbbing, possibly burning)
	Pain localization	Threshold detection Pain intensity
Reflex response	Withdrawal	Guarding and immobility

[a] Respond less strongly to chemical stimuli.

possibly burning pain which follows seconds later and lasts longer is mediated by C fibres.

Peripheral afferent nerve fibres all have their cell bodies in the dorsal root ganglia and terminate in the dorsal horn of the spinal cord (Fig. 3.3).

Dorsal horn

Most afferent fibres enter the spinal cord via the dorsal root. A small proportion enters via the ventral root. The dorsal horn of the spinal cord is divided into five laminae, of which lamina II is known as the *substantia gelatinosa* (Fig. 3.4). The main input to the substantia gelatinosa is from the C fibres. These synapse predominantly with small second order neurones, most of which synapse again within the segment of entry or within the two adjacent segments. Because of their short length they are sometimes called 'interneurones'.

A second group of second order neurones are larger and form two main subgroups. The first is situated in lamina I, which receives input from only a small number of C or A–delta fibres. These are *nociceptor specific neurones* The other subgroup is confined mainly to lamina V. These neurones receive inputs from a large number of sensory nociceptive fibres and from the interneurones arising in the substantia gelatinosa. These multireceptive neurones

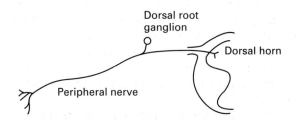

Fig. 3.3   A sensory peripheral nerve.

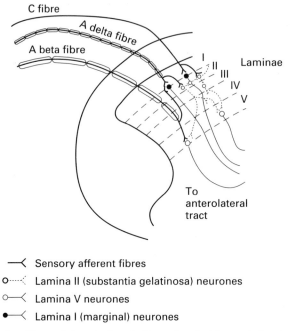

○───< Lamina II (substantia gelatinosa) neurones

○──< Lamina V neurones

●──< Lamina I (marginal) neurones

Fig. 3.4 The dorsal horn of the spinal cord. (Reproduced with permission from Hill 1986.)

are called *wide dynamic range neurones*; they lack spatial discrimination. They are excited by both innocuous (e.g. light touch) and noxious inputs.

The two subgroups subserve different functions. The superficial second order neurones are involved in pain localization; the deeper ones are involved with coding pain intensity. Both, however, cross the spinal cord and ascend in the contralateral anterolateral tract to the brain stem and, in some cases, to the thalamus. While this pattern is true for skin afferents, there may be a different pattern for visceral and some muscle afferents (Hill 1986).

The dorsal horn, particularly the substantia gelatinosa, contains several neurotransmitters including:

- substance P
- glycine
- gamma-aminobutyric acid (GABA)
- enkephalins.

The substantia gelatinosa is one of the densest neuronal areas in the central nervous system (CNS) and is crucial for the reception and modulation of nociceptive messages delivered by peripheral fibres.

Central connections

Nociceptive impulses are subject to modulation (either inhibition or excitation) by descending supraspinal pathways and by large myelinated sensory fibres from the same and neighbouring spinal segments. Onward transmission into spinothalamic and other pathways is therefore modulated by many neuronal influences.

At a higher level the posterior group of thalamic nuclei, the reticular formation and the peri-aqueductal grey matter are important in processing nociceptive information.

NEUROTRANSMITTERS

Pronociceptive transmitters

Two classes of pronociceptive neurotransmitters have been identified (Wilcox 1991):

- neuropeptides
  — neurokinins A & B, and substance P
  — vaso-active intestinal peptide (VIP)
  — calcitonin gene related peptide (CGRP)
- excitatory amino acids
  — glutamate
  — aspartate
  — homocysteate.

Nociceptive fibres, particularly C fibres, contain an abundance of neuropeptides. Most fibres containing substance P also contain glutamate.

Substance P

The 'P' does not stand for pain; it derives from the 'P' in powder, the form in which the peptide was first isolated from horse intestine 60 years ago. Substance P contains 11 amino acids and is synthesized by about 20% of C fibres. It is released into the spinal cord following noxious stimulation, and excites interneurones and other second order neurones. Substance P comes closest to being a specific transmitter for noxious messages. Like most neurotransmitters, it acts at a specific receptor on other nerve cells.

Attempts have been made to deplete substance P. Many people have experienced the effects of capsaicin, the active ingredient in hot pepper. Capsaicin activates substance P containing peripheral nerve fibres. Studies have shown that, when applied to a peripheral nerve of adult rats, capsaicin massively stimulates the fibres. This is followed by prolonged depletion of substance P in the C fibres, with a concomitant decrease in sensitivity. When capsaicin is injected into 2 day-old rats, it is neurotoxic and the substance P containing nerve fibres are permanently destroyed. The rats grow up with a reduced or absent sensitivity to noxious stimuli, although otherwise normal. It is possible that people from cultures which consume very hot, spicy dishes tolerate such food because the C fibres in their tongues were destroyed by repeated exposure to capsaicin as infants.

Excitatory amino acids

Several excitatory amino acid receptors have been identified within the mammalian CNS:

- N–methyl D–aspartate (NMDA) receptor
- nonNMDA receptors.

They are involved in a range of neural activities (Lodge & Collingridge 1991). In the context of pain modulation, most attention hitherto has been directed towards the NMDA receptor (Wilcox 1991, Woolf 1991). Now attention is also being focused on the nonNMDA receptors (Coderre et al 1993).

   The NMDA receptor is closely involved in the development of central (dorsal horn) sensitization (see p. 43). Activation of the postsynaptic NMDA receptor requires the binding of:

- glutamate or aspartate to the receptor
- glycine to an adjacent site as a co-agonist.

This results in a membrane depolarization which removes the magnesium ion block of the resting channel (Fig. 3.5).

   A number of existing drugs have been shown to be noncompetitive NMDA antagonists, for example ketamine, phencyclidine (PCP) — both dissociative anaesthetics — and the benzomorphans (Lodge 1988). These, together with a substance called MK 801, have been used to probe the functions of the receptor.

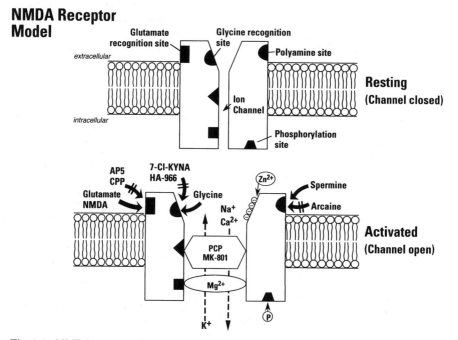

Fig. 3.5 NMDA receptor. (Reproduced with permission from an unpublished concept by Kemp & Foster 1993.)

Antinociceptive transmitters

Opioid peptides

Several naturally occurring peptides with morphine-like properties have been isolated. Three distinct families have been identified (*endorphins, dynorphins, enkephalins*). Each stems from a different prohormone and is preferentially associated with a different class of opioid receptor (Table 3.3):

- endorphins have a high specificity for the mu receptor (main morphine binding site)
- dynorphins for the kappa receptor
- enkephalins for the delta receptor.

All three families of opioid peptides, together with their complementary receptors, are present in the CNS and are concentrated in certain areas, including:

- dorsal horn (spinal cord)
- peri-aqueductal grey matter (brain stem)
- midline raphe nuclei (brain stem).

The opioid peptides form the chemical messengers (neurotransmitters and neurohormones) of a widespread and complex inhibitory signalling system. With respect to pain modulation, the mu receptor is probably the most important (see p. 178). In the dorsal horn, opioid receptors are present in the terminals of A–delta and C fibres and also in the postsynaptic fibres (Fields et al 1980). Endogenous and exogenous opioids act to block both transmitter release from nociceptor afferent terminals and transmitter action postsynaptically. Destruction of nociceptive primary afferents leads to a significant reduction in opioid binding sites in the dorsal horn (Fields et al

Table 3.3 Opioid receptors and their ligands

Receptor	Mu	Kappa	Delta
Endogenous ligands	Beta-endorphin Dermorphin Metorphamide	Dynorphins	Met-enkephalin Leu-enkephalin
Exogenous ligands	Morphine[a] Fentanyl Methadone DAGOL[b]	U50488H[c] U69893 PD117302 Pentazocine	DPDPE[b] DTLET DSTBULET
Antagonists	Naloxone (low dose) Beta-FNA[d]	Naloxone (high dose) Nor-BNI[e]	Naloxone (medium dose) ICI174864

[a] Most clinically used opioids are predominantly mu agonists.
[b] DAGOL, DPDPE, DTLET and DSTBULET are all peptide analogues based on enkephalin.
[c] U50488H, U69893 and PD117302 are nonpeptide kappa agonists.
[d] Beta-FNA is beta-funaltrexamine, an irreversible antagonist.
[e] nor-BNI is nor-binaltorphimine.
From Dickenson 1991b

1980). This may in part explain the reduced opioid responsiveness observed with most neuropathic pains.

Mono-amines

Serotonin is the neurotransmitter for a descending inhibitory pathway running from the peri-aqueductal grey matter in the brain stem to the spinal cord (Mayer & Price 1976). Noradrenaline is the neurotransmitter for a descending inhibitory pathway running from the lateral reticular formation of the midbrain to the spinal cord (Mayer & Price 1976). Both serotonin and noradrenaline are involved in pain modulation.

The following observations emphasize the interrelationship between serotonergic and opioidergic mechanisms in pain modulation:

- electrical stimulation of the peri-aqueductal grey matter in the midbrain produces analgesia in rats (Reynolds 1969)
- increasing the local concentration of serotonin increases the effect of electrical stimulation (Akil & Mayer 1972)
- decreasing the local concentration of serotonin by inhibiting serotonin synthesis decreases the effect of electrical stimulation (Akil & Mayer 1972)
- areas of the brain where electrical stimulation produces analgesia also correspond to the sites of opioid receptors (Pasternak 1980)
- an increase in serotonin levels increases morphine analgesia (Sternbach et al 1976)
- a decrease in serotonin levels decreases morphine analgesia (Sternbach et al 1976)
- destruction of serotonergic pathways blocks the analgesic effect of morphine (Samanin et al 1970, Proudfit & Anderson 1975)
- administration of L-tryptophan, a serotonin precursor, enhances the analgesic effect of morphine in humans (Hosobuchi et al 1980)
- cross-tolerance between stimulation produced analgesia and morphine analgesia has been noted (Mayer & Price 1976).

Opioids and tricyclic antidepressants share a number of pharmacological characteristics in animal studies (Lee & Spencer 1977). Tricyclic antidepressants block the presynaptic re-uptake of serotonin and noradrenaline; they also enhance morphine analgesia (Walsh 1986). Tricyclic antidepressants modify development of morphine tolerance in animals (Spencer 1976). Fluoxetine, a selective serotonin re-uptake inhibitor, enhances the analgesic effect of morphine, methadone and pethidine (Sugrue & McIndewar 1976).

MORPHINE INDUCED ALLODYNIA

Rats given morphine 1–10 µg intrathecally (IT) manifest dose dependent antinociception (Schmauss & Yaksh 1983). In contrast, much higher doses (150 µg) produce a behavioural syndrome characterized by:

- periodic bouts of spontaneous agitation during which the rat scratches and bites at the skin of its caudal dermatomes

- squealing and vigorous efforts to bite and escape when the flank is touched.

Both forms of behaviour are suggestive of allodynia (pain produced by an innocuous stimulus). The phenomenon is not reversed by opioid antagonists and tolerance does not occur (Yaksh et al 1986, Yaksh & Harty 1988). A range of morphine derivatives produce a similar effect (Table 3.4). The sulphated and conjugated metabolites are 10–50 times more potent than morphine itself. This drug induced allodynia (Yaksh & Harty 1988):

- is limited to caudal dermatomes and touching the face or forepaws has no effect (i.e. it is a spinal phenomenon)
- is not antagonized by even high doses of opioid antagonists (i.e. it is not mediated by an opioid receptor)
- does not display cross-tolerance
- does not reflect known opioid potency ratios (more potent opioids such as levorphanol, alfentanil and sufentanil do not produce allodynia).

Although it is possible to postulate which structural characteristics are needed to evoke allodynia, the underlying systems are unknown (Yaksh & Harty 1988). A similar phenomenon is seen with strychnine overdose in humans.

Other animal studies have shown that morphine–3–glucuronide (M3G) antagonizes or attenuates the antinociceptive effect of morphine-6-glucuronide (M6G) (Smith et al 1990, Gong et al 1992). Because M3G does not bind to opioid receptors, this effect must be mediated through a nonopioid mechanism (Labella et al 1979). Allodynia and myoclonus have been noted in humans after high dose IT and IV morphine (Stillman et al 1987, De Conno et al 1991, Sjogren et al 1993). This phenomenon is discussed further in Chapters 4 and 14.

Table 3.4 Morphine induced allodynia in rats

Substances producing allodynia (in order of activity)	Substances without effect
Noroxymorphone-3-glucuronide	Alfentanil
Morphine-3-glucuronide	Codeine
Morphine-3-ethereal sulphate	Dextrorphan
Dihydromorphine	Di-acetylmorphine
Noroxymorphone dihydrate	Levorphanol
Hydromorphone	Methadone
Dihydrocodeine	Nalbuphine
Morphine sulphate	Nalorphine
Dihydro-isomorphine	Naloxone
Morphine hydrochloride	Naltrexone
6-acetylmorphine	Naltrexone-3-glucuronide
N-normorphine	Norpethidine
(+)-morphine	Oxycodone
	Oxymorphone
	Pethidine
	Sufentanil
	Thebaine

From Yaksh & Harty 1988

> **BOX 3.C**
> **USEFUL DEFINITIONS**
>
> **Plasticity**
> The ability of nociceptive neurones to vary their responsiveness to stimuli as a result of:
>
> - prolonged stimulation
> - chemical mediators of inflammation
> - neural injury.
>
> **Sensitization**
> A reduced pain threshold in injured tissue and the surrounding area, or in an area subserved by an injured peripheral nerve or an injured part of the CNS.

NEURAL PLASTICITY

'The transmission of pain should not be viewed as a passive simple process using hard-wired exclusive pathways but as messages arising from the interplay between neuronal systems, both excitatory and inhibitory, at many levels of the central nervous system and which converge particularly on the spinal cord' (Dickenson 1991a).

Plasticity is a word used to describe a general property of the nervous system (Box 3.C), namely the ability to modify function in different circumstances (Coderre et al 1993). The key factors are duration of stimulation and neural sensitization:

- peripheral sensitization (associated with inflammation)
- central sensitization (secondary to peripheral sensitization or neural injury).

Plasticity explains the recurrence of pain after permanent neurodestructive procedures such as spinothalamic tractotomy (cordotomy). Recurrent pain in these circumstances is often more difficult to treat. This makes the timing of such procedures critical; if performed too early, the pain may recur before the patient dies. It may then be necessary to repeat the procedure with the likelihood of decreased efficacy and increased morbidity (McQuay & Dickenson 1990).

NEURAL SENSITIZATION

Both tissue injury and neural injury can produce persistent pain, allodynia and hyperalgesia. There are, however, significant differences in the underlying mechanisms. Tissue injury is typically associated with local inflammation, whereas neural injury commonly leads to neuronal degeneration, neuroma formation and the generation of spontaneous neuronal activity with little or no associated inflammation.

Nociceptive pain produced by tissue injury is influenced significantly by local inflammatory changes, whereas neural injury pain is influenced by pathological changes in function. Although nociceptive and neural injury pain have different peripheral mechanisms, they are both associated with secondary changes in CNS function, notably in the dorsal horn of the spinal cord.

Peripheral sensitization

Tissue injury stimulates:

- synthesis of arachidonic acid metabolites from adjacent membranes, including *prostaglandins* (PGs)
- release of *bradykinin* from its inactive precursor
- release of neuropeptides such as *substance P* and *calcitonin gene related peptide* from C fibres.

This 'inflammatory soup', which also contains *histamine, serotonin, potassium ions* and *hydrogen ions*, activates and sensitizes the peripheral nerve endings causing vasodilatation and plasma extravasation. This results in swelling, tenderness and pain (Table 3.5; Fig. 3.6). In this situation, innocuous stimuli evoke pain (Box 3.D; Fig. 3.7).

Central sensitization

A repetitive transcutaneous stimulus to the receptive field of a C fibre in the rat leads to a dramatic increase in the neuronal response in the dorsal horn of up to 20 times. This phenomenon has been called 'wind up'. It reaches a maximum after 16 seconds. It can also transform 30 seconds of stimulation into several minutes of response.

Nociception associated with wind up is less responsive to opioids (Dickenson & Sullivan 1986). Further, although morphine cannot totally prevent wind up, pretreatment with morphine is more effective than posttreatment. On the other hand, NMDA antagonists prevent wind up, converting the otherwise enhanced response into a steady one (Wilcox 1991).

The NMDA receptor plays a key role in the induction of central sensitization whether triggered by wind up, peripheral sensitization or neural injury (Woolf & Thompson 1991). This receptor-ion channel complex is

Table 3.5   Chemical intermediaries in nociceptive transduction

Substance	Source	Enzyme	Produces pain in man	Effect on primary afferent
Potassium	Injured cells		++	Activate
Serotonin	Platelets		++	Activate
Bradykinin	Plasma kininogen	Kallikrein	+++	Activate
Histamine	Mast cells		+	Activate
Prostaglandins	Arachidonic acid from injured cells	Cyclo-oxygenase	±	Sensitize
Leukotrienes	Arachidonic acid from injured cells	Lipoxygenase	±	Sensitize
Substance P	Primary afferent		±	Sensitize

From Fields 1987

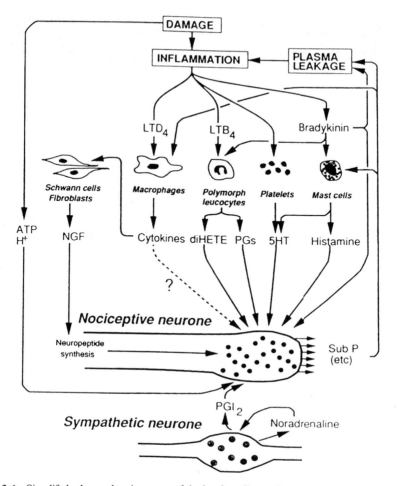

Fig. 3.6 Simplifed scheme showing some of the local mediators that may act on nociceptive nerve terminals under conditions of tissue damage and inflammation, as discussed in text. Abbreviations: LTD_4 = leukotriene D_4; LTB_4 = leukotriene B_4; NGF = nerve growth factor; diHETE = dihydroxy-eicosatetraenoic acid; PGs, prostaglandins E and F_{2x}; 5HT = 5-hydroxytryptamine. (Reproduced with permission from Rang et al 1991.)

not activated at normal resting membrane potentials because the channel is blocked by Mg^{2+} (Fig. 3.5; Mayer et al 1984). When the resting membrane potential is changed by prolonged excitation, the channel unblocks.

Cerebral sensitization

Rats demonstrate a reproducible response to the SC injection of formalin into the hindpaw. Local infiltration with local anaesthetic 25 min after SC formalin results in the abolition of sensation in the paw but the persistence of the behavioural response seen with formalin induced pain (Coderre et al 1990). Such observations have led to the suggestion that the memory of pain contributes to neural sensitization (McQuay & Dickenson 1990). This reflects the phenomenon of somatization seen in humans (see p. 22).

BOX 3. D
EXPERIMENTAL EVIDENCE OF SENSITIZATION AFTER TISSUE INJURY
(Meyer et al 1985)

The following experiment is one of many which demonstrates peripheral sensitization manifesting as *hyperalgesia* and *allodynia*.

Volunteers received a 53°C stimulus to a small area on the palm of the hand near the base of the thumb for 30 seconds. This resulted in a blister after several hours in half the subjects.

Marked primary hyperalgesia was apparent when tested after 10 minutes:

● pain evoked by base temperature (38°C)
● response to original suprathreshold stimuli much increased.

For example, before the burn a 41°C stimulus was not painful; after the burn it was as painful as a stimulus of 49°C beforehand (Fig. 3.7). The threshold for mechanically induced pain was also lowered.

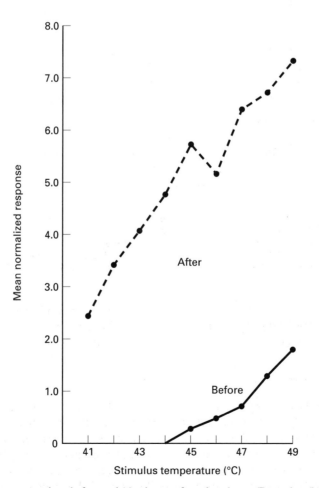

Fig. 3.7   Responses to heat before and 10 minutes after a heat burn. (Reproduced with permission from Meyer et al 1985.)

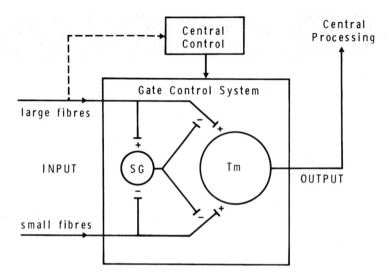

Fig. 3.8 Schematic diagram of the gate control theory of pain. SG represents a substantia gelatinosa cell; Tm, a spinal cord transmission cell. Central control refers to cognitive, motivational, and affective processes which modulate descending pain pathways. Central processing takes place in the reticular formation, thalamus, and limbic system. (+) denotes an excitatory influence; (–) denotes inhibition. (Adapted from Melzack 1973.)

GATE CONTROL THEORY OF PAIN

The gate control theory of pain is summarized in Figure 3.8. Activation of large diameter, low threshold A-beta mechanoreceptors inhibits the response of dorsal horn cells to nociceptive inputs (Wall & Cronly-Dillon 1960, Melzack & Wall 1965). This was the rationale behind the introduction of transcutaneous electrical nerve stimulation (TENS) and dorsal column stimulation. Inhibition is partly presynaptic and partly postsynaptic. The term 'gate control' should be restricted to the rapidly acting mechanisms in the dorsal horn which receive and control the transfer of impulses from the afferent fibres to the transmitting cells.

The gate control theory of pain represented a major advance in scientific thinking about pain (Melzack & Wall 1965). It fitted the facts 30 years ago far better than the discredited specificity and pattern theories of pain. Since then the gate control theory has undergone significant modification (Melzack 1991). Basically, it is an attempt to explain the modulatory functions of the dorsal horn (Fig. 3.8). The original theory has also been extended to embrace 'sensitivity control' and 'connectivity control' (Box 3.E). Sensitivity control is merely a jargonistic way of talking about central (dorsal horn) sensitization. Connectivity control is an attempt to explain the development of pathological 'central pattern generating mechanisms' in neuropathic pain states.

PRE-EMPTIVE ANALGESIA

Following the discovery that prolonged nociception leads to central sensi-

---

BOX 3.E
MECHANISMS WHICH CHANGE THE EXCITABILITY OF DORSAL HORN CELLS
(Wall 1989)

Gate control
Time course = rapid (milliseconds)

- transmitting cells in the dorsal horn affected by peripheral afferents and descending systems
- rapidly inhibitory and excitatory interneurones also acting on transmitting cells
- operates via amino acid neurotransmitters

Sensitivity control
Time course = slow (minutes to hours)

- long latency, long duration changes of excitability triggered by an afferent barrage in unmyelinated afferents, particularly from deep tissue and by descending systems
- probably operates via peptide neurotransmitters

Connectivity control
Time course = prolonged (days to months)

- a latency of days and a duration of months
- the arrival of chemicals transported from the periphery affects neuronal inputs, particularly in unmyelinated C fibres
- may result in 'central pattern generating mechanisms' which account for persistent pain despite deafferentation

---

tization, it was suggested that prophylactic analgesia might be more effective than analgesia given after the onset of pain (Wall 1988, Cousins 1991, Bush 1993). Animal and human studies lend support to this hypothesis. Thus, in the rat, IT morphine before a hindpaw injection of SC formalin produces 70% greater inhibition of C-fibre activity than the same dose after formalin (Dickenson & Sullivan 1987). The same 'before and after' effect was observed with IT local anaesthetic even when given as soon as 5 min after the formalin.

Nociception after formalin lasts only about 1 h. This is a short time scale. A pre-emptive effect, however, has been reported with the use of local anaesthetic in an animal model of neuropathic pain (Selzer et al 1991). This suggests that the pre-emptive effect may be relevant for both nociceptive pain (e.g. postoperative) and neuropathic pain (e.g. phantom limb).

Clinical benefit has been shown with pre-emptive analgesia (Bach et al 1988, McQuay et al 1988, Cousins 1991, Dahl et al 1992a, Bush 1993). In an analysis of the records of nearly 1000 patients who had had orthopaedic surgery, it was found that the median times to the first request for post-operative analgesia after different forms of therapy were:

- general anaesthesia only = <2 h
- opioid premedication and general anaesthesia = >5 h
- local anaesthesia = 8 h
- opioid premedication and local anaesthesia = >9 h.

In addition, whereas 95% of the patients receiving general anaesthesia alone requested analgesics, the percentages in the other three categories were 74%, 82% and 88% (McQuay et al 1988). A study in 60 women using IV patient controlled analgesia (PCA) after abdominal hysterectomy showed that morphine 10 mg IV at the time of induction resulted in a 27% reduction in postoperative morphine requirements (Richmond et al 1993). Pain sensitivity (secondary hyperalgesia) around the wound was also reduced. Another review showed that good pain relief before amputation for limb ischaemia reduces the incidence of postamputation phantom limb pain (Bach et al 1988).

The results of different trials, however, are not consistent. Pre-emptive local anaesthetic block for inguinal herniorrhaphy resulted in reduced pain scores and a delay in requests for analgesia over the initial 6 h postoperative period (Ejlersen et al 1992), but no pre-emptive effect was noted over a longer period (Dierking et al 1992). Patients given epidural fentanyl shortly before thoracotomy reported less pain and used less supplementary analgesic afterwards (Katz et al 1992) but no such effect was observed with pre-emptive epidural bupivacaine and morphine before abdominal surgery (Dahl et al 1992b).

These conflicting findings might possibly relate partly to differences in the effectiveness and duration of the nociceptive blockade by the different interventions. Further, the sensitizing effect of extensive nociceptive stimulation during surgery may be much more difficult to block than the limited chemical or thermal stimuli used in animal models. In addition, it is not known how long afferent blockade must be continued during and after surgery to ensure that central sensitization is prevented and not simply delayed (Bush 1993).

In one study, infiltration with local anaesthetic before general anaesthesia made a measurable difference to the intensity of pain when pressure was subsequently applied to the wound. This difference was found as late as 10 days postoperatively. The comparison was with groups also undergoing hernia surgery but who received either general anaesthesia alone or a spinal injection of local anaesthetic (Tverskoy et al 1990). Another study in hernia patients compared ilio-inguinal block plus spinal anaesthesia with spinal anaesthesia alone and concluded that the ilio-inguinal block provided additional analgesia (Bugedo et al 1990). Pre-operative infiltration of local anaesthetic around the tonsils also reduces postoperative pain (Jebeles et al 1991). On the other hand, nonsteroidal anti-inflammatory drugs (NSAIDs) and paracetamol have no demonstrable pre-emptive effect (McQuay et al 1993).

TYPES OF PAIN

It is clear that all pain cannot be described in terms of a single neural mechanism. As a first step, pain can be divided into (Fig. 3.9; Cervero & Laird 1991):

- physiological
- pathological
- neuropathic.

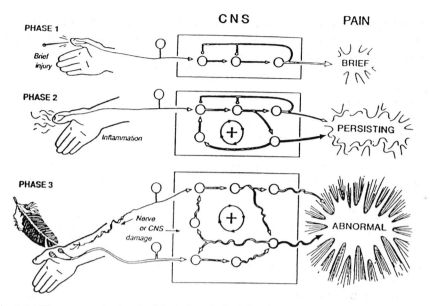

Fig. 3.9 Three types of pain: physiological, pathological and neuropathic. For explanation see text. (Reproduced with permission from Cervero & Laird 1991.)

Physiological pain

The nociceptive system warns of impending injury to the body. In certain circumstances, for example, pain from joints and ligaments indicates a need for a change of posture, and pain in the mouth indicates that the food being chewed is too hot and will burn the mucosa. In other words, physiological pain is protective and is needed for wellbeing and survival. With physiological pain there is a relatively close correlation between the intensity of the stimulus and the intensity of nociception.

The response to a noxious but noninjuring stimulus can be summarized as follows:

- specific spinal cord neurones provide a direct pathway for the transmission of pain related information
- modulation and encoding of the stimulus intensity is provided by wide dynamic range neurones in the dorsal horn.

The mechanisms involved in transmitting and processing a brief noxious stimulus are, therefore, relatively straightforward.

Pathological pain

Persistent noxious stimuli may have two effects on peripheral nociceptors in the affected area (Cervero & Laird 1991):

- nociceptors become sensitized, i.e. the response threshold decreases and the nociceptors can be activated by innocuous stimuli
- a group of silent nociceptors are activated by inflammation.

The afferent flow from an inflamed area will, therefore, increase dramatically as a result of these two mechanisms. Increased excitability occurs in both types of nociceptors after:

- skin burns
- noxious chemical stimulation of the skin or deep tissues
- induction of acute local inflammation.

This leads to an increase in receptive field size and greater spontaneous and evoked firing.

These changes in excitability may last for hours, even in the absence of ongoing stimuli, and are reflected in comparable changes in the dorsal horn (Cervero & Laird 1991). Thus, the CNS moves to a more excitable state as a result of the noxious input generated by tissue injury and inflammation. As healing occurs, recovery to the normal state will take place progressively.

Neuropathic pain

Many changes in the properties of primary afferent neurones have been identified after peripheral nerve injury (Bennett 1990). These changes include:

- spontaneous activity and hyperexcitability in nerve sprouts
- neuroma formation
- ephaptic coupling ('cross-talk') between adjacent nerve fibres.

Thus, as a result of peripheral nerve injury, the CNS receives a large volume of abnormal afferent inflow, and commonly there is a re-organization of central processing. Neuropathic pain is discussed more fully in Chapter 4.

REFERRED PAIN

Patients with ischaemic heart disease commonly experience referred pain in the upper chest, shoulder, neck and arm. This pain, angina pectoris, is the result of myocardial ischaemia but is manifested at other sites. Similarly, visceral pain may not be experienced immediately over the anatomical site. In cancer, referred pain occurs frequently:

- the most common type is that caused by nerve compression
- the most important is that associated with spinal cord compression
- the least well understood is that related to myofascial trigger points.

Referred pain from compression of peripheral nerves, cauda equina or spinal cord is easily understood, as is referred pain from a lesion in the region of the thalamus. Pain associated with myofascial trigger points is discussed in Chapter 4.

With visceral pain, an embryological explanation is at least partly necessary. An example is the presence of pain in the ipsilateral shoulder associated with inflammation of the diaphragm in cholecystitis. Both the diaphragm and the shoulder are innervated by fibres derived from the primitive C4 segment. It is then necessary to postulate that the brain 'misinterprets' the afferent impulses that converge on it from both visceral and somatic structures. The pain from the viscus is represented as having come from the embryologically corresponding somatic area. This is known as the convergence-projection theory (Procacci & Zoppi 1982). Visceral pain is discussed further in Chapter 4.

REFERENCES

Akil H, Mayer D J 1972 Antagonism of stimulation-produced analgesia by pCPA, a serotonin synthesis inhibitor. Brain Research 44: 692

Bach S, Noreng M F, Tjellden N U 1988 Phantom limb pain in amputees during the first 12 months following limb amputation, after pre-operative lumbar epidural blockade. Pain 33: 297–301

Bates M S, Edwards W T, Anderson K O 1993 Ethnocultural influences on variation in chronic pain perception. Pain 52: 101–112

Beecher H K 1946 Pain in men wounded in battle. Annals of Surgery 123: 96–105

Bennett G J 1990 Experimental models of painful peripheral neuropathies. NIPS 5: 128–133

Buchsbaum M S, Davis G C, Bunney W E, 1977 Naloxone alters pain perception and somatosensory evoked potentials in normal subjects. Nature 270: 620–622

Bugedo G J, Carcamo C R, Mertens R A, Dagnino J A, Munoz H R 1990 Preoperative percutaneous ilioinguinal and iliohypogastric nerve block with 0.5% bupivacaine for postherniorrhaphy pain management in adults. Regional Anaesthesia 15: 130–133

Bush D J 1993 Pre-emptive analgesia. British Medical Journal 306: 285–286

Cervero F, Laird J M 1991 A One pain or many pains? a new look at pain mechanisms. NIPS 6: 268–273

Coderre T J, Vaccarino A L, Melzack R 1990 Central nervous system plasticity in the tonic pain response to subcutaneous formalin injection. Brain Research 535: 155–158

Coderre T J, Katz J, Vaccarino A L, Melzack R 1993 Contribution of central neuroplasticity to pathological pain: review of clinical and experimental evidence. Pain 52: 259–285

Cousins M J 1991 Prevention of postoperative pain. In: Bond M R, Charlton J E, Woolf C J (eds). Proceedings of the VIth World Congress on Pain. Elsevier, Amsterdam, pp 41–52

Dahl J B, Erichsen C J, Fuglsang-Fredericksen A, Kehlet H 1992a Pain sensation and nociceptive reflex excitability in surgical patients and human volunteers. British Journal of Anaesthesia 69: 117–121

Dahl J B, Hansen B L, Hjortso N C, Erichsen C J, Moiniche S, Kehlet H 1992b Influence of timing on the effect of continuous extradural analgesia with bupivacaine and morphine after major abdominal surgery. British Journal of Anaesthesia 69: 4–9

De Conno F, Caraceni A, Martini C, Spoldi E, Salvetti M, Ventafridda V 1991 Hyperalgesia and myoclonus with intrathecal infusion of high dose morphine. Pain 47: 337–339

Dickenson A H 1991a Recent advances in the physiology and pharmacology of pain: plasticity and its implications for clinical analgesia. Journal of Psychopharmacology 5: 342–351

Dickenson A H 1991b Mechanisms of the analgesic actions of opiates and opioids. British Medical Bulletin 47: 690–702

Dickenson A H, Sullivan A F 1986 Electrophysiological studies on the effects of intrathecal morphine on nociceptive neurones in the rat dorsal horn. Pain 24: 211–222

Dickenson A H, Sullivan A F 1987 Subcutaneous formalin-induced activity of dorsal horn neurones in the rat: differential response to an intrathecal opiate administered pre or post formalin. Pain 30: 349–360

Dierking G W, Dahl J B, Kanstrupp J, Dahl A, Kehlet H 1992 Effect of pre- vs postoperative inguinal field block on postoperative pain after herniorrhaphy. British Journal of Anaesthesia 68: 344–348

Ejlersen E, Bryde Anderson H, Eliasen K, Mogensen T 1992 A comparison between preincisional and postincisional lidocaine infiltration and postoperative pain. Anesthesia and Analgesia 74: 495–498

Fields H L 1987 Pain. McGraw-Hill, New York

Fields H L, Emson P C, Leigh B K, Gilbert R F T, Iversen L L 1980 Multiple opiate receptor sites on primary afferent fibres. Nature 284: 351–353

Gasser H S, Grundfest H 1939 Axon diameters in relation to the spike dimensions and the conduction velocity in mammalian A-fibers. American Journal of Physiology 127: 393–414

Gong Q-L, Hedner J, Bjorkman R, Hedner T 1992 Morphine-3-glucuronide may functionally antagonize morphine-6-glucuronide induced antinociception and ventilatory depression in the rat. Pain 48: 249–255

Hardy J D, Wolff H G, Goodall H 1952 Pain sensations and reactions. Williams & Wilkins, Baltimore

Hill R G 1986 Current perspectives on pain. Sci Prog Oxford 70: 95–107

Hosobuchi Y, Lamb S, Bascom D 1980 Tryptophan loading may reverse tolerance to opiate analgesics in humans: a preliminary report. Pain 9: 161–169

IASP Subcommittee on Taxonomy 1986 Classification of chronic pain. Pain Suppl 3: 216–221

Jebeles J A, Reilly J S, Gutierrez J F, Bradley E L, Kissin I 1991 The effect of pre-incisional infiltration of tonsils with bupivacaine on the pain following tonsillectomy under general anaesthesia. Pain 47: 305–308

Katz J, Kavanagh B P, Sandler A N et al 1992 Pre-emptive analgesia: clinical evidence of neuroplasticity contributing to postoperative pain. Anesthesiology 77: 439–446

Keele K D 1967 Pain sensitivity and the pain pattern of cardiac infarction. Proceedings of Royal Society of Medicine 60: 417–419

Labella F S, Pinsky C, Havilicek V 1979 Morphine derivatives with diminished opiate receptor potency show enhanced central excitatory activity. Brain Research 174: 263–271

Lee R, Spencer P S J 1977 Antidepressants and pain: a review of the pharmacological data supporting the use of certain tricyclics in chronic pain. Journal of International Medical Research 5 (suppl 1): 146–156

Lloyd D P C, Chang H T 1948 Afferent fibers in muscle nerves. Journal of Neurophysiology 11: 199–207

Lodge D (ed) 1988 Excitatory amino acids in health and disease. John Wiley, Chichester

Lodge D, Collingridge G (eds) 1991 The pharmacology of excitatory amino acids. Elsevier Trends Journal, Cambridge

McQuay H J, Carroll D, Moore R A 1988 Postoperative orthopaedic pain: the effect of opiate premedication and local anaesthetic blocks. Pain 33: 291–295

McQuay H J, Dickenson A H 1990 Editorial: implications of nervous system plasticity for pain management. Anesthesia 45: 101–102

McQuay H J, Jadad A R, Amanor-Boadu S O, Jack T M, Glynn C J 1993 Pre-emptive analgesia: sufficient to change practice? Lancet 342: 434

Mayer D J, Price D D 1976 Central nervous system mechanisms of analgesia. Pain 2: 379–404

Mayer M L, Westbrook G, Guthrie P B 1984 Voltage-dependent blick for Mg^{2+} of NMDA responses in spinal cord neurones. Nature 309: 261–263

Melzack R 1973 The puzzle of pain. Penguin books, Harmondsworth

Melzack R 1991 The gate control theory 25 years later: new perspectives on phantom limb pain. In: Bond M R, Charlton J E, Woolf C J (eds) Proceedings of the VIth World Congress on Pain, Elsevier Science, Amsterdam, pp 9–21

Melzack R, Wall P D 1965 Pain mechanisms: a new theory. Science 150: 971–979

Meyer R A, Campbell J N, Raja S N 1985 Peripheral neural mechanisms of cutaneous hyperalgesia. In: Fields H L, Dubner R, Cervero F (eds) Advances in pain research and therapy, vol 9. Raven Press, New York, pp 53–71

Pasternak G W 1980 Endogenous opioid systems in brain. American Journal of Medicine 68: 157

Portenoy R K 1992 Cancer: pathophysiology and syndromes. Lancet 339: 1026–1031

Procacci P, Zoppi M 1982 Pathophysiology and clinical aspects of visceral and referred pain. In: Bonica J J, Lindblom U, Iggo A (eds) Advances in pain research and therapy, vol 5. Raven Press, New York, pp 643–658

Proudfit H K, Anderson E G 1975 Morphine analgesia: blockade by raphe magnus. Brain Research 98: 612–618

Rang H P, Bevan S, Dray A 1991 Chemical activation of nociceptive peripheral neurones. British Medical Bulletin 47 (3): 534–548

Reynolds D V 1969 Surgery in the rat during electrical analgesia induced by focal brain stimulation. Science 164: 444

Richmond C E, Bromley L M, Woolf C J 1993 Preoperative morphine pre-empts postoperative pain. Lancet 342: 73–75

Samanin R, Gumulka W, Valzelli L 1970 Reduced effect of morphine in midbrain raphe lesioned rats. European Journal of Pharmacology 10: 339–343

Saunders C, Baines M 1983 Living with Dying. The management of terminal disease. Oxford University Press, Oxford

Schmauss C, Yaksh T L 1983 In vivo studies on spinal opiate receptor systems mediating antinociception. II. Pharmacological profiles suggesting a differential association of mu, delta and kappa receptors with visceral, chemical and cutaneous thermal stimuli in the rat. Journal of Pharmacology and Experimental Therapeutics 228: 1–12

Selzer Z, Beilin B Z, Ginzburg R, Paran Y, Shimko T 1991 The role of injury discharge in the induction of neuropathic pain behaviour in rats. Pain 46: 327–336

Shepherd G M 1988 Neurobiology, 2nd edn. Oxford University Press, Oxford

Sjogren P, Jonsson T, Jensen N-H, Drenck N-E, Jensen T S 1993 Hyperalgesia and myoclonus in terminal cancer patients treated with continuous intravenous morphine. Pain 55: 93–97

Smith M T, Watt J A, Cramond T 1990 Morphine-3-glucuronide: a potent antagonist of morphine analgesia. Life Sciences 47: 579–585

Spencer P S J 1976 Some aspects of the pharmacology of analgesia. Journal of International Medical Research 4 (suppl 2): 1–13

Sternbach R A, Janowsky D S, Huey L Y, Segal D S 1976 Effects of altering brain serotonin activity on human chronic pain. In: Bonica J J, Albe-Fessard D (eds) Advances in pain research and therapy, vol 1. Raven Press, New York, pp 601–606

Stillman M J, Moulin D E, Foley K M 1987 Paradoxical pain following high-dose spinal morphine. Pain (suppl 4): S389

Sugrue M F, McIndewar I 1976 Effect of blockade of 5-hydroxytryptamine uptake of drug induced antinociception in the rat. Journal of Pharmacy and Pharmacology 28: 447–448

Tverskoy M, Cozacov C, Ayache M, Bradley E L, Kissin I 1990 Postoperative pain after inguinal herniorrhaphy with different types of anesthesia. Anesthesia & Analgesia 70: 29–35

Wall 1988 The prevention of postoperative pain. Pain 33: 289–290

Wall P D 1989 Introduction. In: Wall P D, Melzack R (eds) Textbook of pain. Churchill Livingstone, Edinburgh, pp 1–18

Wall P D, Cronly-Dillon J R 1960 Pain, itch and vibration. Archives of Neurology 2: 365–375

Walsh T D 1986 Controlled study of imipramiine and morphine in advanced cancer. Proceedings of the American Society of Clinical Oncology 5 (929): 237

Wilcox G L 1991 Excitatory neurotransmitters and pain. In: Bond M R, Charlton J E, Woolf C J (eds). Proceedings of the VIth World Congress on Pain. Elsevier, Amsterdam, pp 97–117

Woolf C J 1991 Central mechanisms of acute pain. In: Bond M R, Charlton J E, Woolf C J (eds). Proceedings of the VIth World Congress on Pain. Elsevier, Amsterdam, pp 25–33

Woolf C J, Thompson W N 1991 The induction and maintenance of central sensitization is dependent on N-methyl-D-aspartic acid receptor activation; implications for the treatment of postinjury pain hypersensitivity states. Pain 44: 293–299

Yaksh T L, Harty G J, Onofrio B M 1986 High doses of spinal morphine produce a nonopiate receptor-mediated hyperaesthesia: clinical and theoretic implications. Anesthesiology 64: 590–597

Yaksh T L, Harty G J 1988 Pharmacology of the allodynia in rats evoked by high dose intrathecal morphine. Journal of Pharmacology and Experimental Therapeutics 244: 501–507

4 | General categories of pain

CLASSIFICATION OF PAIN

Classification of pain into mechanistic categories is still a source of confusion. Division into the three broad categories discussed in Chapter 3, however, is a good start:

- physiological (functional)
- pathological (organic)
- neuropathic.

The Oxford Textbook of Palliative Medicine offers the following classification (Payne & Gonzales 1993):

- somatic
- visceral
- neuropathic
- sympathetically maintained.

This is unsatisfactory because it includes second level categories (somatic v. visceral) with a first level category (neuropathic). Further, given the IASP definition of neuropathy as 'a disturbance of function or pathological change in a nerve', it is difficult not to include sympathetically maintained pain within the broad category of neuropathic pain.

The classification of the Oxford Textbook is unsatisfactory in two other respects, namely, it does not:

- highlight adequately a range of functional muscular pains
- differentiate clearly between nerve compression pain (functional) and neural injury pain (organic).

When these factors are taken into account, a three level classification emerges (Fig. 4.1):

- nociceptive v. neuropathic

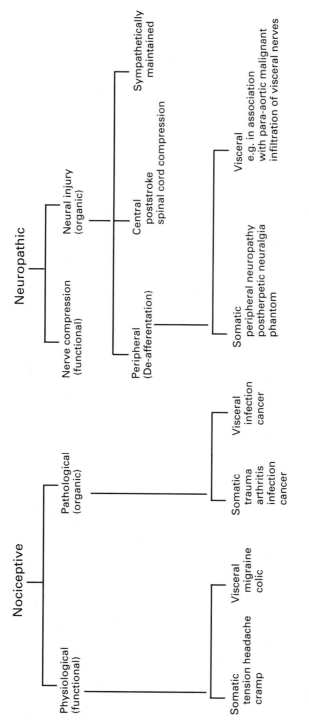

Fig. 4.1 Classification of pain.

- functional v. organic
- somatic v. visceral.

Even with this level of sophistication, however, difficulties arise particularly in relation to nerve compression (see p. 67). As noted in Chapter 3, nociceptive pain is produced by the activation of specific peripheral receptors (nociceptors). In the presence of inflammation, which leads to both peripheral and central sensitization, however, *nonnociceptive* A-beta fibres are also involved.

Discussion of nociceptive pain in this chapter will be largely restricted to functional muscle pain and visceral pain.

FUNCTIONAL MUSCLE PAIN

Cramp

In the physically fit, cramps are uncommon apart from in the calf and foot. In cancer patients, cramps are often seen in muscles overlying or close to painful bone metastases. In the back, for example, partial collapse of a vertebra may result in poor posture and added strain on one set of paravertebral muscles. Anxiety, tension and lack of exercise because of pain and/or weakness also predispose to cramps, notably in the back, chest wall and neck.

A study of 50 cancer patients with severe cramp referred to a neurology consultation service showed, however, that cramp may be a pointer to an underlying condition which requires specific treatment (Table 4.1). In some patients the cramps had been occurring for more than 3 months at the time of referral. Sites of cramp were as follows:

- upper limbs only (6)
- lower limbs only (18)
- upper and lower limbs (21)
- generalized, including trunk (5).

Most patients suffered frequent attacks; nearly half had innumerable episodes every day. Cramps were usually of brief duration (seconds–minutes), but three patients reported sustained painful contractions lasting up to 15 minutes. Nocturnal cramps occurred in over half, with these being predominant in about one third. Fourteen patients had movement or posture induced cramps; 12 of these never had nocturnal cramps. About 80% had a neural cause, either peripheral neuropathy or root/plexus pathology. There were two cases of polymyositis, one of hypomagnesaemia, and nine for whom no cause could be identified. Possibly these were examples of cramp associated anxiety, inactivity and/or myofascial trigger points (see below).

Cramps may be an adverse drug effect (Box 4.A). One report indicated that nearly half of the patients receiving salbutamol had troublesome cramps (Palmer 1978). Most of the hormones used to treat breast cancer can cause cramps, particularly high dose medroxyprogesterone acetate (Siegal 1991). The incidence with corticosteroids is not known. Cramps also occur in

Table 4.1 Classification of causes of muscle cramps in 50 cancer patients

Cause	Number of patients
Complications of malignancy (n = 14)	
Metastatic	
meningeal metastases	6
epidural root compression	3
brachial plexus compression	1
Nonmetastatic (paraneoplastic)	
peripheral neuropathy	2
polymyositis	2
Complications of therapy (n = 21)	
Peripheral neuropathy (vincristine 13, cisplatin 3)	16
Radiation induced plexopathy	3
Arachnoiditis	1
Hypomagnesaemia (cisplatin)	1
Unrelated to malignancy (n = 7)	
Diabetic peripheral neuropathy	3
Spinal degenerative disease	2
Guillain-Barré syndrome (breast cancer)	1
Amitriptyline	1
Unknown cause (n = 2)	
Peripheral neuropathy	2
No pathological condition identified (n = 9)	9
Total	53[a]

[a] Three patients had two causes.
From Steiner & Seigal 1989

BOX 4.A
DRUG-INDUCED CRAMPS (Siegal 1991, Lear & Daniels 1993)

Hormone therapy

- medroxyprogesterone acetate
- other

Prednisolone
Beclomethasone (by inhaler)
$Beta_2$-adrenergic agonists

- salbutamol
- terbutaline

Diuretics
Amphotericin B
Cimetidine
Clofibrate
Lithium
Other

steroid pseudorheumatism (see pp. 95, 436). Important irreversible causes of cramp in cancer include (Siegal 1991):

- radiculopathy
- plexopathy
- peripheral neuropathy.

Bryostatin, a cytotoxic drug, can cause diffuse myalgia which begins 2–3 days after treatment and lasts for up to 5 days.

Myofascial pain

Various terms have been used to describe pain related to muscle trigger points (TPs). They include:

- fibrositis
- muscular rheumatism
- myalgia
- myalgic spots
- myofasciitis
- nonarticular rheumatism.

The IASP (1986) recommends 'myofascial pain' (Box 4.B). Primary fibro-myalgia syndrome (widespread muscle aching and tenderness of more than 3 months duration) is a separate entity.

Trigger points

TPs can develop in any skeletal muscle, although only a minority are commonly involved. The size of a single TP is 3–6 mm (Sola & Bonica 1990). Although TPs can sometimes be palpated, their presence is more commonly established by the pain response of the patient when pressure is applied to them — the so-called jump sign.

BOX 4.B
USEFUL DEFINITIONS

Spasm
A sustained involuntary muscle contraction.

Cramp
A painful spasm.

Myofascial pain
A muscle disorder characterized by the presence of one or more hypersensitive points (trigger points) within muscle and/or the surrounding connective tissue together with pain (often referred into neighbouring areas or the adjacent limb), muscle spasm, tenderness, stiffness, limitation of movement, weakness and, occasionally, autonomic dysfunction.

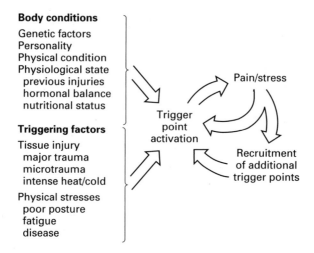

Body conditions

Genetic factors
Personality
Physical condition
Physiological state
    previous injuries
    hormonal balance
    nutritional status

Triggering factors

Tissue injury
    major trauma
    microtrauma
    intense heat/cold

Physical stresses
    poor posture
    fatigue
    disease

Trigger
point
activation

Pain/stress

Recruitment
of additional
trigger points

Fig. 4.2 Factors involved in trigger point activation. (Reproduced with permission from Sola & Bonica 1990.)

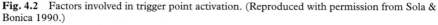

The intensity of myofascial pain ranges from a mild ache to an excruciating pain ± burning pain. The pain is generally periodic but can be persistent, debilitating and limiting.

TP activity may be initiated by one factor but then other factors may contribute to its perpetuation (Fig. 4.2). The ability of these factors to induce pain in an individual is modulated by genetic factors, personality, conditioning and physiological status. Once established, however, a painful event may become self-sustaining.

TPs often remain latent for many years after the original injury. An acute episode of myofascial pain often follows overuse of out of condition muscles, prolonged poor posture, or a period of intense emotional stress. Muscles which are just stiff and tender from exercise do not cause referred pain commonly seen with myofascial pain.

The cardinal features of myofascial pain are:

- the pain consistently relates to the use of specific muscle(s)
- when pressure is applied, tenderness and pain are provoked ('deep allodynia'). The same amount of pressure on the contralateral muscle, if not involved, does not produce pain or tenderness
- stimulation of the TP produces pain which is felt locally and/or referred distally. The referred pain and tenderness are projected in a pattern characteristic of that particular muscle and reproduces part of the patient's complaint. The patterns of referred pain are different from those of nerve root compression but this may not be obvious clinically
- a taut band of muscle passing through the tender spot can be palpated. If the TP is stimulated by snapping palpation or needle penetration a local twitch response of the taut band of muscle is produced
- injection of local anaesthetic into the TP eliminates the pain and tenderness.

The following case history (not of a cancer patient) shows how important knowledge of TPs can be:

■ CASE HISTORY
A future national leader in the USA was injured during World War II and subsequently developed a chronic back disorder from which he suffered for nearly a decade, despite consultation and treatment by some of the most respected orthopaedic surgeons. It was only when someone with expertise in myofascial pain was consulted that the correct diagnosis was made. With TP injection and physical treatments, the pain and suffering decreased and he was able to lead a very active and productive life (Bonica & Sola 1990).

Myofascial pain is the most common musculoskeletal disability of the neck, shoulder girdle and lumbar region (Sola & Bonica 1990). In a survey of 200 unselected young adults, latent TPs were identified in the muscles of the shoulder girdle in 54% of women and 45% of men (Sola et al 1955). In a survey of 1000 ambulatory patients, classic myofascial pain was identified in 32% (36% of women and 26% of men) (Sola & Bonica 1990). Labourers are less likely to develop myofascial pain than sedentary workers (Sola & Bonica 1990). Debilitated cancer patients are almost certainly at greater risk of developing myofascial pain than the general population.

The areas most commonly affected are:

● head and neck
● shoulder girdle
● lumbar region.

Selected TPs and the associated patterns of myofascial pain are shown in Figure 4.3. Myofascial pain is generally eased by a local anaesthetic injection into the TP. Naloxone 10 mg IV reduces the benefit of such an injection (Fine et al 1988). This suggests that an endogenous opioid system is involved in the response obtained by the injection.

VISCERAL PAIN

The following points should be noted about visceral pain (Cervero 1988):

● it cannot be evoked from all viscera
● it is not linked to internal injury
● it is referred to other locations
● it is diffuse and poorly localized
● it may be accompanied by intense motor and autonomic reflexes.

The diffuse localization relates in part to the fact that many visceral afferent fibres end in lamina V of the dorsal horn. The rest end in lamina I, and none in the substantia gelatinosa, i.e. lamina II.

Visceral pain can be evoked by the following stimuli (Ayala 1937):

● spasm of the smooth muscle in hollow viscera

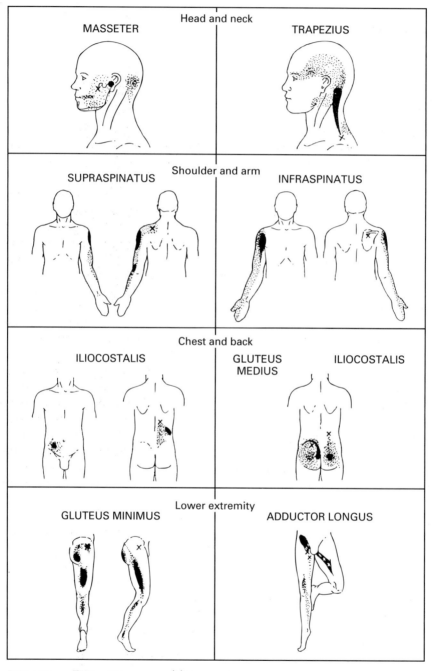

Pain pattern ■▨   Trigger area ✕

Fig. 4.3 Selected trigger points and the associated patterns of local and referred myofascial pain. (Reproduced with permission from Travell & Rinzler 1952.)

- distension of hollow viscera
- ischaemia
- inflammatory states
- chemical stimuli
- traction, compression and twisting of the mesenteries.

Missing from this list are internal injuries produced by cutting, crushing and burning. Unlike the skin, these do not cause visceral pain.

The lack of concordance between injury and visceral pain means that the concept of 'noxious' stimulus needs to be redefined for visceral pain. Thus, a noxious visceral stimulus is not the stimulus which produces injury but the stimulus which evokes pain.

All forms of visceral pain are poorly localized and most are felt in areas considerably larger than the size of the originating viscus. Further, as the pain becomes more intense, so the somatic area in which the pain is felt becomes larger. This suggests that the representation of internal organs within the CNS is imprecise. One exception is the pain of peptic ulcer, which some patients are able to pinpoint to the epigastrium with a fingertip.

Visceral pain is frequently accompanied by skeletal muscle contractures and spasms which last for a considerable amount of time and which contribute greatly to the patient's discomfort. Many forms of visceral pain are accompanied by autonomic reflexes such as tachycardia, a rise in blood pressure and sweating.

Nerve endings in the intestines are located in muscle, whereas in the solid organs (liver, spleen, kidneys) they are found in the capsule. The gastrointestinal tract is insensitive to cutting, tearing and crushing, but is sensitive to distension and to hypersegmentation (Jewell 1983). Intestinal sensory nerves are also stimulated by inflammation, ischaemia and neoplastic infiltration (Table 4.2). In addition, traction on the mesentery or on the peritoneum (via adhesions) causes pain. Because the intestines have a bilateral innervation, it is sometimes stated that intestinal pain is midline or

Table 4.2 Pain from specific viscera

Viscus	Common site of pain
Oesophagus	Retrosternal at site of disease May be referred to the back
Stomach Small intestine	Epigastrium or right upper quadrant May be referred to the back
Colon	Along the line of the colon or in the hypogastrium Often poorly localized May be referred to the back or thighs
Gallbladder Bile duct	Colic in right upper quadrant May be referred to between scapulae and to the right shoulder
Pancreatic	Epigastric: right hypochondrium for the head of the pancreas, left hypochondrium for the tail May be referred to the back in midline

From Jewell 1983

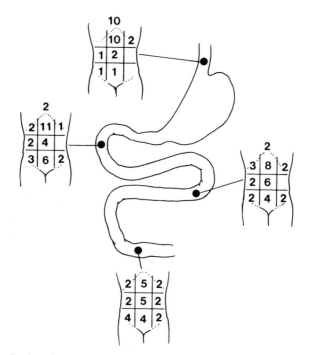

Fig. 4.4   Distribution of abdominal pain induced by balloon inflation in distal oesophagus, second part of duodenum, proximal jejunum, and ileum in 21 patients. Numbers in each sector represent the number of patients perceiving pain at that site. (Reproduced with permission from Moriarty & Dawson 1982.)

symmetrical (Bentley & Smithwick 1940). This is not true of patients with functional abdominal pain (Moriarty & Dawson 1982), nor is it true of cancer patients. Pain from any part of the gastro-intestinal tract may be experienced in most parts of the abdomen (Figs 4.4, 4.5).

The occurrence of abdominal pain in association with oesophageal distension suggests that the mechanism of pain reference is probably not neuro-embryological. The variations seen, however, are consistent with identified alimentary tract trigger points or areas and their known patterns of referral to the abdominal wall.

Although 90% of the nerve fibres in the vagus are sensory, none transmits pain. Abdominal pain is therefore unaltered by vagotomy. The main nociceptive pathways are shown in Table 4.3.

Intestinal pains fall into several distinct categories. There is the gnawing pain associated with hunger and dyspeptic pains associated with hyperacidity, gastric distension or dysmotility. In addition, there is the dull pain of distension, often with associated nausea. There is also the more intense pain called colic ('gripes'). This represents a muscular reaction to persisting distension. Circular and longitudinal muscle coats are probably both involved and the result is a sharp increase in intraluminal pressure, manifesting as severe abdominal pain. This can be overwhelming, particularly in an anxious, fearful patient. It may last a few minutes or several hours. Associated referred pain may be felt in the back and thighs.

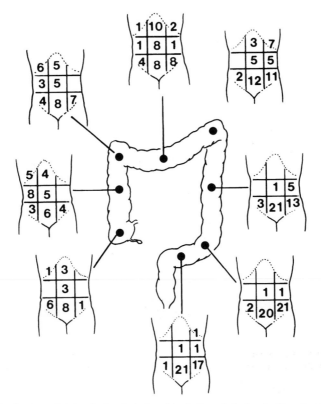

Fig. 4.5 Distribution of abdominal pain induced by balloon inflation in 48 patients investigated for abdominal pain. Numbers in each sector represent the number of patients perceiving pain at that site. (Reproduced with permission from Swarbrick et al 1980.)

Table 4.3 Nerve pathways from the abdominal viscera to the spinal cord

Viscus	Nerve
Oesophagus	Unnamed sympathetic nerves
Liver, spleen	Phrenic nerve (C3–C5)
Gallbladder, pancreas stomach, small intestine }	Coeliac plexus, greater splanchnic nerves (T6–T9)
Appendix, colon, pelvic viscera	Mesenteric plexus, lesser splanchnic nerves (T11–L1)
Kidneys, bladder, rectum	Pelvic nerves (S2–S4)

From Jewell 1983

Patients with irritable bowel syndrome and those who are constipated may also complain of colic. This possibly relates to excessive muscular contraction onto hard faeces. Colic associated with diarrhoea is probably caused by intestinal muscle contracting down on its own lining after the faeces have been evacuated. Some patients experience colic with laxatives. This may be caused by the same mechanism as in diarrhoea, or be more akin to that associated with constipation itself if the faeces are particularly hard and bulky. Colic does not relate to excessively rapid peristalsis. It is physiologically impossible for peristalsis to exceed 30 cm/min.

NEUROPATHIC PAIN

Neuropathic pain results from dysfunction of or injury to the peripheral nervous system (PNS) or the central nervous system (CNS). It may also be associated with overactivity of the sympathetic nervous system. Neuropathic pain is almost always associated with sensory changes (Box 4.C). The exceptions are all nonmalignant conditions:

- trigeminal neuralgia
- glossopharyngeal neuralgia
- metatarsalgia
- tabetic crisis.

This characteristic has given rise to a working definition of neuropathic pain as *pain in an area of abnormal or absent sensation* (Glynn 1989).

BOX 4.C
USEFUL DEFINITIONS

Nociceptor (IASP 1986)
A receptor preferentially sensitive to a noxious stimulus or to a stimulus which would become noxious if prolonged.

Neuropathy (IASP 1986)
A disturbance of function or pathological change in a nerve:

- in one nerve, mononeuropathy
- in several nerves, mononeuropathy multiplex
- if symmetrical and bilateral, polyneuropathy.

Note: Neuritis is a special case of neuropathy and is now reserved for inflammatory processes affecting nerves. Neuropathy is not intended to cover cases like neurapraxis, neurotmesis, or section of a nerve.

Neuralgia (IASP 1986)
Pain in the distribution of a nerve or nerves.

Nociceptive pain
Pain resulting from chemical or physical stimulation of peripheral nerve endings.

Neuropathic pain (Merskey H 1992 Personal Communication)
Pain initiated or caused by a primary lesion or dysfunction in the peripheral or central nervous system.

Peripheral neuropathic pain (Merskey H 1992 Personal Communication)
Pain initiated or caused by a primary lesion or dysfunction in the peripheral nervous system.

Central pain (Merskey H 1992 Personal Communication)
Pain initiated or caused by a primary lesion or dysfunction in the central nervous system.

Several terms have been used to describe pain associated with neural dysfunction:

- neuropathic (Meyerson 1990)
- neurogenic (Bowsher 1989, Meyerson 1990)
- neural lesion (Tasker & Dostrovsky 1989)
- de-afferentation (Wall & Melzack 1989, Bonica 1990)
- dysaesthetic (Tasker 1975, Twycross & Lack 1984).

Neuropathic pain is now the accepted term (Portenoy 1992, Mersky H 1992 Personal Communication). As already noted, neuropathy is defined as a disturbance of function or pathological change in a nerve (IASP 1986). This definition, with the emphasis on dysfunction rather than injury, means that *sympathetically maintained pain* is a type of neuropathic pain.

The classification of neuropathic pain, however, is confused by disagreement about *nerve compression pain*. Some consider nerve compression pain to be nociceptive on the grounds that it is possibly caused by stimulation of the nervi nervorum (nerves to the nerve sheath; Asbury & Fields 1984). Others think that there is insufficient evidence to support this hypothesis (Portenoy 1992). In any case, because nerve compression pain is a form of nerve dysfunction, it can be argued that it is neuropathic by definition whether or not it is also nociceptive (Box 4.C). Thus, in this book, nerve compression pain is classified as neuropathic. It is still important, however, to distinguish between *nerve compression pain* ('functional neuropathic pain') and *neural injury pain* ('organic neuropathic pain').

Nerve compression pain

Nerve compression pain is common in cancer (Twycross & Fairfield 1982). It occurs in the early stages of plexopathy and as a result of metastatic vertebral disease. If a patient survives long enough, reversible nerve compression will progress to irreversible nerve injury.

Nerve compression pain is neurodermatomal in distribution. There may be additional neurological symptoms and signs, but these changes are functional and reversible (Meyerson 1990). Nerve compression pain is generally more opioid responsive than nerve injury pain. A corticosteroid may be needed as a co-analgesic (see pp. 441, 443).

Neural injury pain

In cancer, neural injury pain is usually the result of either treatment or infiltration of a nerve by cancer (Table 4.4). Neurosurgeons have long been aware that procedures which interrupt nociceptive transmission such as rhizotomy and spinothalamic tractotomy (cordotomy) either fail to relieve certain pains or do so only temporarily (Table 4.5).

At one time it was thought that the division between neurosurgical success and failure related to whether the pain was caused by cancer. Failure was considered to be a feature of nonmalignant pain and was attributed to

Table 4.4 Neural injury pain in cancer patients

Caused by cancer	Related to cancer
Plexopathy	Postherpetic neuralgia
Nerve root infiltration	
Spinal cord compression	
Caused by cancer treatment	*Concurrent*
Postoperative incisional pain	Diabetic neuropathy
Phantom limb pain	Poststroke pain
Vinca alkaloid neuropathy	
Platinum drug neuropathy	
Radiation induced plexopathy	

Table 4.5 Response of neural injury pain to local anaesthetic and neurodestructive procedure

Procedure	Response
Local anaesthetic	65% complete relief
	24% partial relief
Percutaneous cordotomy	50% mild benefit
Thalamic surgery	32% benefit
Percutaneous intercostal neurectomy	25% benefit
Spinal cord transection	0% benefit

From Tasker 1987

the plasticity of the nervous system, enabling it to circumvent the interruption given sufficient time. It was, however, noted over 50 years ago that resistance to surgical intervention was seen with neural injury pains in general and not just with nonmalignant pain or selected types of nonmalignant pain (Livingston 1943). Further, even then, it was suggested that neuropathic pain related to some form of perturbation in the CNS which, once established, persisted despite subsequent interventions.

Pathophysiology

Neural injury does not always result in pain. For example:

- postherpetic neuralgia is rare in young people but becomes more common with increasing age
- apparently identical peripheral nerve lesions will result in pain in only a minority of patients
- animal experiments suggest that the propensity to develop neuropathic pain may be genetic (Devor 1989).

A loss of afferent input at any level within the nervous system induces a cascade of anatomical, neurochemical and physiological changes, which extend centrally from the site of injury (Wall 1984). It is not necessary to choose between a peripheral and a central mechanism for neural injury pain. Almost certainly, both the PNS and CNS are involved, each with a separate but interrelated role. The primary pathophysiological process appears to be neuronal hyperexcitability. This is probably the result of abnormal remodelling of the axonal membrane at the cut nerve end (Devor 1989).

A number of phenomena have been noted in experimentally produced neuromas in rats:

- the sprouts of up to 30% of damaged sensory axons, both myelinated and unmyelinated, generate activity in the absence of any apparent stimulation (Wall & Gutnick 1974, McMahon 1990)
- some 50% of the sprouts also become mechanosensitive (Scadding 1981). Light touch or pressure frequently elicits a discharge lasting many seconds in injured axons
- some 15% of injured axons begin to respond to the injection of adrenaline and related sympathomimetics into nearby arteries. Such a challenge usually elicits a discharge lasting many seconds
- 'cross talk' develops between neighbouring denuded sprouts (ephaptic transmission), i.e. electrical activity in one axon terminal may excite an adjacent axon by the direct flow of current, and not by the release of a neurotransmitter (Devor 1989).

Normal nerves are capable of generating rhythmic discharges only at specialized terminal structures; injured nerves acquire this capability at ectopic sites. When an ectopic capability is established, there may be spontaneous discharges and/or sensitivity to a range of depolarizing stimuli, i.e. mechanical, chemical and metabolic. The end result of these changes is a new CNS steady state in which there is (Wall 1989, Tasker & Dostrovsky 1989):

- hyperexcitability
- spontaneous activity
- an expanded receptive field.

One way of integrating the data from animal studies is shown in Figure 4.6.

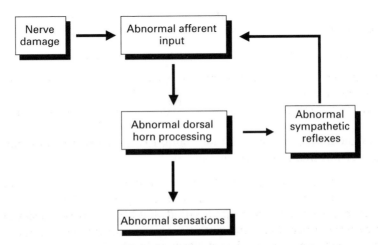

Fig. 4.6 A general scheme to explain how nerve injuries may lead to persistent sensory abnormalities. (Reproduced with permission from McMahon 1990.)

In this model, a positive feedback has been included via the sympathetic nervous system. Such a feedback would help to explain the explosive and self-sustaining nature of the disorder (McMahon 1990). This model is probably not relevant for many patients with neural injury pain because, in them, regional sympathetic blockade has little effect. It is probable, therefore, that neuropathic pain syndromes are caused by a range of neurophysiological disturbances. There may also be variable degrees of dorsal horn sensitization, with or without the development of 'central generating mechanisms'. It is not surprising, therefore, that response to treatment is variable.

Few neuropathic pains respond completely to morphine but many respond to an antidepressant ± an anticonvulsant, or to an oral local anaesthetic congener. A minority need other measures such as epidural morphine and bupivacaine ± clonidine (see p. 365), and some respond well to SC ketamine (see p. 476). As already noted, neurodestructive procedures are not always of benefit (Table 4.5). Only 50% of patients derived even mild benefit from percutaneous cordotomy compared with a good response in over 80% of patients with nociceptive pain (Tasker 1987).

Some operations are complicated by the subsequent development of chronic incisional pain. This is not necessarily associated with the severing of a major nerve trunk; it can result from an incision involving only small nerve branches (Meyerson 1990). It is often said that the pain is caused by neuroma formation in scar tissue. A neuroma is present, however, in only a minority of cases. Genetic susceptibility may be the reason why some patients develop this form of neural injury pain.

Characteristics of neural injury pain

When describing neuropathic pain, it is necessary to be familiar with a number of terms (Box 4.D).

Central pain, e.g. poststroke pain, may well be indistinguishable from nociceptive pain — an aching pain of variable intensity. Typically, however, there is:

- a history of a cerebrovascular accident
- no local disease to account for the pain
- an area of altered sensation incorporating the painful area but commonly extending beyond it.

Peripheral neural injury pain is more common. Its characteristics are exemplified in postherpetic neuralgia and diabetic neuropathic pain. Pain in postherpetic neuralgia typically has the following characteristics (Raftery 1979):

- a superficial burning or stinging sensation with a neurodermatomal distribution (almost always present)
- allodynia and hyperalgesia (almost always present)

BOX 4.D
USEFUL DEFINITIONS (IASP 1986)
[Sections in parenthesis are author's notes]

Alloydnia
Pain due to a stimulus which does not normally provoke pain. [i.e. *an exaggerated response with a reduction in pain threshold*]

Causalgia
A syndrome of sustained burning pain, allodynia, and hyperpathia after a traumatic nerve lesion, often combined with vasomotor and sudomotor dysfunction and later trophic changes.

Dysaesthesia
An unpleasant abnormal sensation, whether spontaneous or evoked.

Note: Compare with pain and with paraesthesia. Special cases of dysaesthesia include hyperalgesia and allodynia. A dysaesthesia should always be unpleasant and a paraesthesia should not be unpleasant.

Hyperaesthesia
Increased sensitivity to stimulation, excluding the special senses.

Note: Hyperaesthesia may refer to various modes of cutaneous sensibility including touch and thermal sensation without pain, as well as to pain. The word is used to indicate both diminished threshold to any stimulus and an increased response to stimuli that are normally recognized. Allodynia is suggested for pain after stimulation which is not normally painful. Hyperaesthesia includes both allodynia and hyperalgesia, but the more specific terms should be used wherever they are applicable.

Hypo-aesthesia
Decreased sensitivity to stimulation, excluding the special senses.

Hyperalgesia
An increased response to a stimulus which is normally painful. [i.e. *an exaggerated response with a normal pain threshold*]

Note: Can be differentiated into inflammatory and neuropathic hyperalgesia. The former can be further divided into primary (at the site of the injury) and secondary (in the surrounding area). Hyperalgesia evoked by innocuous stimuli is called *allodynia*.

Hyperpathia
A painful syndrome, characterized by an increased reaction to a stimulus, particularly a repetitive stimulus, as well as an increased threshold . [i.e. *an exaggerated response with an increased pain threshold*]

- spontaneous stabbing pains (less frequent)
- a deep ache (less frequent).

In contrast, in diabetic neuropathic pain, aching pain may be the most prominent feature (Kastrup et al 1986). Thus, to limit the diagnosis of peripheral neural injury pain to cases of superficial burning pain ± stabbing pain will mean that some cases of nerve injury pain will go unrecognized. This is particularly relevant with the postoperative incisional pain syndromes.

There are three varieties of allodynia. These may co-exist in the same patient:

- mechanical (pain triggered by touch, wind or clothing)
- cold (pain exacerbated by cold)
- movement (related to dysfunction of the muscle spindles).

Some patients with marked allodynia cannot bear clothing against the affected area, or find that water running over the area when washing provokes a marked exacerbation. Also there may be evidence of sympathetic dysfunction manifesting as (Bowsher 1990):

- cutaneous vasodilation
- increased skin temperature
- altered pattern of sweating.

Neuropathic pain with associated sympathetic dysfunction is distinct from sympathetically maintained pain. The extent of the sympathetic contribution can be quantified only by performing a diagnostic sympathetic block with local anaesthetic and noting any change in pain and sensation.

Sympathetically maintained pain

Sympathetically maintained pain (SMP) is a relatively uncommon sequel to tissue injury or sympathetic nerve injury (Roberts 1986). The incidence of SMP in cancer patients is not known. In a series of nearly 300 cancer pain patients referred to a Pain Relief Clinic, about 5% were diagnosed as having SMP (Churcher 1990). These patients, however, were highly selected.

The essential features of SMP are (Churcher & Ingall 1987):

- pain (often burning)
- sensory disorder
- pain relief and reversal of sensory disorder by sympathetic block.

It has been suggested that SMP results from sensitization of the wide dynamic range neurones in lamina V of the dorsal horn, and that mechanoreceptors, not nociceptors, are the afferent fibres which evoke the pain (Roberts 1986). As with neural injury pain, there may be a genetic propensity for SMP. It has also been suggested that SMP is a disorder of peripheral $alpha_1$-adrenergic receptors (Davis et al 1991).

Another hypothesis relates SMP to failed natural opioid modulation in regional sympathetic ganglia (Hannington-Kiff 1991). Whichever hypothesis one accepts, it is important to remember that neural injury or a history of major injury is unnecessary. In causal terms, therefore, it helps to think in terms of 'irritation' and/or stimulation of the regional sympathetic nerves rather than a precise injury.

In cancer patients, SMP is more common in the lower limb. Typically it is seen with para-aortic lymphadenopathy, and is usually associated with cancer of the cervix or rectum (Churcher 1990). In addition to pain exacerbated by cold, patients may give a history of muscle fatigue and weakness. In later stages, a cool painful limb with other signs of sympathetic overdrive is a more common finding than the hot foot which results from autosympathectomy (Watson & Evans 1986).

■ CASE HISTORY

A 38 year-old woman presented with burning, tight circumferential pain over the thigh of 1 year's duration. This followed a course of chemotherapy for cancer of the cervix. Her pain was exacerbated by cold weather or by limb dependency. Examination showed a cool limb with allodynia, hyperpathia and uniform hypoalgesia to pinprick. Symptoms were relieved and physical signs reverted to normal following a lumbar sympathetic block with local anaesthetic (Churcher 1990).

Patients with a pleural mesothelioma sometimes present with a mixed picture of neural injury pain and SMP. Contact with even light clothes is uncomfortable (allodynia), and there may be excessive sweating on the affected side, together with a depressed pinprick response on sensory testing. Contact thermography can be used to provide evidence of sympathetic overactivity in these patients (Churcher 1990).

■ CASE HISTORY

A 75 year-old woman gave a 1 year history of a painful arm together with a cold sensation and sensitive skin. Cancer of the breast had been treated by radiotherapy 4 years previously. A cold arm, a mild Horner's syndrome and tapering, partly flexed fingers were present on examination. Allodynia and hyperpathia were present below the elbow. She had trophic skin changes on her hand, wasting of the hypothenar muscles and extreme tenderness to pressure over the heads of the metacarpals. Her pain and tenderness was relieved by local anaesthetic stellate ganglion block (Churcher 1990).

Burning pain spreading up the line of the carotid vessels and over the hemicranium (worse when lying down) is sometimes seen in patients with malignant glands in the neck. They dislike brushing their hair on the painful side (Churcher 1990).

Differential diagnosis

It is necessary to differentiate between the burning pain of neural injury and the burning pain of SMP (Table 4.6). This can be difficult because:

• features are not constant
• some are common to both conditions
• sometimes they co-exist.

The distribution of SMP, however, does not correspond with the dermatomal pattern of the peripheral nerves. Instead it reflects the pattern of sympathetic

Table 4.6 Comparison of neural injury and sympathetically maintained pain (SMP)

	Neural injury	SMP
Cause	nerve destruction	nerve irritation
Pattern	dermatomal (if peripheral)	vasotopographic
Concomitants		
stabbing pain	common	unusual
allodynia	+	+/–
hyperpathia	+/–	+/–
deep pressure	comforts	tender near joints (common)
pinprick	diminished (usually)	diminished (usually)
muscle atrophy	+	+/–
muscle fatigue	–	+/–
trophic changes	late	early[a]
limb temperature	normal/cold	usually colder[b]
Tricyclic drug	good relief (often)	little or no relief
Sympathetic block	no relief	partial or complete relief[c]

[a] Trophic changes may affect skin, subcutaneous tissues and/or nails; may be atrophic (e.g. shiny taut skin, hair loss) or hypertrophic (e.g. hyperkeratosis).
[b] If in doubt, temperature changes can be confirmed with a thermo-couple. Valid only if the pulses are equal in both the affected and normal limbs, and no history of deep venous thrombosis. In some patients the temperature may vary with warm episodes and sweating.
[c] Sensory abnormalities revert to normal.

vascular innervation (Fig. 4.7). Radiographs of the limb show osteoporosis and an isotope bone scan may contain 'hot spots'. These may be mistaken for osteolytic metastases (Mackinnon & Holder 1984, Churcher 1988).

If SMP is suspected, a sympathetic block with local anaesthetic should be arranged. This not only confirms the diagnosis but often gives relief which outlasts the duration of action of the local anaesthetic. If symptoms return, lumbar sympathectomy under radiographic control is a safe procedure with minimal adverse effects. It is unwise to perform a permanent sympathetic (stellate ganglion) block for arm pain because of the likelihood of damage to surrounding structures.

MORPHINE INDUCED PAIN

Pain with allodynia and myoclonus have been noted in humans after:

- high dose intrathecal (IT) morphine (Stillman et al 1987, De Conno et al 1991)
- high dose IV morphine (Sjogren et al 1993).

■ CASE REPORT

Three male cancer patients aged 61–74 years with lower body pain had analgesic infusion pumps implanted with catheters in the lumbosacral intrathecal space. Morphine was infused at a constant rate (80, 120 and 200 mg/day) and boluses were given for exacerbations of pain. Five episodes of intense pain in the lower limbs accompanied by allodynia occurred within 30 minutes of a bolus of morphine (4–45 mg) (Stillman et al 1987).

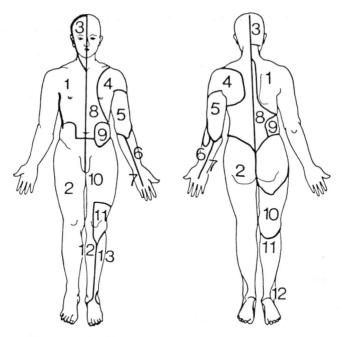

Fig. 4.7 Arterial supply to the skin.
 1 subclavian artery = cervicothoracic sympathetic outflow = upper quadrant of the body
 2 iliac arteries = lumbar sympathetic outflow = lower quadrant of the body
 3 common carotid artery
 4 axillary artery
 5 brachial artery
 6 radial artery
 7 ulnar artery
 8 thoracic aorta
 9 abdominal aorta
10 femoral artery
11 popliteal artery
12 posterior tibial artery
13 anterior tibial artery
(Reproduced with permission from Gerbershagen 1979.)

This phenomenon has been termed 'paradoxical pain' (Stillman et al 1987). Unfortunately, the term has been defined in a number of different ways, including nociceptive pain not responsive to morphine (Bowsher 1993). Ambiguity destroys the usefulness of the term (Hanks et al 1993, Hardy 1993), and it should be discarded.

It has been suggested that this phenomenon sometimes relates to a genetic inability to convert morphine to morphine-6-glucuronide (M6G), an active metabolite of morphine (Morley et al 1992). This results in higher concentrations than normal of morphine-3-glucuronide (M3G), a metabolite which is possibly a nonspecific CNS stimulant at high concentrations (Gong et al 1992). Given the results of animal studies, however, it seems likely that the phenomenon would occur in all patients at even higher dose levels (see p. 40).

Other paradoxical reactions to opioids or opioid antagonists include those described below.

Poststroke pain

This may be relieved by repeated high doses of naloxone (a pure opioid antagonist) but uninfluenced by morphine (Budd 1985, Ray & Tai 1988).

Biliary colic induced or exacerbated by morphine

This is secondary to morphine induced constriction of the sphincter of Oddi (Gaensler et al 1948, Alper & Van Dam 1959). The pain is relieved by naloxone (Lang & Pilon 1980).

Headache associated with raised intracranial pressure

An opioid induced increase in pCO_2 leads to reflex cerebral vasodilatation, a further increase in intracranial pressure and increased headache (Kepes 1952, Keats 1954, Swerdlow et al 1955). In practice, however, this sequence of events is rarely seen because the dose of the opioid is usually more than enough to compensate for any increased headache.

REFERENCES

Alper M H, Van Dam L D 1959 Morphine, biliary spasm, and nalorphine. Anesthesiology 20: 713–714
Asbury A K, Fields H L 1984 Pain due to peripheral nerve damage: An hypothesis. Neurology (Cleveland) 34: 1587–1590
Ayala M 1937 Douleur sympathique et douleur viscerale. Revue Neurologique 68: 222–242
Bentley F H, Smithwick R H 1940 Visceral pain produced by balloon distension of the jejunum. Lancet ii: 389–391
Bonica J J 1990 The management of pain, 2nd edn. Philadelphia, Lea & Febiger
Bonica J J, Sola A E 1990 Other painful disorders of the low back. In: Bonica J J (ed) The management of pain, 2nd edn. Lea & Febiger, Philadelphia, pp 1484–1514
Bowsher D 1989 Pathways and mechanisms. In: Swerdlow M, Charlton J E (eds) Relief of intractable pain, 4th edn. Elsevier, Amsterdam, pp 1–22
Bowsher D 1990 How physiology of neurogenic pain dictates management. Geriatric Medicine Sept: 33–40
Bowsher D 1993 Paradoxical pain. British Medical Journal 306: 473–474
Budd K 1985 The use of the opiate antagonist, naloxone, in the treatment of intractable pain. Neuropeptides 5: 419–422
Cervero F 1988 Visceral pain. In: Dubner R, Gebhart F G, Bond M R (eds) Proceedings of the Vth World Congress on Pain. Elsevier Science Publishers, Amsterdam, pp 216–226
Churcher M D 1988 Sympathetic dependent pain mimicking tumour spread. The Pain Clinic 2: 169–171
Churcher M D 1990 Cancer and sympathetic dependent pain. Palliative Medicine 4: 113–116
Churcher M D, Ingall J R F 1987 Sympathetic dependent pain. The Pain Clinic 1: 217–218
Davis K D, Treede R B, Raja S N, Meyer R A, Campbell J N 1991 Topical application of clonidine relieves hyperalgesia in patients with sympathetically maintained pain. Pain 47: 309–317
De Conno F, Caraceni A, Martini C, Spoldi E, Salvetti M, Ventafridda V 1991 Hyperalgesia and myoclonus with intrathecal infusion of high dose morphine. Pain 47: 337–339
Devor M 1989 The pathophysiology of damaged peripheral nerves. In: Wall P D, Melzack R (eds) Textbook of pain, 2nd edn. Churchill Livingstone, Edinburgh pp 63–81

Fine P G, Milano R, Hare B D 1988 The effects of myofascial trigger point injections are naloxone reversible. Pain 32: 15–20

Gaensler E A, McGowan J M, Henderson F F 1948 A comparative study of the action of demerol and opium alkaloids in relation to biliary spasm. Surgery 23: 211–220

Gerbershagen H U 1979 Blocks with local anaesthetics in the treatment of cancer pain. In: Bonica J J, Ventafriddda V (eds) Advances in pain research and therapy, vol 2. Raven Press, New York, pp 311–323

Glynn C 1989 An approach to the management of the patient with deafferentation pain. Palliative Medicine 3: 13–21

Gong Q-L, Hedner J, Bjorkman R, Hedner T 1992 Morphine-3-glucuronide may functionally antagonize morphine-6-glucuronide induced antinociception and ventilatory depression in the rat. Pain 48: 249–255

Hanks G W C, O'Neill W M, Fallon M T 1993 Paradoxical pain. British Medical Journal 306: 793

Hannington-Kiff J G 1991 Does failed natural opioid modulation in regional sympathetic ganglia cause reflex sympathetic dystrophy? Lancet 338: 1125–1127

Hardy P A J 1993 Paradoxical pain. British Medical Journal 306: 793–794

IASP Subcommittee on Taxonomy 1986 Classification of chronic pain. Pain Suppl 3: 216–221

Jewell D 1983 Symptomatology of gastrointestinal disease. In: Weatherall D J, Ledingham J G G, Warrell D A (eds) Oxford Textbook of Medicine. Oxford University Press, Oxford, pp 12.11–12.17

Kastrup J, Angelo H R, Petersen P, Dejgard A, Hilsted J 1986 Treatment of chronic painful diabetic neuropathy with intravenous lidocaine infusion. British Medical Journal 292: 173

Keats A S 1954 Effect of nalorphine and morphine on cerebrospinal fluid pressure in man. Federal Proceedings 13: 374

Kepes E R 1952 Effect of demerol on the cerebrospinal fluid pressure. Anesthesiology 13: 281–286

Lang D W, Pilon R N 1980 Naloxone reversal of morphine-induced biliary colic. Anesthesia and Analgesia 59: 619–620

Lear J, Daniels R G 1993 Muscle cramps related to corticosteroids. British Medical Journal 306: 1169

Livingston W K 1943 Pain mechanisms: A physiologic interpretation of causalgia and its related states. MacMillan, New York

Mackinnon S E, Holder L E 1984 The use of three-phase radionuclide bone scanning in the diagnosis of reflex sympathetic dystrophy. Journal of Hand Surgery 9a: 556–563

McMahon S B 1990 The pathophysiological consequences of nerve injury. Intractable Pain Society 8 (1): 19–27

Meyerson B A 1990 Neuropathic pain: An overview. In: Lipton S, Tunks E, Zoppi M (eds) Advances in pain research and therapy, vol 13. Raven Press, New York, pp 193–199

Moriarty K J, Dawson A M 1982 Functional abdominal pain: further evidence that whole gut is affected. British Medical Journal 284: 1670–1672

Morley J S, Miles J B, Wells J C, Bowsher D 1992 Paradoxical pain. Lancet 340: 1045

Palmer K N V 1978 Muscle cramp and oral salbutamol. British Medical Journal 2: 833

Payne R, Gonzales G 1993 Pathophysiology of pain in cancer and other terminal diseases. In: Doyle D, Hanks G W, MacDonald N (eds) Oxford textbook of palliative medicine. Oxford University Press, Oxford, pp 140–148

Portenoy R K 1992 Cancer: pathophysiology and syndromes. Lancet 339: 1026–1031

Raftery H 1979 The management of postherpetic pain using sodium valproate and amitriptyline. Irish Medical Journal 72: 399–401

Ray D A A, Tai Y M A 1988 Infusions of naloxone in thalamic pain. British Medical Journal 296: 969–970

Roberts W J 1986 A hypothesis on the physiological basis for causalgia and related pains. Pain 24: 297–311

Scadding J W 1981 Development of ongoing activity, mechanosensitivity and adrenaline sensitivity in severed peripheral nerve axons. Experimental Neurology 73: 345–363

Siegal T 1991 Muscle cramps in the cancer patient: causes and treatment. Journal of Pain and Symptom Management 6: 84–91

Sjogren P, Jonsson T, Jensen N-H, Drenck N-E, Jensen T S 1993 Hyperalgesia and myoclonus in terminal cancer patients treated with continuous intravenous morphine. Pain 55: 93–97

Sola A E, Bonica J J 1990 Myofascial pain syndromes. In: Bonica J J (ed) The management of pain, 2nd edn. Lea & Febiger, Philadelphia, pp 352–367

Sola A E, Rodenberger M L, Gettys D B 1955 Incidence of hypersensitive areas in posterior shoulder muscles. American Journal of Physiological Medicine 34: 585

Steiner I, Siegal T 1989 Muscle cramps in cancer patients. Cancer 63: 574–577

Stillman M J, Moulin D E, Foley K M 1987 Paradoxical pain following high-dose spinal morphine. Pain suppl 4: S389

Swarbrick E T, Hegarty J E, Bat L et al 1980 Site of pain from the irritable bowel. Lancet ii: 443–446

Swerdlow M, Foldes F F, Siker E 1955 The effects of nisentil hydrochloride and levallorphan tartrate on cerebrospinal fluid pressure. British Journal of Anaesthesia 27: 244–249

Tasker R R 1975 Percutaneous cordotomy. Comprehensive Therapy 1: 51–56

Tasker R 1987 The problem of deafferentation pain in the management of the patient with cancer. Journal of Palliative Care 2 (2): 8–12

Tasker R R, Dostrovsky J O 1989 Deafferentation and central pain. In: Wall P D, Melzack R (eds) Textbook of pain, 2nd edn. Churchill Livingstone, Edinburgh pp 154–180

Travell J, Rinzler S H 1952 The myofascial genesis of pain. Postgraduate Medicine (Minneapolis) 11 May: 425–434

Twycross R G, Fairfield S 1982 Pain in far-advanced cancer. Pain 14: 303–310

Twycross R G, Lack S A 1984 Therapeutics in terminal care. Pitman books, London

Wall P D 1984 Mechanisms of acute and chronic pain. In: Kruger L, Liebeskind J C (eds). Advances in pain research and therapy. vol 6. Raven Press, New York, pp 95–104

Wall P D 1989 Introduction. In: Wall P D, Melzack R (eds) Textbook of pain, 2nd edn. Churchill Livingstone, Edinburgh pp 1–18

Wall P D, Gutnick M 1974 Ongoing activity in peripheral nerves: The physiology and pharmacology of impulses originated from a neuroma. Experimental Neurology 43: 580–593

Wall P D, Melzack R (eds) 1989 Textbook of pain, 2nd edn. Churchill Livingstone, Edinburgh

Watson C P N, Evans R J 1986 Intractable pain with cancer of the rectum. Pain Clinic 1: 29–34

Cancer pain syndromes I

A series of pain syndromes unique to cancer have been described (Foley 1979, Portenoy 1989, Bonica 1990). Some are uncommon and others rare. Pattern recognition is the key to diagnosis.

METASTASES TO BASE OF SKULL

Loosely speaking, the base of the skull is the area behind the nose and above the pharynx. There are several syndromes associated with metastases to this area. They share certain features:

- paraesthesia, dysaesthesia or pain
- dysfunction of one or more cranial nerves
- limited diagnostic help from plain radiographs.

The cranial nerves are affected as they pass through or emerge from various foramina in the middle and posterior cranial fossae (Table 5.1). The commonest causes are cancers spreading directly from the nasopharynx and bone metastases from cancers of the breast, bronchus and prostate.

Although headache features prominently in the classical descriptions of

Table 5.1 Foramina in base of skull through which cranial nerves pass

Foramen	Cranial nerve
Middle fossa	
Rotundum	V^2
Ovale	V^3
Posterior fossa	
Jugular	IX, X, XI
Anterior condylar (hypoglossal) canal	XII

Table 5.2 Pain syndromes caused by invasion of skull

Syndrome	Pathophysiology	Characteristics of pain	Concomitants
Cavernous sinus	Metastasis to cavernous sinus	Frontal headache	Dysfunction of cranial nerves III-VI (diplopia, ophthalmoplegia, papilloedema)
Sphenoid sinus	Metastasis to the sphenoid sinus	Frontal headache radiating to temple with intermittent retro-orbital pain	Dysfunction of cranial nerve VI (diplopia) and nasal stuffiness
Clivus syndrome	Metastasis to clivus of sphenoid bone and basilar part of occipital bone	Vertex headache exacerbated by neck flexion	Dysfunction of cranial nerves VII & IX–XII (facial weakness, hoarseness, dysarthria, dysphagia, trapezius muscle weakness). Begins unilaterally but extends bilaterally
Jugular foramen	Metastasis to jugular foramen	Occipital pain exacerbated by head movement, radiating to the vertex and to shoulder and arm	Dysfunction of cranial nerves IX–XII (hoarseness, dysarthria, dysphagia, trapezius muscle weakness)
Occipital condyle	Metastasis to occipital condyle	Localized occipital pain exacerbated by neck flexion	Dysfunction of cranial nerve XII (paralysis of tongue ⟶ dysarthria and buccal dysphagia), weakness of sterno-mastoid muscle, stiff neck

Sources: Foley 1979, Portenoy 1989, Bonica 1990

these syndromes (Table 5.2), some patients complain only of paraesthesia or dysaesthesia and numbness in the distribution of one or more cranial nerves. When pain is present, this may precede any other symptoms and signs by weeks or months. Sometimes the syndromes occur bilaterally.

Involvement of hypoglossal nerve (XII) indicates involvement of the neighbouring hypoglossal canal. An associated Horner's syndrome indicates extracranial involvement of the sympathetic nerves in proximity to the jugular foramen:

- ipsilateral ptosis
- constricted pupil
- enophthalmos
- reduced facial sweating.

Radiographic investigation is often unrewarding. A plain radiograph is normally no help, but an isotope bone scan may identify skull metastases. Computed tomography (CT) may help (Fig. 5.1). In a quarter of cases, none of these help, and the diagnosis has to be made on clinical evidence only (Greenberg et al 1981). Indeed, if classical, radiographic investigation can be bypassed and palliative radiotherapy proceeded with.

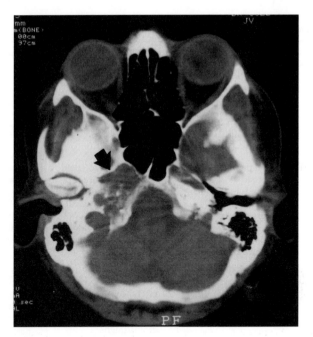

Fig. 5.1 This middle aged woman who had had breast cancer 4 years earlier presented with paralysis of the right VI and XII nerves. CT shows metastatic erosion of the apex of the right petrous bone (arrow).

METASTASES TO VERTEBRAE

Metastases to vertebral bodies often cause midline pain (Table 5.3). Pain from a vertebral pedicle (a common site for a metastasis) may be associated with unilateral nerve root pain. Epidural extension of a paravertebral tumour can also cause unilateral root pain. Disease progression may lead to vertebral body collapse, unilateral or bilateral root pain and paraplegia or tetraplegia. Common differential diagnoses to consider in cancer patients complaining of neck or back pain are:

- degenerative disc disease
- osteoporosis.

Degenerative disc disease is rare at C7, T1 or LI. Radiographic differentiation of osteoporosis from bone metastases may be difficult, particularly in the presence of vertebral body collapse. Ordinary and computed tomography usually allow a distinction to be made. In osteoporotic vertebral body collapse, tomography usually shows intact vertebral end plates and symmetrical collapse. In metastatic disease, there is:

- erosion of the vertebral end plates
- destruction of one or more pedicles
- asymmetrical collapse of the vertebral body.

Because the image is based on a signal which reflects tissue chemistry,

Table 5.3 Pain syndromes caused by vertebral metastases, spinal cord compression and meningeal involvement

Syndrome	Pathophysiology	Characteristics of pain	Concomitants
Vertebrae			
Fracture of odontoid process of C1	Metastasis of odontoid process of C1 $\longrightarrow$ pathological fracture and subluxation $\longrightarrow$ compression of spinal cord	Severe neck pain radiating to occiput and vertex of skull, exacerbated by movements of neck, particularly flexion	Progressive sensory, motor and autonomic dysfunction beginning in upper limb
C7–T1 metastasis	Haematogenous spread of cancer of breast and bronchus; or tumour in paravertebral space $\longrightarrow$ spread to adjacent vertebra and epidural space	Constant aching pain in paraspinal area radiating to both shoulders; unilateral radicular pain (C7–T1) radiating to shoulder and medial aspect of arm	Often tenderness on percussion of spinous process; paraesthesia and numbness in fingers 4 & 5; progressive weakness of triceps and hand
Lumbar metastasis	Common site of metastasis from breast, prostate, and other tumours	Aching pain in midback with reference to one or both sacro-iliac joints; radicular pain in groins/thighs	Pain may be exacerbated by sitting or lying down and relieved by standing or vice versa
Sacral metastasis	Common site of metastasis from breast, prostate, and other tumours	Aching pain in the sacral and/or coccygeal region exacerbated by sitting and relieved by walking	Peri-anal sensory loss; bowel and bladder dysfunction; impotence; may be exacerbated by sitting or lying down and relieved by walking
Spinal cord compression and meninges			
Epidural spinal cord compression	Tumour compression of spinal cord; usually related to vertebral metastasis and collapse	Aching pain and tenderness in the region of involved vertebrae, radicular pain, and garter or cuff distribution of pain in legs	Motor weakness progressing to paraplegia; sensory loss; loss of bowel and bladder function
Meningeal carcinomatosis	Tumour infiltration of the cerebrospinal meninges	Headache, with or without neck stiffness; and pain in the low back and buttocks	Malignant cells in CSF

Sources: Foley 1979, Portenoy 1989, Bonica 1990

magnetic resonance imaging (MRI) is the technique of choice when a metastasis alters tissue chemistry without producing any structural change (Fig. 5.2).

With C7-T1 metastases, an associated Horner's syndrome suggests paravertebral disease with involvement of the sympathetic chain. With lumbar metastases, occasionally there will be little local pain. Instead, pain is referred to the sacro-iliac joint and/or superior posterior illiac crest. Thus, when investigating sacro-iliac pain, it is important to take radiographs of the whole of the lumbar spine.

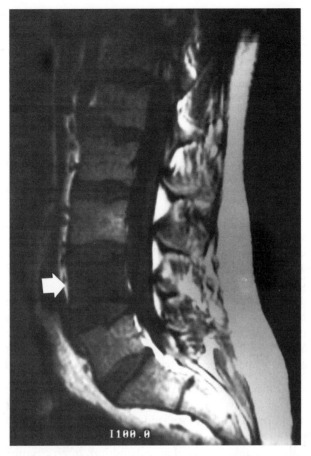

Fig. 5.2 An example of the ability of MRI to detect metastatic disease in bone marrow. This 28 year-old man presented with unremitting low back pain. Clinical examination and conventional radiographs were normal, as was CT. MRI shows an abnormal signal throughout the L4 vertebral body (arrow). Biopsy showed nonHodgkin's lymphoma.

SPINAL CORD COMPRESSION

Spinal cord or cauda equina compression occurs in 1–2% of all cancer patients (Table 5.3). It usually results from the distortion of a vertebral body or pedicle by metastasis. Collapse of the vertebral body is not always a feature; in some cases the compression is caused by nonvertebral epidural metastases. About 70% occur in the thoracic region, 30% in the lumbar and 10% in the cervical spine (Closs & Bates 1987). Multiple sites of compression occur in about 20% of cases (Gilbert et al 1978). Cancer of the breast and bronchus and lymphoma account for 40% of cases of spinal cord compression (Table 5.4).

The first symptom is usually pain which may have been present from as little as 1 day to as much as 2 years. It is generally exacerbated by coughing, sneezing, and straining. The nature of the pain varies according to the site of compression. Local pain is not always present, and may be masked by

Table 5.4 Primary tumour in 1038 cases of spinal cord compression

Primary tumour	Percentage
Bronchus	15
Breast	14
Lymphoma	11
Unknown	9
Sarcoma	8
Myeloma	7
Prostate	7
Kidney	6
Gastro-intestinal	4
Miscellaneous	18

From Black 1979

previously prescribed analgesics. Local tenderness is common. Root pain is often unilateral in cervical or lumbar compression, but is generally bilateral in patients with a thoracic lesion, particularly if associated with epidural spread.

Some patients experience more pain when lying flat (therefore worse at night) whereas, with peripheral nerve compression, rest usually reduces pain intensity (therefore nights are not disturbed by pain). With thoracic cord compression, almost all patients have an upgoing plantar response.

Several pains may be associated with paraplegia (Guttman 1973):

- local vertebral metastatic pain which may radiate laterally
- spasm of the quadratus lumborum muscles, unilateral or bilateral
- nerve root compression pain localized at the level of the cord lesion, unilateral or bilateral
- pain in the legs, nondermatomal in distribution, often circumferential like a garter, cuff or incomplete stocking
- visceral pain caused by a distended bladder or bowel.

More than one quarter of paraplegics with partial or total spinal cord lesions complain of burning, tingling pain (dysaesthesia) in segments of the body below the level of the lesion. These pains are sometimes replaced by:

'Severe crushing pressure, by vice-like pinching sensations, by streams of fire running down the leg to the feet and out of the toes, or by a pain produced by the pressure of a knife being buried in the tissue, twisted around rapidly, and finally withdrawn all at the same time' (Davis & Martin 1974).

These pains may occur after total or partial spinal cord lesions at any level, although it has been suggested that they occur most after lesions of the cauda equina (Davis & Martin 1947, Botterell et al 1954, Guttman 1973). The onset of such pains may be immediate or, more commonly, is delayed for months or years. The pain recurs indefinitely in the most severely affected. Because there is often a long latent period, few patients with malignant paraplegia experience them.

A plain radiograph of the whole spine is essential. In 80% of cases it

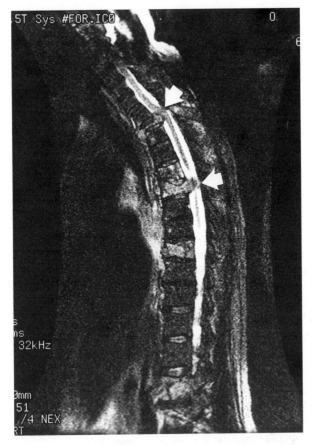

Fig. 5.3 An example of the value of MRI as a noninvasive alternative to myelography in patients with suspected spinal cord compression. This patient with cancer of the prostate had symptoms which appeared clinically to refer to the lower thoracic region. Sagittal MRI shows altered signal intensity in the bodies of T4, 7, 8, and 11. These indicate active metastases. At two levels (T4 and T8) there has been partial vertebral collapse and tumour extension into the canal, producing significant cord compression (arrows). The patient therefore required radiotherapy covering both levels.

will reveal bone destruction — loss of a pedicle or vertebral body collapse (usually sparing the intervertebral disc) at one or more levels. It may also reveal a soft tissue mass adjacent to the vertebrae. An obviously collapsed vertebra, however, may not be the site of the cord compression. A myelogram gives valuable information concerning the site and extent of the compression. Nowadays myelography is often combined with CT. Plain CT is of little use, however, except to confirm vertebral disease. MRI is the investigation of choice (Fig. 5.3). This must not delay treatment and to be helpful it needs to be readily available.

MENINGEAL CARCINOMATOSIS

Meningeal carcinomatosis occurs as a result of metastatic spread into the

CSF. Numerous metastatic seedlings develop on the meninges of both the brain and the spinal cord. There may also be concomitant invasion of the CNS. In one survey, meningeal infiltration by cancer occurred in about 10% of patients with disseminated cancer (Posner & Chernik 1978). In another survery, 90% of cases related to (Wasserstrom et al 1982):

- breast cancer (> 50%)
- lung cancer (> 25%)
- melanoma (12%).

Lymphoma is another relatively common site. Symptoms and signs can be grouped into those involving:

- brain (Table 5.5)
- cranial nerves (Table 5.6)
- spinal nerves (Table 5.7).

Most patients have symptoms and signs in more than one area at the time of diagnosis. Initial cytological examination of the CSF was diagnostic in just over half the cases, and eventually became positive in over 90% (Wasserstrom et al 1982).

Table 5.5   Meningeal metastases from solid tumours in 90 patients — cerebral signs and symptoms

Symptoms		Signs	
Headache	30	Mental change	28
Mental change	15	Seizures	5
Difficulty walking	12	generalized (3)	
Nausea/vomiting	10	focal (2)	
Unconsciousness	2	Papilloedema	5
Dysphasia	2	Diabetes insipidus	2
Dizziness	2	Hemiparesis	1
		Total: 45 patients	

From Wasserstrom et al 1982

Table 5.6   Meningeal metastases from solid tumours in 90 patients — cranial nerve symptoms and signs

Symptoms		Signs	
Diplopia	18	Ocular muscle paresis	18
Hearing loss	7	(III, IV, VI)	
Visual loss	5	Facial weakness (VII)	15
Facial numbness	5	Diminished hearing (VIII)	9
Decreased taste	3	Optic neuropathy (II)	5
Tinnitus	2	Trigeminal neuropathy (V)	5
Hoarseness	2	Hypoglossal neuropathy (XII)	5
Dysphagia	1	Blindness	3
Vertigo	1	Diminished gag (IX, X)	3
		Total: 50 patients	

From Wasserstrom et al 1982

Table 5.7 Meningeal metastases from solid tumours in 90 patients — spinal symptoms and signs

Symptoms		Signs	
Lower motor neurone weakness	34	Reflex asymmetry	64
Paraesthesia	31	Weakness	54
Back/neck pain	23	Sensory loss	24
Radicular pain	19	Straight-leg raising	11
Bowel/bladder dysfunction	12	Decreased rectal tone	10
		Neck rigidity	7

Total: 74 patients

From Wasserstrom et al 1982

Headache and back pain are the most common initial presentations. The headache is often severe and may well be associated with symptoms and signs of meningeal irritation (i.e. nausea, vomiting, photophobia and neck rigidity). In another survey, radicular pain in the buttocks and legs occurred in one third of cases (Olson et al 1974). Helpful radiological investigations are:

- myelography
- CT myelography
- MRI with gadolinium enhancement (Fig. 5.4).

UNILATERAL FACIAL PAIN IN CANCER OF BRONCHUS

Several cases of unilateral ear and facial pain associated with cancer of the bronchus have been reported (Bindoff & Heseltine 1988). The characteristic features of the pain are that it:

- is unilateral
- is initially localized in or around the ear
- is later more diffuse
- has no detectable local cause.

The pain is a form of referred pain, relating to a sensory branch of the vagus (nerve of Arnold) which conveys messages from part of the external auditory canal and a small area of skin behind the ear.

■ CASE HISTORY
A 39 year-old woman complained of right sided facial pain increasing over 4 months. Initially, it was deep in the ear and the right side of her throat. The pain later spread to involve the whole right side of her face, with no triggering factors and no relief from nonopioid analgesics. She smoked up to 10 cigarettes a day. She subsequently had haemoptysis. A chest radiograph showed a right upper lobe shadow and a prominent right hilum. Biopsy confirmed cancer. Radiotherapy to the right upper lobe and hilum resulted in complete relief of pain (Bindoff & Heseltine 1988).

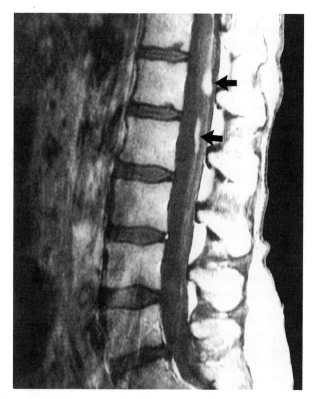

Fig. 5.4   MRI used to detect cauda equina infiltration. This patient with a previous history of breast cancer presented with severe sciatica. MRI was the investigation of choice, because of its ability to distinguish between degenerative disc disease and root compression by vertebral metastases. If neither possibility is demonstrated, gadolinium-enhanced MRI is required in case the symptoms are caused by metastases in the spinal canal. In this patient enhanced images showed two plaques of tumour (arrows) infiltrating the roots of the cauda equina.

Finger clubbing may provide a clue to diagnosis in this syndrome (Schoenen et al 1992).

BRACHIAL PLEXOPATHY

Painful brachial plexopathy occurs in cancer patients for four reasons (Kelly & Payne 1991):

- stretch injury during surgery
- transient inflammatory plexopathy (idiopathic or radiation-induced)
- metastasis
- progressive radiation fibrosis.

Brachial plexopathy is a common complication of Pancoast's tumour (superior pulmonary sulcus syndrome), breast cancer, and lymphoma. Compared with radiation plexopathy, recurrent tumour is more often associated with:

- earlier onset

- severe pain
- Horner's syndrome.

The differential diagnosis is discussed further on page 95.

LUMBOSACRAL PLEXOPATHY

Lumbosacral plexopathy (LSP) presents with sacral and leg pain, and associated weakness. Variable features include (Jaeckle et al 1985):

- leg oedema
- mass palpable PR
- hydronephrosis.

Three syndromes have been described (Jaeckle et al 1985):

- upper (L1-L4) 31%
- lower (L4-S3) 51%
- upper and lower (L1-S3) 18%.

Most patients report an insidious development of pelvic pain and root or nerve pain radiating into the leg, followed weeks or months later by sensory symptoms and weakness. Bladder dysfunction and impotence are unusual.

Lumbar plexopathy ('upper lumbosacral plexopathy') may be caused by tumour at one of several sites:

- intrathecal (meningeal carcinomatosis)
- epidural (epidural extension of paravertebral tumour, e.g. lymphoma)
- epidural (associated with spinal cord compression)
- paravertebral, i.e. at exit foramina from spinal canal (paravertebral tumour, e.g. lymphoma)
- psoas muscle (malignant psoas syndrome, e.g. melanoma, gynaecological cancers, psoas muscle sarcoma)
- renal bed (recurrence of renal cancer)
- retroperitoneum (lymphadenopathy overlying psoas muscle associated with spread of cancer of colon, stomach, adrenal gland and pancreas)
- retroperitoneum (sarcoma).

A comparable range of possibilities exists for sacral plexopathy. CT is a key investigation. The density of muscle and tumour is similar, however, and the diagnosis may be made on the basis of an enlarged 'muscle' mass. MRI will clarify if the diagnosis is in doubt.

Renal bed recurrence

Local recurrence of renal cancer after nephrectomy may cause ipsilateral lumbar back pain and L1 and/or L2 nerve compression pain in the ipsilateral groin and/or upper thigh. There is often associated numbness and weakness of iliopsoas muscle manifesting as impaired flexion of the thigh. Activity typically exacerbates the pain. Radiographic investigation may be difficult.

Bowel prolapses into the renal bed after nephrectomy and interferes with ultrasound. CT is the best imaging technique in this situation.

Malignant psoas syndrome

The features of this syndrome are (Stevens & Gonet 1990):

- clinical evidence of lumbar plexopathy
- painful fixed flexion of the ipsilateral thigh with exacerbation of pain when extension of the hip is attempted (= a positive psoas test)
- CT evidence of ipsilateral psoas major muscle enlargement (Fig. 5.5).

Ultrasound is, in fact, better than CT because muscle and cancer have different echogenicity. MRI will also distinguish. A painful fixed flexion deformity is also seen with more distal muscle infiltration, i.e. of the iliacus within the pelvis.

Proximally, the psoas major muscle is attached to vertebrae T12–L5. The ventral rami of nerves L1–3 and most of nerve L4 transverse the paravertebral belly of the psoas muscle. Branches give rise to iliohypogastric (L1), ilio-inguinal (L1) and genitofemoral (L1–2) nerves which descend superficially on the surface of the muscle posterior to the iliac fascia and the para-aortic and iliac lymph nodes.

PERIPHERAL NEUROPATHY

The incidence of peripheral neuropathy as a nonmetastatic (paraneoplastic) manifestation of malignant disease is between 1% and 5% (Kelly & Payne 1991). It is highest in lung cancer, followed by cancer of the stomach, colon and breast (McLeod 1984). A pure sensory neuropathy may be caused by an auto-immune dorsal root ganglionitis. This is most commonly associated with small cell lung cancer but is seen occasionally with cancer of the breast, ovary, and colon (Kelly & Payne 1991).

Cancer may also directly invade a peripheral nerve. Examples include:

- chest wall or rib lesions which infiltrate intercostal nerves
- paraspinal masses which entrap one or more nerves as they emerge from intervertebral foramina.

CT or MRI usually identifies the tumour. As already noted, paraspinal tumours may extend into the epidural space and lead also to spinal cord compression.

POSTOPERATIVE PAIN SYNDROMES

Chronic neuropathic pain is an uncommon complication of surgical treatment. In most patients, nerve section results only in anaesthesia in the distribution of the nerve. In a small proportion, nerve section also results in pain (Table 5.8). This occurs more frequently after:

- thoracotomy
- mastectomy

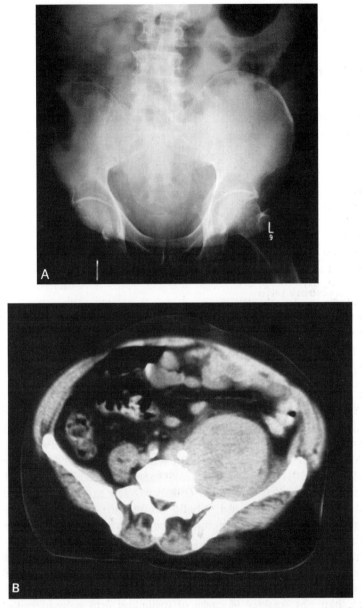

Fig. 5.5 Plain radiograph (A) and CT (B) in a patient with severe pain in anterior left thigh and associated fixed thigh flexion. CT shows massive expansion of the left psoas muscle in the left iliac fossa caused by infiltration by tumour. No abnormality was detectable on the plain radiograph.

- radical neck dissection
- amputation.

Postthoracotomy pain

Pain develops 1–2 months after thoracotomy. Although neuropathic, it is

Table 5.8   Postoperative cancer pain syndromes

Syndrome	Pathophysiology	Characteristics of pain	Concomitants
Postthoracotomy Postmastectomy Postradical neck resection	Severance of nerves during operation ⟶ neuropathic response	Continuous, burning or aching pain +/– bouts of stabbing pain in the areas supplied by affected nerves, exacerbated by touch and movement	Allodynia in the scar; hyperaesthesia in the adjacent area; neuroma uncommon
Postamputation pain	Neuropathic	Constant aching or burning pain in stump and/or in phantom limb	Palpation of trigger points in stump precipitates or exacerbates pain

Sources: Foley 1979, Portenoy 1989, Bonica 1990

commonly aching in character. The pain occurs in an area of sensory loss and the patient may complain of intermittent stabbing pains. Allodynia is usually present, although it may not be prominent.

Postmastectomy pain

Postmastectomy pain has been divided into three types, acute, subacute and late (IASP 1986). Such a classification, however, is not helpful. It is better to classify the pain according to cause (Vecht 1990):

- postaxillary dissection pain
- postmastectomy scar pain
- phantom breast pain.

Postaxillary dissection pain usually develops less than 6 months after mastectomy and relates to section of the intercostobrachial nerve (T1–2) close to the lateral chest wall during axillary lymph node dissection (Granek et al 1982, Vecht 1990). The pain is typically superficial and burning in character, and there is associated numbness (Fig. 5.6). The area affected is the inner aspect of the upper arm and a band around the ipsilateral chest wall at the level of the axilla. There may be intermittent stabbing pains, which occasionally is the dominant feature.

Some patients with postaxillary dissection pain have associated paraesthesiae in the hand. These may be caused by an otherwise subclinical lesion to the brachial plexus. Postaxillary dissection pain accounts, however, for less than one quarter of cases of ipsilateral arm pain in breast cancer (Table 5.9).

Postmastectomy pain which does not affect the axilla may be either a postoperative scar pain or a phantom breast sensation (Jamison et al 1979). These affect the chest wall in the area of the amputated breast. With neuropathic postoperative scar pain, a woman may be unable to wear a breast prosthesis because of associated allodynia. Clothing often has to be loose for the same reason.

If recurrence is suspected, it is important to investigate with CT and/or MRI. MRI is probably better.

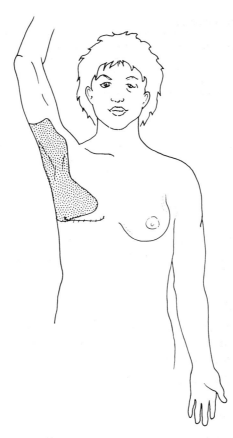

Fig. 5.6 The intercostobrachial nerve can be injured during breast surgery. The nerve has a variable distribution to the skin of the axilla and anterolateral chest wall.

Table 5.9 Causes of ipsilateral arm pain in 38 patients with breast cancer

Cause	Number of patients
Lesions of the brachial plexus	17
tumour infiltration (8)	
radiofibrosis (5)	
lymphoedema (entrapment) (1)	
transient neuritis (3)	
Cervical radiculopathy	4
vertebral metastasis (4)	
Carpal tunnel syndrome	4
with lymphoedema (2)	
without lymphoedema (2)	
Postsurgical pain	8
postaxillary dissection pain (7)	
Adhesive capsulitis of shoulder	5

From Vecht 1990

Postradical neck dissection pain

This is characterized by ipsilateral neck pain (C3 distribution) which is usually superficial and burning (+ allodynia ± stabbing pains). Sometimes it is predominantly aching in character.

Postamputation pain

After amputation of a limb, the patient may complain of either stump pain or phantom limb pain (Table 5.7). These are distinct from phantom limb sensation, which is experienced by all amputees.

TREATMENT RELATED PAIN

Pains related to anticancer treatment are summarized in Table 5.10.

Mucositis

Mucositis is a painful condition caused by mucosal injury and inflammation of the mouth and pharynx, and sometimes the oesophagus, ± secondary infection, secondary to local radiotherapy or to certain forms of chemo-

Table 5.10 Treatment related cancer pain syndromes

Syndrome	Pathophysiology	Characteristics of pain	Concomitants
Postchemotherapy			
Mucositis	Ulceration of buccal and pharyngeal mucosa	Severe pain exacerbated by drinking, eating and talking	
Peripheral neuropathy	Caused by vinca alkaloids	Constant symmetrical burning pain in the hands and/or feet	Allodynia
Steroid pseudorheumatism	Caused by rapid withdrawal of corticosteroids	Diffuse myalgia and arthralgia	Fatigue and general malaise
Aseptic necrosis of humoral/femoral head	Complication of chronic corticosteroid therapy	Aching pain in shoulder or hip	Limitation of joint movement
Postradiation therapy			
Radiation fibrosis of brachial or lumbosacral plexus	Fibrosis of connective tissue surrounding nerves with consequent neural injury	Increasingly severe burning pain in the arm or leg	Allodynia; numbness motor weakness (usually C5–6 distribution in the arm)
Radiation myelopathy	Damage to spinal cord; causes pain in less than 20%	Pattern similar to spinal cord compression; local back pain, radicular pain and/or neuropathic pain referred distally	Other sensory and motor symptoms and signs of myelopathy

Sources: Foley 1979, Portenoy 1989, Bonica 1990

therapy. Occasionally the pain is so severe that ingestion of food and fluids is impossible. In one series of patients who had undergone bone marrow transplantation for aplastic anaemia and leukaemia, 62% had moderate to severe pain for 2–4 weeks and 22% had mild discomfort (Sullivan et al 1984). The pain usually develops 2–3 days after transplantation. Local radiation can also cause colorectal mucositis (colitis, proctitis).

Steroid pseudorheumatism

Patients receiving corticosteroids for rheumatoid arthritis occasionally develop a syndrome comprising diffuse pains in muscles, tendons, joints and bones, associated with malaise, asthenia, pyrexia, and, sometimes, neuropsychological disturbances. Patients may experience cramps, and the muscular pain may have a burning quality about it, particularly in the intercostals. This syndrome, called steroid pseudorheumatism, is sometimes seen in cancer patients:

- receiving 100 mg of prednisolone daily (equivalent to about 14 mg of dexamethasone) for several days in association with chemotherapy
- with spinal cord compression given dexamethasone 100 mg daily for several days (Greenberg et al 1979)
- on relatively high doses of dexamethasone to reduce intracranial pressure caused by brain metastases
- on reduction from high dose to low dose
- on reduction of an average maintenance dose after a prolonged course.

Avascular bone necrosis

Aseptic necrosis of the head of the humerus or femur may develop in patients receiving a corticosteroid. Pain in the shoulder or hip and leg is the most common presentation. There is progressive limitation of joint movements. Radiographic changes may not be apparent for weeks or months. MRI is the investigation of choice in the early stage (Fig. 5.7). Aseptic necrosis is more common in patients with lymphoma (see p. 433).

Radiation plexopathy

From time to time a patient presents with pain in the arm associated with other symptoms and signs which suggest compression of, or damage to, the brachial plexus. In the majority, there is clear evidence of metastatic disease from a cancer of the head and neck, breast or bronchus. Sometimes, there is no such evidence and, in a patient who has had previous radiotherapy to this area, the question arises as to whether the plexopathy could be caused by postradiation fibrosis.

The distinction is important because, if metastatic, hormonal treatment or chemotherapy may be beneficial. Difficulty arises when evidence of postradiation tissue damage is present, but recurrence is also possible. Only surgical exploration and/or the passage of time will confirm the cause. After

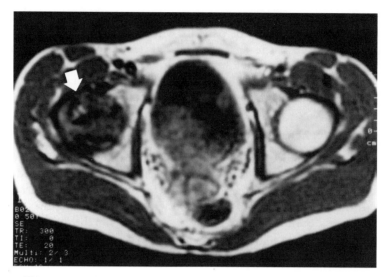

Fig. 5.7 This 32 year-old man developed pain in the right hip some months after chemotherapy for teratoma of the testicles. An axial MRI section of the pelvis shows normal medullary bone in the head of the left femur but a dramatically altered signal intensity in the right femoral head (arrow), because of replacement of normal fatty marrow by necrotic bone. MRI usually gives obvious and unequivocal findings in avascular bone necrosis, making it the technique of choice.

5 years of progressive plexopathy without evidence of metastasis, the likelihood of recurrence becomes progressively less and the value of the time factor as a criterion for radiation plexopathy becomes correspondingly more. The two conditions, however, can differ in a number of respects (Table 5.11), including the presence or absence of pain (Kori et al 1981).

■ CASE HISTORY

A 76 year-old woman who had had a left mastectomy for cancer nearly 40 years before, began to experience pain in the left arm. It increased in extent and intensity over 18 months and was associated with loss of function in the hand and forearm. The arm then swelled up and, although no masses were palpable, a presumptive diagnosis of recurrent breast cancer was made. Treatment with tamoxifen was commenced. Within 3 months the swelling resolved, but the neurological signs and symptoms did not. The pain had changed to a more superficial, burning discomfort with marked allodynia. She was treated with a tricyclic antidepressant and regular oral morphine. This achieved a moderate degree of relief. Tamoxifen induced a prolonged remission and the patient lived at home with her equally elderly husband until she died of other causes about 5 years later. Earlier treatment with tamoxifen might well have prevented the pain and disability.

Radiation myelopathy

Pain is an early symptom in 15% of patients with radiation myelopathy, i.e. postradiation spinal cord ischaemia (Jellinger & Sturm 1971). The pain

Table 5.11   Characteristics of pain in 100 patients with brachial plexopathy

	Tumour group (n = 78)	Radiation group (n = 22)
Presenting symptom	82%	18%
Location	Shoulder, upper arm, elbow; radiates to fingers 4 & 5	Shoulder, wrist, hand
Nature	Aching pain in shoulder; lancinating pain in elbow and ulnar aspect of hand; occasional dysaesthesia, burning, freezing sensations	Aching pain in shoulder; tightness and heaviness in arm and hand; paraesthesiae in C5, 6 distribution
Severity	Moderate – severe; 98% severe	Mild – moderate; only 35% severe
Course	Progressive neurological dysfunction, atrophy and weakness C7–T1 distribution; pain persistent	Progressive weakness in C5, 6 distribution; pain stabilizes or improves with appearance of weakness

From Kori et al 1981

may be localized to the area of spinal cord injury or may be referred pain, with dysaethesiae below the level of injury. Clinically, the neurological symptoms and signs usually begin with a Brown-Sequard syndrome (ipsilateral motor paresis with contralateral sensory loss at a cervical or thoracic level) and progress to a complete transverse myelopathy.

Diagnosis is by exclusion. The differential diagnosis includes:

- intramedullary tumour
- epidural spinal cord compression
- arteriovenous malformation
- transverse myelitis.

Investigation begins with plain radiographs of the spine; these are usually normal. Myelography, if done, is usually also normal. MRI will either be normal or show atrophic changes.

Radiation induced peripheral nerve tumours

A painful enlarging mass in an area which has been radiated some years before is likely to be a late local recurrence. Rarely it turns out to be a radiation induced tumour of the nerve sheath (Schwannoma). Such tumours have been reported 4–20 years after radiation therapy (Foley et al 1975). They cause pain and progressive neurological deficit in the distribution of the involved nerve (usually the brachial or lumbar plexus). The diagnosis is established by biopsy. The most important differential diagnoses are:

- radiation fibrosis
- recurrent tumour.

Ultrasound can often distinguish between a scar (contracted) and a tumour (expanded). If doubt persists, MRI should be undertaken.

REFERENCES

Bindoff L, Heseltine D 1988 Unilateral facial pain in patients with lung cancer: a referred pain via the vagus? Lancet i: 812–815

Black P 1979 Spinal metastasis: current status and recommended guidelines for management. Neurosurgery 5: 726–746

Bonica J J 1990 The management of pain, 2nd edn. Lea & Febiger, Philadelphia

Botterell E H, Callaghan J C, Jonsse A T 1954 Pain in paraplegia: clinical management and surgical treatment. Proceedings of the Royal Society of Medicine 47: 281–288

Closs S, Bates T D 1987 The management of malignant spinal cord compression. Bailliere's Clinical Oncology 1 (2): 431–441

Davis L, Martin J 1947 Studies upon spinal cord injuries. II. The nature and treatment of pain. Journal of Neurosurgery 4: 483–491

Foley K M 1979 Pain syndromes in patients with cancer. In: Bonica J J, Ventafridda V (eds) Advances in pain research and therapy, vol 2. Raven Press, New York, pp 59–75

Foley K M, Woodruff J M, Ellis F, Posner J B 1975 Radiation-induced malignant and atypical schwannomas. Neurology 25: 354

Gilbert T W, Jae-HO K, Posner J B 1978 Epidural spinal cord compression from metastatic tumour: diagnosis and treatment. Annals of Neurology 3: 40–51

Granek I, Ashikari R, Foley K M 1982 Postmastectomy pain syndrome: clinical and anatomic correlates. Proceedings of the American Society of Clinical Oncology 1: 152

Greenberg H S, Kim J-H, Posner J B 1979 Epidural spinal cord compression from metastatic tumour: results with a new treatment protocol. Annals of Neurology 8: 361–366

Greenberg H S, Deck M D F, Vikram B, Chu F C H, Posner J B 1981 Metastasis to the base of the skull: clinical findings in 43 patients. Neurology 31: 530–537

Guttman L 1973 Spinal injuries: comprehensive management and research. Blackwells, Oxford

International Association for the Study of Pain 1986 Classification of chronic pain. Pain 3 (suppl): S1–S225

Jaeckle K A, Young D F, Foley K M 1985 The natural history of lumbosacral plexopathy in cancer. Neurology 35: 8–15

Jamison K, Wellisch D K, Katz R L, O'Pasnau R O 1979 Phantom breast syndrome. Archives of Surgery 114: 93–95

Jellinger K, Sturm K W 1971 Delayed radiation myelopathy in man. Journal of the Neurolological Sciences 14: 389–408

Kelly J B, Payne R 1991 Pain syndromes in the cancer patient. Neurologic Complications of Systemic Cancer 9 (4): 937–953

Kori S H, Foley K M, Posner J B 1981 Brachial plexus lesions in patients with cancer: 100 cases. Neurology (NY) 31: 45–50

McLeod J G 1984 Carcinomatous neuropathy. In: Dyck P J, Thomas P K, Lambert E H et al (eds) Peripheral neuropathy. W B Saunders, Philadelphia, p 2180

Olson M E, Chernik N L, Posner J B 1974 Infiltration of the leptomeninges by systemic cancer: a clinical and pathologic study. Archives of Neurology 30: 122–137

Portenoy R K 1989 Cancer pain: epidemiology and syndromes. Cancer 63: 2298–2307

Posner J B, Chernik N L 1978 Intracranial metastases from systemic cancer. Advanced Neurology 19: 579–592

Schoenen J, Broux R, Moonen G 1992 Unilateral facial pain as the first symptom of lung cancer: are there diagnostic clues? Cephalagia 12: 178–179

Stevens M J, Gonet Y M 1990 Malignant psoas syndrome: recognition of an oncologic entity. Australasian Radiology 34: 150–154

Sullivan K M, Syrjala K, Flournoy N, Chapman C R, Storb R, Thomas E D 1984 Pain following intensive chemoradiotherapy and bone marrow transplantation. Pain 2 (suppl): S215

Vecht C J 1990 Arm pain in patient with breast cancer. Journal of Pain and Symptom Management 5: 109–117

Wasserstrom W R, Glass J P, Posner J B 1982 Diagnosis and treatment of leptomeningeal metastasis from solid tumors. Cancer 49: 759–772

CHAPTER 6 | Cancer pain syndromes II

In this chapter, various other pain syndromes which are seen in cancer patients are described. Some are clearly not specific to cancer but pattern recognition is just as important for diagnosis and appropriate treatment.

INFECTION

Infection was the cause of pain in 4% of nearly 300 patients referred to a pain relief service in a cancer hospital (Gonzalez et al 1989). Infection in or around a tumour can lead to a rapid increase in pain, but is not always thought of as a possible cause. One report, however, describes seven patients with head and neck cancer in whom infection was responsible for some or all of their pain (Bruera & MacDonald 1986).

All the patients had large tumour masses with ulceration and necrosis, together with swelling, induration, and erythema of the surrounding tissue. In each case, pain had previously been relieved with an oral opioid, and then increased considerably over a few days. In three of the patients there was a change in the appearance of the tumour, two had a leucocytosis and one was febrile. Empirical treatment with antibiotics resulted in pain relief within 3 days in all seven patients.

FRACTURED RIB SYNDROME

Pathological fractures of the ribs are relatively common in cancer of the breast and prostate, and also occur in other cancers which metastasize to bone. A rib fracture may well be painless at rest, particularly if a patient is already taking analgesics. The rectus abdominis muscles, however, are attached to the inner aspect of the lower ribs. Thus, when the body is moved from a sitting to lying position, or vice versa, these muscles tug on the fractured bone and cause transient severe pain. Deep breaths, coughing, laughing and twisting the trunk also cause severe pain. The diagnosis may not be made, however, because the patient simply complains of a new severe chest pain. If alert to this possibility, the doctor will ask the appropriate questions and elicit the classical features of the syndrome.

FUNCTIONAL INTESTINAL PAINS

Squashed stomach syndrome

This is seen frequently in advanced cancer and warrants special mention. In this syndrome, epigastric pain is caused by relative gastric distension. This often occurs in patients with a grossly enlarged liver, whether or not there is any associated gastric abnormality. It is important to recognize the cause of the postprandial discomfort because explanation to the patient is crucial in management (Box 6.A). Some patients, particularly those with an endo-oesophageal tube, also experience retrosternal (oesophageal) pain secondary to acid regurgitation.

BOX 6.A
SYMPTOMS OF SQUASHED STOMACH SYNDROME

Early satiation
Epigastric fullness
Epigastric discomfort/pain
Flatulence
Hiccup
Nausea
Vomiting (particularly postprandial)
Heartburn

Constipation

Although severe constipation is often painless, in some patients it causes a lot of pain. Constipation can cause intestinal (abdominal) colic and, if there is faecal impaction, rectal (deep perineal) colic. Constipation can also cause pain in the right iliac fossa. This is caused by gaseous caecal distension secondary to constipation. Hard retained faeces are usually palpable in the descending colon. Sometimes the transverse colon is palpable too. The caecum is tender on palpation. Identical caecal symptoms and signs are also seen in obstruction of the colon. Careful history taking and clinical evaluation usually enables the two conditions to be differentiated.

■ CASE HISTORY
A 79 year-old man with known cancer of the stomach had an emergency operation for strangulated left inguinal hernia. It was decided to continue nursing the patient on the surgical ward because of his poor prognosis. The nurses insisted on morphine being prescribed because he continued to complain of central abdominal pain. About 6 weeks later, as he had not died,

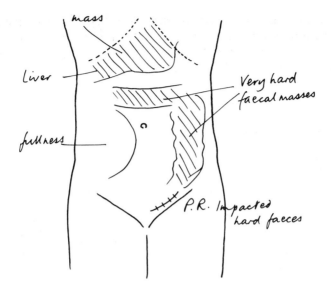

Fig. 6.1 Abdominal findings in a 79 year-old man with cancer of the stomach when admitted from a university teaching hospital to a palliative care unit two and a half weeks before death.

the patient was transferred to a palliative care unit. Abdominal and rectal examination confirmed constipation with faecal impaction (Fig. 6.1). Rectal and oral laxative measures were instituted and the morphine curtailed over the course of a week. The patient was encouraged to sit out of bed and he was helped to begin walking again. He died of a pulmonary embolus some days later.

Irritable bowel syndrome

Irritable bowel syndrome (IBS) is a term used to describe several functional motility disorders of the gastro-intestinal tract (Read 1985, Thompson 1993). About 10% of the population are affected. This means that IBS will be seen in cancer patients relatively commonly.

Common features are abdominal pain and a variable pattern of defaecation (Box 6.B). Upper gastro-intestinal symptoms such as postprandial fullness and heartburn are also common, and stress the diffuse nature of the functional disturbance. Symptoms may be intermittent or continuous. Descriptions of the pain include colic, cramping, stabbing, aching, burning, and 'like a blockage'. Some patients complain of a continuous dull ache with intermittent attacks of colic. Many patients have periods free of symptoms.

Balloon distension of the pelvic colon produces pain more consistently in patients with IBS than in healthy controls (Ritchie 1973). It is reasonable, therefore, to think of IBS as an oversensitive gastro-intestinal tract in which normal alimentary sensations are perceived as pain. Most cancer patients with IBS will have had the condition diagnosed many years before and will not confuse the pain of IBS with cancer pain. This is not always the case, however, as the following account illustrates.

BOX 6.B
SYMPTOMS OF IRRITABLE BOWEL SYNDROME

Abdominal pain in various sites, commonly in left iliac fossa

Pain often exacerbated by distension

- spontaneous
- barium enema
- sigmoidoscopy

Relief of pain with

- defaecation
- passage of flatus

Bowel habit alternating between frequent passage of loose faeces and constipation with small pellets or 'ribbon' stools

More frequent and looser faeces at the onset of bouts of pain
Passage of mucus with faeces
Feelings of incomplete rectal evacuation

■ CASE HISTORY

A 78 year-old man with cancer of the prostate was referred to a palliative care unit for pain relief. He experienced intermittent abdominal pain which caused him and his family great distress. He had been prescribed a strong opioid to use 'as required'. He became housebound and increasingly dependent. He took several different laxatives for increasingly troublesome constipation. If he did not defaecate before noon, he became visibly anxious and experienced progressively more intense cramping abdominal pain. He insisted on suppositories (bisacodyl 10 mg) rather than wait for a spontaneous bowel action later in the day. The pain was eased by defaecation and, to a lesser extent, by the opioid.

A carefully taken history and clinical examination strongly suggested that the patient was not suffering from cancer pain but from functional bowel pain. The situation was made worse by debility and drug related constipation. With perseverance, the patient's pattern of defaecation was steadily improved and the opioid stopped. His family still acted, however, as if he was imminently dying and often sat with him in silence and in tears. After 1 year, the patient and family reluctantly accepted that he had 'grumbling cancer' rather than terminal cancer. He continued to rehabilitate slowly, and began to drive his car again. The whole family, however, continued to need close supervision to prevent recidivism.

HEPATIC PAIN

Pain is not a constant feature of hepatomegaly. In 90 patients with advanced cancer and hepatomegaly, less than 40% had right hypochondrial pain (Table 6.1). If pancreatic cancer patients are excluded (the pain could be pancreatic rather than hepatic), the figure drops to about one third.

Table 6.1 Right hypochondrial pain in 90 patients with hepatomegaly

Primary site	Number of patients	% with pain
Bronchus	19	26
Colon	14	36
Stomach	12	42
Breast	11	27
Rectum	8	25
Pancreas	5	100
Others	12	17
Unknown	9	89
Total	90	39

Source: Baines & Kirkham 1989

The most common pain associated with hepatomegaly is an aching right hypochondrial pain (Box 6.C). In some patients this is exacerbated by standing or prolonged walking. This is probably caused by traction on the hepatic ligaments.

Patients occasionally develop rapidly increasing right upper quadrant pain, and present with an 'acute abdomen'. In far advanced cancer, the most likely cause of such pain is haemorrhage into a hepatic secondary with acute distension of the pain sensitive liver capsule. The dose of morphine generally needs to be doubled or trebled to relieve the pain. (This will diminish as the haematoma resolves and/or the capsule adapts, and analgesic requirements usually return to prehaemorrhage levels within a week.)

Patients with gross hepatomegaly sometimes complain of discomfort in the lower rib cage, often bilaterally. This may relate to outward pressure on the rib cage. The use of a nonopioid, for example paracetamol, often gives significant relief.

A few patients complain of intermittent sharp pains in the right hypochondrium. These are probably caused by the enlarged liver pinching the parietal peritoneum between itself and the lower border of the rib cage. Explanation, and a change of position and local massage when afflicted usually provides relief. Some patients with hepatomegaly also complain of backache. This is caused by postural factors and is comparable to the backache of pregnancy.

BOX 6.C
PAINS ASSOCIATED WITH HEPATOMEGALY

Hepatomegaly
Traction on hepatic ligaments (when standing or walking)
Intrahepatic haemorrhage
Outward pressure on rib cage
Pinching of abdominal wall
Lumbar spinal strain (as in pregnancy)

PANCREATIC PAIN

As with other primary sites, pain is not a constant feature in pancreatic cancer. Pain relates to obstruction of the pancreatic ducts, and to infiltration of pancreatic connective tissue, capillaries and/or afferent nerves. It occurs in about 90% of patients with cancer of the head of the pancreas, particularly if the growth is near the ampulla of Vater (Macfarlane & Thomas 1964). Jaundice is a common accompanying feature. On the other hand, pain occurs in only 10% of patients with cancer of the pancreatic body and tail, and is generally a late feature.

Pancreatic pain is usually upper abdominal. It is often said that the pain will be on the right side with cancer of the head of the pancreas and on the left with cancer of the tail. This is not always the case (Table 6.2). The patient usually experiences constant pain which becomes increasingly severe over a period of time. As with other causes of epigastric pain, in some patients the pain is eased by bending forward and exacerbated by lying supine.

Pain may also be experienced in the back. It is typically midline in the upper lumbar or lower thoracic region. It may spread laterally, particularly if severe. Unless there is co-existent degenerative spinal disease, there is no bone tenderness or restriction of spinal movement. The presence of back pain may indicate:

- referred pain from the pancreas itself
- spread into the retroperitoneum and para-aortic nodes
- penetration into paravertebral muscles.

Table 6.2   Site of pain in 32 patients with cancer of pancreas

Site	Percentage[a]
Right upper quadrant	38
Left upper quadrant	28
Circumferential (at level of pancreas)	25
Epigastrium	19
Left lower quadrant	19
Right lower quadrant	13
Back only	6

[a] 41% of patients had multiple sites of pain.
From Krech & Walsh 1991

INTRAPELVIC PAIN

Intrapelvic pain was present in 11% of a series of 350 patients with advanced cancer (Baines & Kirkham 1989). In over half the pain was associated with recurrent cancer of the colon or rectum. A quarter had malignancies of the female reproductive tract, and 1% had extra-abdominal primaries.

The pattern of pain associated with intrapelvic malignant disease varies (Box 6.D). Central hypogastric pain is relatively common in cancers of the bladder and uterus. It is also seen in patients with colorectal cancer, particularly if adherent to or invading the bladder or uterus. More common

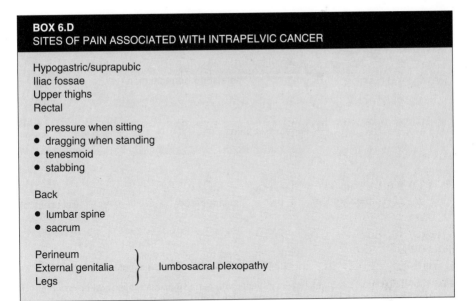

BOX 6.D
SITES OF PAIN ASSOCIATED WITH INTRAPELVIC CANCER

Hypogastric/suprapubic
Iliac fossae
Upper thighs
Rectal

- pressure when sitting
- dragging when standing
- tenesmoid
- stabbing

Back

- lumbar spine
- sacrum

Perineum
External genitalia } lumbosacral plexopathy
Legs

is pain in the iliac fossae. This is typically unilateral and associated with local recurrence adherent to the lateral pelvic wall. Sometimes the patient becomes bedbound because walking exacerbates the pain. This suggests attachment to, or infiltration of, the ipsilateral iliopsoas muscle by the cancer.

Presacral recurrence often leads to lumbosacral plexopathy (see p. 89). Pain may be felt in the perineum or external genitalia rather than in the legs. Severe intrapelvic pain often radiates to the upper thighs in a diffuse manner. Pain may also be referred to the lumbar region as in some non-malignant gynaecological disorders.

Rectal pain is another type of intrapelvic malignant pain. It may be experienced even if the rectum has been excised surgically. If a local recurrence is present the patient may complain of discomfort on sitting. This may be mild and described as a feeling of 'pressure', or it may be severe enough to prevent the patient from sitting down. The reverse is also seen; no pain when sitting but an increasingly severe dragging pain when standing for more than a few minutes or after walking 50–100 m. This type of pain may relate to a deeper recurrence with adherence to myofascial structures.

'Tenesmoid pain' (a painful sensation of rectal fullness) is occasionally a problem. It is similar to the discomfort felt by normal subjects when experiencing an intense urgent desire to defaecate. Usually such pain is related to local tumour in the unresected rectum, or to involvement of the presacral plexus by recurrence tumour. Rarely, it represents a phantom phenomenon after rectal excision. Severe stabbing pains ('like a red hot poker') are occasionally reported. These may relate to spasm of the rectum or the pelvic floor. This type of pain may make the patient distraught.

A review of perineal pain after perineal resection for rectal cancer showed that most early onset pains (within a few weeks of surgery) were neuropathic,

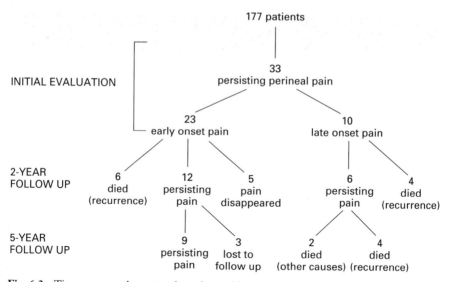

Fig. 6.2   Time course and outcome in patients with perineal pain after perineal resection of cancer of the rectum. (Reproduced with permission from Boas et al 1993.)

and that late onset pain (more than 3 months) invariably indicated recurrence (Fig. 6.2). In over 60% the early onset pain was described as shooting, bursting, or a tight ache. In most the intensity was mild to moderate, intermittent and spontaneous. Only 1/23 patients obtained good relief from nonopioids and opioids. The late onset pain was mainly sharp aching, often severe and continuous, located deeper within the pelvis and, in 80%, exacerbated by pressure and sitting (Boas et al 1993). In contrast to the early onset group, over half of the patients responded well to nonopioids and opioids.

Phantom bladder pain is rare. It probably occurs only after cystectomy when, before surgery, the patient has had considerable bladder pain either from the tumour itself or from intractable cystitis. Phantom bladder symptoms (bladder distension and a desire to void) are described more often. They occur after cystectomy, cord transection and in patients on haemodialysis (Dorpat 1971).

BLADDER SPASM

Spasm of the detrusor muscle manifests as a deep painful sensation lasting for several minutes or up to half an hour in the suprapubic region, and/or referred to the tip of the penis. Frequency depends on the cause (Box 6.E). Irritation of the trigone by infection or cancer may act as a trigger. Investigation may include:

- bacterial cultures (to identify infection)
- cystoscopy (to detect intravesical cancer)
- magnetic resonance imaging (MRI) (to detect intramural and extravesical cancer).

BOX 6.E
CAUSES OF BLADDER SPASMS IN CANCER

Cancer
Intravesical   ⎱ of bladder or prostate
Intramural   ⎰ or other intrapelvic tumours
Extravesical

Cancer treatment
Radiation fibrosis
Indwelling catheter

- without retention (mechanical irritation)
- with partial retention (catheter sludging)
- secondary to infection

Concurrent
Infection (cystitis)
Anxiety

LYMPHOEDEMA

The reported incidence of pain in lymphoedema varies from 9–63% (Stillwell 1969, Markowski et al 1981, Brismar & Ljungdahl 1983, Corneillie et al 1984, Kissin et al 1986, Badger et al 1988, Alliot et al 1990, Vecht 1990). At a specialist lymphoedema clinic, the incidence when first seen was 57% (Table 6.3). Although many patients had more than one pain, they were categorized according to the dominant one (Table 6.4).

Tissue pressure pain was characterized by a deep ache with or without tightness, which tended to be exacerbated by:

- hot weather (because of increased swelling)
- exercise.

Pain, therefore, increases during the day. Analgesics are relatively ineffective but supporting the arm usually helps (Carroll & Rose 1992). Patients may have difficulty sleeping unless a comfortable position can be found and

Table 6.3 Incidence of tightness and pain in 100 lymphoedema patients

Group	Number of patients	Tightness (%)	Pain (%)
Noncancer	22	23	64
Active cancer	46	43[a]	67[b]
Inactive cancer	32	21[a]	37[b]
Total	100	32	57

[a] p = <0.05, comparison of two proportions (Armitage 1971).
[b] p = <0.01.
From Badger et al 1988

Table 6.4   Types of pain in patients with lymphoedema

Type	Number of patients
Tissue pressure	25
Muscle tension	15
Neuropathic	12[a]
Inflammation and/or infection	5
None	43

[a] All cancer patients, including 10 with active disease; in 3 patients pain caused by cervical spondylosis.
From Badger et al 1988

maintained. Muscle tension pain results from the weight of the limb pulling down on supporting muscles and ligaments.

BREAKTHROUGH PAIN

The term breakthrough pain has become part of the vocabulary associated with chronic pain (Box 6.F). The essence of breakthrough pain is its unpredictability. Because it is predictable, movement related pain ('incident pain'), is best not called breakthrough pain. In practice, it often is. In one study, incident pain occurred in about 20% of patients (Bruera et al 1992).

In a review of 41 patients with either incident or breakthrough pain, the median number of pain episodes in 24 h was four (Table 6.5). Only five patients had more than 10 episodes. The maximum number was reported by a patient with cancer of the bronchus who experienced stabbing pain whenever he coughed because of a rib fracture. About one quarter of the pains were neuropathic.

The median duration of breakthrough pain was 30 min (ranging from

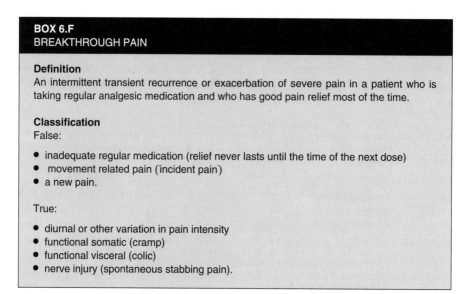

BOX 6.F
BREAKTHROUGH PAIN

Definition
An intermittent transient recurrence or exacerbation of severe pain in a patient who is taking regular analgesic medication and who has good pain relief most of the time.

Classification
False:

- inadequate regular medication (relief never lasts until the time of the next dose)
- movement related pain ('incident pain')
- a new pain.

True:

- diurnal or other variation in pain intensity
- functional somatic (cramp)
- functional visceral (colic)
- nerve injury (spontaneous stabbing pain).

Table 6.5 Precipitating events for incident and breakthrough pain in 41 patients

Incident ('volitional')	
Movement in bed	7
Walking	4
Cough	6
Sitting	2
Standing	2
Touch	1
	22
Breakthrough ('nonvolitional')	
Bowel distension	4
Ureteric distension	1
Medication regurgitated	1
Precipitant not identified	23
	29
Total	51

Source: Portenoy & Hagen 1990

1 min to 4 h). Time to maximum intensity varied, but was less than 3 min in about half. Pain usually recurred in the same location. All but two represented a transient exacerbation of a known underlying cancer pain. In about one third of the patients, the pain occurred towards the end of the interval between regular analgesic doses, indicating a need for an increase in the dose of morphine.

REFERENCES

Alliot F, Miserey G, Cluzan R 1990 Secondary upper limb lymphoedema can be painful and disturb the quality of life. World Lymphology Conference, Tokyo

Armitage P 1971 Statistical methods of medical research. Blackwells, Oxford, p 129

Badger C M A, Mortimer P S, Regnard C F B, Twycross R G 1988 Pain in the chronically swollen limb. In: Partsch H (ed) Progress in Lymphology – XI. Elsevier Science Publishers BV, Amsterdam, pp 243–246

Baines M, Kirkham S R 1989 Carcinoma involving bone and soft tissue. In: Wall P D, Melzack R (eds) Textbook of pain. Churchill Livingstone, Edinburgh, pp 590–597

Boas R A, Schug S A, Acland R H 1993 Perineal pain after rectal amputation: a 5 year follow up. Pain 52: 67–70

Brismar B, Ljungdahl I 1983 Postoperative lymphoedema after treatment of breast cancer. Acta Chirurgica Scandinavica 149: 687–689

Bruera E, MacDonald R N 1986 Intractable pain in patients with advanced head and neck tumors: a possible role of local infection. Cancer Treatment Reports 70: 691–692

Bruera E, Fainsinger R, MacEachern T, Hanson J 1992 The use of methylphenidate in patients with incident cancer pain receiving regular opiates: a preliminary report. Pain 50: 75–77

Carroll D, Rose K 1992 Treatment leads to significant improvement: effect of conservative treatment in pain in lymphoedema. Professional Nurse October: 32–36

Corneillie P, Gruwez J A, Lerut T, Van Elst F 1984 Early and late postoperative sequelae after surgery for carcinoma of the breast. Acta Chirurgica Beligium 84: 227–231

Dorpat T L 1971 Phantom sensations of internal organs. Comprehensive Psychiatry 12: 27–35

Gonzalez G R, Foley K M, Portenoy R K 1989 Evaluative skills necessary for a cancer pain consultant. Presented at the American Pain Society Meetings, Phoenix, Arizona, October 26–29

Kissin M W, Querci della Rovere G, Easton D, Westbury G 1986 The risk of lymphoedema following treatment of breast cancer. British Journal of Surgery 73: 580–584

Krech R L, Walsh D 1991 Symptoms of pancreatic cancer. Journal of Pain and Symptom
    Management 6: 360–367
Macfarlane D A, Thomas L P 1964 Textbook of Surgery. Churchill Livingstone, Edinburgh
Markowski J, Wilcox J P, Helm P A 1981 Lymphoedema incidence after specific
    postmastectomy therapy. Archives of Physical Medicine and Rehabilitation 62: 922–926
Portenoy K R, Hagen N A 1990 Breakthrough pain: definition, prevalence and characteristics.
    Pain 41: 273–281
Read N W 1985 Irritable bowel syndrome. Grune & Stratton, London
Ritchie J 1973 Pain from the pelvic colon by inflating a balloon in the irritable colon syndrome.
    Gut 14: 125–132
Stillwell G K 1969 Treatment of postmastectomy lymphoedema. Modern Treatment
    6: 369–412
Thompson W G 1993 Irritable bowel syndrome: pathogenesis and management. Lancet
    341: 1569–1572
Vecht C J 1990 Arm pain in the patient with breast cancer. Journal of Pain and Symptom
    Management 5: 109–117

Evaluation

PQRST CHARACTERISTICS

Traditionally, doctors are taught to evaluate pain by determining its PQRST characteristics (Table 7.1). A blind belief in the efficacy of so simple an approach, however, may hinder rather than help the doctor when evaluating pain in cancer patients. Determination of the PQRST characteristics is only the beginning; it provides a *description* of the pain but no more.

Evaluation implies the ability to make a diagnosis and decide on an initial plan of management. Among other things, this demands an understanding of:

- the pathological processes which give rise to pain (see p. 48)
- the phenomenon of referred pain (see p. 50)
- neuro-anatomy.

When complete, an evaluation should allow the physician to say whether the pain:

- is caused by the cancer or by another disorder
- constitutes a specific cancer pain syndrome
- is nociceptive, neuropathic or mixed nociceptive-neuropathic.

In addition, provisional conclusions about the patient's psychological state

Table 7.1 The PQRST characteristics of pain

P	Palliative factors	'What makes it less intense?'
	Provocative factors	'What makes it worse?'
Q	Quality	'What is it like?'
R	Radiation	'Does it spread anywhere else?'
S	Severity	'How severe is it'
T	Temporal factors	'Is it there all the time, or does it come and go?'

From Gray 1977

and social circumstances should have been reached. With patients thought to be somatizers, it may be necessary to obtain the help of a clinical psychologist or psychiatrist (Creed & Guthrie 1993).

SETTING THE CLINICAL SCENE

The following case history is a good example of pain in advanced cancer.

■ CASE HISTORY

A 63 year-old woman with a history of epigastric pain was found at laparotomy to have cancer of the pancreas with liver metastases. When seen 10 days postoperatively by a palliative care doctor she was receiving morphine 25 mg q4h PO. This failed to provide adequate relief. She was drowsy, mentally distressed and complained of insomnia. It was explained that (Fig. 7.1):

- some of her pains were muscular
- she probably had pain from a fractured rib
- her abdominal incision would probably be uncomfortable on movement for several weeks, but would improve steadily
- some of the abdominal pain was probably caused by constipation
- certain pains respond better to aspirin and nondrug measures than to morphine.

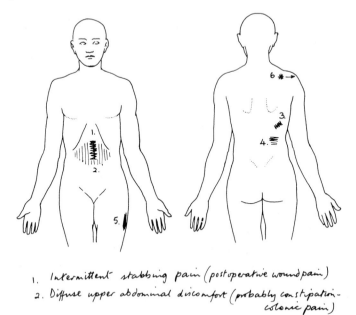

1. Intermittent stabbing pain (postoperative wound pain)
2. Diffuse upper abdominal discomfort (probably constipation - colonic pain)
3. Rib pain (? cracked)
4. Muscle spasm
5. meralgia paraesthetica
6. T.P. pain (supraspinatus)

Fig. 7.1   Pain chart of 63 year-old woman with cancer of tail of the pancreas, 10 days postoperatively. (Reproduced with permission from Twycross & Lack 1986.)

The following measures were taken:

- she was prescribed aspirin q4h
- the nurses were advised about the nature of the rib pain
- the dose of morphine was reduced and a night sedative introduced
- a laxative was prescribed and rectal measures planned for the following day.

The next day she was dramatically improved following a good night, and had minimal pain. Her morphine was reduced further and, after 3 days, she was taking only 5 mg q4h with 15 mg nocte.

This case history re-inforces the following points:

- not all pains in cancer are malignant in origin
- cancer patients with pain often have more than one pain
- muscular pains may be as severe as (or even more severe than) much pain caused directly by the cancer
- some pains, however intense, do not benefit by the use of incremental doses of morphine
- careful clinical evaluation is necessary before commencing treatment
- explanation is an essential modality of treatment
- re-evaluation after initiating treatment is necessary to confirm or modify the initial evaluation
- re-evaluation may lead to changes in treatment in the light of initial results and/or adverse drug effects.

DIAGNOSTIC PROBABILITIES

Pain in cancer may be:

- caused by the cancer itself (by far the most common)
- related to the cancer or debility (e.g. muscle spasm, constipation, bedsores)
- related to cancer treatment (e.g. chronic postoperative scar pain, chemotherapy mucositis)
- caused by a concurrent disorder (e.g. arthritis, spondylosis).

The causes of pain in a series of 100 cancer pain patients are given in Table 7.2. Eighty of these patients had two or more pains; 34 had four or more (Fig. 7.2). The average was three pains. Cancer was the sole cause of pain in only 41 patients. In nine, none of the pains was caused by cancer; in two of these, constipation was the sole cause of pain. Myofascial trigger point pain occurred in 12 patients and accounted for 24 pains.

In palliative care, as far as possible, doctors need to develop the skill of determining the cause of the pain on the basis of:

- diagnostic probability
- pattern recognition.

Time and energy consuming investigations are increasingly contra-indicated

Table 7.2   Causes of pain in 100 cancer pain patients

	Number of pains	Number of patients
Caused by cancer		
Bone	58	31
Nerve compression	56	31
Soft tissue infiltration	35	31
Visceral involvement	33	31
Raised intracranial pressure	2	2
Myopathy	2	2
	186 (61%)	91
Related to cancer or debility		
Muscle spasm	14	11
Constipation	11	11
Capsulitis of shoulder	4	4
Lymphoedema	4	3
Bedsore	1	1
Postherpetic neuralgia	1	1
Pulmonary embolus	1	1
Bladder spasm (catheter)	1	1
	37 (12%)	33
Related to treatment		
Postoperative	8	7
Colostomy	2	2
Nerve block	2	1
Postoperative adhesions	1	1
Postradiation fibrosis	1	1
Oesophageal	1	1
	15 (5%)	12
Concurrent disorders		
Myofascial	24	12
Spondylosis	12	11
Osteo-arthritis	4	3
Ischial tuberosity	2	1
Migraine	2	2
Sacro-iliac	1	1
Miscellaneous	20	15
	65 (22%)	45
Total	303 (100%)	100

Modified from Twycross & Fairfield 1982

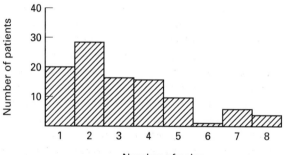

Fig. 7.2   Number of pains experienced by 100 consecutive cancer patients with pain on admission to Sobell House. (Reproduced with permission from Twycross & Fairfield 1982.)

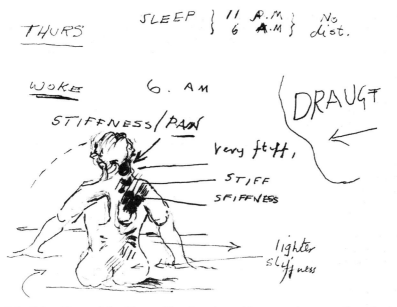

Fig. 7.3 Pain self-portrait by 65 year-old male patient with pancreatic cancer. Sites of pain indicate that pain was probably muscular in origin. Explanation, massage and diazepam at night prescribed. (Reproduced with permission from Twycross & Lack 1986.)

as a patient moves closer to death. With experience, the correct diagnosis can often be made by asking the patient to identify the site of the pain and to describe it fully. A comprehensive list of all possible causes of pain would be too long to be helpful. What is required is an informed imagination, making use of, for example, the information given in Table 7.2.

Awareness of the common muscle pain syndromes is necessary to prevent many erroneous conclusions (Fig. 7.3). Knowledge of the patterns of metastatic spread is also helpful (Fig. 7.4). When pain is wrongly assumed to be cancerous in origin, it tends to be invested with all the negative implications of cancer pain. This makes the pain worse.

■ CASE HISTORY

A 4 year-old child with an inoperable pontine glioma experienced increasing pain in the head and occipital region. She lay flat all the time because elevation of the head caused a marked increase in pain. With this history, it was necessary to postulate a local source of pain (possibly caused by postradiation meningeal adhesions) in addition to the diffuse headache of secondary hydrocephalus (which would have been helped by a more erect posture). The diffuse pain was relieved by small, regular doses of morphine, but not until she was transferred from a King's Fund to an Ellison bed (which elevates head, neck and trunk in unison) was it possible for the child to sit up without pain. Subsequently, it became possible to transfer the child from bed to a high-backed, reclining chair and eventually to lift her onto her mother's lap. This suggested that some of the pain had been caused by spasm of the neck muscles, and that the confidence engendered by the ability to sit up in bed allowed additional manoeuvres to be undertaken without pain.

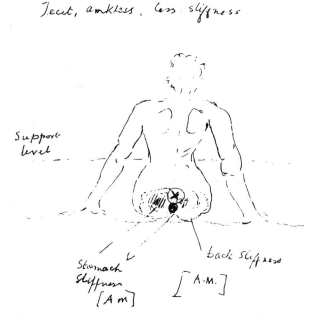

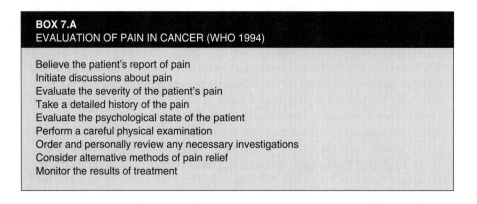

Fig. 7.4 Second self-portrait by patient with pancreatic cancer. Myofascial pains have now resolved. New pain probably also nonmalignant because of unlikelihood of sacral bone metastases in pancreatic cancer. Pain therefore considered to relate to lying in bed for long periods. Analgesics were not prescribed. Explanation, sheepskin and progressive mobilization resulted in relief. (Reproduced with permission from Twycross & Lack 1986.)

SYSTEMATIC EVALUATION

From the history and clinical examination, supplemented if necessary by radiograph, scan, or other investigation, it should be possible to develop a clear mental picture of the physical mechanisms underlying the patient's pain (Box 7.A). Then, evaluation completed and diagnosis made, treatment is started. Doctors are familiar with this sequence of events in relation to

---

BOX 7.A
EVALUATION OF PAIN IN CANCER (WHO 1994)

Believe the patient's report of pain
Initiate discussions about pain
Evaluate the severity of the patient's pain
Take a detailed history of the pain
Evaluate the psychological state of the patient
Perform a careful physical examination
Order and personally review any necessary investigations
Consider alternative methods of pain relief
Monitor the results of treatment

acute abdominal pain for example, but often fail to apply the same logical approach when evaluating pain in advanced cancer. Yet, evaluation in this area needs to be equally thorough.

A body chart on which to record pain data is a great help in elucidating a complex situation (Fig. 7.5). Formal pain scales, discussed in Chapter 8,

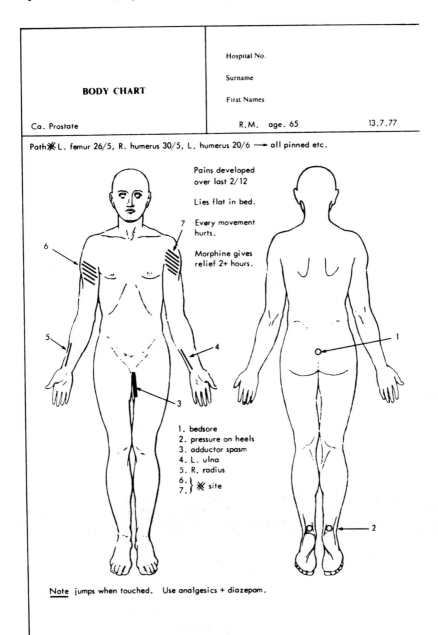

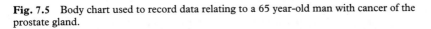

Fig. 7.5 Body chart used to record data relating to a 65 year-old man with cancer of the prostate gland.

can help but are not essential. It is often helpful, however, to use a number of descriptive words, for example pressure and aching, and to ask the patient to relate the present pain to past pain such as a toothache.

Children under 8 years generally cannot use the same scales or verbal processes as adults. Young children may be able to communicate the intensity of their pain by using a series of faces ranging from smiling to crying, and selecting the face that best matches the pain (Fig. 7.6; Bieri et al 1990). Alternatively, if the child says he hurts, he may be presented with four coins or pebbles and asked to indicate how many pieces of hurt he feels, with four objects being the worst hurt. A similar approach can be used with illiterate patients (Fig. 7.7), and in situations where communication

0   1   2   3   4   5

1. Explain to the child that each face is for a person who feels happy because he has no pain (hurt, or whatever word the child uses) or feels sad because he has some or a lot of pain.

2. Point to the appropriate face and state, "This face is. . .":
0—"very happy because he doesn't hurt at all."
1—"hurts just a little bit."
2—"hurts a little more."
3—"hurts even more."
4—"hurts a whole lot."
5—"hurts as much as you can imagine, although you don't have to be crying to feel this bad."

3. Ask the child to choose the face that best describes how he feels. Be specific about which pain (e.g. "shot" or incision) and what time (e.g. now? earlier before lunch?).

Fig. 7.6   A series of faces (happy ⟶ unhappy) can be used by a child to quantify pain. (Reproduced with permission from McCaffery & Beebe 1989.)

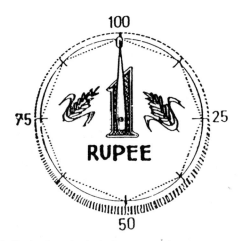

Fig. 7.7   Evaluation of pain by 'Rupee Scale' (100 paise = 1 rupee).

BOX 7.B
ESTIMATING PAIN INTENSITY IN THE ABSENCE OF DIRECT COMMUNICATION (WHO 1994)

Observations of caregivers, e.g. parents, spouse
Vocalizations, e.g. groaning
Facial expression, e.g. furrowed brow
Changes in physiological responses, e.g. increase in pulse rate and increase or decrease in blood pressure
Response to a trial dose of analgesic

---

is difficult because of the lack of a common language (Box 7.B; Prkachin 1992).

Because most patients with advanced cancer have pain, it should be asked about at the initial consultation if the patient does not mention it spontaneously. However, direct questioning may not produce a truthful answer because patients often put on a brave face for a doctor. This is more likely if relatives are present during the interview.

Unlike patients with acute pain, most cancer patients in pain do not groan audibly, or appear restless and in distress. When seen by a doctor the patient may simply say, 'I have terrible pain' and volunteer no further information. The pain does, however, disturb sleep, limit activity, and affect mental concentration. Intensity of pain must be assessed, therefore, not only by the patient's appearance and description, but also by discovering the following details:

- what drugs have failed to relieve
- whether sleep is disturbed
- in what ways activity is limited.

Helpful questions include:

'How long is it since you went out?'
'What are you doing around the house?'
'Have you had to give up any hobbies or anything else you usually do because of the pain?'

Making notes should be kept to a minimum when talking with patients. Receiving the doctor's full attention is therapeutic, and a vital part of pain management. The body chart should, however, be completed in conjunction with the patient who can then verify its accuracy. An overprinted body chart is useful to help standardize the data obtained (Fig. 7.8).

If possible, the patient's spouse or key caregiver should be interviewed. Sometimes it is only their comments which reveal the true picture. Usually, when the pain is relieved, the patient will concur spontaneously with the spouse's earlier opinion.

Information about past illnesses, the current level of anxiety and depression, suicidal thoughts, and the degree of functional incapacity helps to detect

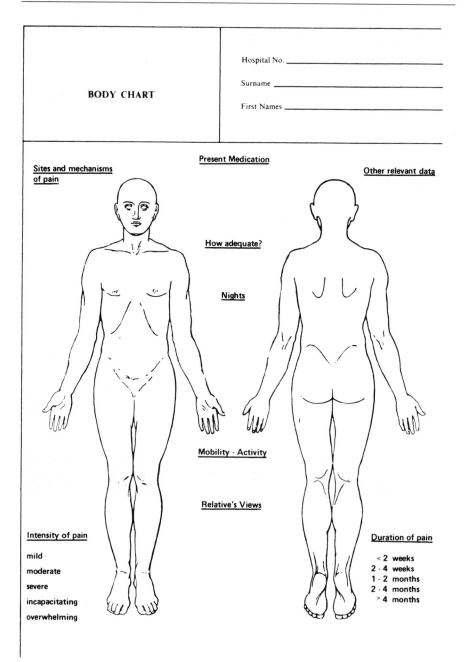

BODY CHART

Hospital No. _____

Surname _____

First Names _____

Sites and mechanisms of pain

Present Medication

Other relevant data

How adequate?

Nights

Mobility - Activity

Relative's Views

Intensity of pain

mild

moderate

severe

incapacitating

overwhelming

Duration of pain

< 2 weeks
2 - 4 weeks
1 - 2 months
2 - 4 months
> 4 months

Fig. 7.8 Overprinted body chart used at Sobell House for recording pain data.

patients who may require more specific psychological support. Depression occurs in up to 25% of cancer patients (Massie 1990). Other common psychiatric syndromes are also seen in patients with cancer pain. Detecting these is an important part of the total evaluation.

HISTORY OF ANALGESIC MEDICATION

A detailed history of analgesic medication is part of evaluation, and takes time to obtain. Whereas, on referral, details of past anticancer treatment are usually available, it is uncommon to receive much information about past analgesics and their effects. An analgesic medication history includes:

- a list of drugs
- dose
- route of administration
- regular or 'as needed'
- interval between doses
- patient's view on drug efficacy
- adverse effects
- duration of use of drug
- reason for discontinuation.

RADIOLOGICAL INVESTIGATIONS

Investigations should be reserved for cases where there is doubt about the cause of pain, or where a decision about further anticancer treatment depends upon the precise localization of the disease. Although plain radiographs are a useful screening procedure, they should not be used to overrule a clinical diagnosis if negative (Box 7.C). They are inadequate in areas of the body where bone shadows overlap such as the base of the skull, C2, C7, T1 vertebral bodies and the sacrum.

BOX 7.C
DIAGNOSTIC RADIOLOGY AND CANCER PAIN

A 40–60% change in bone density is necessary to detect changes on plain radiographs; pain can occur with less than this.

Plain radiographs are inadequate to evaluate where bone shadows overlap:

- base of skull
- C7, C8, T1 veretbrae
- sacrum.

Ordinary tomography of a vertebral body may distinguish between osteoporotic collapse and a metastasis.

Plain radiographs detect only 80% of osseous metastases.

Bone scans detect 95% of metastases.

Bone scans are sometimes negative in myeloma

Bone scan may show presence of a metastasis 3–6 months before plain radiograph.
CT not often more helpful than isotope bone scan, but is procedure of choice for evaluation of retroperitoneal, paravertebral, pelvic and skull base areas.

It is sometimes necessary to proceed with treatment on the basis of clinical judgement alone.

Although it is more sensitive than a plain radiograph, an isotope bone scan — which detects increased vascularity — does not necessarily establish a diagnosis of bone metastasis. The following can also give a positive bone scan:

- osteoporosis
- collapsed vertebral bodies
- disuse atrophy
- Paget's disease
- osteomyelitis.

Poor specificity is less of a problem in known advanced cancer. Local pain and the known presence of metastases elsewhere increases the likelihood that a positive scan reflects malignant disease (McKillop & McDougall 1980). On the other hand, a negative bone scan does not rule out metastasis. Further, in a previously irradiated site, a bone scan is often negative despite active disease.

Computed tomography (CT) has been found particularly useful in evaluating the cranial vault, orbits, base of the skull, cervicothoracic junction and brachial plexus area of the spine, thoracic and lumbar vertebrae and the pelvic bones and sacrum (Kori et al 1981).

CT and magnetic resonance imaging (MRI) are the most sensitive diagnostic procedures for evaluating cancer patients with pain. CT provides a detailed visualization of bone and soft tissue and is most useful in defining early bony changes. MRI is particularly useful in evaluating vertebral body involvement, epidural spinal cord compression, and parenchymal brain metastases. CT is also useful in directing needle placement for biopsy and for procedures such as coeliac axis plexus block.

Treatment with analgesic drugs while establishing the cause of the pain often markedly improves a patient's ability to undergo the necessary investigations. Thus, because pain relief does not obscure the diagnosis, analgesics should not be withheld while the cause of the pain is being established.

BONE PAIN

The majority of bone metastases are not painful. Those which are cause pain in various ways. These include local bone pain, radiation into surrounding tissues, referred pain, nerve compression, muscle spasm, and associated myofascial pain.

Local bone pain ranges from a dull ache to a deep oppressive intense pain. It is often worse on movement and on weightbearing. Sometimes it is worse at night. With a pathological rib fracture, the pain is most intense when changing from a sitting to a supine posture or vice versa, or when the trunk is rotated laterally. In long bones, weightbearing may cause additional pain as a result of microscopic buckling.

Certain cancers are more likely to produce bony metastases (Box 7.D) and 80% are in the axial skeleton (Schutte 1979). Metastases in the hands and feet are usually associated with a bronchogenic primary. A normal bone

---

BOX 7.D
PRIMARY SITES COMMONLY ASSOCIATED WITH BONE METASTASES

Myeloma	Prostate
Melanoma	Kidney
Breast	Thyroid
Bronchus	

---

radiograph with abnormal scan is highly suggestive of malignant disease, especially if there is no history to suggest local trauma or osteitis secondary to infection or radiation. On the other hand, in multiple myeloma the bone scan is less reliable than plain radiographs for detecting bone lesions. A scan may also be difficult to interpret after radiotherapy.

NERVE PAIN

Trunk and extremities

Pain relating to nerve compression or damage is perceived in a relatively constant part of the body surface (Fig. 7.9). Access to a dermatomal map is important as few doctors remember the complete pattern. There is inevitably some variation.

Diagnosis is easier when there are other signs or symptoms of nerve impairment, such as numbness, weakness and altered tendon reflexes. However, pain usually precedes other sensory and motor changes by weeks or months. Patients often describe less intense nerve compression pain as a constant ache. Some experience intermittent stabbing or shooting pains on movement. When compression progresses to nerve injury, the patient may complain of superficial burning pain ± allodynia.

Metastatic involvement of the spine is the most common cause of nerve root compression pain in patients with advanced cancer. Sometimes, a plain radiograph of the appropriate part of the spine is all that is necessary to confirm the presence of a secondary deposit in the relevant vertebra(e). A normal report should not, however, be regarded as conclusive. Inevitably, some radiographs are initially misread, often because the radiologist is not given sufficient clinical information. 'Normal' radiographs should be reviewed with a radiologist if the history and clinical findings suggest root compression. Sometimes an isotope bone scan is indicated but nerve root compression by a bone metastasis is unlikely if, after review, the radiograph is still considered normal. It requires a relatively large lesion with distortion of the bone architecture to produce compression of a neighbouring nerve.

CT may be necessary in a small number of patients. Although in relation to nerve compression, it is unlikely that CT will detect a relevant bone lesion if an isotope scan has not. CT will, however, detect otherwise undetectable soft tissue metastases, such as a neoplastic mass in the neck compressing one or more nerves of the brachial plexus, or a retroperitoneal mass affecting lumbar nerve roots. It is possible for a patient to develop nerve compression

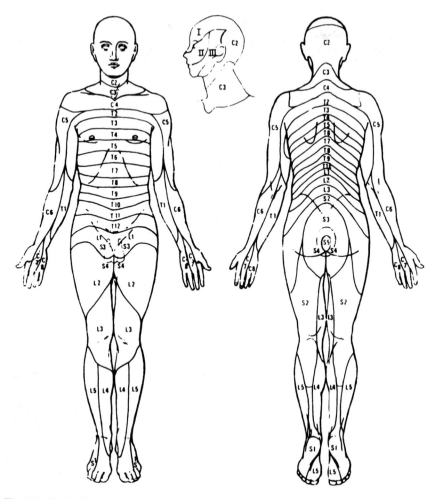

Fig. 7.9 Body chart showing dermatomes, i.e., areas in which pain is experienced if the corresponding nerve is compressed or damaged.

months, occasionally years, before a soft tissue mass becomes clinically detectable. CT can help to prevent the long latent period which may exist between the onset of the pain and the institution of appropriate treatment.

Cervical plexopathy

The cervical plexus is formed of the upper four cervical nerves (Fig. 7.10). The superficial branches are primarily sensory. They comprise the:

- *greater occipital nerve;* this is part of the posterior primary ramus of C2 and of C3 and subserves the occipital portion of the neck and the scalp as far forward as the vertex
- *small occipital nerve;* this supplies the skin behind the ear
- *greater auricular nerve;* this subserves pain sensation from the skin in the region of the angle of the jaw, the lower ear lobe and over the mastoid

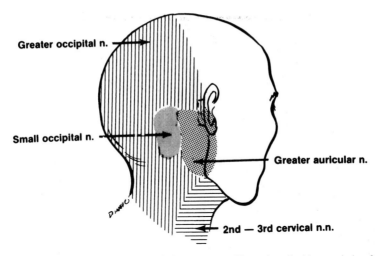

Fig. 7.10 Sensory distribution of cervical plexus nerves. (Reproduced with permission from Boop & Fischer 1981.)

- *superficial cervical nerve;* this subserves anterior and lateral parts of the neck.

The sensory fibres of cranial nerves V, VII, IX and X and of the cervical plexus, enter the CNS in a common tract of descending fibres and grey matter which is continuous down to the C4 level of the spinal cord. This tract is called the *spinal tract of the trigeminal.* As these fibres descend in the tract they send collaterals to all levels of the nucleus. There is ample opportunity for these sensory nerves to overlap in function centrally. Referred pain patterns may be explicable on this basis. Alteration of the input to this central neural pool may result in changes in other areas. For example, cervical nerve blocks sometimes reduce the pain of a facial neuralgia.

Pain in the ear may be very difficult to elucidate because there are so many nerves supplying the area:

- *trigeminal (auriculotemporal)*
- *facial (nervus intermedius*; Fig. 7.11*)*
- *vagus* (Fig. 7.12)
- *glossopharyngeal* (Fig. 7.11)
- *greater auricular nerve.*

From the middle ear and medial aspect of the tympanic membrane, sensory fibres originate in the tympanic branch of the glossopharyngeal nerve (cranial IX). This branch (Jacobson's nerve) also subserves sensation from the mastoid cells and upper Eustachian tube. Other sensory fibres in the glossopharyngeal nerve come from the soft palate, tonsillar region, posterior one third of the tongue, and posterior pharynx down to the epiglottis (Fig. 7.11).

The vagus (cranial X) conveys sensation via the superior laryngeal nerve from the epiglottis and adjacent region of the pharynx and from the vallecula.

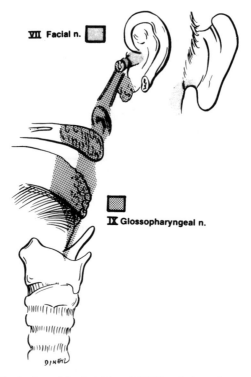

Fig. 7.11   Sensory distribution of the facial (cranial VII) and glossopharyngeal nerves (cranial IX). (Reproduced with permission from Boop & Fischer 1981.)

The recurrent laryngeal nerve supplies the larynx below the vocal folds (Fig. 7.12). The vagus also conducts sensation from a small area of the external auditory canal posteriorly and from adjacent skin of the external ear (Fig. 7.12). It is this branch which probably explains why occasional patients with nonmetastatic bronchogenic cancer experience unilateral facial pain (see p. 87).

RE-EVALUATION

The dictum 'Review! Review! Review!' is basic to cancer pain management. With cancer, one is dealing with a progressive process. This means that new pains may develop or old pains re-emerge. It should not be assumed that a fresh complaint of pain merely calls for an increase in the dose of an analgesic. A new complaint of pain demands re-evaluation, an explanation to the patient and, only then, modification of drug therapy or other intervention.

The probability that the initial prescription will be inadequate increases with the intensity of pain. Patients should be re-evaluated within 1–2 h if the pain is overwhelming, or after 1–2 days if severe or moderate. If troublesome adverse effects result, treatment may need to be modified. In

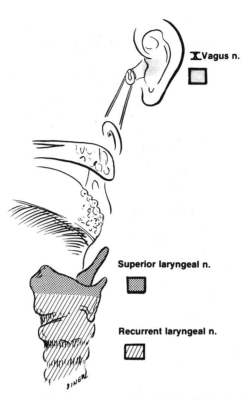

Vagus n.

Superior laryngeal n.

Recurrent laryngeal n.

Fig. 7.12 Sensory distribution of the vagus nerve (cranial X). (Reproduced with permission from Boop & Fischer 1981.)

addition, the relief of the major pain may allow a second less severe pain to surface.

■ CASE HISTORY

An 85 year-old man with cancer of the prostate and right femoral metastatic pain was treated with aspirin and morphine. The next day he indicated that, although less severe, pain was still present. Further questioning revealed that the site of pain was now retrosternal and epigastric; he had no femoral pain at all. The dose of morphine was left unaltered, and the prescription of an antacid resulted in complete relief.

In the case of the man with seven pains (Fig. 7.5), it was necessary to review progress in relation to each pain. On the second day, he was reluctant to admit that several pains were less intense but, as judged by his reactions to passive movement, they undoubtedly were. Possibly his reluctance was due to a shifting baseline of reference. It was necessary to point out the objective difference observed and to encourage him to recognize that the pains were beginning to ease. It was a case of 'chipping away' at his total pain until, after a week, he was sufficiently more comfortable to be able to sit up in bed.

REFERENCES

Bieri D, Reeve R A, Champion G D, Addicoat L, Ziegler J B 1990 The faces pain scale for the self-assessment of the severity of pain experienced by children: development, initial validation, and preliminary investigation for ratio scale properties. Pain 41: 139–150.

Boop W C, Fisher J A 1981 Methods of pain control. In: Suen Y Y, Myers E N (eds) Cancer of the head and neck. Churchill Livingstone, New York, pp 821–838

Creed F, Guthrie E 1993 Techniques for interviewing the somatising patient. British Journal of Psychiatry 162: 467–471

Gray J 1977 A pain in the neck — and shoulder. Pain Topics 1: 6

Kori S H, Krol G, Foley K M 1981 Computed tomographic evaluation of bone and soft tissue metastases. In: Weiss L, Gilbert H A (eds) Bone metastases. GK Hall, Boston, 245–257

Massie M J 1990 Depression. In: Holland J C, Rowland J H (eds) Handbook of Psychooncology. Oxford University Press, Oxford, pp 283–290

McCaffery M, Beebe A 1989 Pain: clinical manual for nursing practice. C V Mosby Co, St Louis

McKillop J H, McDougall I R 1980 The role of skeletal scanning in clinical oncology. British Medical Journal 281: 407–409

Prkachin K M 1992 The consistency of facial expressions of pain: a comparison across modalities. Pain 51: 297–306

Schutte H E 1979 The influence of bone pain on the results of bone scans. Cancer 44: 2039–2043

Twycross R G, Fairfield S 1982 Pain in far-advanced cancer. Pain 14: 303–310

Twycross R G, Lack S A 1986 Alimentary symptoms in far-advanced cancer. Churchill Livingstone, Edinburgh

World Health Organization 1994 WHO Revised Method for Relief of Cancer Pain

Measurement of pain

EVALUATING PAIN IN CLINICAL PRACTICE

'English, which can express the thoughts of Hamlet and the tragedy of Lear, has no words for the shiver and the headache. . . The meerest school girl when she falls in love has Shakespeare and Keats to speak for her; but let a sufferer try to describe a pain in his head to a doctor and language at once runs dry' (Virginia Woolf).

The multidimensional nature of cancer pain has already been emphasized. There is no instrument which adequately assesses the different dimensions of cancer pain together with its intensity. Despite Virginia Woolf's comment, measurement of pain in clinical practice depends largely on verbal dialogue between the patient and the doctor or nurse. Thus, in practice, I seldom ask patients to grade their pain as mild, moderate or severe. If complained about, the pain is 'troublesome' and calls for a therapeutic response. I then seek to discover what treatments have been tried and what benefit they gave, if any. Then, on the basis of what the patient has told me, I develop a therapeutic strategy.

A rating scale is mandatory, of course, in research projects (Max et al 1991), and ideally when clinical data are being collected for audit. A scale also helps clinically if there is a large caring team. A series of numbers will immediately tell any member of the team the 'natural history' of the patient's pain over previous weeks and months. At some centres in the UK, nurses keep pain records routinely (Walker et al 1987). The Royal London Hospital pain observation chart is one example. Another widely used chart is that of the Burford Nursing Development Trust.

When scales are used, they should be completed by the patient and not by someone else. As noted in Chapter 1, close relatives record more pain than the patients themselves (Morris et al 1986).

RATING SCALES

Several different types of rating scales are in current use. These can be broadly classified as:

- categorical (verbal rating scale)
- visual analogue scale (VAS, linear analogue)
- 'verbal analogue'
- 'numerical analogue'.

In addition to being simple, any measure of a subjective state or symptom which a person records must be valid, reliable and sensitive (Max et al 1991). Symptoms, however, defy absolute measurement; only their indicants can be evaluated (Aitken & Zealley 1970). This means that there can be no absolute arbiter of validity. Although the indicants may be quantifiable, they can never do more than reflect the subjective experience.

Several errors tend to occur when rating scales of any type are used, including (Hamilton 1968):

- bias, i.e. a tendency to rate high or low
- halo effect, i.e. a tendency to rate all variables either high or low.

The impact of such errors will be reduced by comparing within-patient differences rather than single scores.

Five criteria are generally considered when evaluating rating scales (Jensen et al 1986):

- ease of administration and scoring
- rate of incorrect use
- sensitivity (number of categories available)
- sensitivity (statistical power)
- correlation of results with those obtained using other scales.

In order to evaluate six commonly used rating scales, 75 patients with chronic pain were asked to use all six to record present, least, most and average intensities of pain. It was found that all six scales gave similar results (Jensen et al 1986). Choice of scale, therefore, is a matter of the investigator's personal preference.

In single dose trials, measurements are commonly made every 30–60 min. This permits the development of a time-response curve and determines duration of effect. Several abbreviations are now widely used in relation to such trials, sometimes without explanation (Table 8.1).

Categorical scales

The oldest and perhaps most widely used scale is the four point intensity scale (none, mild, moderate, severe). This is variously called a *categorical*, *interval*, *ordinal* or *verbal rating* scale. A scale of this type can be criticized on the grounds that it is not sensitive enough. For example, a patient in whom an analgesic reduces pain from 'more than severe' to 'below severe but above

Table 8.1 Abbreviations commonly used in analgesic trial reports

Abbreviation	Meaning	Definition
PID	Pain intensity difference	A later score subtracted from the baseline score
SPID	Summed pain intensity differences	Sum of PID at agreed time intervals over an agreed period of time
TOTPAR	Total pain relief	Sum of pain relief scores at agreed time intervals over an agreed period of time
VAS	Visual analogue scale	
VRS	Verbal rating scale (i.e. categorical scale)	

moderate' is forced to choose severe both times (Max & Laska 1991). To try to resolve this dilemma, many centres include a fifth option, namely, *excruciating*.

A second criticism is that the numerical scores (0, 1, 2, 3) ascribed to the different categories for analytical and statistical purposes assume that the intervals between the categories are equal steps. It has been suggested that there is a greater difference between severe and moderate than between moderate and mild, and between mild and none (Lasagna 1960). In over 200 patients, however, a comparison with the 100 mm VAS showed the four point scale to be remarkably linear (Fig. 8.1). A similar linearity was found with a six point scale in 85 cancer patients (Tamburini et al 1987). There were, however, anomalous results in a few patients:

- one patient described slight pain (category 1) as more intense than troublesome pain (category 2)
- two patients placed excruciating pain (maximum verbal category) beyond the end of the VAS ('pain as bad as could be')
- three patients placed two of the verbal category words at the same point on the VAS.

In contrast, in a second study of 116 normal volunteers, it was shown that words assigned the same value on different categorical scales (e.g. *mild, slight, little*) were not placed on identical points on a VAS (Table 8.2). Even the most commonly used words, mild (23), moderate (46) and severe (88), were not linear (Sriwatanakul et al 1982).

Although developed after the categorical scale, the VAS is now commonly used as the 'gold standard' for comparative purposes (Ohnhaus & Adler 1975, Wallenstein et al 1980, Littman et al 1985).

Categorical pain relief scales

In postoperative pain trials in the past, patients were often asked whether their pain had been 'at least 50% relieved'. Although only a two point scale, it was said to be a useful measure. Now it has been superseded by categorical and VAS pain relief scales. The 50% relief approach, however, is useful in

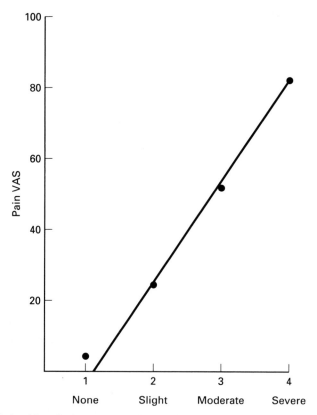

Fig. 8.1 Relationships of pain category scale to VAS pain ratings made by 264 patients in analgesic studies. The four categories are spaced in a roughly even manner, although the spacing between 'none' and 'slight' pain is somewhat smaller than the other two intervals. (Reproduced with permission from Wallenstein et al 1980.)

Table 8.2 VAS values assigned to terms used on different categorical pain scales

Categorical scale score	Categorical scale term	VAS value	Evaluation of differences (unpooled t tests)
1	Little	12	
	Slight	12	
	Mild	23	$p < 0.001$
2	Some	21	
	Moderate	46	$p < 0.001$
3	A lot	74	
	Severe	88	$p < 0.001$
4	Terrible	88	
	Very severe	94	$p < 0.01$

From Sriwatanakul et al 1982

clinical practice with patients who find it difficult to express themselves. If they reply 'less than 50%', they can be asked whether more than 25% etc. If they reply 'more than 50%', they can be asked whether 75% and so on.

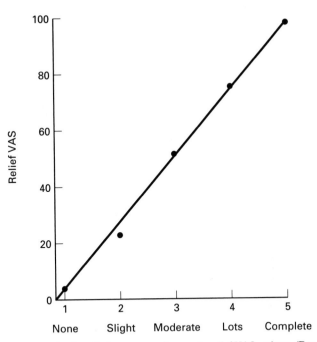

Fig. 8.2 Relationship of pain relief category scale to pain relief VAS ratings. (Reproduced with permission from Wallenstein 1984.)

Pain relief scales rely on a patient's memory of how intense the pain was at a point in the past compared with how intense the pain is now. This is not difficult in a single dose study lasting 4–6 h, but may affect accuracy in longer term studies. When compared with a VAS, the five point pain relief scale is remarkably linear (Fig. 8.2). A categorical pain relief scale is more sensitive to small reductions in pain than a categorical pain scale (Max & Laska 1991).

Visual analogue scales

In 1920 'a new method for securing the judgement of superiors (foremen) on subordinates (workmen)' called a graphic rating scale (GRS) was developed in the USA (Fig. 8.3). Several other possible uses for the GRS were subsequently suggested, including psychological evaluation and measuring the effect of drugs and other variables on efficiency (Freyd 1923). The advantages of graphic rating were considered to be its simplicity:

- easy to understand and complete
- freedom from direct quantitative terms
- enhanced sensitivity by allowing the rater to discriminate as finely as he wished.

The GRS is only 'pseudographic', however, if a rater always places a mark midway over one of the verbal descriptions. To reduce the possibility of this

13. How flexible is he?

Hidebound Runs in a rut	Slow to take up new ideas	Progressive tendencies	Quick to pick up new ways and habits	Is always adapting himself and taking up new ideas

18. Is he quiet or talkative?

Seldom talks When questioned answers briefly	Does not uphold his end of the conversation	Moderately talkative	More than upholds his end of the conversation	Great talker always going

Fig. 8.3 Examples of horizontal graphic rating scales. (Reproduced with permission from Freyd 1923).

happening, raters were specifically warned against this (Champney 1941). In time, new rating scales were created which were relatively clear of verbal explanation by using a vertical 'thermometer' rather than an horizontal 'yardstick'.

The visual analogue scale (VAS) represents a further evolutionary step (Clark & Spear 1964, Joyce 1966, Aitken 1969, Revill et al 1976). The two ends of a VAS are labelled to correspond with the minimum and maximum extremes which can be experienced but there are no intermediate cues (Fig. 8.4). Intermediate points are nonverbal so as to reduce the opportunity for widely differing interpretations by patients. The nonverbal nature of the scale circumvents the potential difficulty of equalizing the intervals on a categorical scale. A horizontal rather than a vertical line is preferred by significantly more patients (Sriwatanakul et al 1983).

As with the GRS, there are certain rules 'based on experience' which should be observed when constructing a VAS. The choice of words to anchor the ends of the scale is very important (Levy 1969). It is only too easy to construct a VAS which, in practice, is merely a two point scale. Properly constructed, however, a standard 100 mm VAS with provision for 101 possible scores is much more sensitive than a four point scale (FPS). It possibly has a place, therefore, in situations where symptoms are minimal or completely relieved but differences are being looked for with different drugs or with different doses of the same drug.

A VAS for pain has been compared with a FPS in patients with chronic arthritis (Joyce et al 1975). Of patients who stated a preference, 32 out of 52 said they preferred the VAS because it was 'more accurate', 'more sensitive' or 'gave better indication of the pain'. The rest preferred the FPS because it was 'easier', 'more definite' or 'needed less imagination'. The difference was not statistically significant.

Pain as bad as could possibly be ——————————————————— Completely painfree

Fig. 8.4 Pain visual analogue scale.

In another trial in patients with rheumatoid arthritis (Berry & Huskisson 1972), severity of pain was evaluated on a weekly basis using both VAS and FPS. There was a highly significant concordance between the results from the two methods (r = 0.79, p < 0.01). Because the patients used them simultaneously, however, this was hardly surprising. A similar result was obtained in noncancer patients both for pain and other symptoms (Clark & Spear 1964, Woodforde & Merskey 1972).

Because patients are not used to expressing the intensity of their symptoms in this way, the initial explanation by the research assistant generally needs to be 'painstaking' (Huskisson 1974). Even so, most patients are said to have no difficulty in understanding the analogue concept of the line (Zealley & Aitken 1969, Huskisson 1974, Joyce et al 1975). This is not, however, for elderly patients (Deschamps et al 1988). Certainly, at a palliative care unit, patients generally had difficulty completing a VAS for mood (Twycross 1977). This probably related to the fact that the scale was 'bipolar', i.e. ranging from depression through normal mood to elation, whereas the VAS for pain and other symptoms was 'unipolar', i.e. ranging from normal to most extreme. In addition, several patients interpreted 'could not be happier' as 'as happy as could be in the circumstances'.

The VAS has four other drawbacks:

- it cannot be used by confused or sedated patients (Jadad & McQuay 1993)
- it requires intact visual and motor function
- its use involves two steps, i.e. the estimate by the patient and the measurement by the researcher
- the length changes if photocopied; this makes comparison difficult between distances measured on the original and on photocopied duplicates (Bloomfield & Hanks 1981).

Some centres have modified the format of the VAS in order to facilitate its use, and some have used longer scales, i.e. 20 cm or 50 cm (Jadad & McQuay 1993). Others have gone further and reverted, in effect, to an old style GRS. The Brief Pain Inventory has numbers 0 to 10 printed along the horizontal line in addition to the two sets of extreme words (see below).

Some centres have introduced a VAS *pain relief* scale. Used in conjunction with an ordinary VAS pain scale, it is more sensitive in detecting differences between drugs and between different doses of the same drug (Wallenstein 1991).

MEMORIAL PAIN ASSESSMENT CARD (MPAC)

This is used at the Memorial Sloan-Kettering Cancer Center, New York (Fig. 8.5). It is a folded card measuring approximately 14×21 cm (size A5), and features a jumbled categorical scale and three VAS (Fishman et al 1987):

- pain intensity
- pain relief
- mood.

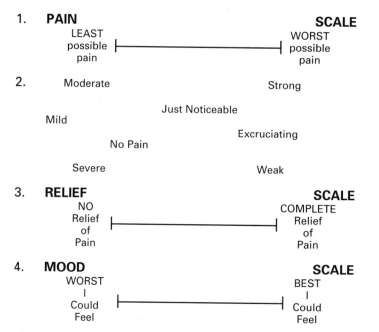

Fig. 8.5 Memorial Pain Assessment Card; items 1 & 4 = outside, and items 2 & 3 = inside.

With practice, most patients take less than 20 seconds to complete the card. This makes it practical for serial measurements.

BRIEF PAIN INVENTORY (BPI)

The BPI was developed by the Pain Research Group, Department of Neurology, University of Wisconsin for research purposes (Daut et al 1983). It generates a mass of data, and analysis of repeated use becomes extremely time consuming. The incorporation of *interference factors* into the inventory is good clinical sense (see Fig 1.4 p. 10). They reflect the sort of questions an astute doctor would ask a patient with pain. Even so, it is too cumbersome for routine clinical use. A short form is available (Fig. 8.6). This is perhaps the most which is feasible in daily clinical practice. The Pain Disability Index is a similar tool (Tait et al 1987).

QUALITY OF LIFE QUESTIONNAIRE

A broad based quality of life questionnaire has been developed. It is intended for use in any clinical setting. The items of the questionnaire have been refined by several years of research (Padilla & Grant 1985, Aaronson 1988, Ferrell et al 1989a, 1989b). Items 1–10 measure aspects of physical wellbeing and items 11–16 measure psychosocial wellbeing.

WEEKLY RECORD OF PAIN INTENSITY AND DURATION

For many years, the Division of Pain Therapy and Palliative Care, National

Brief Pain Inventory (Short Form)

Date: ___/___/___ Time: ______

Name: ______ ______ ______
Last First Middle Initial

1) Throughout our lives, most of us have had pain from time to time (such as minor headaches, sprains, and toothaches). Have you had pain other than these everyday kinds of pain today?

1. Yes 2. No

2) On the diagram, shade in the areas where you feel pain. Put an X on the area that hurts the most.

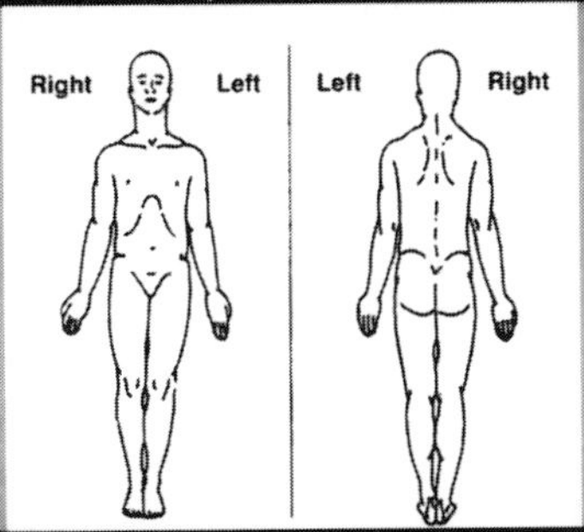

3) Please rate your pain by circling the one number that best describes your pain at its **worst** in the last 24 hours.

0	1	2	3	4	5	6	7	8	9	10
No Pain										Pain as bad as you can imagine

4) Please rate your pain by circling the one number that best describes your pain at its **least** in the last 24 hours.

0	1	2	3	4	5	6	7	8	9	10
No Pain										Pain as bad as you can imagine

5) Please rate your pain by circling the one number that best describes your pain on the **average**.

0	1	2	3	4	5	6	7	8	9	10
No Pain										Pain as bad as you can imagine

6) Please rate your pain by circling the one number that tells how much pain you have **right now.**

0	1	2	3	4	5	6	7	8	9	10
No Pain										Pain as bad as you can imagine

Fig. 8.6 Shortened version of Brief Pain Inventory. (Reproduced with permission from the Pain Research Group, Department of Neurology, University of Wisconsin.)

Cancer Institute, Milan, has made a weekly evaluation of patients' pain (Ventafridda et al 1983). The aim is to obtain a single integral score for both pain intensity and duration over each 24 h period. Intensity is measured using a six point scale:

- no pain = 0
- slight (*lieve*) 1
- moderate or troublesome (*molesto*) = 2.5
- severe or exhausting (*esaurisce*) = 5

- terrible (*terribile*) = 7.5
- excruciating/killing (*micidiale*) = 10.

The patient and family are instructed as to how to fill in the form which also includes:

- number of hours slept
- number of painfree hours
- number of hours in which pain was experienced.

Functional status is also recorded (Karnofsky & Burchenal 1949), together with the time spent standing, sitting and lying down. A record of medication is also kept with any adverse effects. The results are then transferred by a trained assistant into the Division's records. The 'integrated pain score' is obtained in the following way:

- record the number of hours in each pain category
- multiply by score for that category
- add the products obtained
- divide the weekly total by seven to obtain the mean daily score (Table 8.3).

Scores of up to 240 are possible, although in practice few exceed 100. It takes about 1 min with a calculator to obtain the integrated score.

A daily integrated pain score has been compared with a daily VAS (Ventafridda et al 1983). In addition to completing a 24 h record, 39 patients were asked to indicate their average pain during the same period on a single VAS. There was a statistically significant correlation between the VAS and the integrated score (Fig. 8.7). This, however, creates an interesting dilemma. On the one hand, it is difficult to accept that a *single retrospective* VAS truly reflects data obtained on an hourly contemporary basis over 24 h. On the other hand, if it does, it is difficult to justify the continued use of the more complex and time consuming hourly record.

A second report from Milan compared the integrated score with a VAS, a numerical scale (0–10), a categorical scale and the Italian Pain Questionnaire — the Italian version of the McGill Pain Questionnaire (see below). The various scores showed 'a high degree of association' (De Conno et al 1992).

Table 8.3 Example of daily integrated pain score

| | Asleep | Pain | | | | | | Integrated score |
		None	Slight	Moderate	Severe	Terrible	Killing	
Hours	6	7	4	0	4.5	2	0.5	
Pain value	0	0	1	2.5	5	7.5	10	
Products	0	0	4	0	22.5	15	5	46.5

From Ventafridda et al 1983

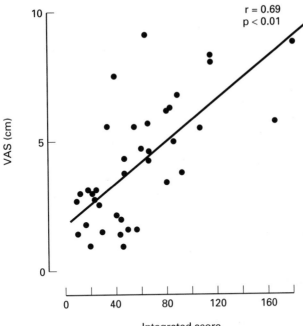

Fig. 8.7   Correlation between the integrated pain score and a VAS (39 patients). (Reproduced with permission from Ventafridda et al 1983.)

McGILL PAIN QUESTIONNAIRE

Categorical rating scales and VAS measure the intensity or *quantity* of pain. The McGill Pain Questionnaire (MPQ) aims primarily to evaluate the *quality* of pain (Fig. 8.8). The MPQ includes a body image to indicate pain location, and has 78 words divided into 20 subclasses (Fig. 8.8). These can be grouped into four subscales which reflect four major dimensions:

- sensory
- affective
- evaluative (cognitive)
- miscellaneous.

All but the miscellaneous group were derived theoretically (Melzack & Torgerson 1971).

The MPQ is usually completed with the help of a research assistant. In each subclass, the patient is requested to choose the one word which best describes his present pain, and to ignore any subclass which is not applicable. The MPQ is scored in two ways:

- number of words chosen
- numerical value of words chosen.

A short form of the MPQ has been developed with 15 words (Melzack 1987, Dudgeon et al 1993).

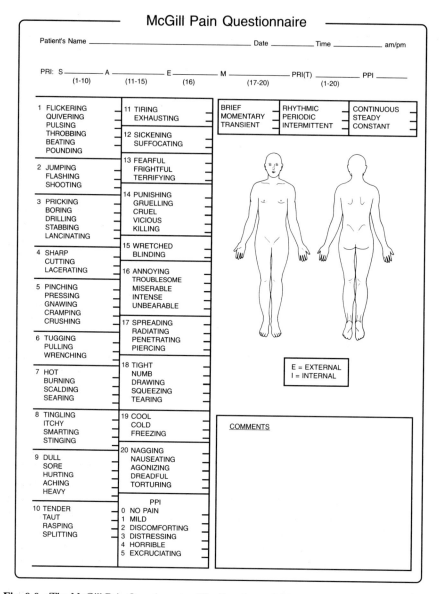

Fig. 8.8 The McGill Pain Questionnaire. The descriptors fall into four major groups: sensory = 1–10; affective = 11–15; evaluative = 16; miscellaneous = 17–20. The rank value for each descriptor is based on its position in the word subclass. The sum of the rank values is the pain rating index (PRI). The present pain intensity (PPI) is based on a scale of 0–5. (Reproduced with permission from Melzack 1983.)

History of MPQ

The MPQ originally included 102 words ('pain descriptors') derived from written descriptions of clinical pain which were grouped according to similarity of meaning. Twenty university graduates (14 men and 6 women, mean age 30 years) were then asked their opinion regarding the ordering of the words. Subsequently, each word was rated on a seven point scale within its subclass by 140 psychology students (90% men), 20 doctors and 20 patients. The average age of the three groups was 20, 26 and 31 years respectively (Melzack et al 1985).

Thus, the population used to design the MPQ was predominantly young well educated males not experiencing pain. This may explain the choice of some descriptors which are either difficult to understand and/or are not often used spontaneously by patients with chronic pain (Deschamps et al 1988). Indeed, more than one third of the psychology students required an explanation for such words as *lancinating*, *searing*, *rasping* and *wrenching* (Klepac et al 1981).

The MPQ scoring system assumes that the descriptors within a subclass are equidistant on an interval scale. This is not the case (Reading et al 1982). A word such as *numb* (subclass 18) does not seem to fit into a valid interval intensity scale. Also, *taut* (subclass 10) and *tight* (subclass 18) would generally be regarded as synonymous (Deschamps et al 1988).

Further, the MPQ does not give equal consideration to the three dimensions it claims to examine. The number of subclasses for sensory, affective and evaluative aspects of pain are unequal. The Pain Rating Index (PRI) is predominantly a reflection of the sensory component. In addition, the number of words within a subclass ranges from two to six. It follows that an equal PRI may not represent equal pain intensity — compare *quivering* in subclass 1 and *blinding* in subclass 15 (Fig. 8.7).

Meta-analysis of MPQ

A meta-analysis of 51 studies incorporating over 3600 subjects with seven painful conditions has been undertaken in an attempt to estimate normative mean scores for pain quality and intensity (Wilkie et al 1990). In all seven conditions, the estimated mean scores were less than 50% of the maximum (Table 8.4). Chronic painful conditions tended to score higher affective scores. Of the 78 MPQ words, only 19 were selected by more than 20% of subjects (Box 8.A). Working from the published data, it was not possible to identify different word patterns for the seven conditions nor detect differences in scores (Wilkie et al 1990).

The 19 commonly used words came from 14/20 word subclasses, and included:

- sensory = 9
- affective = 4
- evaluative = 3
- miscellaneous = 3

Twelve of the 19 words are included in the short MPQ.

Although two words (*shooting* and *sharp*) were selected frequently by subjects with all painful conditions, no word was specific for any one condition.

Table 8.4 McGill Pain Questionnaire mean scores by painful condition

| | Maximum possible score | Painful condition | | | | | | | |
		Cancer	Low back	Chronic mixed	Postoperative	Obstetrics & gynaecology	Dental	Experimental	Total
Pain rating index									
Sensory	42	12	16	15	14	16	11	12	14
Affective	14	5	6	4	2	3	2	2	3
Evaluative	5	3	2	3	2	2	3	3	3
Miscellaneous	17	5	6	5	4	5	4	6	5
Total	78	24	28	25	21	25	18	20	23
Number of words chosen	20	9	10	11	9	7	8	9	9
Present pain index	5	2.2	2.3	2.6	1.6	2.4	2.2	2.2	2.3

From Wilkie et al 1990

BOX 8.A
MPQ WORDS CHOSEN BY OVER 20% OF 3600 SUBJECTS (Wilkie et al 1990)

Aching	Sickening
Burning	Terrifying
Gnawing	Tiring
Heavy	Annoying
Sharp	Intense
Shooting	Unbearable
Stabbing	Nagging
Tender	Tight
Throbbing	Torturing
Exhausting	

The MPQ does not, therefore, help in diagnosis. Thus, in summary, the MPQ (Wilkie et al 1990, Holroyd et al 1992):

- is time consuming
- is used uncritically by many investigators
- has a spurious validity conferred on it by virtue of the reputation of its originator
- requires reconstruction using patients of various educational backgrounds and ages
- needs an equal number of words in each subclass
- needs an equal number of subclasses in each subscale
- should be used only as a research tool with a clear understanding of its limitations
- should not be used in monitoring/auditing pain relief in cancer patients.

UNAIDED USE OF VERBAL DESCRIPTORS

Whatever its limitations, the MPQ has stimulated people to consider ways of broadening the scope of pain evaluation beyond intensity alone, and to consider further the 'language of pain'. The MPQ not only permits the use of descriptors, but offers a list of 78 words. However, is this the best way to use descriptors? What about spontaneous choice?

In one study, some 300 cancer patients who had reported pain within the previous month completed a three page questionnaire (Tearnan & Cleeland 1990). Among other things, they were asked to describe the pain in their own words. A total of 129 different words were used, with a mean of two words per patient. Ten words accounted for two thirds of the total (Box 8.B).

Using the MPQ as a guide, words were grouped into three major semantic classes (sensory, affective, evaluative). The reliability of the grouping was demonstrated by a 98% agreement between two independent observers as to the classification of each word. Of the words used, the words were classified as follows:

- sensory 87%

BOX 8.B

WORDS ACCOUNTING FOR TWO THIRDS OF ALL WORDS CHOSEN BY 302 CANCER PATIENTS TO DESCRIBE THEIR PAIN (Tearnan & Cleeland 1990)

Ache	Dull
Sharp	Continual
Stabbing	Hurting
Burning	Pressure
Throbbing	*Shooting*

Dull and ache were often used as a single word; i.e. 'dull ache'
Words in italics also appear in the MPQ
'Pressure' is comparable to 'heavy' in the MPQ

- evaluative 11%
- affective 2%.

Eleven categories were then formed to describe the sensory words (Table 8.5). Constrictive pressure was the most diverse with 15 words, and location the least with two, namely, *deep* and *surface*.

The infrequent use of affective words prevented further analysis. It was, however, possible to classify the evaluative words into high and low intensity. Patients used high intensity words (e.g. *severe, horrendous, unbearable*) more frequently than low intensity ones (68% v. 32%). There was an association between patients with high intensity pain and words in the high evaluative group. (e.g. *severe, unbearable, hell, excruciating, strong, intense* and *bad*). Interestingly, *ache* was used more frequently by the high intensity pain patients, with *dull ache* being the typical choice for low intensity pain patients.

Frequency and range of word use did not differ across the cancer diagnostic categories. Further, no differences were identified between patients grouped according to the anatomical site of the pain (i.e. soft tissue, bone, nerve).

This study confirms the limitation of verbal descriptors as aids to diagnosis

Table 8.5 Categorization of sensory words used by 302 cancer patients to describe their pain

Category	Percentage[a]
Dullness (e.g. dull ache)	26
Punctate pressure (e.g. stabbing)	12
Constrictive pressure (e.g. pressure, cramping)	11
Incisive pressure (e.g. sharp)	11
Periodicity (e.g. continual)	8
Thermal (e.g. burning)	8
Tenderness (e.g. hurts, sore)	6
Temporal (e.g. throbbing)	4
Spatial (e.g. shooting)	4
Traction (e.g. pulling, twisting)	3
Location (e.g. deep)	1

[a] Percentage of all words chosen (n = 232).
From Tearnan & Cleeland 1990

of causes and mechanisms of pain. It also indicates that, if verbal descriptors are to be included, a checklist is necessary to maximize the patients' response.

CONCLUSION

A rating scale is mandatory in research. It is also of value in clinical practice, particularly when there is a large caring team. A straightforward, easily understood scale is best. The short form of the Brief Pain Inventory is an attractive tool for use in chronic pain patients (including cancer patients) because it:

- encompasses a 24 h period
- elicits variation in pain intensity.

REFERENCES

Aaronson N K 1988 Quality of life: what is it? How should it be measured? Oncology 2 (5): 69–74

Aitken R C B 1969 Measurement of feelings using visual analogue scales. Proceedings of the Royal Society of Medicine 62: 989–992

Aitken R C B, Zealley A K 1970 Measurement of moods. British Journal of Hospital Medicine 4: 215–224

Berry H, Huskisson E C 1972 Treatment of rheumatoid arthritis: a trial of meprothixol. Clinical Trials Journal 9: 13

Bloomfield S S, Hanks G W 1981 The visual analogue scale. British Journal of Clinical Pharmacology 11: 98

Champney H 1941 The measurement of parent behaviour. Child Development 12: 131

Clark P R F, Spear F C 1964 Reliability and sensitivity in the self-assessment of well-being. Bulletin of the British Psychological Society 17: 18a

Daut R L, Cleeland C S, Flanery R C 1983 Development of the Wisconsin brief pain questionnaire to assess pain in cancer and other disease. Pain 17: 197–210

De Conno F, Caraceni A, Martini C, Ventafridda V 1992 Multidimensional pain measurement in cancer patients. Poster presentation. 2nd European Congress on Palliative Care, Brussels

Deschamps M, Band P R, Coldman A J 1988 Assessment of adult cancer pain: shortcomings of current methods. Pain 32: 133–139

Dudgeon D, Raubertas R F, Rosenthal S N 1993 The short-form McGill Pain Questionnaire in chronic cancer pain. Journal of Pain and Symptom Management 8: 191–195

Ferrell B, Wisdom C, Wenzle C 1989a Quality of life as an outcome variable in management of cancer pain. Cancer 63: 2321–2329

Ferrell B, Wisdom C, Wenzle C, Brown J 1989b Effects of controlled-release morphine on quality of life for cancer pain. Oncology Nursing Forum 16: 521–526

Fishman B, Pasternak S, Wallenstein S L, Houde R W, Holland J C, Foley K M 1987 The Memorial Pain Assessment Card. A valid instrument for the evaluation of cancer pain. Cancer 60: 1151–1158

Freyd M 1923 The graphic rating scale. Journal of Educational Psychology 14: 83–102

Grossman S A, Sheidler V R, McGuire D B, Geer C, Santor D, Piantadosi S 1992 A comparison of the Hopkins pain rating instrument with standard visual analogue and verbal descriptor scales in patients with cancer. Journal of Pain & Symptom Management 7: 196–203

Hamilton M 1968 Some notes on rating scales. The Statistician 18: 11

Holroyd K A, Holm J E, Keefe F J et al 1992 A multi-center evaluation of the McGill Pain Questionnaire: results from more than 1700 chronic pain patients. Pain 49: 301–311

Huskisson E C 1974 Measurement of pain. Lancet ii: 1127–1131

Jadad A R, McQuay H J 1993 The measurement of pain. In: Pynsent P B, Fairbank J C T, Carr A (eds) Outcome measures in orthopaedics. Butterworth-Heinemann, Oxford, pp 16–29

Jensen M P, Karoly P, Braver S 1986 The measurement of clinical pain intensity: a comparison of six methods. Pain 27 117–126

Joyce C R B 1966 The assessment of drugs with behavioural effects. In: Trounce J R (ed) Second Symposium on Advanced Medicine. Pitman, London, p 370

Joyce C R B, Zutshi D W, Hrubes V, Mason R M 1975 Comparison of fixed interval and visual analogue scales for rating chronic pain. European Journal of Clinical Pharmacology 8: 415–420

Karnofsky D A, Burchenal J H 1949 The clinical evaluation of chemotherapeutic agents in cancer. In: McLeod C M (ed) Evaluation of chemotherapeutic agents. Columbia University Press, New York, pp 191–205

Klepac R K, Dowling J, Rokke P, Dodge L, Schafer L 1981 Interview vs. paper-and-pencil administration of the McGill Pain Questionnaire. Pain 11: 241–246

Lasagna L 1960 The clinical measurement of pain. Annals of New York Academy of Science 86: 28–37

Levy R 1969 Measurement of mood (discussion). Proceedings of the Royal Society of Medicine 62: 996

Littman G S, Walker B R, Schneider B E 1985 Reassessment of verbal and visual analog ratings in analgesic studies. Clinical Pharmacology and Therapeutics 38: 16–23

Max M B, Laska E M 1991 Single dose analgesic comparisons. In: Max M B, Portenoy R K, Laska E M (eds) Advances in pain research and therapy, vol 18. Raven Press, New York, pp 55–95

Max M B, Portenoy R K, Laska E M (eds) 1991 Advances in pain research and therapy, vol 18. Raven Press, New York

Melzack R 1983 The McGill Pain Questionnaire. In: Melzack R (ed) Pain measurement and assessment. Raven Press, New York, pp 41–48

Melzack R 1987 The short-form McGill Pain Questionnaire. Pain 30: 191–197

Melzack R, Torgerson W S 1971 On the language of pain. Anesthesiology 34: 50–59

Melzack R, Katz J, Jeans M E 1985 The role of compensation in chronic pain: analysis using a new method of scoring the McGill Pain Questionnaire. Pain 23: 101–112

Morris J N, Mor V, Goldberg R J, Sherwood S, Greer D S, Hiris J 1986 The effect of treatment setting and patient characteristics on pain in terminal cancer patients: A report from the National Hospice Study. Journal of Chronic Diseases 39: 27–35

Ohnhaus E E, Adler R 1975 Methodological problems in the measurement of pain: a comparison between the verbal rating scale and the visual analogue scale. Pain 1: 379–384

Padilla G, Grant M 1985 Quality of life as a cancer nursing outcome variable. Advanced Nursing Science 8 (1): 45–60

Reading A E, Everitt B S, Sledmere C M 1982 The McGill Pain Questionnaire: a replication of its construction. British Journal of Clinical Psychology 21: 339–349

Revill S I, Robinson J O, Rosen M, Hogg M I J 1976 The reliability of a linear analogue for evaluating pain. Anaesthesia 31: 1191–1198

Sriwatanakul K, Kelvie W, Lasagna L 1982 The quantification of pain: an analysis of words used to describe pain and analgesia in clinical trials. Clinical Pharmacology and Therapeutics 32: 143–148

Sriwatanakul K, Kelvie W, Lasagna L, Calimlim J F, Weis O F, Mehta G 1983 Studies with different types of visual analog scales for measurement of pain. Clinical Pharmacology and Therapeutics 34: 234–239

Tait R C, Pollard A C, Margolis R B et al 1987 The pain disability index: psychometric and validity data. Archives of Physical Medicine and Rehabilitation 68: 439–441

Tamburini M, Selmi S, De Conno F, Ventafridda V 1987 Semantic descriptors of pain. Pain 25: 187–193

Tearnan B H, Cleeland C S, 1990 Unaided use of pain descriptors by patients with cancer pain. Journal of Pain and Symptom Management 5: 228–232

Twycross R G 1977 Choice of strong analgesic in terminal cancer: diamorphine or morphine? Pain 3: 93–104

Ventafridda V, De Conno F, Di Trapani P, Gallico S, Guarise G, Rigamonti G, Tamburini M 1983 A new method of pain quantification based on a weekly self-descriptive record of the intensity and duration of pain. In: Bonica J J, Lindblom U, Iggo A (eds) Advances in pain research and therapy vol 5. Raven Press, New York, pp 891–895

Walker V A, Dicks B, Webb P 1987 Pain assessment charts in the management of chronic cancer pain. Palliative Medicine 1: 111–116

Wallenstein S L 1984 Scaling clinical pain and pain relief. In: Bromm B (ed) Pain measurement in man: neurophysiological correlates of pain. Elsevier, Amsterdam, pp 389–396

Wallenstein S L 1991 Commentary. The VAS relief scale and other analgesic measures:

carryover effect in parallel and crossover studies. In: Max M, Portenoy R, Laska E (eds) Advances in pain research and therapy, vol 18. Raven Press, New York, pp 97–103

Wallenstein S L, Heidrich G, Kaiko R, Houde R W 1980 Clinical evaluation of mild analgesics; the measurement of clinical pain. British Journal of Clinical Pharmacology 10: 319S–327S

Wilkie D J, Savedra M C, Holzemer W L, Tesler M D, Paul S M 1990 Use of the McGill Pain Questionnaire to measure pain: a meta-analysis. Nursing Research 39: 36–41

Woodforde J M, Merskey H 1972 Some relationships between subjective measures of pain. Journal of Psychosomatic Research 16: 167–172

Zealley A K, Aitken R C B 1969 Measurement of mood. Proceedings of the Royal Society of Medicine 62: 993–995

General strategy

MULTIMODAL MANAGEMENT

The use of analgesics and pain relief are not synonymous. The fact that pain is a somatopsychic experience immeasurably widens the scope for intervention. Management will include attention to factors such as anxiety, depression, fatigue, boredom and loneliness (Table 9.1). Further, because all pains do not respond equally to analgesics (Schulze et al 1988, Hanks 1991), their use can never be more than part of a multimodal approach to management (Box 9.A).

CONCEPT OF OPIOID RESISTANT PAIN

A pain may be said to be opioid resistant if:

- there is little or no relief despite a progressive increase in opioid dose
- there are intolerable adverse effects despite the use of standard measures to control them.

Table 9.1 Nondrug factors affecting pain threshold

Threshold lowered	Threshold raised
Discomfort	Relief of other symptoms
Insomnia	Sleep
Fatigue	Sympathy
Anxiety	Understanding
Fear	Companionship
Anger	Creative activity
Sadness	Relaxation
Depression	Reduction in anxiety
Boredom	Elevation of mood
Mental isolation	
Social abandonment	

BOX 9.A
PAIN MANAGEMENT IN CANCER

Examination

- to establish trust
- to confirm site
- to identify cause

Explanation

- to reduce psychological impact of pain

Modification of pathological process

- radiation therapy
- hormone therapy
- chemotherapy
- surgery
- correction of hypercalcaemia
- pituitary ablation with alcohol

Elevation of pain threshold

- nondrug methods (Table 9.1)
- primary analgesics
- secondary analgesics
- psychotropic drugs

Interruption of pain pathways

- local anaesthesia:
  lignocaine
  bupivacaine
- neurolysis:
  chemical (alcohol, phenol, chlorocresol)
  cold (cryotherapy)
  heat (thermocoagulation)

Modification of lifestyle

- avoid pain-precipitating activities

Immobilization

- rest
- cervical collar
- surgical corset
- moulded plastic splints
- slings
- orthopaedic surgery

There are exceptions to this working definition. A patient with postradical neck dissection pain who obtained little relief from morphine 35 g/24 h by IV infusion could be considered to have opioid resistant pain, despite the absence of intolerable adverse effects. (The patient subsequently had complete relief with amitriptyline 75 mg nocte.)

Controversy continues about whether certain pains are intrinsically resistant to opioids, for example neuropathic pain (Arner & Meyerson 1988, Bowsher 1990, Portenoy et al 1990, Wall 1990). Three questions need to be considered:

- does opioid resistant pain exist?
- if so, is it relative rather than absolute, i.e. would a higher dose of morphine achieve relief?
- is it predictable on the basis of the type of pain?

The concept of opioid resistance stems from clinical observation and is supported by animal studies (Woolf & Wall 1986, McQuay & Dickenson 1990). Studying the phenomenon under controlled conditions, however, is not easy. If opioid resistance is a relative rather than an absolute phenomenon, imposition of dose limits in a study might produce a false negative result, particularly if subjects had been previously receiving opioids and had developed some tolerance, i.e. there was a shift to the right in the dose-response curve. To circumvent this problem IV patient controlled analgesia (PCA) has been used. With this approach, response to morphine was seen under double-blind conditions in three out of six patients with neuropathic pain compared to all four patients with nociceptive pain (Jadad et al 1992).

A response to opioids by neuropathic pain was also shown in a controlled trial in patients with postherpetic neuralgia (Rowbotham et al 1991). Lignocaine $\leqslant$ 450 mg and morphine $\leqslant$ 25 mg were given by IV infusion over 1 h. Both drugs were equally effective — but only partially (Fig. 9.1).

The results of another study suggested that only the patient's affective response to the neuropathic pain was altered by morphine, leaving the sensory dimension unchanged (Kupers et al 1991). Such a view would fit with the results of an open study in which 16 patients with neuropathic pain were

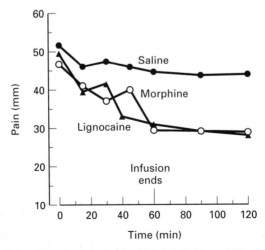

Fig. 9.1   Mean pain intensity scores during the 60-min infusion and 60-min postinfusion observation period. (Reproduced with permission from Rowbotham et al 1991.)

given IV morphine 3–4 mg every 10 min up to a total of 18–20 mg (Tasker et al 1983). Relief was graded as follows:

- complete 2
- partial 7
- none 7.

In eight patients, naloxone 400 μg IV was subsequently given, including five who had obtained pain relief. The fact that naloxone did not reverse the analgesia suggests that the relief was mediated by a nonopioid mechanism (Tasker et al 1983).

In another study, a response to opioids was observed in neuropathic pain with IV opioid infusions (Portenoy et al 1990). In at least one patient, however, 'maximum pain relief' coincided with 'maximum sedation'. In such patients, opioids are unlikely to be a realistic option.

The concept of opioid resistance is important. The situation in relation to neuropathic pain, however, is more complex and less clear cut than previously thought. Indeed, neuropathic pains are generally more responsive if treated with spinal morphine (Moulin et al 1985, Ottesen et al 1990).

EDMONTON STAGING SYSTEM FOR CANCER PAIN

Several attempts have been made to identify which pains are less responsive to analgesics (Mercadante et al 1992). The Edmonton staging system for cancer pain identifies seven possible predictive factors (Box 9.B). This permits the classification of pain into three stages:

- stage 1 = good prognosis
- stage 2 = intermediate prognosis
- stage 3 = poor prognosis.

Results from a group of 52 cancer pain patients are shown in Table 9.2, and appear to confer a high measure of validity on the staging system. However, while the predictors highlight problem areas, it is difficult to imagine such a detailed system being used routinely in clinical practice. A working classification of pain based on anticipated response to opioids is needed (Box 9.C).

OPIOID RESPONSIVE PAINS

Six important principles govern the use of analgesics in the management of opioid responsive pains. These collectively comprise the WHO Method for Relief of Cancer Pain (Box 9.D).

Oral medication

Morphine and other strong opioids are effective by mouth. Thus, apart from the last few hours or days of life, few patients require injections to relieve their pain. A larger dose is needed by mouth, however, because of reduced bio-availability. Thus, the dose needs to be *doubled* when converting from the

BOX 9.B
POSSIBLE PREDICTORS OF POOR RESPONSE TO ANALGESICS
(Bruera et al 1989)

Pain mechanism

- neuropathic pain
- muscle spasm
- pain without clinically identifiable mechanism

Pain characteristics

- incident pain (i.e. aggravated by movement, swallowing, micturition, defaecation)
- superficial burning pain
- spontaneous stabbing/shooting/lancinating pain

Previous opioid exposure

- patients already receiving high doses of opioids, e.g. more than morphine 300 mg PO/ 24 h, or equivalent, when referred

Impaired cognitive function

- impaired cognitive function may make evaluation of pain and response to treatment difficult (Massie et al 1983, Bruera et al 1987)

Psychological distress

- anxiety, depression and/or hostility may make treatment more difficult (Massie et al 1983, Bruera et al 1987)

Rapid escalation of dose

- suggests opioid resistance for either physical or psychological reasons

History of drug addiction or alcoholism

- evaluation of pain and response to treatment is more difficult if the patient is seeking solace through drugs

Table 9.2   Final pain relief according to original pain stage

Stage	Number of patients (%)		Total
	Good relief	Poor relief	
1	18 (82)	4 (18)	22
2	4 (50)	4 (50)	8
3	2 (9)	20 (91)	22
Total	24	28	52

Chi-squared of the distribution = 23.47 ($p < 0.0001$).
From Bruera et al 1989

SC route (Kalso & Vainio 1990), and *trebled* from the IV route (Consensus Statement 1994). Patients with intractable vomiting as well as pain will need parenteral medication — both anti-emetic and analgesic. Once the vomiting has been controlled it is generally possible to revert to the oral route.

BOX 9.C
OPIOID RESISTANT CANCER PAIN: CLINICAL CLASSIFICATION

Pseudoresistant

- underdosing
- poor alimentary absorption (*rare*)
- poor alimentary absorption because of vomiting
- ignoring psychological aspects of care

Semiresistant

- soft tissue
- muscle infiltration ⎫
- bone metastasis ⎬ associated with local inflammation
- neuropathic (some) ⎭
- raised intracranial pressure
- activity related

Resistant

- neuropathic (some)
- muscle spasm

BOX 9.D
WHO METHOD FOR RELIEF OF CANCER PAIN (WHO 1986)

'The right drug in the right dose at the right time intervals'

- by the mouth
- by the clock
- by the ladder
- for the individual
- use of adjuvant medication
- attention to detail

Suppositories are a useful alternative, particularly in the home. The dose of morphine PO and PR is the same (Pannuti et al 1982, Kaiko et al 1989).

Regular medication

'Regular' medication (syn: time contingent, scheduled) means that a patient receives a drug at specific stated times. In contrast, 'as needed' medication (syn: as required, *pro re nata*) means that the doctor prescribes a drug to be given at the discretion of a nurse or on request by the patient.

In a study of patients with persistent pain, mostly cancer, it was found that when analgesics were prescribed 'as needed' they were seldom and sometimes never used, despite the fact that patients were known to be in pain (Hunt et al 1977). Great reliance was placed by the nurses on patients either asking for analgesics or admitting to needing them when asked on a routine drug round.

Even postoperatively with diminishing pain, 'as needed' IM medication is generally unsatisfactory, or at best, less satisfactory than continuous IV administration (Nayman 1979, Rutter et al 1980, Working Party 1990). The reasons given for an alternative approach in the management of postoperative pain are even more compelling in cancer (Box 9.E).

To allow pain to re-emerge before administering the next dose not only causes unnecessary suffering but also encourages tolerance. 'As needed' medication, therefore, has no place in the treatment of persistent pain (Fig. 9.2). Continuous pain requires regular prophylactic therapy. The next dose is given before the effect of the previous one has worn off and, therefore, before the patient may think it necessary.

For codeine and morphine 'q4h' is optimal. If a strong analgesic other than morphine is used, the doctor must be familiar with its pharmacology. Pethidine is generally effective for only 2–3 h, although it is commonly given q4–6h (Marks & Sachar 1973). On the other hand, levorphanol and phenazocine are satisfactory when given q6h; and buprenorphine and methadone q8h. With methadone, with a plasma halflife of over 2 days when taken regularly PO, there is a likelihood of cumulation leading to worsening adverse effects, particularly in the elderly and debilitated (Twycross 1977).

BOX 9.E
LIMITATIONS OF 'AS NEEDED' ANALGESICS (Working Party Report 1990)

Pharmacokinetic factors

- variation in time taken to achieve peak plasma concentration
  (IM pethidine = 10–90 min; IM morphine = 4–60 min)
- variation in peak plasma concentration (IM pethidine = 4–fold; IM morphine = 5–fold)

Pharmacodynamic factors

- variation in minimum effective analgesic concentration (varies 4–fold for several opioids)

Staff factors

- shortage of nurses causes delay between recurrence of pain and a request for an analgesic being made
- auxiliary nurses are not allowed to administer drugs
- fear of causing respiratory depression or 'addiction' makes many nurses frightened to administer strong opioids until 'absolutely necessary'
- patients may not be asked about their pain (Donovan et al 1987)

Patient factors

- some patients may believe that pain is both inevitable and untreatable
- some patients do not appreciate that the onus is on them to ask for an analgesic
- fears concerning 'addiction' may cause the patient to suffer in silence (Levin et al 1985)

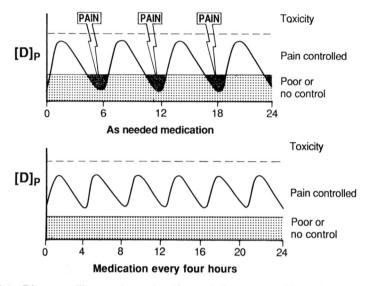

Fig. 9.2   Diagram to illustrate the results of 'as needed' compared with regular 4-hourly morphine sulphate. [D]p = plasma concentration of drug. (Reproduced with permission from Twycross & Lack 1983.)

Analgesic ladder

The WHO analgesic ladder has three steps (Fig. 9.3). It is necessary to be familiar with one or two alternatives for patients who cannot tolerate the standard preparations, i.e. aspirin, codeine, morphine. Aspirin has two alternatives: paracetamol (which has no anti-inflammatory effect) and the non-steroidal anti-inflammatory drugs (NSAIDs). For step 2, many centres in the UK use dextropropoxyphene in preference to codeine.

From a pharmacological point of view, step 2 is unnecessary. Codeine is essentially a prodrug of morphine (see p. 236). Small doses of morphine can therefore substitute for codeine — or indeed other weak opioids. Thus, in the Philippines, weak opioids are not included in the official Guidelines on Cancer Pain Relief (Philippines Cancer Control Programme 1991). In most countries, however, it is easier to obtain and prescribe a weak opioid than a strong opioid because of Controlled Drug regulations. This makes step 2 a practical necessity.

Spinal analgesia can be regarded as a fourth step. Some centres introduce SC morphine as an intermediate step between strong opioids and spinal analgesia. This is incorrect; SC morphine represents an alternative third step in patients who cannot take oral morphine. It does not offer intrinsic additional benefit. Other parallel steps include other drugs ('secondary analgesics') used for pains which do not respond to nonopioid and opioid analgesics ('primary analgesics').

The use of morphine is determined by analgesic need and not by the doctor's estimate of life expectancy — which is often wrong. The right dose of morphine is the one which gives adequate relief for 4 h without intolerable

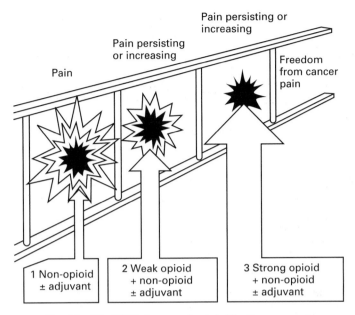

Fig. 9.3 The WHO 3 step analgesic ladder for cancer pain.

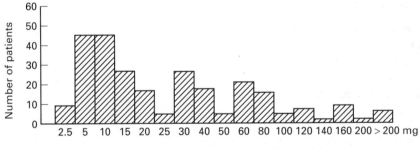

Maximum 4-hourly dose of oral morphine sulphate

Fig. 9.4 Maximum doses of oral morphine sulphate given q4h to 254 cancer patients at Sobell House, 1982. Median dose 15 mg; maximum dose 1800 mg. 67% = 30 mg, 91% ≤ 100 mg, 2% ≥ 200 mg.

adverse effects. 'Maximum' or 'recommended' doses, derived mainly from postoperative parenteral single dose studies, are not applicable for cancer pain. Because the effective dose of oral morphine ranges from as little as 5 mg q4h to more than 1 g q4h (Fig. 9.4), step 3 can be thought of as a ladder in itself.

The following points should be noted:

- it is pharmacological nonsense to prescribe simultaneously two weak opioids or two strong opioids
- it is sometimes justifiable for a patient on a strong opioid to be given another weak or strong opioid as a second 'as needed' analgesic for occasional, troublesome pain. Generally, however, if pain breaks through

the 'analgesic cover', patients should be advised to take an extra dose of their regular medication

- avoid short acting preparations like dextromoramide, pentazocine and pethidine
- do not prescribe a mixed agonist-antagonist (e.g. pentazocine) with an agonist (e.g. morphine). It is unnecessary and may result in antagonism
- 'keep it simple': a doctor's analgesic ladder, including alternatives, should comprise no more than eight or nine drugs. It is better to know and understand a few drugs than to have a fleeting acquaintance with the whole range.

Some doctors still tend to indulge in pharmacological roulette and 'kangaroo' from weak opioid to weak opioid or from strong opioid to strong opioid. A patient obtains relief with, for example, hydromorphone 2 mg q4h. The pain recurs, and the medication is changed to morphine instead of adjusting upwards the dose of the previously satisfactory analgesic. This is done, presumably, on the grounds that the hydromorphone has 'failed'. No thought is given to the fact that when using a strong opioid agonist, the dose can be adjusted upwards considerably.

What makes 'kangaroo jumping' with strong opioids more hazardous is the widespread belief that morphine (or diamorphine) is the most potent strong opioid. Therefore, regardless of dose, doctors believe these drugs must be more effective. It is no wonder that both doctor and patient despair when morphine proves no better, and sometimes worse, than the previously used analgesic.

Individual dose titration

The concept of individual analgesic requirements is still foreign to many doctors and nurses. Published data show, however, that individual requirements vary considerably both postoperatively (Catling et al 1980) and in advanced cancer (Twycross 1974, Vijayaram et al 1990, Brescia et al 1992).

The aim, therefore, is to titrate the dose of the analgesic against the pain, gradually increasing the dose until the patient is painfree. At lower doses, increments are generally greater in terms of percentage than when adjusting to a higher dose. For example 5 mg $\rightarrow$ 10 mg is a 100% increases, whereas:

10 mg $\longrightarrow$ 15 mg
20 mg $\longrightarrow$ 30 mg
40 mg $\longrightarrow$ 60 mg

are all 50% increases. Most patients never need more than 200 mg/24 h. The majority continue to obtain relief with doses as small as 10–30 mg q4h.

Many patients are denied relief because of a failure to optimize the dose of the prescribed analgesic. There is little justification for this because relief is not an 'all or none' phenomenon. The patient's response to a suboptimal dose in terms of degree and duration of relief guides the doctor in the process of dose titration.

When pain recurs or a new pain develops, some patients are advised to reduce the interval between doses of morphine from 4 h to 3 h, or even 2 h. This is bad practice. It is better to increase the dose and maintain a q4h regimen.

Some doctors find it disturbing to prescribe large doses of morphine because they were taught that the lethal dose of morphine is 1 mg/kg body weight (Goldstein et al 1974). This has no relevance, however, to the use of morphine in cancer patients because:

- the dose is titrated against the patient's pain
- the usual route of administration is oral and not by injection
- patients receiving high doses are not 'opioid naive', i.e. there is almost certainly some tolerance.

Adjuvant medication

Adjuvant (concomitant) medication is the norm (Box 9.F).

Laxatives

Laxatives are always necessary when a patient is prescribed morphine unless there is a definite reason for not doing so, for example steatorrhoea or an ileostomy (Twycross & Harcourt 1991). Experience at many centres strongly suggests that a combination of a contact laxative (peristaltic stimulant) and a surface-wetting agent (faecal softener) achieves the best results, for example standardized senna (up to 75 mg a day) and docusate (up to 600 mg a day). Combination preparations reduce the number of tablets/capsules the patient has to swallow (e.g. co-danthrusate in the UK and casanthranol-docusate in the USA). More than one third of inpatients with terminal cancer continue

---

BOX 9.F
ADJUVANT DRUGS FOR ANALGESIC LADDER

Control of adverse effects

- laxative
- anti-emetic

Psychotropic medication

- night sedative
- anxiolytic
- antidepressant

Co-analgesic

- corticosteroid

to need rectal measures (suppositories, enemas or manual evacuations) in addition to oral laxatives (Twycross & Lack 1986).

Anti-emetics

About two thirds of patients prescribed morphine need an anti-emetic (Hanks 1982). Haloperidol 1–1.5 mg stat and nocte is the anti-emetic of choice if nausea or vomiting is induced by an opioid. In some patients haloperidol is ineffectual because of morphine induced delayed gastric emptying. Thus, if a patient does not respond to haloperidol and the pattern of vomiting is suggestive of gastric stasis, a gastrokinetic anti-emetic (metoclopramide or domperidone) should be substituted.

Psychotropic drugs

Psychotropic drugs should *not* be prescribed routinely. If the patient is very anxious, however, an anxiolytic should be prescribed for a week or more (e.g. diazepam 5–10 mg nocte). If a patient remains depressed after 2 weeks of satisfactory pain relief, an antidepressant should be considered.

Many patients benefit from the use of a night sedative (e.g. temazepam, chloral hydrate). Discomfort is worse at night when the patient is alone with his pain and his fears. The cumulative effect of many sleepless, pain-filled nights is a substantial lowering of the patient's pain threshold with a concomitant increase in pain intensity.

It is sometimes necessary to use morphine at night in patients well controlled by a weak opioid during the day; or to use a considerably larger dose of morphine at bedtime to relieve pains which are particularly troublesome when lying down for a prolonged period.

In the past, aqueous morphine was often prescribed with a second drug, either cocaine (a stimulant) or a phenothiazine (an anxiolytic-sedative). Sometimes both were given — which is pharmacological nonsense. Increasing the dose of morphine would be hazardous in these circumstances if, by increasing the volume of the mixture to be taken, the quantity of the second drug was increased automatically. Depending on which second drug was given, this could lead either to agitation or to somnolence. Psychotropic drugs, therefore, should be given separately; and the dose of each drug adjusted individually according to need (see p. 401).

Attention to detail

Attention to detail is an essential skill in cancer pain management. It is, however, difficult to describe succinctly. It certainly means not making assumptions. Thus, in the following cases, asking the patient to identity precisely where the pain was resulted in a proper evaluation and the institution of appropriate treatment:

- 'I have low back pain'
  assumption: patient has lumbar pain possibly related to spondylosis
  reality: patient has sacral pain caused by a bone metastasis

- 'I have pain in my left shoulder'
  assumption: patient has a new pain, possibly metastatic
  reality: patient has recurrent pain in rhomboid muscle related to a
  myofascial trigger point
- 24 h after starting analgesics: 'I still have pain'
  assumption: need to increase dose of morphine
  reality: original pain completely relieved; new pain caused by aspirin
  related gastritis.

Attention to detail means precision in taking a drug history. Thus, if a patient says, 'I take morphine every 4 hours', the doctor asks, 'Tell me when you take your first dose . . . your second dose . . . etc'. When this is done, it often turns out that the patient is taking morphine q.i.d rather than q4h, and possibly 'as needed' rather than prophylactically. On one occasion, 'every 4 hours' meant 0800, 1200, 1600, 2000 h. Perhaps it was not surprising that this patient woke in excruciating pain at about 0300 h — so much so that she dreaded going to bed at night.

Attention to detail means the provision of precise guidelines for drug regimens. 'Take as much as you like, as often as you like' is a recipe for minimum relief, maximum adverse effects and considerable anxiety. Further, when the prescription of an additional drug is considered, it is important to ask if it is possible:

- to stop one or more of the preparations the patient is already taking
- to substitute one drug for any two of those presently or about to be prescribed.

Attention to detail also means being equally thorough when re-evaluating a patient and monitoring treatment. Finally, attention to detail means being prepared to address psychosocial issues, including responding honestly and gently to a patient's request for more information about his condition.

OPIOID RESPONSIVE PAIN BUT DO *NOT* USE OPIOIDS

There are some pains which may well respond to opioids but for which opioids are contra-indicated, namely, functional gastro-intestinal pains:

- squashed stomach syndrome
- constipation pain
- irritable bowel syndrome.

These functional pains require more specific treatment. Indeed, despite initial relief, the use of opioids ultimately makes matters worse (Glare & Lickiss 1992). Squashed stomach syndrome is discussed further in Chapter 23.

OPIOID SEMIRESPONSIVE PAINS

Generally, these require:

- opioid
- second drug ('co-analgesic')
- ± nondrug treatment

Severe metastatic bone pain is a good example of opioid semiresponsive pain. Indeed, an opioid alone may be less effective than a NSAID in this situation. Thus, when a NSAID in maximum dose fails to relieve adequately, the opioid should be *added* to, not substituted for, the NSAID. At the same time, palliative radiotherapy should be considered (see p. 487). Soft tissue and muscle infiltration pains require a similar drug approach.

With neuropathic pain, the situation is more complex. For an evolving nerve compression-nerve injury syndrome associated with tumour progression, a combination of primary and secondary analgesics will almost certainly be needed, e.g. morphine ± NSAID and a tricyclic antidepressant ± anticonvulsant. Alternative approaches include spinal analgesia with morphine and bupivacaine ± clonidine (Box 9.G).

OPIOID RESISTANT PAINS

Pains which are intrinsically resistant need a completely different approach. Such pains include:

- cramp (see Chapters 4 & 23)
- some neuropathic pains (Box 9.G).

BOX 9.G
APPROACH TO NEUROPATHIC PAIN

Nerve compression pain is generally more responsive to opioids than neural injury pain.

A combination of morphine and a corticosteroid may well relieve nerve compression pain resistant to morphine alone.

Most pure neural injury pains (e.g. chronic postoperative scar pains, postherpetic neuralgia) are best treated with secondary analgesics in the first instance:

- antidepressant (see p. 409) } generally regarded as drugs of choice
- anticonvulsant (see p. 468) }
- alprazolam (see p. 406)
- mexiletine (see p. 463)
- flecainide (see p. 464).

Spinal analgesia (see p. 365) will be needed for some patients, particularly those with cancer related plexopathy:

- morphine
- morphine and bupivacaine
- morphine and clonidine
- morphine, bupivacaine and clonidine.

SC ketamine with PO/SC morphine is an alternative to spinal analgesia (see p. 476).

Nondrug treatments include:

- TENS (see p. 528)
- dorsal column stimulation (see p. 518)
- hypnosis (see p. 542).

ANXIETIES ABOUT PRESCRIBING

'Freedom from any anxiety prescribing may amount to dangerous ignorance'
(Julian & Herxheimer 1977).

Most doctors have anxieties about prescribing just as many patients have anxieties about the drugs they take. Unless doctors recognize their own anxieties, they are unlikely to be able to understand or to deal sensibly with those of the patient. Some of the more common fears held by doctors, patients and families about strong opioids are discussed in Chapter 20. A recognition that such fears are generally groundless or exaggerated helps to allay anxiety. Even so, in the individual patient, there remains the possibility that what a doctor prescribes may harm rather than help the patient. It is not possible, for example, to predict who will have anaphylactic shock after receiving aspirin or penicillin. It is normal and necessary to be anxious about prescribing.

The doctor should *not* spell out all the 'small print' adverse reactions. If he does, compliance will be much reduced. The following information, however, is necessary:

- common adverse effects
- advice about alcohol and driving
- a 'hot line' for emergency advice.

SUPERVISION

Supervision is necessary to achieve maximum relief with minimum adverse effects. Sometimes, treatment may need to be reviewed within hours; certainly after one or two days; and always at the end of the first week. Subsequent follow up varies according to psychological and therapeutic need. New pains may develop and old pains re-emerge. A fresh complaint of pain demands re-evaluation, and not just a message to increase pain medication — even though this may be an important short term measure.

The time scale with morphine resistant neuropathic pain is different. Occasionally relief is apparent within days but, more typically, it is achieved over two to three weeks, sometimes longer. This is because most doctors do not give patients a loading dose of a tricyclic agent. Instead they build the dose up week by week. Generally, therefore, the patient will be initially receiving a suboptimal dose. The patient and family should be warned about this. As always, however, the first aim is improved sleep and correction of physical and mental exhaustion.

Even if maximum pain intensity remains unchanged for some time, pain-free intervals of lengthening duration may develop. Recognizing this provides an important boost to morale which, in turn, helps further to reduce pain intensity.

With somatizers, a long time scale is also necessary. The help of a psychologist or psychiatrist with a knowledge of and interest in palliative care will probably be necessary (Bass & Benjamin 1993).

DRUGS AT HOME

Regimens should be simple to understand and easy to administer (Griffiths 1990). Generally, it is necessary to adopt a q4h regimen only if ordinary morphine tablets or solution are being used. For other patients, 'with meals and at bedtime' is usually adequate. Variations include:

- on waking, after lunch and tea, and bedtime
- after breakfast and at bedtime.

If some drugs are best given before meals and others after, it is advisable to forsake pharmacological purity and to opt for one or other time so as to avoid an impossibly complex schedule. It is necessary to look at boxes and other containers to check that the pharmacist has not given the patient contrary or complicating advice (Fig. 9.5).

With a q4h regimen, the first and last doses are linked to the patient's waking and bedtime. The additional times during the day are usually 1000 h, 1400 h and 1800 h unless the patient wakes exceptionally late. When writing out the list of drugs and doses for the patient (and family) to work from, it is helpful to add what the different drugs are for, even if this is obvious.

Capsules should be described as capsules and tablets as tablets, not vice

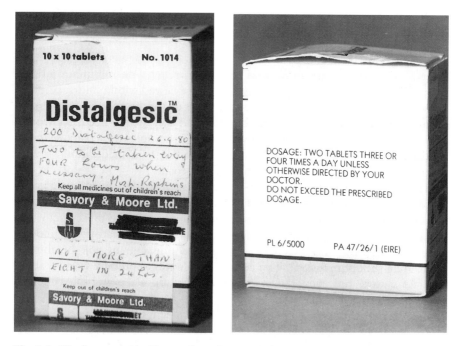

Fig. 9.5   The front and side of a container of a commonly used nonopioid–weak opioid combination tablet. The family practitioner prescribed two tablets q4h. The pharmacist added 'when necessary' and the conflicting 'not more than 8 in 24 hours'. To be helpful, he should have covered the manufacturer's advice on the side of the box as the doctor had clearly prescribed more than this. The pharmacist's additions caused the patient's family much concern and uncertainty.

versa. Doses should not be described simply as 'spoonfuls'. Patients have been known to use a tablespoon (15 ml) instead of a teaspoon (3.5–5 ml). A plastic beaker/cup with each 5 ml clearly marked is generally the best way for the patient to self-administer liquid preparations. If the above recommendations are carried out, some patients can cope immediately with a new regimen. Often, however, a patient is found to be in confusion when visited the next day by a home care nurse. For patients in hospital or a palliative care unit, self-medication before discharge is good practice, and may forestall many of the potential difficulties.

Ingenuity may be needed to ensure compliance, as demonstrated by the example of Mrs D (Ajemian & Mount 1980). Poor vision and lack of co-ordination made it impossible for her to handle her medication the normal way. Large colour coded cards were marked with the medication times. Each day when the nurse came, she put out the medication for the next 24 h, arranged in a minidispensary on a small table beside the patient's chair (Fig. 9.6). Several commercial systems are available.

The relative or friend giving medication may also be elderly or infirm. On one home care programme, a third of the 'primary care persons' (closest caregivers) were over 65, including 4% who were over 80, and a third were not in good health themselves (Lack & Buckingham 1978). Medication, therefore, must be as straightforward as possible for their sake also.

Getting through the night may need careful planning. For example:

- the 0200 h dose prepared and left by the bedside (sometimes with an alarm clock set)
- a double dose of morphine at bedtime
- using a m/r morphine preparation.

One wife who nursed her husband with lung cancer did not sleep in a bed for over a month because her nights were broken by the frequent need for analgesics (Wilkes 1965). Short acting opioids such as dextromoramide and pethidine are rarely satisfactory. A regular 'in between' tablet (in effect a q2h regimen) is also impossible to maintain for long.

Studies show that compliance is improved if time is taken to explain what each preparation is for (MacDonald et al 1977). A list of medication serves

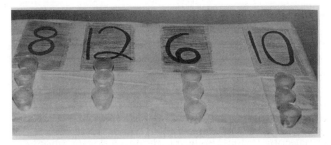

Fig. 9.6 A minidispensary arranged by the home care nurse for a patient with poor vision and inco-ordination. (Reproduced with permission from Ajemian and Mount 1980.)

as re-inforcement when written with doses, times to be taken and purpose of prescription. Verbal and written instructions should include the following:

- drugs, their names and what each is for
- which are to be taken regularly and which are to be taken when a problem arises
- adverse effects and what to do if they occur
- what to do if vomiting begins and medicines cannot be taken, or if the patient is unable to swallow
- what to do if supplies unexpectedly run out
- how to measure liquid medicines
- how to keep track of whether a tablet has been taken
- keeping medicines away from children.

In short, the doctor has to educate the patient about his medication (Box 9.H). Ideally, even when the patient handles his own medication, the family should be included because this helps to create an atmosphere of co-operation and support.

BOX 9.H
PATIENTS' QUESTIONS ABOUT ANALGESICS

Which of my medicines are for pain?
How should I take them?
Do these drugs have adverse effects?
Isn't morphine dangerous?
If I take morphine, will I get addicted?
How much is it safe for me to take?
What if the dose doesn't relieve my pain?
Can I take different pain medicines on the same day?
What about nonprescription pain killers — may I use them?
Will I need injections when my pain gets worse?
What can I do about drowsiness?
What can I do about constipation?
Should I eat fibre?
What can I do about nausea?
What happens if I stop taking the morphine?
How do antidepressants help relieve my pain?
Can I take alcohol?
What is the difference between aspirin and paracetamol?
Can cancer patients take aspirin?
How should I take aspirin to reduce its adverse effects?
I can't take aspirin; what other medicines contain aspirin?
What shall I do if I am still in pain and my doctor says there's nothing more he can do?

PREREQUISITES FOR SUCCESS

As already noted in Chapter 1, it is not difficult to achieve a good result in most cancer patients. It does, however, require a doctor who:

- appreciates that pain is a somatopsychic experience

- carefully evaluates the cause(s) of pain
- adopts a multimodal approach, combining nondrug with drug measures
- differentiates between 'opioid responsive', 'opioid semiresponsive' and 'opioid resistant' pains
- uses the right drug in the right dose at the right time intervals
- recognizes that the effective dose of a strong opioid varies widely
- closely monitors patients receiving opioids, and treats adverse drug effects, particularly constipation and nausea and vomiting
- works closely with, and listens to, the nurses and other caregivers.

REFERENCES

Ajemian I, Mount B M 1980 Terminal care-essence. In: Ajemian I, Mount B M (eds) The Royal Victoria Hospital manual on palliative/hospice care. Arno Press, New York, p 5

Arner S, Meyerson B A 1988 Lack of analgesic effect of opioids on neuropathic and idiopathic forms of pain. Pain 33: 11–23

Bass C, Benjamin S 1993 The management of chronic somatisation. British Journal of Psychiatry 162: 472–480

Bowsher D 1990 How physiology of neurogenic pain dictates management. Geriatric Medicine Sept: 33–40

Brescia F J, Portenoy R K, Ryan M, Krasnoff L, Gray G 1992 Pain, opioid use, and survival in hospitalized patients with advanced cancer. Journal of Clinical Oncology 10: 149–155

Bruera E, Chadwick S, Weinlick A et al 1987 Delirium and severe sedation in patients with terminal cancer. Cancer Treatment Reports 7: 787–788

Bruera E, MacMillan K, Hanson J, MacDonald R N 1989 The Edmonton staging system for cancer pain: preliminary report. Pain 37: 203–209

Catling J A, Pinto D M, Jordan C, Jones J G 1980 Respiratory effects of analgesia after cholecystectomy: comparison of continuous and intermittent papaveretum. British Medical Journal 281: 478–480

Consensus Statement 1994 Use of morphine for cancer pain. European Association for Palliative Care.

Donovan B D, Dillon P, McGuire L 1987 Incidence and characteristics of pain in a sample of medical-surgical inpatients. Pain 30: 67–78

Glare P, Lickiss J N 1992 Unrecognized constipation in patients with advanced cancer: a recipe for therapeutic disaster. Journal of Pain and Symptom Management 7: 369–371

Goldstein A, Aronow L, Sumner M 1974 Principles of drug action, 2nd edn. Wiley & Sons, New York, pp 586–591

Griffith S 1990 A review of the factors associated with patient compliance and the taking of prescribed medicines. British Journal of General Practitioners 40: 114–116

Hanks G W 1982 Antiemetics for terminal cancer patients. Lancet i: 1410

Hanks G W 1991 Opioid responsive and opioid non-responsive pain in cancer. British Medical Bulletin 47: 718–731

Hunt J M, Stollar T D, Littlejohns D W, Twycross R G, Vere D W 1977 Patients with protracted pain: a survey conducted at the London Hospital. Journal of Medical Ethics 3: 61–73

Jadad A R, Carroll D, Glynn C J, Moore R A, McQuay H J 1992 Morphine sensitivity of chronic pain: a double-blind randomised crossover study using patient-controlled analgesia. Lancet i: 1367–1371

Julian P, Herxheimer A 1977 Doctors' anxieties in prescribing. Journal of the Royal College of General Practitioners 27: 662–665

Kaiko R F, Healy N, Pav J, Thomas G B, Goldenheim P D 1989 The comparative bioavailability of MS Contin tablets (controlled release oral morphine) following rectal and oral administration. In: Twycross R D (ed) The Edinburgh Symposium on Pain Control and Medical Education. Royal Society of Medicine, London, pp 235–241

Kalso E, Vainio A 1990 Morphine and oxycodone in the management of cancer pain. Clinical Pharmacology and Therapeutics 47: 639–646

Kupers R C, Konings H, Adriaensen H, Gybels J M 1991 Morphine differentially affects the sensory and affective pain ratings in neurogenic and idiopathic forms of pain. Pain 47: 5–12

Lack S A, Buckingham R W 1978 First American Hospice: Three Years of Home Care. Van Dyck, New Haven

Levin D N, Cleeland C S, Dar R 1985 Public attitudes towards cancer pain. Cancer 56: 2337–2339

MacDonald E T, MacDonald J B, Phoenix M 1977 Improving drug compliance after hospital discharge. British Medical Journal 2: 618–621

McQuay H J, Dickenson A H 1990 Implications of nervous system plasticity for pain management. Anaesthesia 45: 101–102

Marks R M, Sachar E J 1973 Undertreatment of medical inpatients with narcotic analgesics. Annals of Internal Medicine 78: 173–181

Massie M J, Holland J, Glass E 1983 Delirium in terminally ill cancer patients. American Journal of Psychiatry 140: 1048–1050

Mercadante S, Maddaloni S, Roccella S, Salvaggio L 1992 Predictive factors in advanced cancer pain treated only by analgesics. Pain 50: 151–155

Moulin D E, Max M B, Kaiko R F et al 1985 The analgesic efficacy of intrathecal D-Ala^2-D-Leu^5-enkephalin in cancer patients with chronic pain. Pain 23: 213–221

Nayman J 1979 Measurement and control of postoperative pain. Annals of the Royal College of Surgeons of England 61: 419–426

Ottesen S, Minton M, Twycross R G 1990 The use of epidural morphine at a palliative care centre. Palliative Medicine 4: 117–122

Pannuti F, Rossi A P, Iafelice G et al 1982 Control of chronic pain in very advanced cancer patients with morphine hydrochloride administered by oral, rectal and sublingual route. Clinical report and preliminary results on morphine pharmacokinetics. Pharmacological Research Communications 14: 369–380

Philippines Cancer Control Program 1991 Guidelines on cancer pain relief. Department of Health, Republic of the Philippines

Portenoy R K, Foley K M, Inturrisi C E 1990 The nature of opioid responsiveness and its implications for neuropathic pain: new hypotheses derived from studies of opioid infusions. Pain 43: 273–286

Rowbotham M C, Reisner-Keller L A, Fields H L 1991 Both intravenous lidocaine and morphine reduce the pain of postherpetic neuralgia. Neurology 41: 1024–1028

Rutter P C, Murphy F, Dudley H A F 1980 Morphine: controlled trial of different methods of administration for postoperative pain relief. British Medical Journal 280: 12–13

Schulze S, Roikjaer O, Hasselstrom L, Jensen N H, Kehlet H 1988 Epidural bupivacaine and morphine plus systemic indomethacin eliminates pain but not systemic response and convalescence after cholecystectomy. Surgery 103: 321–327

Tasker R R, Tsuda T, Hawrylyshyn P 1983 Clinical neurophysiological investigation of deafferentation pain. In: Bonica J J, Lindblom U, Iggo A (eds) Advances in pain research and therapy, vol 5. Raven Press, New York, pp 713–738

Twycross R G 1974 Clinical experience with diamorphine in advanced malignant disease. International Journal of Clinical Pharmacology, Therapy & Toxicology 9: 184–198

Twycross R G 1977 A comparison of diamorphine with cocaine and methadone. British Journal of Clinical Pharmacology 4: 691–692

Twycross R G, Lack S A 1983 Symptom Control in Far-Advanced Cancer: Pain Relief. Pitman, London

Twycross R G, Lack S A 1986 Control of Alimentary Symptoms in Far-Advanced Cancer. Churchill Livingstone, Edinburgh

Twycross R G, Harcourt J M V 1991 Use of laxatives at a palliative care centre. Palliative Medicine 5: 27–33

Vijayaram S, Ramamani P V, Chandrashekhar N S et al 1990 Continuing care for cancer pain relief with oral morphine solution. Cancer 66: 1590–1595

Wall P D 1990 Neuropathic pain. Pain 43: 267–268

Weber F H, McCallum R W 1992 Clinical approaches to irritable bowel syndrome. Lancet 340: 1447–1452

Wilkes E 1965 Terminal care at home. Lancet i: 799–801

Woolf C J, Wall P D 1986 Morphine-sensitive and morphine-insensitive actions of C-fibre input on the rat spinal cord. Neuroscience Letters 64: 221–225

Working Party of the Commission on the Provision of Surgical Services 1990 Pain after Surgery. Royal College of Surgeons of England & College of Anaesthetists, London

World Health Organization 1986 Cancer Pain Relief. World Health Organization, Geneva

Classification and mechanisms of action

DRUGS AND PAIN

Many drugs influence pain (Table 10.1). Some affect it indirectly, such as antibiotics in cystitis or sinusitis and penicillamine or gold in rheumatoid arthritis. These drugs act by modifying the pathological process and fall outside the definition of analgesic (Box 10.A). Spasmolytics comprise another category of drug which relieves pain indirectly; in this case by relaxing muscle (Table 10.2).

Table 10.1 Drugs and pain relief

Type	Mode of action
Nonsteroidal anti-inflammatory drug (NSAID)	Reduction of inflammation and peripheral neural sensitization
Analgesic	Reduction in pain perception by the activation of one or more inhibitory mechanisms
Antidepressant	Enhancement of CNS descending inhibitory pathways; and by alleviation of depression
Anticonvulsant	Membrane stabilizing effect and/or facilitation of GABA inhibitory mechanisms
Anxiolytic	Reduction of skeletal muscle spasm; and by reduction of anxiety
Spasmolytic	Reduction of muscle spasm
Corticosteroids	Reduction of inflammation and peripheral neural sensitization; reduction in neural hyperexcitability (local effect only); and possibly by modifying affective component
Antirheumatoid drugs	Modification of pathological process; secondary reduction of inflammation and peripheral neural sensitization
Antibiotics	Modification of pathological process; secondary reduction of inflammation and peripheral neural sensitization

BOX 10.A
USEFUL DEFINITIONS

Analgesic
A drug which reduces the perception of pain without loss of consciousness.

Primary analgesic
A drug which is marketed primarily for relief of pain.

Secondary analgesic
A drug which relieves pain but which is marketed primarily for some other purpose.

Table 10.2 Spasmolytic drugs

Muscle	Drug
Somatic	Muscle relaxants: musculotropic — dantrolene GABA facilitation — baclofen — diazepam
Smooth	Antispasmodics: musculotropic — alverine — mebeverine — peppermint oil anticholinergic — dicyclomine — hyoscine *butylbromide* — propantheline
Cardiac	Calcium channel blockers: verapamil nifedipine diltiazem

Analgesic drugs are the commonest treatment for pain. In 1990, total sales worldwide, including nonprescription ('over the counter') preparations, amounted to £5.4 billion and accounted for 7% of all pharmaceutical sales. Nonopioids accounted for the vast majority (Table 10.3). Growth in sales is fairly steady at 8% per annum for all classes of analgesic. This, however, is less than for drugs generally (Rang 1992).

CLASSIFICATION OF ANALGESICS

Analgesics are now generally classified as nonopioid and opioid. The nonopioids subdivide into nonsteroidal anti-inflammatory drugs (NSAIDs) and 'simple analgesics'. NSAIDs share three properties:

- analgesic
- anti-inflammatory
- antipyretic.

Table 10.3   Worldwide analgesic sales in 1990

Class of drug	Percentage of total[a]
NSAID	48
Other nonopioid[b]	34
Opioid	9
Muscle relaxant	8
Antimigraine	2

[a] Rounded to nearest whole number.
[b] Mainly paracetamol.
From Rang 1992

Table 10.4   Classification of drugs used in rheumatoid arthritis

Type of drug	Example
Simple analgesics	Paracetamol/acetaminophen Codeine
Analgesics with anti-inflammatory properties	Aspirin NSAIDs
Pure anti-inflammatory drugs	Corticosteroids

Compounds with more specific action in rheumatoid arthritis	Gold
	Penicillamine
	Immunosuppressive drugs:
	  azathioprine
	  methotrexate

In contrast, simple analgesics are simply analgesic (e.g. nefopam) or analgesic and antipyretic (e.g. paracetamol/acetaminophen). The use of the phrase 'simple analgesic' stems from the classification of drugs used in rheumatoid arthritis (Table 10.4). Rheumatologists have traditionally placed codeine and other weak opioids in this category. While this is correct in one sense (*all* opioids are simple analgesics, i.e. have no anti-inflammatory effects), the inclusion of codeine and similar drugs in this category serves to obscure the fact that they are opioids.

In the past, opioids were classified as:

- opium and opium alkaloids (i.e. codeine, morphine, etc.)
- opiates (semisynthetic derivatives of an opium alkaloid, e.g. diamorphine, buprenorphine)
- opioids (synthetic drugs, e.g. pethidine, methadone).

The synthetic opioids were subdivided according to chemical structure. Now, however, 'opioid' is used as a generic term and includes all drugs with morphine-like actions (Box 10.B). Classification on the basis of chemical structure, however, does have its uses. For example, in cases of morphine intolerance, awareness of chemical differences permits the choice of a chemically distinct alternative. On the other hand, some patients who have unacceptable adverse effects with morphine do not manifest the same effects with oxycodone even though it is chemically closely related (Kalso & Vainio 1990).

BOX 10.B
USEFUL DEFINITIONS

Opioid
A generic term for all substances which bind specifically to endogenous opioid receptors and produce some agonist actions. Such drugs may or may not have a pharmacological profile similar to that of morphine.

Alkaloid
An organic base, usually of vegetable origin, containing nitrogen as a component of a heterocyclic ring structure e.g. atropine, cocaine, morphine, nicotine.

Receptor affinity ('potency')
A term used to describe the power of attraction between the drug and the drug receptor. Affinity determines the dose of drug required to produce a certain level of biological effect.

Intrinsic activity ('efficacy')
The degree to which the drug is able to stimulate a receptor and thereby produce a biological effect. Intrinsic activity is a basic property of all drugs which act through receptors.

Agonist
A drug which when bound to the receptor stimulates the receptor to the maximum level. By definition the intrinsic activity of a full agonist is unity, e.g. morphine.

Antagonist
A drug which when bound to the receptor fails to produce any stimulation of that receptor, e.g. naloxone. By definition the intrinsic activity of a pure antagonist is zero.

Partial agonist
A drug which when bound to the receptor stimulates the receptor to a level below the maximum level, e.g. buprenorphine (partial mu agonist). By definition the intrinsic activity of a partial agonist lies between zero and unity.

Mixed agonist-antagonist
A drug which acts simultaneously on different receptor subtypes, with the potential for agonist action on one or more subtypes and antagonist action on one or more subtypes, e.g. pentazocine (partial mu agonist + kappa agonist + weak delta antagonist).

Ligand
A substance which binds to a receptor. (The use of this term circumvents the need to say whether the substance is an agonist or an antagonist.)

The best classification is probably one based on receptor affinity:

- agonist
- partial agonist
- mixed agonist-antagonist
- antagonist.

In practice, however, the terms 'weak opioid' (codeine etc.) and 'strong opioid' (morphine etc.) continue to have wide currency. Because of this, they will be used here even though, within a class of drugs, potency and efficacy comprise a spectrum and cannot be rigidly divided into subclasses. Thus, in the Revised Method for Relief of Cancer Pain (WHO 1994), the following classification has been adopted:

- opioids for mild to moderate pain
- opioids for moderate to severe pain.

The terms 'mild analgesics' for nonopioids and 'strong analgesics' for opioids are still sometimes used. Their use must be discouraged, however, because there are occasions when morphine (a 'strong analgesic') does not relieve pain which aspirin (a 'mild analgesic') does. Further, parenteral NSAIDs are frequently used to relieve biliary and ureteric colic (Broggini et al 1984, Lundstam et al 1985, Hetherington & Philip 1986, Thompson et al 1989) and postoperative pain (Nuutinen et al 1986) because they are as effective as opioids.

MECHANISMS OF ACTION OF ANALGESICS

It is often stated that aspirin and NSAIDs act peripherally and opioids centrally, i.e. within the CNS. Paracetamol and nefopam also act centrally but by nonopioid mechanisms. The reality is, however, more complex (Ferreira 1981). NSAIDs appear to act at several sites, some peripheral and some central. The same appears to be true of the opioids but with the central actions predominating.

Nonopioids

Peripheral action

It is generally considered that the analgesic effect of NSAIDs results from their ability to inhibit cyclo-oxygenase, with a consequential reduction in tissue prostaglandins (PGs) (Fig. 10.1). As noted in Chapter 3, tissue injury leads to the release of various chemical mediators, including:

- bradykinin
- histamine
- PGs
- serotonin
- substance P.

In a series of experiments it was shown that a combination of bradykinin, histamine and PGE_1 caused moderately severe pain when injected into the skin of the fore-arm (Ferreira 1972). Alone, none caused pain; nor did the combination of bradykinin and histamine, although either with PGE_1 caused some pain. These results led to the suggestion that PGs sensitize nociceptive nerve endings to various other mediators. NSAIDs inhibit PG synthesis and it was concluded, therefore, that NSAID analgesia results from this.

NSAIDs are 99% bound to albumin in plasma. Protein bound NSAIDs escape from the circulation, however, into the inflamed tissue as a result of

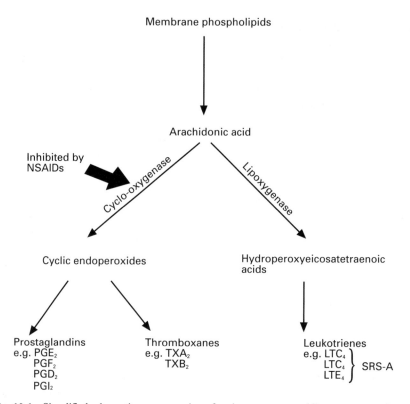

Fig. 10.1 Simplified schematic representation of cyclo-oxygenase and lipoxygenase pathways leading to the production of PGs, thromboxanes and leukotrienes from arachidonic acid. (Reproduced with permission from Clissold 1986.)

increased capillary permeability. Enzymes released from lysosomes in inflamed tissue then disrupt the carrier protein and release the NSAID (Togl-Leimuller et al 1986). This creates a concentration gradient in the inflamed tissue which results in cumulation of unbound NSAID locally. Thus, in the acidic inflamed environment, undissociated lipid soluble NSAID predominates. This facilitates transport into the cells. At intracellular pH, however, the dissociated water soluble form predominates. This creates a second concentration gradient into the cell where NSAIDs act as inhibitors of microsomal cyclo-oxygenase (McCormack & Brune 1991).

There is, however, no close relationship between the effectiveness of a drug as a cyclo-oxygenase inhibitor in vitro and its anti-inflammatory effect in vivo. Some compounds, including chlorpromazine and several of the tricyclic antidepressants, inhibit cyclo-oxygenase but are not anti-inflammatory (Famaey 1978) while benzofen has anti-inflammatory properties but is not a cyclo-oxygenase inhibitor.

Further, the alkaline derivatives of NSAIDs, e.g. antipyrine and indoxole are almost as potent inhibitors of cyclo-oxygenase as their acidic counterparts, phenylbutazone and indomethacin, but have only a minimal anti-inflammatory effect (Ham et al 1972). Some anti-inflammatory drugs are more selective than others with respect to cyclo-oxygenase inhibition. Indomethacin and the fenamates are relatively broad spectrum inhibitors, whereas phenylbutazone selectively inhibits PGE_2 and slightly *stimulates* the synthesis of PGF_2. Fenamates not only inhibit PG synthesis but also antagonize some of the effects of already synthesized PG, possibly by interfering with PG binding at their cellular receptor sites.

NSAIDs are effective analgesics, however, in conditions where there is little or no inflammation. Further, a comparison of NSAIDs in postdental extraction pain shows a clear dissociation between efficacy as an analgesic and potency as an inhibitor of cyclo-oxygenase (Table 10.5). Thus, azapropazone 400 mg and oxaprozin 1.2 g both achieve a significantly superior analgesic effect to aspirin after 30 and 60 min respectively even though they are weak cyclo-oxygenase inhibitors (Shimura 1972, Winter & Post 1983). On the other hand, even though it is rapidly absorbed after oral administration, diclofenac 100 mg is no better than aspirin 650 mg, and diclofenac 50 mg cannot be distinguished from placebo (Frame & Rout 1986, Adair et al 1988, Clark et al 1989, Nelson et al 1989).

Yet, as already noted, diclofenac is a highly potent cyclo-oxygenase inhibitor which is particularly effective in treating biliary and renal colic — conditions in which PGs are known to play an important role.

Further evidence for an alternative or dual mechanism of action comes from tests involving SC formalin. In humans, SC formalin causes an intense, sharp burning pain for 4–5 min followed by a throbbing ache for 30–60 min. A similar biphasic pattern is observed in mice. Licking of the injected paw is observed for up to 5 min and between 20–30 min after the formalin injection. Using this test, the effects of an intraperitoneal injection of aspirin 0–400 mg/kg, indomethacin 0–40 mg/kg or placebo control were compared. Aspirin had a dose dependent antinociceptive effect during both early and late phases, whereas indomethacin was effective only during the late phase.

Similar findings have been reported for aspirin in a study investigating the antinociceptive action of aspirin and tenoxicam in adjuvant induced arthritis in rats (Braga et al 1987). IV aspirin produced a marked antinociceptive effect at about 8 min. The antinociceptive effect of IV tenoxicam was apparent only at about 30 min (Braga et al 1987).

Table 10.5 Analgesic efficacy in dental pain of orally administered NSAIDs relative to aspirin 650 mg

Significantly superior	Not significantly different	Significantly inferior
Azapropazone (3)	Diclofenac (1)	Fenbufen (1)
Diflunisal (3)	Etodolac (1)	Nabumetone (1)
Flurbiprofen (1)	Sulindac (1)	
Ketoprofen (2)		
Naproxen (3)		
Oxaprozin (3)		
Tolmetin (3)		

Numbers in parentheses indicate capacity to inhibit prostaglandin synthesis: 1 = potent; 2 = moderate; 3 = week. Compounds are listed alphabetically.
From McCormack & Brune 1991

In chemically induced chronic hyperalgesia in the paw of the rat, a dissociation between antinociceptive and anti-inflammatory effects has been shown (Marquez & Ferreira 1987). Antinociception was observed with a plantar injection of dipyrone but not after indomethacin. At clinical doses, dipyrone is a weak inhibitor of PG synthesis and is almost devoid of anti-inflammatory activity (McCormack & Brune 1991).

The 'down regulation' of sensitized nociceptors by dipyrone has been further demonstrated in vivo following IV administration (He et al 1990), and in humans under experimental conditions following oral administration (Handwerker et al 1990). In both studies it was concluded that the effects of dipyrone on nociceptive pathways, both peripheral and central, did not include an anti-inflammatory component.

A pure analgesic effect (i.e. independent of an anti-inflammatory effect) has been shown for the NSAID azapropazone in volunteers subjected to focused ultrasound to the proximal interphalangeal joint of the index finger (Wright & Davies 1989, Wright et al 1989).

With NSAIDs, therefore, it is important to distinguish between:

- an anti-inflammatory effect
- an analgesic effect
- an analgesic effect secondary to an anti-inflammatory effect.

Most studies do not make such distinctions. Nonetheless, the assumption that all NSAIDs relieve pain only through inhibition of cyclo-oxygenase is not in accord with published data.

Central action

NSAIDs can be detected in CSF after oral administration (Gaucher et al 1983). Central effects have been reported for most NSAIDs (Box 10.C; Rainsford 1984). Flurbiprofen, for example, has occasionally caused (Enevoldson & Wiles 1990):

- tremor
- ataxia

BOX 10.C
CENTRAL EFFECTS OF NSAIDS (Enevoldson & Wiles 1990, Zoppi & Zamponi 1990)

Antipyresis

Salicylates stimulate brain serotonin turnover

Naloxone inhibits the early phase of diclofenac analgesia

Adverse effects include dizziness, drowsiness, slurred speech, particularly in the elderly

Visual hallucinations reported with indomethacin

Parkinsonism caused by flurbiprofen, indomethacin and sulindac

Parkinsonism improved by diflunisal

- myoclonus
- akathisia (motor restlessness)
- hypertonia
- Parkinsonism.

Further it has been shown that diclofenac (Sacerdote et al 1985, Vescovi et al 1987):

- stimulates beta-endorphin release from the pituitary gland
- increases beta-endorphin concentration in the hypothalamus
- decreases opioid withdrawal symptoms.

In the light of these observations, it is not surprising that pretreatment with naloxone delays the onset of diclofenac analgesia (Fig. 10.2). A central analgesic action has also been shown in humans with ketoprofen (Willer et al 1989).

In rats, fenamates produce dose related central excitation, whereas ibuprofen and indomethacin produce dose related central sedation (Wallenstein 1985). In humans, acute poisoning with mefenamic acid is characterized by central excitation, whereas acute poisoning with ibuprofen and indomethacin is characterized by central sedation (Vale & Meredith 1986).

In animal studies, three supraspinal structures have been identified as possible sites responsible for the central analgesic effect of NSAIDs:

- thalamus

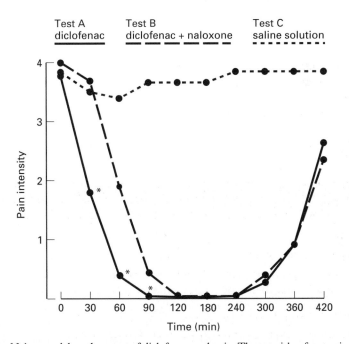

Fig. 10.2 Naloxone delays the onset of diclofenac analgesia. The asterisk refers to significant differences between test A and test B pain scores ($p < 0.05$). (Reproduced with permission from Vescovi et al 1987.)

Table 10.6   Inhibition of prostaglandin formation

	Dog spleen ID_{50} μg/ml[a]	Rabbit brain ID_{50} μg/ml[a]
Indomethacin	0.06	1.3
Aspirin	6.6	11.0
Paracetamol	100.0	14.0

[a] ID_{50} = dose required for 50% inhibition.
From Flower & Vane 1972

Table 10.7   Central antinociceptive effects of selected analgesics

Substance	Spinal cord		Thalamus
	Direct	Indirect	
Morphine	Depression	Activation of inhibition from peri-aqueductal grey	Depression
Dipyrone } Aminophenazone }	Excitation	Activation of inhibition from peri-aqueductal grey	Depression
Lysine-aspirin } Paracetamol }	Nil	Nil	Depression

From Carlsson et al 1988

- hypothalamus
- peri-aqueductal grey matter in the brain stem.

It has been suggested that the effects at the three sites may interact with each other (Willer et al 1989).

Paracetamol has been shown to depress evoked nociceptive activity in the thalamus of the rat (Carlsson & Jurna 1987), and to inhibit brain PG synthesis (Table 10.6). This latter action has been shown to be responsible for the antipyretic effect of the drug (Flower & Vane 1972).

Other experiments show that dipyrone has spinal as well as supraspinal sites of action (Table 10.7). The spinal actions provide an explanation for the antinociceptive effects of dipyrone on chemically induced hyperalgesia in the rat.

Opioids

As noted in Chapter 3, four main subtypes of opioid receptors have been postulated, and are designated mu, kappa, delta and epsilon (Table 10.8). The so-called sigma receptor (Martin 1984) possibly does not exist as such. Endogenous opioids (beta-endorphin, enkephalins, dynorphin) and exogenous opioids (morphine and other opioid drugs) exert their effects by interacting with these receptors. Any given opioid may interact to a variable extent with all receptor subtypes as either an agonist, a partial agonist, mixed agonist-antagonist or an antagonist (Vaught 1991). Published sources, how-ever, do not always give the same pattern of receptor affinity for opioid

Table 10.8 Tentative classification of opiate receptor subtypes and actions

Subtype	Prototypic	Proposed actions
Mu		
mu$_1$	Opioid drugs and most opioid peptides	Supraspinal analgesia including: peri-aqueductal grey nucleus raphe magnus locus coeruleus Prolactin release Free feeding and deprivation induced feeding Acetylcholine turnover in the brain Catalepsy
mu$_2$	Morphine	Respiratory depression Growth hormone release (?) Dopamine turnover in the brain Gastro-intestinal tract motility Guinea pig ileum bio-assay Feeding Most cardiovascular effects
Delta	Enkephalins	Spinal analgesia Dopamine turnover in the brain Mouse vas deferens bio-assay Growth hormone release (?) Feeding
Kappa	Ketocyclazocine Dynorphin	Spinal analgesia Inhibition of antidiuretic hormone release Sedation Feeding
Epsilon	Beta-endorphin	Rat vas deferens bio-assay Hormone (?)

From Pasternak 1988

drugs. A major problem is that affinity studies are generally done on isolated pieces of animal tissue in an organ bath. The results of these in vitro studies may well not reflect in vivo reality.

A second problem is that many articles still quote data from before the identification of the delta receptor, and from the period when the postulated sigma receptor was thought to be a distinct opioid specific entity. This has led to 'copy cat' reproduction of outdated material. The table of receptor selectivity shown here differs in several respects from more traditional representations (Table 10.9). Most commonly used opioid analgesics have the same profile as morphine.

Opioid analgesia is mediated through mu, delta and kappa receptors (Vaught 1991). Because of the development of highly specific opioid agonists and antagonists, the contribution of each receptor subtype can be evaluated. Mu receptor activation inhibits nociception over a broader range of intensities and stimulation modalities than at the delta and kappa receptors.

In animals, mu receptors seem to be the most important supraspinally, and delta and kappa receptors spinally. Thus, in animal studies, opioid peptides which bind strongly to delta receptors are more potent at spinal level than morphine which binds relatively poorly (Yaksh 1983). This differentiation, however, is not true in man. Even so, such findings may have implications for the development of opioid drugs for spinal application.

Table 10.9 Receptor selectivity of opioid analgesics

Drug	Receptor type		
	Mu	Kappa	Delta
Morphine	A	a	a
Buprenorphine	pA	Ant	A
Butorphanol	pA	A	Ant
Fentanyl	A	a	a
Levorphanol	A	x	A
Methadone	A	x	A
Nalbuphine	Ant	pA	ant
Oxymorphone	A	a	a
Pentazocine	pA	A	ant
Pethidine	a	–	–
Naloxone	Ant	Ant	Ant

A = strong agonist; a = weak agonist; Ant = strong
antagonist; ant = weak antagonist;
pA = partial agonist; x = negligible activity; – = no activity.
Sources: Hill 1992, Corbett et al 1993

Current evidence does not support the hypothesis that different opioid receptor subtypes are related to the relief of a specific type of somatic pain, namely, pain caused by a thermal, chemical or mechanical stimulus (Fields et al 1991). In man, kappa agonists ('kappa preferring opioids') have limited analgesic potency compared to mu agonists.

Mu receptor

The mu receptor is by far the most extensively investigated and understood. Mu receptors predominate in the brain stem and subcortical regions of the brain but, in animals, are infrequently found in the spinal cord (Pasternak 1988). Mu receptors, however, are well represented in the spinal cord in man. Two major adverse effects of opioids are linked predominantly to mu receptors, namely, respiratory depression and decreased gastro-intestinal motility.

Blocking mu receptors with mu selective antagonists in experimental animals blocks morphine analgesia for more than 24 h (Pasternak et al 1980a, 1980b). Mu blockade also reduces the analgesic effect of many different opioid drugs and opioid peptides (Pasternak 1988).

Two subclasses of mu receptors (mu_1 and mu_2) have been identified. Almost all the analgesic effects of opioids are derived from agonist activation of mu_1 receptors (Hayes & Vogetang 1991). Mu_1 stimulation also causes prolactin release, hypothermia, and catalepsy (Anonymous 1990).

Mu_2 receptor activation results in most of the adverse effects of opioids. This receptor has a lower affinity for mu agonists than the mu_1 receptor (Pasternak 1988). The effects of ligand binding to this receptor are:

• respiratory depression
• gastro-intestinal stasis
• urinary retention

- bradycardia
- miosis
- euphoria
- physical dependence.

Mu_2 receptors also mediate most features of morphine withdrawal (Pasternak 1988). The development of a mu_1 selective agent would clearly be of clinical benefit.

Kappa receptor

The kappa receptor is found predominately in cortical and spinal locations, and is the preferred site of the endogenous dynorphins. The effects on spinal transmission predominate (Jaffe & Martin 1985). Kappa agonists (not clinically available) exert their effects in a mu tolerant individual, thereby showing that kappa stimulation is separate from mu stimulation (Jaffe & Martin 1990). In animal studies, kappa receptor activation does not block thermal pain (Hayes & Vogetang 1991).

The analgesic effect of pentazocine is predominantly mediated by the kappa receptor. Sedation and miosis are associated with kappa receptor activation, and are seen in patients taking pentazocine. Respiratory depression is also observed, but both this effect and the miosis are considerably less intense than that seen with mu receptor agonism (Shook et al 1990).

Delta receptor

The delta opioid receptor is also responsible for analgesia. In animals, these receptors mediate spinal analgesia. Both enkephalins and beta-dynorphins bind to these receptors; the enkephalins are more selective. Delta receptors are also located diffusely in the cerebral cortex and may act synergistically with mu receptors (Pasternak 1988, Hayes & Vogetang 1991). The adverse effect most commonly associated with delta receptors is respiratory depression (Anonymous 1990). This is less than with mu activation but more than with kappa. Research is hampered because of the lack of a highly selective agonist which crosses the blood-brain barrier.

Delta preferring agonists produce moderate analgesia in a range of tests (Vaught 1991). It is not clear how much of this is mediated via delta receptors and how much via mu receptors because all presently available delta ligands have some mu receptor activity. More selective ligands such as DPDPE are relatively less analgesic. On the other hand, in mu tolerant animals, delta mediated antinociception can be observed at both supraspinal and spinal levels. A similar effect with a delta preferring agonist, a modified leu-enkephalin (DADL), has been demonstrated in man (Moulin et al 1985).

Differences in affinity for different opioid receptor subtypes has been demonstrated in an experiment with mice. One group was made tolerant to morphine and the other to levorphanol. The effect of the alternative opioid was then tested. Levorphanol-tolerant mice were also morphine-tolerant whereas morphine-tolerant mice were not tolerant to levorphanol. This response was explained by assuming that levorphanol is a strong agonist at both mu and delta receptors but morphine is a strong agonist at the mu receptor and a weak agonist at the delta receptor (Moulin et al 1988).

Differences in affinity for different opioid receptor subtypes may well, therefore, have useful clinical applications. DADL is a pentapeptide which preferentially binds to mu$_1$ receptors with an affinity equal to that of morphine but to delta receptors with an affinity nine times greater than morphine (Wolozin & Pasternak 1981). One patient with a sacral chordoma who was not responding to intrathecal (IT) morphine obtained excellent pain relief with IT DADL (Onofrio & Yaksh 1983). A subsequent controlled trial compared IT morphine with IT DADL in 10 cancer patients with lumbosacral plexopathy (Moulin et al 1985). Both drugs were equally effective although some patients had a better response with one rather than the other. Despite this outcome, the anecdotal report of greater benefit in the patient with the sacral chordoma should not be totally disregarded.

Epsilon receptor

The epsilon receptor is highly selective for the beta-endorphins but lacks affinity for enkephalins. It is not related to analgesia. Little is known about the epsilon receptor function and its role remains unclear.

Sigma receptor

The sigma receptor is unrelated to analgesia. The effects of sigma activation are psychotomimetic (dysphoria, hallucinations). Pentazocine is an agonist for this receptor. A more useful effect is respiratory stimulation, in contrast to depression with delta receptors (Anonymous 1990). Because the sigma receptor is not blocked by naloxone, strictly speaking it is not an opioid receptor.

Further, as already noted, the sigma receptor possibly does not exist as such. The psychotomimetic effects of opioids might relate to a phencyclidine-like effect at the NMDA receptor-ion complex (Lodge 1988).

Site of analgesic action of opioid drugs

Systemically administered opioids act at various sites both in the CNS and in the periphery (Fields et al 1991).

Peripheral action Opioid receptors have been demonstrated in peripheral afferent nerve fibres (Fields et al 1980, Young et al 1980, Laduron 1984). Local administration of hydrophilic opioid agonists (which have a limited ability to cross the blood-brain barrier) reduces the hypersensitivity to a noxious stimulus in inflamed tissue. Studies using selective agonists and antagonists indicate that these peripheral analgesic effects are mediated by mu, delta and kappa opioid receptors (Stein et al 1989). The cellular mechanism underlying these effects is not known. An effect on the local release of sensitizing agents of the peripheral afferent terminal, however, is a reasonable hypothesis (Hargreaves et al 1988, Fields et al 1991, Stein 1993). Awareness of peripheral opioid receptors has led to several clinical applications, principally in orthopaedic surgery (Feldman 1993).

CNS action Microinjection studies have shown that there are several discrete brain regions where locally applied opioids will induce a powerful change in an animal's response to a noxious thermal, mechanical or chemical stimulus. The use of intracerebroventricular and spinal opioids in man has confirmed the central action of opioids (Yaksh et al 1988). Several different mechanisms may underlie the antinociceptive effect of opioids in the CNS (Fields et al 1991).

REFERENCES

Adair S F, Mehlisch D R, Brandes S, Brown P, Burton C 1988 Diclofenac sodium (voltaren) shows analgesic efficacy in dental pain model. Journal of Clinical Pharmacology 28: 915
Anonymous 1990 Analgesics: opioid analgesics. In: Drug evaluation subscription. American Medical Association 1: 1–2
Braga P C, Biella G, Tiengo M 1987 Effects of tenoxicam on nociceptive thalamic neuronal firing in arthritic rats. Drugs Under Experimental Clinical Research XIII: 389–398
Broggini M, Corbetta E, Grossi E, Borghi C 1984 Diclofenac sodium in biliary colic: a double blind trial. British Medical Journal 288: 1042
Carlsson K-H, Jurna I 1987 Central analgesic effect of paracetamol manifested by depression of nociceptive activity in thalamic neurones of the rat. Neuroscience Letters 77: 339–343
Carlsson K-H, Monzel W, Jurna I 1988 Depression by morphine and non-opioid analgesic agents, metamizol (dipyrone), lysine acetylsalicylate, and paracetamol, of activity in rat thalamus neurones evoked by electrical stimulation of nociceptive afferents. Pain 32: 313–326
Clark M S, Tomasetti B J, Mehlisch D R 1989 Diclofenac sodium (voltaren) shows analgesic efficacy in dental pain model. Journal of Dental Research (Special Issue) 68: 918
Clissold S P 1986 Aspirin and related derivatives of salicylic acid. Drugs 32 (Suppl 4): 8–26
Corbett A D, Paterson S J, Kosterlitz H W 1993 Selectivity of ligands for opioid receptors. In Herz A (ed) Opioids I. Springer-Verlag, London, pp 657–672
Enevoldson T P, Wiles C M 1990 Acute Parkinsonism associated with flurbiprofen. British Medical Journal 300: 540–541
Famaey P 1978 Recent developments about non-steroidal anti-inflammatory drugs and their mode of action. General Pharmacology 9: 155–161
Feldman S H 1993 Peripheral opiate receptors. Anaesthesia 48: 171–172
Ferreira S H 1972 Prostaglandins, aspirin-like drugs and analgesia. Nature: New Biology 240: 200–203
Ferreira S H 1981 Peripheral and central analgesia. Pain supplement 1: 54
Fields H L, Emson P, Leigh B, Gilbert R, Iversen L 1980 Multiple opiate receptor site on primary afferent fibers. Nature 284: 351–353
Fields H L, Cox B M, Foley K M et al 1991 Group report: strategies for improving the pharmacological approaches to the maintenance of analgesia in chronic pain. In: Basbaum A I, Besson J-M (eds) Towards a new pharmacotherapy of pain. John Wiley, Chichester, pp 205–226
Flower R J, Vane J R 1972 Inhibition of prostaglandin synthetase in brain explains the anti-pyretic activity of paracetamol. Nature 240: 410–411
Frame J W, Rout P G J 1989 A comparison of ibuprofen and dihydrocodeine in relieving pain following wisdom teeth removal. British Journal of Dentistry 166: 121–124
Gaucher A, Netter P, Faure G, Schoeller J P, Gerardin A 1983 A diffusion of oxyphenbutazone into synovial fluid, synovial tissue, joint cartilage and cerebrospinal fluid. European Journal of Clinical Pharmacology 25: 107–112
Ham E A, Cirillo V J, Zametti M, Shen T Y, Kuehl F A 1972 Studies on the mode of action of

non-steroidal anti-inflammatory agents. In: Ramwell P W, Phariss B B (eds). Prostaglandins in Cellular Biology. Plenum Press, New York, pp 345–352

Handwerker H O, Beck A, Forster C, Gall Th, Magerl W 1990 Analgesic effects of dipyrone as compared to placebo. In: Brune K (ed) New pharmacological and epidemiological data in analgesics research. Birkhauser, Cambridge, Mass, pp 19–28

Hargreaves K M, Dubner R, Joris J 1988 Peripheral actions of opiates in the blockade of carrageenan-induced inflammation. In: Dubner R, Gebhart F G, Bond M R (eds) Proceedings of the Vth World Congress on Pain. Elsevier Science, Amsterdam, pp 55–60

Hayes S R, Vogetang J 1991 Opiate receptors and analgesia: an update. Journal of Post Anesthesia Nursing 6: 125–128

He X, Neugebauer V, Schaible H G, Schmidt R F 1990 New aspects of the mode of action in dipyrone. In: Brune K (ed) New pharmacological and epidemiological data in analgesics research. Birkhauser, Cambridge, Mass, pp 9–18

Hetherington J W, Philip N H 1986 Diclofenac sodium versus pethidine in acute renal colic. British Medical Journal 92: 237–238

Hill R G 1992 Multiple opioid receptors and their ligands. Frontiers of Pain 4: 1–4

Jaffe J H, Martin W R 1985 Opioid analgesics and antagonists: In: Gilman A G, Goodman L S, Rall T W, Murad F (eds) Goodman and Gilman's the pharmacological basis of therapeutics, 7th edn. Macmillan, New York, pp 485–504

Kalso E, Vainio A 1990 Morphine and oxycodone in the management of cancer pain. Clinical Pharmacology and Therapeutics 47: 639–646

Laduron P 1984 Axonal transport of opiate receptors in the capsaicin sensitive neurones. Brain Research 294: 157–160

Lodge D (ed) 1988 Excitatory amino acids in health and disease. John Wiley, Chichester

Lundstam S, Ivarsson L, Lindblad L, Kral J G 1985 Treatment of biliary pain by prostaglandin synthetase inhibition with diclofenac sodium. Current Therapeutic Research 37 (3): 435–439

McCormack K, Brune K 1991 Dissociation between the antinociceptive and anti-inflammatory effects of the nonsteroidal anti-inflammatory drugs: a survey of their analgesic efficacy. Drugs 41: 533–547

Marquez J O, Ferreira S H 1987 Regional dipyrone nociceptor blockade: a pilot study. Brazilian Journal of Medical Biological Research 20: 441–444

Martin W R 1984 Pharmacology of opioids. Pharmacological Reviews 35: 283–323

Moulin D E, Max M B, Kaiko R F et al 1985 The analgesic efficacy of intrathecal D-Ala^2-D-Leu^5-enkephalin in cancer patients with chronic pain. Pain 23: 213–221

Moulin D E, Ling G S F, Pasternak G W 1988 Unidirectional analgesic cross-tolerance between morphine and levorphanol in the rat. Pain 33: 233–239

Nelson S L, Adair S F, Brahim J S 1989 Dental pain trial measures analgesia of diclofenac sodium. Journal of Dental Research (Special Issue) 68: 224

Nuutinen L S, Wuolijoki E, Pentikainen I T 1986 Diclofenac and oxycodone in treatment of postoperative pain: a double-blind trial. Acta Anaesthesiologica Scandinavica 30: 620–624

Onofrio B M, Yaksh T L 1983 Intrathecal delta-receptor ligand produces analgesia in man. Lancet i: 1386–1387

Pasternak G W 1988 Multiple morphine and enkephalin receptors and the relief of pain. Journal of the American Medical Association 259: 1362–1367

Pasternak G W, Childer S R, Snyder S H 1980a Opiate analgesia; evidence for mediation by a subpopulation of opiate receptors. Science 208: 514–516

Pasternak G W, Childer S R, Snyder S H 1980b Naloxonazone, a long-acting opiate antagonist: effects in intact animals and on opiate receptor binding in vitro. Journal of Pharmacology and Experimental Therapeutics 214: 455–462

Rainsford K D 1984 Side-effects of anti-inflammatory/analgesic drugs: epidemiology and gastrointestinal tract. Trends in Pharmacological Sciences 5: 156–159

Rang H P 1992 Abstract for International Conference on Pain, London

Sacerdote P, Monza G, Mantegazza P, Panerai A E 1985 Diclofenac and pirprofen modify pituitary and hypothalamic beta-endorphin concentrations. Pharmacological Research Communications 17: 679–684

Shimura K 1972 Clinical effects of azapropazone in the field of oral surgery. Kiso to Rinsho 6: 2339–2349

Shook J E, Watkins W D, Canaporesi E M 1990 Differential roles of opioid receptors in respiration, respiratory disease and opiate-induced respiratory depression. American Reviews of Respiratory Disease 142: 859–909

Stein C 1993 Peripheral mechanisms of opioid analgesia. Anesthesia and Analgesia 76: 182–191

Stein C, Millan M J, Shippenberg T S, Peter K, Herz A 1989 Peripheral opioid receptors mediating antinociception in inflammation. Evidence for involvement of mu, delta and kappa receptors. Journal of Pharmacology and Experimental Therapy 284: 1269–1275

Thompson J F, Pike J M, Chumas P D, Rundle J S H 1989 Rectal diclofenac compared with pethidine injection in acute renal colic. British Medical Journal 299: 1140–1141

Togl-Leimuller A, Egger G, Porta S 1986 Albumin as one-way transport vehicle into sites of inflammation. Experimental Pathology 30: 91–96

Vale J A, Meredith T J 1986 Acute poisoning due to nonsteroidal anti-inflammatory drugs. Medical Toxicology 1: 12–31

Vaught J L 1991 What is the relative contribution of mu, delta and kappa opioid receptors to antinociception and is there cross-tolerance? In: Basbaum A I, Besson J-M (eds) Towards a new pharmacotherapy of pain. John Wiley, Chichester, pp 121–136

Vescovi P, Passeri M, Gerra G, Grossi E 1987 Naloxone inhibits the early phase of diclofenac analgesia in man. The Pain Clinic 1: 151–155

Wallenstein M C 1985 Differential effects of prostaglandin synthetase inhibitors on EEG in rats. European Journal of Pharmacology 111: 201–209

Willer J-C, De Broucker T, Bussel B, Roby-Brami A, Harrewyn J-M 1989 Central analgesic effect of ketoprofen in humans: electrophysiological evidence for a supraspinal mechanism in a double-blind and cross-over study. Pain 38: 1–7

Winter Jr L, Post A 1983 Double-blind comparison of single oral doses of oxaprozin, aspirin and placebo for relief of post-operative oral surgery pain. Journal of International Medical Research 11: 308–314

Wolozin B L, Pasternak G W 1981 Classification of multiple morphine and enkephalin binding sites in the central nervous system. Proceedings of the National Academy of Science (Wash) 78: 6181–6185

World Health Organization 1994 Revised Method for Relief of Cancer Pain and other symptoms management. WHO, Geneva (In Press)

Wright A, Davies I ab I 1989 The recording of brain evoked potentials resulting from intra-articular focused ultrasonic stimulation: a new experimental model for investigating joint pain in humans. Neuroscience Letters 97: 145–150

Wright A, Davies I ab I, Walker F S, Riddell J G 1989 Azapropazone analgesia in a joint pain model. Abstract 93. British Journal of Rheumatology 28: 53

Yaksh T L 1983 In vivo studies on spinal opiate receptor systems mediating antinociception: I. mu and delta-receptor profiles in the primate. Journal of Pharmacology and Experimental Therapeutics 226: 303–316

Yaksh T L, Al-Rodhan N R F, Jensen T S 1988 Sites of action of opiates in production of analgesia. In: Fields H L, Besson J-M (eds) Progress in brain research, vol 77. Elsevier, Amsterdam, pp 371–394

Young W, Wamsley J, Zaren M, Kuhar M 1980 Opioid receptors undergo axonal flow. Science 210: 76–78

Zoppi M, Zamponi A 1990 Anti-inflammatory drugs. In: Lipton S, Tunks E, Zoppi M (eds) Advances in pain research and therapy, vol 13. Raven Press, New York, pp 329–335

CHAPTER 11 | Nonopioids I

INTRODUCTION

This chapter discusses aspirin, paracetamol, selected nonsteroidal anti-inflammatory drugs (NSAIDs) and nefopam. Adverse effects of the NSAIDs are discussed mainly in Chapter 12.

The importance of NSAIDs in cancer pain management has been highlighted in two surveys. The first reviewed the analgesic needs of 292 patients for 8 weeks after referral (Ventafridda et al 1987). At first, half of the patients needed only a NSAID. After 8 weeks, however, only 7.5% of the surviving patients obtained relief with a NSAID alone.

The second survey monitored the analgesic needs of over 1000 patients until they died. Analgesics were administered for more than 55 000 days (mean = 52 days/patient); nonopioids were used on over 47 000 days, i.e. 86% of the total (Table 11.1). Drugs of choice were flurbiprofen 150–300 mg/day and m/r diclofenac 150–300 mg/day. Other nonopioids were used only when patients were already taking them when first evaluated. They were given PO, PR or via a nasogastric tube for 95% of the time. Dipyrone (metamizole) was

Table 11.1 Use of nonopioids in 1070 patients with advanced cancer

Mode	Number of days (rounded)
Nonopioid alone	7 000
+ Weak opioid	15 000
+ Strong opioid	24 000
+ Spinal opioid	1 000
No nonopioid	8 000
Total	55 000

From Grond et al 1991

used when parenteral medication was necessary (Grond et al 1991). Dipyrone is not available in the UK or the USA.

A NSAID is generally essential for the relief of metastatic bone pain and soft tissue infiltration pain. Some NSAIDs are also very effective in biliary and ureteric colic (Anonymous 1987, Thompson et al 1989).

ASPIRIN

■ DRUG PORTRAIT

Aspirin (acetylsalicylic acid) is a semisynthetic derivative of salicylic acid, a naturally occurring substance. It is the 'parent' NSAID. In small doses, aspirin is simply analgesic and antipyretic. In large doses (> 3.6 g/day), it also has an anti-inflammatory effect. Aspirin appears to act at more than one site and by more than one mechanism (Morley 1975, Ferreira 1981). Its primary action is at the site of pain.

Aspirin is readily absorbed from the upper gastro-intestinal tract. About two thirds reaches the systemic circulation unchanged; one third is hydrolyzed during absorption by esterases in the gut wall, plasma or liver. Considerable variation exists between patients in plasma concentration after identical doses. At low doses, increments result in proportional increases in blood level. Doses up to 1200 mg, possibly 1800 mg, provide increasing relief. Aspirin has a plasma halflife of 15–20 min. It is rapidly hydrolyzed to salicylate by plasma and hepatic esterases. The salicylate remains detectable in the plasma for several hours and is responsible for part of the effects of aspirin. 80% of the salicylate is converted to salicylurate by conjugation with glycine. This is then excreted in the urine. In overdose, this pathway becomes saturated, and a small increase in dose results in a relatively large increase in plasma concentration. A single dose is effective for 4–6 h.

Aspirin was first marketed in 1898 and it remains the world's most extensively used nonprescription analgesic, although it has been overtaken by paracetamol in some countries. Although paracetamol has a lower ceiling effect, aspirin and paracetamol have similar dose-response and time-effect curves at standard doses (Fig. 11.1).

The fact that aspirin remains so popular highlights its general acceptability when used for acute pains such as headache, toothache, sprains and bruises. Aspirin is not innocuous, however, as Chapter 12 amply demonstrates.

Aspirin in small doses is not anti-inflammatory. 600 mg produces relief which begins within 30 min of taking it; this lasts for ≤ 6 h. Further doses have the same effect. In patients with a normal plasma albumin, a daily intake of ≥ 3.6 g is probably necessary for a significant anti-inflammatory effect. Several days are required to achieve maximum benefit.

It is not known how much aspirin itself reaches sites of inflammation. From animal studies with chemically induced inflammation it is known that aspirin has an effect in certain models where sodium salicylate does not. Further, some of the adverse effects of aspirin — hypersensitivity, gastric injury, anaemia, and impairment of platelet function — are largely linked to

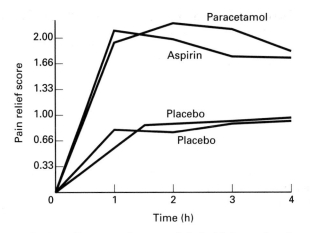

Fig. 11.1   Composite time-effect curves from two clinical trials in postdental extraction pain comparing aspirin 650 mg with placebo, and paracetamol 650 mg with placebo. (Reproduced with permission from Cooper 1981.)

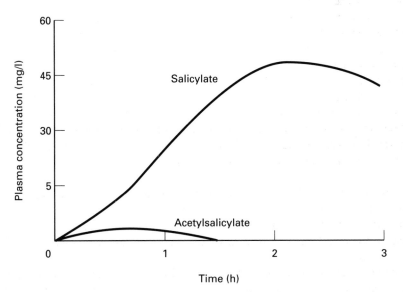

Fig. 11.2   Blood levels of acetylsalicylic acid after oral ingestion of 650 mg of aspirin. (Reproduced with permission from Leonards 1976.)

the presence of the acetyl radical. It seems, therefore, that the initial effect of aspirin is mediated via the intact molecule, and the continuing effect is mediated by salicylate (Fig. 11.2).

Aspirin and salicylate are uricosuric in doses of >5 g/day. Doses of 2–3 g/day usually do not alter urate excretion, whereas doses of 1–2 g/day may lead to an increased plasma urate concentration because of a competitive effect on tubular secretion (Flower et al 1980). Both medium and low doses block the uricosuric effect of probenecid.

Aspirin is rapidly hydrolyzed in vivo to salicylic acid and acetate, and many of its pharmacological actions are attributable to the salicylic acid moiety. Hydrolysis is not, however, a prerequisite for activity; aspirin itself has some unique properties (Flower et al 1980). Thus, aspirin inhibits cyclo-oxygenase by irreversible acetylation, whereas salicylic acid has no acetyl-ating capacity. Even so, the two drugs produce comparable inhibition of prostaglandin (PG) synthesis in vivo. This suggests that aspirin probably inhibits cyclo-oxygenase by more than one mechanism.

Aspirin and some other salicylate derivatives (e.g. choline magnesium trisalicylate, salsalate) are hydrolyzed to salicylic acid in the body. Thus once absorbed and hydrolyzed the pharmacokinetic properties of these drugs are those of salicylic acid. Diflunisal, another salicylate derivative, is not hydrolyzed to salicylic acid.

Orally administered aspirin is rapidly and usually completely absorbed from the stomach and upper small intestine as either aspirin or salicylic acid. Several factors affect the rate of absorption (Box 11.A). Of these, drug formulation is the major determinant because it controls the rate of tablet dissolution (Levy & Hollister 1965), a necessary preliminary before absorption (Table 11.2).

Gastro-intestinal pH has a major influence on aspirin absorption. First, the low pH in the stomach facilitates the rapid absorption of lipophilic unionized aspirin. Then, in the small intestine, the higher pH aids the dissolution of solid aspirin tablets.

BOX 11.A
FACTORS AFFECTING ASPIRIN AND SALICYLATE ABSORPTION (Clissold 1986)

Drug formulation
pH of stomach contents
Rate of gastric emptying
Food
Concurrent administration of other drugs
Nervous state
Posture
Exercise
Disease states associated with altered gastro-intestinal transit time

---

Table 11.2 Absorption characteristics of aspirin tablets

Preparation	Time to peak concentration	
	Aspirin	Salicylic acid
Dispersible	15–40 min	30–60 min
Standard	25–60 min	45–120 min
M/r tablets	1–2 h	4–12 h
Enteric coated	4–6 h	8–14 h

From Clissold 1986

Aspirin is 70% protein bound in the plasma, compared with 85% of salicylic acid. Distribution of salicylic acid occurs by pH dependent passive diffusion. This limits its ability to cross the blood-brain barrier (Flower et al 1980). The elimination of salicylic acid is complex and utilizes five different pathways. Metabolism occurs mainly in the endoplasmic reticulum and the liver. As urinary pH increases the urinary excretion of free salicylic acid increases, and the fraction of a dose excreted as unchanged drug may increase from 50% to 85%. In addition, more tends to be excreted unchanged at higher doses.

Unlike cells, platelets cannot resynthesize cyclo-oxygenase. Thus, the impact of a single dose of aspirin lasts the lifetime of the platelet. This is the explanation behind once a day treatment with aspirin in prophylaxis against thrombosis.

Preparations of aspirin

Aspirin is available in a wide range of 'over the counter' preparations (Box 11.B). Because of the use of brand names, the patient may not always know that he is taking aspirin, and may not think it important to tell his doctor that he is taking nonprescription analgesics. In other words, a patient can be taking aspirin without his doctor being aware of it.

Aspirin BP, USP

The rate of absorption varies according to formulation. Some 'over the counter' preparations made by wet compression consist of large less soluble particles and cause more gastric erosions and occult blood loss. More expensive formulations made by dry granulation ('slugging') are less gastrotoxic.

BOX 11.B
UK BRAND NAMES FOR ASPIRIN (Pal 1986)

Actron	Fynnon Calcium Aspirin
Alka-Seltzer	Genasprin
Anadin	Hypon
Antoin	Laboprin
Askit	Mrs Cullen's Powders
Aspergum	Myolgin
Aspro	Nu-Seal
Beecham Powders	Paynocil
Breoprin	Phensic
Caprin	Powerin
Claradin	Safapryn
Codis	Solmin
Cojene	Solphin
Disprin	Veganin
Duralin	

Dispersible Aspirin BP

This is a combination of aspirin, calcium carbonate and citric acid. When the tablet is dropped into water the calcium carbonate and citric acid react with effervescence and disperse the aspirin into a fine suspension. Dispersible aspirin is more rapidly absorbed (Fig. 11.3) and produces only half as much occult bleeding.

Buffered aspirin

This is a mixture of aspirin and antacids. Effervescent buffered aspirin (Alka-Seltzer) contains enough sodium bicarbonate to exacerbate congestive cardiac failure in susceptible patients. This makes it undesirable for long term use.

By neutralizing some of the gastric acid, buffered aspirin reduces the amount of mucosal injury by aspirin and gastric acid. Compared with dispersible aspirin, a buffered preparation (Bufferin, USA) produces only one third as much occult blood loss. Buffered preparations are more slowly absorbed from the stomach than dispersible and effervescent forms (Fig. 11.3). On the other hand, they speed up gastric emptying.

Glycine-aspirin (Paynocil, UK)

This is highly soluble and will dissolve on the tongue or in the mouth. It can, of course, also be swallowed. Because of the rapid dissolution time,

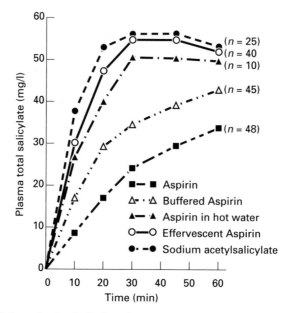

Fig. 11.3   Total plasma levels of salicylate after ingestion of various aspirin preparations. Total dose was equivalent to 640 mg of aspirin in all cases. (Reproduced with permission from Leonards 1963.)

small particle size and rapid absorption, glycine-aspirin causes relatively few gastric erosions.

Enteric coated aspirin

Enteric coated aspirin releases the aspirin only in the relatively alkaline environment of the small intestine. Absorption may not be complete in patients with a rapid intestinal transit time. The size of the tablet may be a deterrent to its use.

Esterified aspirin

Benorylate is an ester of aspirin and paracetamol (Fig. 11.4). It is absorbed intact and hydrolyzed within 15 min in the bloodstream to the two constituent substances. It need be given, however, only b.i.d. The most convenient formulation is a suspension containing 4 g/10 ml. This is equivalent to about 2.3 g of aspirin and 1.9 g of paracetamol. Benorylate causes less faecal blood loss than dispersible aspirin. Tablets containing 750 mg are also available.

Injectable aspirin

A preparation of injectable aspirin is available in some countries (not in

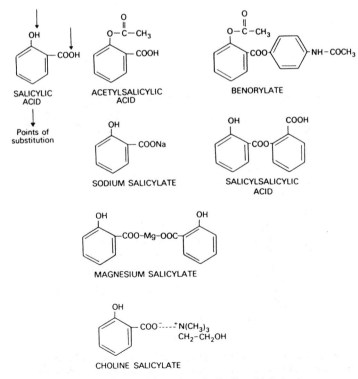

Fig. 11.4 Chemical formulae of salicylic acid derivatives.

the UK or the USA). Lysine-aspirin is prepared in freeze-dried ampoules, each containing 900 mg (equivalent to aspirin 500 mg). In a trial in patients undergoing major gynaecological surgery, 1.8 g of IM lysine-aspirin was shown to be as effective as 10 mg of IM morphine hydrochloride (Kweekel-De Vries et al 1974).

Aspirin suppositories

Aspirin suppositories can be used in patients no longer able to tolerate oral preparations of aspirin. Both 300 and 600 mg sizes are available in the UK; a wider range of strengths is available in the USA. The dose is the same as PO.

NONACETYLATED SALICYLATES

Several nonacetylated salicylates are available (Box 11.C). None interferes with platelet function in normal therapeutic doses. This means that they are safer to use in patients with a bleeding tendency who need a NSAID.

Sodium salicylate is no longer used in the UK. It is less potent than aspirin when used as an occasional analgesic. It is less irritant to the stomach but causes sodium loading if used chronically.

Salsalate

This was the first of the modified salicylates to be introduced. It is an ester of two molecules of salicylic acid (Fig. 11.4). Salsalate is completely absorbed

---

BOX 11.C
SALICYLIC ACID DERIVATIVES

Aspirin (acetylsalcylic acid)
Enteric coated
Buffered
Cation aspirin

- glycine-aspirin
- lysine-aspirin

Benorylate (esterified aspirin-paracetamol)

Nonacetylated salicylates
Cation salicylates

- choline salicylate
- magnesium salicylate
- choline-magnesium trisalicylate

Salsalate (salicylsalicylic acid)
Diflunisal

from the gastro-intestinal tract. It is rapidly hydrolyzed to two molecules of salicylic acid in the body. Only about 10% is conjugated before hydrolysis. The plasma halflife of salsalate is about 1 h. Peak salsalate concentrations are obtained after about 1.5 h; and peak salicylic acid concentrations after 2–4 h. It is insoluble in gastric juice and causes little gastric bleeding. It is relatively slow in onset compared with other NSAIDs but lasts longer; b.i.d. administration is generally sufficient.

Choline salicylate

Choline salicylate is a crystalline powder which is very soluble in water (Fig. 11.4). It is marketed in the USA as Arthropan, an aqueous mint flavoured solution, containing 870 mg/5 ml. This is approximately equivalent to aspirin 650 mg. It causes less gastric injury (Simon & Mills 1980a). It is useful for patients who have difficulty swallowing tablets. In the UK, choline salicylate is available only as a dental gel (8.7%), and is used for treating painful conditions of the mouth.

Choline magnesium trisalicylate

This is a mixture of choline salicylate and magnesium salicylate (Fig. 11.4). Each tablet contains 500 mg of salicylate and a dose schedule of 1–1.5 g b.i.d. is recommended. The plasma halflife varies in a dose dependent manner. At the lower dose the mean plasma halflife of trisalicylate is about 8 h; at the higher dose it is 18 h.

Diflunisal

This is a salicylic acid derivative with a plasma halflife of about 10 h. It is given b.i.d. It causes less faecal blood loss than equivalent doses of aspirin. It also produces a significant decrease in plasma uric acid concentration. Diflunisal affects platelet function only in doses > 500 mg b.i.d..

Diflunisal is well absorbed after oral administration, and peak plasma concentration is attained after about 2 h. Steady state concentration is reached after 3–4 days with a dose of 125 mg b.i.d., after 7–9 days with 500 mg b.i.d. With each doubling of dose, the plasma concentration increases about three times. Bio-availability is reduced by aluminium containing antacids, although this effect is less marked in nonfasting subjects. Concomitant administration of diflunisal with aspirin 2.4 g/day significantly decreases the plasma concentration of diflunisal (Brogden et al 1980).

Diflunisal is not metabolized to salicylic acid. The parent compound is conjugated to glucuronide and excreted in the urine. In renal impairment the terminal halflife increases from 10 h to 115 h when creatinine clearance falls below 2 ml/min. Gastrotoxicity is less common than with aspirin.

Diflunisal has been evaluated in various situations (Brogden et al 1980, Cooper 1983). In postdental extraction pain, diflunisal 250–1000 mg had a greater and longer effect than aspirin 650 mg (Fig. 11.5). Peak analgesic

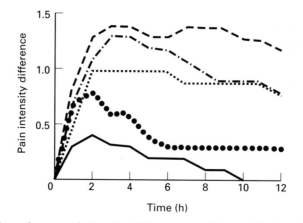

Fig. 11.5   Change in mean pain intensity difference score with time following administration of placebo (—, n = 38), aspirin 650 mg (●, n = 42), diflunisal 250 mg (•••, n = 39), diflunisal 500 mg (-•-, n = 41), and diflunisal 1000 mg (---, n = 41) in 201 patients with postoperative pain following oral surgery. (Reproduced with permission from Forbes et al 1982b.)

effects of diflunisal 500 and 1000 mg are greater than paracetamol 600 mg and paracetamol 600 mg + codeine 60 mg (Forbes et al 1982a). Diflunisal 500 mg is also superior to codeine 60 mg in relieving postdental extraction pain. It is as effective as pentazocine 50 mg in patients with cancer pain.

PARACETAMOL

■ DRUG PORTRAIT

Paracetamol (acetaminophen) is a synthetic nonopioid analgesic. It is also a pharmacologically active metabolite of acetanilide and phenacetin. Like aspirin it is antipyretic. Unlike aspirin, it has no anti-inflammatory effect in most circumstances. As an analgesic it acts centrally, inhibiting brain cyclo-oxygenase (Flower & Vane 1972). It is absorbed mainly from the small intestine. Peak plasma concentrations are achieved in 30–60 min. Paracetamol readily crosses the blood-brain barrier. CSF concentrations peak at 2 h and thereafter remain almost equal to plasma concentrations. The plasma halflife is 2–3 h. Plasma protein binding is negligible, about 10% (Levy 1981).

25% of the population are slow absorbers. When sorbitol is included in the formulation, this figure drops to 10% (Gwilt 1963). Drugs that delay gastric emptying delay absorption. Paracetamol 500–650 mg is definitely more effective than 300 mg, but the effect of 1 g is not always clearly distinguishable from 500–650 mg. Within this range it is equipotent with aspirin.

Paracetamol is metabolized in the liver and mostly excreted in the urine as sulphate or glucuronide. The metabolic pathways are saturable and, in overdosage, an intermediate metabolite causes acute hepatic necrosis which may be fatal (Davis et al 1976). Paracetamol is *not* converted to aniline or paraphenetidin, toxic metabolites of acetanilide and phenacetin respectively (Margetts 1976). A single dose is effective for 4–6 h.

Although paracetamol was known to have analgesic properties in 1893, it was not marketed until the 1950s (Clissold 1986). In 1963, paracetamol was added to the British Pharmacopoeia, since when its popularity as an 'over the counter' analgesic has increased progressively. It is now more popular than aspirin in the UK.

Although paracetamol is a cyclo-oxygenase inhibitor, the drug is not anti-inflammatory in most circumstances. This paradox may be explained by a differential effect on cyclo-oxygenase from different tissues. As noted in Chapter 10, rabbit and dog brain cyclo-oxygenases are sensitive to inhibition by paracetamol while dog spleen cyclo-oxygenase is not (Flower & Vane 1972). Paracetamol has an anti-inflammatory effect in postdental extraction pain; it is more effective than aspirin in reducing both pain and swelling (Skjelbred et al 1977).

Studies indicate that a regular intake of paracetamol 2 g/day may result in an increase in prothrombin time, and necessitate a reduction in the dose of concurrently administered coumarin anticoagulants (Boeijinga et al 1982). The underlying mechanism is not clear, but may relate to interference with the hepatic synthesis of factors II, VII, IX and X.

The other main distinguishing features of paracetamol are that:

- it usually can be taken by those hypersensitive to aspirin
- it does not injure the gastric mucosa
- it is well tolerated by patients with peptic ulcers
- it does not affect plasma uric acid concentration
- it has no effect on platelet function
- liquid preparations are stable
- adverse effects are minor and minimal.

The small differences in absorption observed between commercial preparations of paracetamol are overshadowed by individual differences. Some people are slow absorbers (Prescott & Nimmo 1971). The addition of sorbitol to the formulation improves the rate of absorption in most slow absorbers, possibly by enhancing gastric emptying or increasing the rate of dissolution. Sorbitol is not present in paracetamol BP but is included in several proprietary preparations in the UK (e.g. Panasorb, Panadeine Co., Solpadeine and Panadol Soluble).

Paracetamol can be given by suppository. Rectal bio-availability is 68–88% of oral bio-availability, and the peak plasma concentration is delayed.

Adverse effects

Paracetamol is a very safe drug when used in doses up to 1 g q4h. Unlike phenacetin, paracetamol does not cause methaemoglobinaemia, and haematological disturbances such as thrombocytopenia and agranulocytosis are extremely rare. Allergic reactions to paracetamol are rare but sporadic cases of urticaria, bronchospasm and anaphylaxis have been reported (Stricker et al 1985). Symptoms usually appear within 1 h of ingestion. Only 5% of people, who are sensitive to aspirin, however, have a cross-sensitivity to paracetamol (Settipane 1981).

Sporadic cases of paracetamol related cholestatic jaundice have been reported (Waldum et al 1992, Wong et al 1993).

In overdose, paracetamol causes severe hepatocellular necrosis. Hepato-toxicity is caused by the formation in the hepatic parenchymal cell of a minor metabolite with high alkylating activity (Prescott 1980). This binds covalently to cell constituents causing damage and necrosis. The small amount of this metabolite formed with therapeutic doses is rapidly detoxified by conjugation with reduced glutathione. With toxic doses, glutathione is depleted and the excess metabolite is free to damage hepatic cells.

In adults, the threshold dose for liver toxicity is about 250 mg/kg (equal to about 15 g in a 60 kg person), whereas the maximum single therapeutic dose is about 15 mg/kg, i.e. 1 g (Prescott 1986). The smallest reported fatal overdose is 18 g. Many have survived with doses of up to 25 g. Above this level, death is increasingly likely unless specific treatment is instituted, though survival has been reported after 75 g. Antidotes such as IV acetylcysteine or oral methionine (both precursors of glutathione) protect the liver if given within 10–12 h of paracetamol ingestion. In fact, acetylcysteine may be effective for 24 h or even longer (BNF 1993).

There is, however, considerable individual variation in susceptibility to the toxicity of paracetamol after overdosage (Mitchell 1977). Some patients may be at greater risk because of increased activity of the specific iso-enzyme responsible for the metabolic activation of paracetamol or decreased capacity for glutathione synthesis resulting from malnutrition. Chronic alcoholics are more vulnerable but, even so, with therapeutic doses, it is not possible to reach the threshold for toxicity (Prescott 1986).

On the other hand, chronic hepatic necrosis has been reported in a man who took paracetamol 4 g/day for a year (Bonkowsky et al 1978), and in another patient paracetamol 2.9 g/day exacerbated chronic active hepatitis and cirrhosis (Johnson & Tolman 1977). Even so, the recommendation of the British National Formulary (BNF) to limit the maximum dose of para-cetamol to 4 g/day is unnecessarily cautious. At many palliative care units, this dose is regularly exceeded.

NONSTEROIDAL ANTI-INFLAMMATORY DRUGS (NSAIDs)

Aspirin and salicylic acid were the only NSAIDs until phenylbutazone was marketed in 1952 and indomethacin in 1964. Since then the number has rapidly increased (Box 11.D). As noted in Chapter 10, by modifying the inflammatory process, NSAIDs cause a reduction in local heat, swelling and stiffness. They also relieve pain, partly in consequence of the anti-inflammatory effect. NSAIDs are not disease specific and do not modify the disease process other than by reducing inflammation. NSAIDs are more effective than corticosteroids in treating neoplastic fever (Warshaw et al 1981, Chang 1988). NSAIDs vary widely in their pharmacokinetic characteristics (Table 11.3).

In single dose studies, NSAIDs demonstrate a plateau effect beyond which increasing amounts produce little or no additional relief. They are generally

BOX 11.D
CLASSIFICATION OF NSAIDS

Salicylates (see Box 11.C)
Aspirin
Salicylates

Propionates
Fenbufen
Fenoprofen
Flurbiprofen
Ibuprofen
Ketoprofen
Ketorolac
Naproxen
Tiaprofenic acid

Acetates
Alclofenac
Diclofenac
Etodolac
Indomethacin
Sulindac
Tolmetin

Fenamates
Flufenamic acid
Mefenamic acid

Oxicams
Piroxicam
Tenoxicam

Pyrazolones
Azapropazone
Oxyphenbutazone
Phenylbutazone

Butazones
Nabumetone

Table 11.3 NSAID pharmacokinetics

Drug	Halflife (h)	Protein binding (%)	Urinary excretion (%)	Active metabolite
Aspirin	0.25	70	< 5	+
Azapropazone	13	99	60	−
Diclofenac	1.5	99	< 5	?
Diflunisal	5–20[a]	99	5	−
Etodolac	3	99	5	
Fenbufen	10	99	5	+
Fenoprofen	3	99	5	?
Flufenamic acid	9	90	< 5	
Flurbiprofen	3.5	99	10	
Ibuprofen	2.5	99	< 5	
Indomethacin	5	90	15	
Ketoprofen	1–5	95	25	
Ketorolac	5	99	60	
Mefenamic acid	3.5	high	10	
Nabumetone	26	99	< 5	+
Naproxen	14	99	10	
Phenylbutazone	70	99	< 5	+
Piroxicam	45	99	10	
Salicylate	2–30[a]	85	10	
Sulindac	7	96	< 5	+
Tenoxicam	72	99	< 5	
Tiaprofenic Acid	2	98		
Tolmetin	1	99	5	

[a] Dose dependent elimination.
From Rawlins 1993

well tolerated by mouth. Gastrotoxicity is usually less than with aspirin, and occult bleeding is often within the normal range. A patient who cannot tolerate one NSAID may find another more acceptable. Most NSAIDs cause constipation when taken regularly, although diflunisal, flurbiprofen, indomethacin and ketorolac can cause diarrhoea and mefenamic acid commonly does so. Like aspirin, NSAIDs interfere with platelet function and prolong bleeding time. Unlike aspirin, this effect is reversible. NSAIDs commonly cause sodium and water retention, and thereby reduce the effect of diuretics. NSAIDs exhibit a number of important pharmacokinetic interactions (Table 11.4).

Most NSAIDs are highly bound to plasma protein (mainly albumin) but they are not all bound primarily to the same sites. At normal plasma concentrations, each drug binds preferentially to one of three major sites which may be designated diazepam, digoxin and warfarin sites (Busson 1984). The secondary and tertiary sites are occupied only at higher plasma concentrations. Thus, with normal doses, a drug is unlikely to displace other drugs bound to these sites. This explains why ibuprofen, for example, can usually be prescribed safely with coumarin anticoagulants and oral hypoglycaemics but aspirin cannot.

Choice of NSAID

In rheumatoid arthritis and related arthropathies, it is accepted that considerable variation exists between patients both with respect to response and to tolerability. Even if a controlled trial shows that one drug is more efficacious than another, the 'better' drug may not be better for a given individual. This variability is particularly marked with the weaker propionic acid derivatives. As yet, no such variability has been shown in metastatic bone pain, but that is not to say it does not exist.

Comments on individual NSAIDs are included for the following reasons:

- ibuprofen — widely used and available 'over the counter'
- flurbiprofen — NSAID of choice at Sobell House
- naproxen — NSAID of choice at many centres
- dipyrone — not available in the UK and USA but used extensively in many countries
- indomethacin — widely available and still used at some centres
- mefenamic acid — broader mechanism of action
- diclofenac — used increasingly and available as an injection
- ketorolac — an alternative parenteral NSAID
- benzydamine — used as an oral rinse and topically.

Ibuprofen

■ DRUG PORTRAIT

Ibuprofen was the first of the propionic acid derivatives to be introduced. It is widely available throughout the world and, because it is well tolerated, can

Table 11.4 Pharmacokinetic interactions with NSAIDs

Drug affected	NSAIDs implicated	Effect	Approach to management
NSAID affecting other drug			
Oral anticoagulants	Azapropazone Oxyphenbutazone Phenylbutazone	Inhibition of metabolism of warfarin, increasing anticoagulant effect	Avoid this group of NSAIDs; monitor where unavoidable (*note* pharmacodynamic interactions also)
Lithium	Probably all NSAIDs (? except sulindac, aspirin)	Inhibition of renal excretion of lithium, increasing lithium serum concentrations and increasing risk of toxicity	Use sulindac or aspirin if NSAID unavoidable; monitor lithium concentration and reduce dose accordingly
Oral hypoglycaemic agents	Azapropazone Oxyphenbutazone Phenylbutazone	Inhibition of metabolism of sulphonylurea drugs, prolonging halflife and increasing risk of hypoglycaemia	Avoid this group of NSAIDs
Phenytoin	Oxyphenbutazone Phenylbutazone	Inhibition of metabolism of phenytoin, increasing plasma concentration and risk of toxicity	Avoid this group of NSAIDs
	Other NSAIDs	Displacement of phenytoin from plasma protein	Careful interpretation of phenytoin concentration; measurement of unbound concentration may be helpful
Methotrexate	Probably all NSAIDs	Reduced clearance of methotrexate (mechanism unclear) increasing plasma concentration and risk of severe toxicity	Simultaneous dosing is contra-indicated; NSAIDs between cycles of chemotherapy probably safe
Sodium valproate	Aspirin	Inhibition of valproate metabolism increasing plasma concentration	Avoid aspirin; monitor plasma concentration with other NSAIDs
Digoxin	All NSAIDs	Potential reduction in renal function (particularly in very young and very old) reducing digoxin clearance and increasing plasma concentration and risk of toxicity (No interaction if renal function normal)	Avoid NSAIDs if possible; if not, check digoxin plasma concentration and plasma creatinine
Aminoglycosides	All NSAIDs	Reduction in renal function in susceptible individuals, reducing aminoglycoside clearance and increasing plasma concentration	Monitor plasma concentration and adjust dose

Table 11.4 (contd)

Drug affected	NSAIDs implicated	Effect	Approach to management
Other drug affecting NSAID			
Antacids	Indomethacin ? other NSAIDs	Variable effects of different preparations: — aluminium containing antacids reduce rate and extent of absorption of indomethacin — sodium bicarbonate increases rate and extent of absorption of indomethacin	No action required unless reduction in absorption results in poor response to NSAID; dose may need to be increased
Probenecid	Probably all NSAIDs	Reduction in metabolism and renal clearance of NSAIDs and glucuronide metabolites which are hydrolyzed back to parent drug	May be used therapeutically to increase the response to NSAID
Barbiturates	Phenylbutazone ? other NSAIDs	Increased metabolic clearance of NSAID	May require higher dose of phenylbutazone
Caffeine	Aspirin	Increased rate of absorption of aspirin	No action required
Cholestyramine	Naproxen ? other NSAIDs	Anion exchange resin binds NSAIDs in gut reducing rate (? and extent) of absorption	Separate dosing times by 4 h; may need higher dose of NSAID
Metoclopramide	Aspirin	Increased rate and extent of absorption of aspirin in patients with migraine	May be used therapeutically

From Tonkin & Wing 1988 (modified)

be purchased without prescription. Ibuprofen is also safe in overdose. No deaths have been reported with ibuprofen alone, even with a single dose of 40 g (Busson 1984). Ibuprofen is rapidly absorbed after oral administration; peak plasma concentrations occurring within 2 h. The plasma halflife is about 2 h. With chronic pain, ibuprofen generally needs to be taken q.i.d.

In doses up to 1200 mg/day, ibuprofen acts predominantly as an analgesic. Its anti-inflammatory properties are more evident at higher doses. Doses of 2400 mg/day are well tolerated by most patients. Tablets are available in 200, 400 and 600 mg size. Mg for mg, ibuprofen is three times more potent than aspirin, i.e. 200 mg is equivalent to 600 mg of aspirin. Thus higher doses of ibuprofen will have a greater analgesic effect than standard doses of aspirin.

Flurbiprofen

■ DRUG PORTRAIT

Flurbiprofen is a strong NSAID. It is rapidly absorbed following oral administration, with peak plasma concentrations 90 min after a single dose. Although the plasma halflife is under 4 h, flurbiprofen is best given b.i.d. (Kowanko et al 1981). It is excreted in the urine both as unchanged drug and a number of hydroxylated metabolites. Usual doses are 50–100 mg b.i.d.

Flurbiprofen is the NSAID of choice at Sobell House. The maximum effective dose in metastatic bone pain has not been established. Occasionally, massive fluid retention has occurred in patients receiving 100 mg t.i.d. Flurbiprofen causes diarrhoea in some patients.

Considerable emphasis has been placed on the extremely good showing of flurbiprofen as an in vitro inhibitor of PG synthesis (Table 11.5). In vitro and in vivo are not the same, however, nor is potency synonymous with efficacy. The poor position held by aspirin in the league table indicates that such studies are not a guide to clinical efficacy. It is wrong to conclude that flurbiprofen is clinically superior to all other NSAIDS. In various animal and clinical studies, flurbiprofen has been shown to be 8–20 times more potent than aspirin.

Table 11.5 Relative molar potencies of NSAIDs for 50% inhibition of PGE_2 synthesis in vitro

Drug	Molar potency relative to aspirin
Flurbiprofen	5610
Indomethacin	257
Naproxen	45
Ibuprofen	22
Phenylbutazone	3
Aspirin	1
Salicylic acid	< 0.02
Paracetamol	< 0.01

From Crook et al 1976

Flurbiprofen has been used in cases of instability of the detrusor of the urinary bladder. A number of PGs stimulate contraction of the human bladder muscle in vitro. Animal studies indicate that PGs are produced naturally by the detrusor and increase tone and spontaneous activity. In man, frequency, urgency and urge incontinence were all significantly reduced by flurbiprofen 50 mg t.i.d. compared with placebo (Cardozo et al 1980). Flurbiprofen was well tolerated by most patients.

Naproxen

■ DRUG PORTRAIT

Naproxen is a propionic acid derivative and a strong NSAID. It is readily absorbed when given orally. Naproxen is also absorbed rectally but peak concentrations in plasma are achieved more slowly. The plasma halflife is about 14 h. Naproxen and its metabolites are almost entirely excreted in the urine. Usual doses are 250–500 mg b.i.d.

Naproxen is the NSAID of choice at many centres. Plasma concentrations do not increase at doses greater than 500 mg b.i.d., because of the rapid urinary excretion and the extent of plasma binding (Simon & Mills 1980b). Higher plasma concentrations can be obtained, however, on a q6h regimen to a maximum of about 1400 mg/day, but whether this results in improved pain relief has yet to be determined (Sevelius et al 1980).

Naproxen sodium is also available; 550 mg is equivalent to 500 mg naproxen. Naproxen sodium is more rapidly absorbed, and results in higher plasma concentrations, and an earlier onset of action (Sevelius et al 1980).

Dipyrone

■ DRUG PORTRAIT

Dipyrone (metamizol) is a unique NSAID in that it has an antispasmodic effect in addition to analgesic, antipyretic and weak anti-inflammatory properties. Its effect on the sphincter of Oddi is comparable to that of hyoscine butylbromide (Brandstatter 1983, Brandstatter et al 1990). It has central effects (both spinal and supraspinal) and also relieves experimentally induced hyperalgesia in animals (see p. 176). Dipyrone inhibits cyclo-oxygenase most markedly in brain tissues (Brune 1980). Postoperatively, IM dipyrone 2.5 g is equivalent to pethidine 100 mg.

Like most NSAIDs, dipyrone has a reversible effect on platelet function. It is not available in some countries including the UK and the USA because of fears about agranulocytosis. Formulations vary from country to country but include tablets, drops, syrup, suppositories and ampoules for injection. The maximum recommended oral dose is 1 g (2 tablets) q.i.d.

Dipyrone is a widely used nonopioid analgesic. The combination of central and peripheral actions makes it an attractive option. Unfortunately, concern about agranulocytosis has led to its withdrawal in some countries. In 1978, however, the *International Agranulocytosis and Aplastic Anaemia Study* was commissioned by the manufacturers. The results were published in 1991 (Kaufman et al 1991). The epidemiological data was collected from several centres throughout Europe and from Israel. An unexplained dichotomy emerged. The relative risk of developing agranulocytosis while taking dipyrone was increased 13 and 23 times in Germany and Spain respectively, but was not significantly increased elsewhere. Most cases of agranulocytosis associated with dipyrone occured in the first 2 weeks of use. The incidence of agranulocytosis did not fall after dipyrone was withdrawn from Sweden.

The excess risk of agranulocytosis with dipyrone is less than 1 case/million weeks of use. In comparison, the excess risk of serious gastro-intestinal bleeding with aspirn is 8 cases/million weeks of use (Kaufman et al 1991). Both adverse effects carry a mortality risk of about 10%. Dipyrone is, therefore, significantly safer than aspirin. Further, as already noted, dipyrone has a broader mode of action and can be given by injection.

Indomethacin

■ DRUG PORTRAIT
Indomethacin is a strong NSAID. It is rapidly absorbed from the gastro-intestinal tract, when give orally or as a suppository. The plasma halflife is 5 h. Indomethacin and its metabolites are excreted mainly in the urine and, to a lesser extent, in the faeces. Usual doses are 75–200 mg/day given in divided doses.

In addition to inhibiting cyclo-oxygenase, indomethacin has been shown to exert anti-inflammatory effects in other ways. For example, in rats it interferes with the migration of leucocytes into inflammatory sites. It also increases the intracellular concentration of cyclic AMP by inhibition of phosphodiesterase. (Cyclic AMP stabilizes lysosomal membranes in polymorphonuclear leucocytes and macrophages.)

Indomethacin can produce almost every alimentary tract symptom from angular stomatitis to pruritis ani. Gastric toxicity is the most common. Headache occurs in about 50% of patients when the total daily dose exceeds 100 mg. In cancer patients this may be masked if the patient is also receiving an opioid. Indomethacin, like flurbiprofen, is of benefit in detrusor instability but, in a dose of 100 mg b.i.d., headache and nausea occurred in 60% of cases (Cardozo & Stanton 1980).

Other central nervous system (CNS) effects are dizziness, drowsiness, dysphoria, delirium, hallucinations, depression, seizures and syncope. Taken with haloperidol, indomethacin may cause profound drowsiness (Bird et al 1983).

Mefenamic acid

■ DRUG PORTRAIT
Mefenamic acid is a derivative of fenamic acid. It inhibits cyclo-oxygenase like other NSAIDs but also blocks PG receptors in the cell wall (Tolman & Partridge 1975). It is well absorbed from the gastro-intestinal tract, and the

plasma halflife is 3–4 h. In man 20% of the drug is excreted in the faeces. Usual doses are 250–500 mg t.i.d.

Mefenamic acid is the most commonly used fenamate. The major gastro-intestinal adverse effect is diarrhoea, which occurs in over 10% of patients.

In some countries its use is not recommended for more than 1 week because of the likelihood of adverse gastro-intestinal effects and nephro-toxicity (Abruzzo 1981). It is not superior to aspirin. At some centres, mefenamic acid is used in conjunction with other NSAIDs, presumably with the hope that there will be an additive effect because of its dual mechanisms of action.

Diclofenac

■ DRUG PORTRAIT

Diclofenac is a well tolerated NSAID. About 10% of patients experience adverse effects but these are usually mild and transient. In only 2% does the drug need to be withdrawn, usually because of gastric intolerance (Todd & Sorkin 1988). Mean plasma halflife is about 1.5 h. Age and renal or hepatic impairment do not have any significant effect on plasma concentrations of diclofenac, although metabolite concentrations are increased in severe renal failure. The principal metabolite, hydroxydiclofenac possesses little anti-inflammatory effect. Diclofenac does not interact with coumarin anticoagulants or oral hypoglycaemic agents. Diclofenac is available as both tablets and suppositories. Diclofenac can also be given by injection (75 mg in 3 ml). Tablets are either enteric coated or m/r. Peak plasma concentration may be delayed for several hours if taken after food. Diclofenac is rapidly and completely absorbed after oral administration (John 1979). Naloxone delays the onset of diclofenac induced analgesia.

For cancer pain, diclofenac usually needs to be given q8h to maintain optimum 'round the clock' relief. M/r preparations are designed to provide relief for 24 h but sometimes are best given b.i.d. The manufacturer's licence is for 100–150 mg/day. Many patients have been prescribed 200 mg/day (i.e. 100 mg b.i.d.), however, with no adverse effects but with greater benefit.

Although diclofenac is a potent reversible inhibitor of *induced* platelet aggregation, at usual oral therapeutic doses it has no effect on platelet adhesiveness or bleeding time (Todd & Sorkin 1988). IV diclofenac, however, does have a measurable effect on bleeding time although most subjects remain within the normal range.

Many established NSAIDs manifest rare or severe adverse effects which are never, or hardly ever, observed with diclofenac. For example, acute pancreatitis has been reported with sulindac and aseptic meningitis with ibuprofen but not with diclofenac. Cutaneous reactions and photosensitivity are likewise rare with diclofenac.

IM diclofenac is more effective than various opioid-spasmolytic combinations in biliary and renal colic (Lundstam et al 1982, Thompson et al

1989). If administered by SC infusion, it must be given alone because it is immiscible with other drugs.

Ketorolac

■ DRUG PORTRAIT

Ketorolac is structurally related to the acetate NSAIDs tolmetin and indomethacin but is described as a cyclic propionate (Buckley & Brogden 1990, Litvak & McEvoy 1990). It is available as ketorolac trometamol (tromethamine) which is more water soluble. Over 99% of the oral dose is absorbed and systemic bio-availability is over 80%. Peak plasma levels are reached after 30 min by the oral route, and after 45 min IM.

The plasma halflife of ketorolac is about 5 h by both PO and IM routes. In the elderly this increases to 6–7 h (Greenwald 1992). About 75% of a dose is excreted in the urine within 7 h, and over 90% within 2 days (Litvak & McEvoy 1990), nearly two thirds as unmodified ketorolac. The rest is excreted in the faeces. Because of adverse reactions, mainly gastric haemorrhage, the original dose recommendations have been revised, with an emphasis on short term use. In the UK, ketorolac is available in 10 mg tablets and in ampoules containing either 10 mg/ml or 30 mg/ml. In the USA it is available in two strengths 15 mg/ml and 60 mg/2 ml. The duration of useful analgesia is 6–8 h. Ketorolac is used mainly as a postoperative analgesic.

The analgesic and anti-inflammatory activity of ketorolac resides mainly in the laevorotatory isomer. The analgesic effect is far greater than the antipyretic and anti-inflammatory properties. In animal studies, ketorolac is about 350 times more potent than aspirin as an analgesic but only 20 times more potent as an antipyretic (Greenwald 1992). As an anti-inflammatory ketorolac is about half as potent as indomethacin and twice as potent as naproxen. Like most NSAIDs, ketorolac inhibits platelet aggregation.

Oral ketorolac has been evaluated in postdental extraction pain. Ketorolac 10 mg PO was significantly superior to aspirin 650 mg for peak and total effects and superior to paracetamol 600 mg and codeine 60 mg for total effect (Forbes et al 1990a). Ketorolac 10 mg and 20 mg and ibuprofen 400 mg provided equal relief (Forbes et al 1990b). In another postoperative study, ketorolac 10 mg PO and naproxen sodium 550 mg PO gave equal relief, and both were better than morphine 10 mg IM (Brown et al 1990).

Ketorolac is used by some palliative care units when a parenteral NSAID is indicated, with misoprostol 200 µg t.i.d. PO (Pye & Trotman 1993). It is compatible with both physiological saline and 5% dextrose. It is precipitated by morphine, pethidine, hydroxyzine and promethazine. It should, therefore, be drawn up in a separate syringe (Litvak & McEvoy 1990). It does not irritate tissue and can be given SC.

Benzydamine

■ DRUG PORTRAIT

Benzydamine is a unique NSAID with local anaesthetic properties. It is absorbed transdermally, and is concentrated in inflamed tissue. Benzydamine stabilizes cell membranes and thereby reduces the response to inflammatory mediators.

Benzydamine oral rinse or spray is a useful local analgesic in oropharyngeal mucositis caused by radiotherapy and chemotherapy (Kim et al 1985, Epstein et al 1989). Benzydamine has also been used as a 3% aqueous cream to relieve the pain of decubitus ulcers (Jepson 1992). After applying the cream, the pressure sore and inflamed area was enclosed in a semipermeable film held loosely in place by adhesive tape. In a preliminary study, 17 patients (aged 54–91 years) with 30 ulcers were treated. All were confined to chairs or bed and all but four had advanced malignant disease. After 48 h all were painfree, 29 within 24 h. The surrounding inflammation was much reduced.

TRANSDERMAL NSAIDs

The rationale behind transdermal NSAIDs is local benefit without systemic adverse effects. Several transdermal preparations are available:

- ibuprofen cream
- felbinac gel
- piroxicam gel.

In contrast to other transdermal systems (e.g. fentanyl, hyoscine, nitrates), the aim is to limit systemic availability. Can this be achieved? Fat solubility is necessary for satisfactory penetration of the skin but rapid transfer into the systemic circulation from skin capillaries usually prevents local accumulation. There is some evidence to suggest, however, that topically applied salicylates and certain other NSAIDs (e.g. diclofenac, ibuprofen, indomethacin) can achieve high local SC concentrations (Chlud & Wagener 1987). In synovial fluid and peri-articular tissues, these may approach the therapeutically effective concentrations expected from the oral administration of the same drugs.

In the UK, ibuprofen cream is available without prescription. Application to the skin produces plasma concentrations which are 5% of those obtained with oral administration, whereas the muscle and fascial concentrations are 25 times greater (Mondino et al 1983, Kageyama 1987). A randomized placebo-controlled double-blind trial in 80 patients with sprains and bruises showed that patients treated with transdermal ibuprofen fared significantly better in terms of (Peters et al 1987):

- speed of resolution
- relief of pain
- reduction in swelling
- return of function.

Evidence of benefit is less clear in relation to felbinac and piroxicam (Anonymous 1990). Topical gels have not been compared with standard oral formulations. The use of transdermal NSAIDs other than ibuprofen, therefore, cannot be recommended.

PRURITUS AND PAIN IN EN CUIRASS BREAST CANCER

From time to time a patient with breast cancer complains of both pruritus and pain in association with en cuirass breast cancer.

■ CASE HISTORY

A 73 year-old woman with recurrent breast cancer experienced pain in the affected area over the right breast and chest wall. At the time of referral, symptoms had been present for about a year. Several opioids had already been tried but stopped because of vomiting. She had also had various nerve blocks, including intrathecal blocks with either phenol or chlorocresol. After these, the pain was no better and she experienced in addition some weakness and discomfort in the right thigh. She became depressed and distressed by the lack of success.

It was considered that 'the major problem is psychogenic'. Two weeks after starting mianserin 10 mg t.i.d. she was noted to be generally better and eating well, but still in pain. When admitted to a palliative care unit, the patient was taking only mianserin and flurazepam as a night sedative. Treatment was started with co-proxamol 2 tablets q4h and the mianserin was continued as a single 30 mg dose at bedtime. As the co-proxamol did not provide much relief, flurbiprofen 100 mg t.i.d. was added. Within 2–3 days the chest wall and arm became almost completely free of pain and pruritus. Her mood improved and she became more active and completely independent. She was discharged after 2 weeks. Apart from a second short admission for other reasons, she spent nearly 2 months at home essentially painfree before she deteriorated rapidly and died, probably as a result of a cerebral metastasis.

Certain PGs intensify both pain and pruritus (Editorial 1980). The concurrence of both symptoms in patients with cutaneous metastases from breast cancer, therefore, is understandable. Although the relative and absolute intensity of the pain and pruritus varies, much relief has been obtained in several patients with this syndrome with either flurbiprofen or naproxen.

NEFOPAM

■ DRUG PROTRAIT

Nefopam is a synthetic nonopioid analgesic. It is the only member of the benzoxazocine class of analgesics. It is chemically related to orphenadrine and diphenhydramine, but does not have antiParkinsonian or antihistaminic properties. It is centrally acting, although its mechanism of action is not known. Nefopam causes a reduction in the ventilatory response to carbon dioxide, which is not dose dependent (Bhatt et al 1981). It has no effect on opioid withdrawal (Gasser & Bellville 1975), and its effects are not reversed by naloxone. It does not inhibit cyclo-oxygenase. It lowers normal body temperature but its action on fever has not been evaluated. It has anticholinergic and sympathomimetic effects which are not usually noticeable unless other drugs with similar properties are taken concurrently.

Nefopam is available as a tablet and an injection. The plasma concentration and the analgesic effect peak after about 2 h when given PO and about 1.5 h after IM injection. The oral to parenteral potency ratio is 1:3. The plasma halflife is about 5 h. Nefopam is excreted mostly as an inactive metabolite in the urine. In the UK, nefopam is available as a 30 mg tablet and a 20 mg injection. The manufacturers recommend an initial oral dose of 60 mg q8h (30 mg in elderly patients), or 20 mg IM q6h. Usual oral doses are 30–90 mg q8h.

Most clinical trials have been in patients with nonmalignant pain. Nefopam 15 mg IM is approximately equivalent to 50 mg of pethidine (Tigerstedt et al 1977). There is probably a low ceiling effect. In one study, nefopam 30 mg IM was no more effective than 15 mg, although it lasted longer and was associated with a higher frequency of adverse effects (Sunshine & Laska 1975). In another study, nefopam 22 mg IM was more effective than 11 mg, and the higher dose was comparable to morphine 4 mg IM (Beaver & Feise 1977). In patients with episiotomy pain, nefopam 45 mg and 90 mg PO gave comparable analgesia to dextropropoxyphene hydrochloride 65 mg (Bloomfield et al 1980). A relatively low ceiling effect may explain why the reported potency ratio of nefopam to morphine varies between 1:1.66 and 1:3 (Sunshine & Laska 1975, Beaver & Feise 1977).

The main adverse effects are dryness of the mouth and insomnia. Other reported adverse effects include nausea, nervousness and lightheadedness. Less frequently, vomiting, blurred vision, drowsiness, sweating, tachycardia and headache occur. These effects are dose related and usually transient. Nefopam may colour urine pink. In overdose, nefopam causes CNS excitation. This should be treated with diazepam PO/PR or midazolam SC.

The following precautions should be noted:

- because nefopam is anticholinergic it should be used with caution in patients with glaucoma or hesitancy of micturition
- because nefopam enhances motor neurone activity, patients with epilepsy should not take it
- in dogs, high doses of nefopam increase the hepatotoxicity of high doses of paracetamol.

Although this latter effect is not seen with therapeutic doses, it is probably wise to monitor liver function if nefopam and paracetamol are prescribed concurrently in patients with known hepatic dysfunction.

Unlike other nonopioids, nefopam is a step 2 analgesic, i.e. an alternative to a weak opioid when the latter are not available or cause unacceptable adverse effects.

REFERENCES

Abruzzo J L 1981 Anti-inflammatory and antirheumatic drugs. Annals of Internal Medicine 94: 270–271
Anonymous 1987 NSAIDs for renal and biliary colic: intramuscular diclofenac. Drug and Therapeutics Bulletin 25: 85–86
Anonymous 1990 More topical NSAIDs: worth the rub? Drugs and Therapeutics Bulletin 28: 27–28
Beaver W T, Feise G A 1977 A comparison of the analgesic effect of intramuscular nefopam and morphine in patients with postoperative pain. Journal of Clinical Pharmacology 17: 579–591
Bhatt A M, Pleuvry B J, Maddison S E 1981 Respiratory and metabolic effects of oral nefopam in human volunteers. British Journal of Clinical Pharmacology 11: 209–211
Bird H A, Le Gallez P, Wright V 1983 Drowsiness due to haloperidol/indomethacin in combination. Lancet i: 830–831
Bloomfield S S, Barden T P, Mitchell J 1980 Nefopam and propoxyphene in episiotomy pain. Clinical Pharmacology and Therapeutics 27: 502–507
Boeijinga J J, Boerstra E E, Ris P, Breimer D D, Jeletich-Bastiaanse A 1982 Interaction between paracetamol and coumarin anticoagulants. Lancet i: 506
Bonkowsky H L, Mudge G H, McMurtry R J 1978 Chronic hepatic inflammation and fibrosis due to low doses of paracetamol. Lancet i: 1016–1018
Brandstatter G 1983 Pharmacological pressure reduction in the human common bile duct. Zeitschrift fuer Gastroenterologie 21: 168–174
Brandstatter G, Kratochvil P, Kalhammer R, Schinzel S 1990 The effect of metamizol on motility of sphincter of Oddi. Poster presented at World Congresses of Gastroenterology, Digestive Endoscopy, and Colo-proctology.
British National Formulary 1993 Emergency treatment of poisoning. In: British National Formulary, No. 25. British Medical Association, London, pp 15–22
Brogden R W, Heel R C, Pakes G E, Speight T M, Avery G S 1980 Diflunisal: a review of its pharmacological properties and therapeutic use in pain and musculoskeletal strains and sprains and pain in osteoarthritis. Drugs 19: 84–106
Brown C R, Moodie J E, Dickie G et al 1990 Analgesic efficacy and safety of single dose oral and intramuscular ketorolac tromethamine for postoperative pain. Pharmacotherapy 10: 59s–70s
Brune K 1980 Biodistribution of mild analgesics. British Journal of Clinical Pharmacology 20: 279
Buckley M M-T, Brogden R N 1990 Ketorolac: a review of its pharmacodynamic and pharmacokinetic properties, and therapeutic potential. Drugs 39: 86–109
Busson M 1984 Update on ibuprofen: review article. Journal of International Medical Research 14: 53–62
Cardozo L D, Stanton S L 1980 A comparison between bromocriptine and indomethacin in the treatment of detrusor instability. Journal of Urology 124: 281–282
Cardozo L D, Stanton S L, Robinson H, Hole D 1980 Evaluation of flurbiprofen in detrusor instability. British Medical Journal 280: 281–282
Chang J C 1988 Antipyretic effect of naproxen and corticosteroids on neoplastic fever. Journal of Pain and Symptom Management 3: 141–144
Chlud K, Wagener H H 1987 Percutaneous nonsteroidal anti-inflammatory drug (NSAID) therapy with particular reference to pharmacokinetic factors. EULAR Bulletin 2: 40–43
Clissold S P 1986 Paracetamol and phenacetin. Drugs 32 (suppl 4): 46–59
Cooper S A 1981 Comparative analgesic efficacies of aspirin and acetaminophen. Archives of Internal Medicine 141: 282–285
Cooper S A 1983 New peripherally-acting oral analgesic agent. Annual Review of Pharmacology and Toxicology 23: 617–647
Crook D, Collins A J, Bacon P A, Chan R 1976 Effect of aspirin-like drug therapy. Prostaglandin synthetase activity from human rheumatoid synovial microsomes. Annals of the Rheumatic Diseases 35: 327–332
Davis M, Labadarios D, Williams R S 1976 Metabolism of paracetamol after therapeutic and hepatotoxic doses in man. Journal of International Medical Research 4 (suppl 4): 40–45
Editorial 1980 Itch. Lancet ii: 568–569
Epstein J B, Stevenson-Moore P, Jackson S et al 1989 International Journal of Radiation, Oncology, Biology and Physics 16: 1571–1575

Ferreira S 1981 Peripheral and central analgesia. Abstracts 3rd World Congress on Pain, Edinburgh

Flower R J, Vane J R 1972 Inhibition of prostaglandin synthetase in brain explains the antipyretic actions of paracetamol. Nature 240: 410–411

Flower R J, Moncada S, Vane J R 1980 Analgesic-antipyretics and anti-inflammatory agents; drugs employed in the treatment of gout. In: Gilman A G, Goodman L S, Gilman A (eds) Goodman and Gilman's the pharmacological basis of therapeutics, 6th edn. Macmillan, New York, pp 682–728

Forbes J A, Beaver W T, White E H, White R W, Neilson G B, Shackleford R W 1982a A new oral analgesic with an unusually long duration of action. Journal of the American Medical Association 248: 2139–2142

Forbes J A, Calderazzo J P, Bowser M W, Foor V M, Shackleford R W, Beaver W T 1982b A 12 hour evaluation of the analgesic efficacy of diflunisal, aspirin, and placebo in post-operative dental pain. Journal of Clinical Pharmacology 22: 89–96

Forbes J A, Butterworth G A, Burchfield W H, Beaver W T 1990a Evaluation of ketorolac, aspirin, and an acetaminophen-codeine combination in postoperative oral surgery pain. Pharmacotherapy 10: 77s–93s

Forbes J A, Kehm C J, Grodin C D, Beaver W T 1990b Evaluation of ketorolac, ibuprofen, acetaminophen and an acetaminophen-codeine combination in postoperative oral surgery pain. Pharmacotherapy 10: 94s–105s

Gasser J C, Bellville J W 1975 Respiratory effects of nefopam. Clinical Pharmacology and Therapeutics 18: 175–179

Greenwald R A 1992 Ketorolac: an innovative nonsteroidal analgesic. Drugs of Today 28: 41–61

Grond S, Zech D, Schug S A, Lynch J 1991 Validation of World Health Organization guidelines for cancer pain relief during the last days and hours of life. Journal of Pain and Symptom Management 6: 411–422

Gwilt J R 1963 The absorption characteristics of paracetamol tablets in man. Journal of Pharmacy and Pharmacology 15: 445–453

Jepson B A 1992 Relieving the pain of pressure sores. Lancet 339: 503–504

John V A 1979 The pharmacokinetics and metabolism of diclofenac sodium (Voltarol) in animals and man. Rheumatology & Rehabilitation Suppl 2: 22–37

Johnson G K, Tolman K G 1977 Chronic liver disease and acetaminophen. Annals of Internal Medicine 87: 302–304

Kageyama T 1987 European Journal of Rheumatology and Inflammation 8: 114–115

Kaufman D W, Kelly J P, Levy M, Shapiro S 1991 The drug etiology of agranulocytosis and aplastic anaemia. Oxford University Press, New York

Kim J H, Chu F, Lakshmi V, Houde R 1985 A clinical study of benzydamine for the treatment of radiotherapy induced mucositis of the oropharynx. International Journal of Tissue Reaction 7: 215–218

Kowanko I C, Pownall R, Knapp M S, Swannell A J, Mahoney P G C 1981 Circadian variations in the signs and symptoms of rheumatoid arthritis and in the therapeutic effectiveness of flurbiprofen at different times of day. British Journal of Clinical Pharmacology 11: 477–484

Kweekel-De Vries W J, Spierdijk J, Mattie H, Herman J M H 1974 A new soluble acetylsalicylate derivative in the treatment of postoperative pain. British Journal of Anaesthesia 46: 133–135

Leonards J R 1963 The influence of solubility on the rate of gastrointestinal absorption of aspirin. Clinical Pharmacology and Therapeutics 4: 476–479

Leonards J R 1976 Are all aspirins alike? Australian and New Zealand Journal of Medicine 6 (suppl. 1): 8–13

Levy G 1981 Comparative pharmacokinetics of aspirin and acetaminophen. Archives of Internal Medicine 141: 279–281

Levy G, Hollister L E 1965 Dissolution rate limited absorption in man. Journal of Pharmaceutical Sciences 54: 1121–1125

Litvak K M, McEvoy G K 1990 Ketorolac: an injectable nonnarcotic analgesic. Clinical Pharmacy 9: 921–935

Lundstam S O A, Leissner K-H, Wahlander L A, Kral J G 1982 Prostaglandin-synthetase inhibition with diclofenac sodium in treatment of renal colic: comparison with use of a narcotic analgesic. Lancet i: 1096–1097

Margetts G 1976 Phenacetin and paracetamol. Journal of International Medical Research 4 (suppl 4): 55–70

Mitchell J R, McMurtry R J, Stratham C N, Nelson S D 1977 Molecular basis for several drug-induced nephropathies. American Journal of Medicine 62: 518–526

Mondino A, Zanolo G, Giachetti C, Testaguzza F, Engels B, Wagener H H 1983 Med Welt 34: 1052–1054

Morley J 1975 Mode of action of aspirin. In: Dale T L C (ed) Proceedings of the Aspirin Symposium. Ratleigh Printers, Rochford, pp 19–22

O'Hara D A, Fragen R J, Kinzer M, Pemberton D 1987 Ketorolac tromethamine as compared with morphine sulfate for treatment of postoperative pain. Clinical Pharmacology and Therapeutics 41: 556–561

Pal B 1986 General practitioners' awareness of availability of NSAIDs without prescription. The Practitioner 230: 75–78

Peters H, Chlud K, Berner G et al 1987 Percutaneous kinetics of ibuprofen (German). Acta Rheumatologica 12: 208–211

Prescott L F 1980 Hepatotoxicity of mild analgesics. British Journal of Clinical Pharmacology 10: 373S–379S

Prescott L F 1986 Effects of non-narcotic analgesics on the liver. Drugs 32 (suppl 4): 129–147

Prescott L F, Nimmo J 1971 Genetic inequivalence: clinical observations. Acta Pharmacologica (Kbh) 29: 288–303

Pye K, Trotman I 1993 Use of ketorolac by continuous subcutaneous infusion for the control of cancer-related pain. Presented at the Palliative Care Research Forum, London

Rawlins M D 1993 Non-opioid analgesics. In: Doyle D, Hanks G W C, MacDonald N (eds) Oxford Textbook of Palliative Medicine. Oxford Medical Publications, Oxford, pp 182–187

Settipane G A 1981 Adverse reactions to aspirin and related drugs. Archives of Internal Medicine 141: 328–332

Sevelius H, Runkel R, Segre E, Bloomfield S S 1980 Bioavailability of naproxen sodium and its relationship to clinical analgesic effects. British Journal of Clinical Pharmacology 10: 259–263

Simon L S, Mills J A 1980a Nonsteroidal anti-inflammatory drugs. Part 1. New England Journal of Medicine 302: 1179–1185

Simon L S, Mills J A 1980b Nonsteroidal anti-inflammatory drugs: Part 2. New England Journal of Medicine 302: 1237–1243

Skjelbred P, Album B, Lokken P 1977 Acetylsalicylic acid vs paracetamol: effects on postoperative course. European Journal of Clinical Pharmacology 12: 257–264

Stricker B H C H, Meyboom R H B, Lindquist M 1985 Acute hypersensitivity reactions to paracetamol. British Medical Journal 291: 938–939

Sunshine A, Laska E 1975 Nefopam and morphine in man. Clinical Pharmacology and Therapeutics 18: 530–534

Thompson J F, Pike J M, Chumas P D, Rundle J S H 1989 Rectal diclofenac compared with pethidine injection in acute renal colic. British Medical Journal 299: 1140–1141

Tigerstedt I, Sepponen J, Tammisto T, Turunen M 1977 Comparison of nefopam and pethidine in postoperative pain. British Journal of Anaesthesia 49: 1133–1138

Todd P A, Sorkin E M 1988 Diclofenac sodium: a reappraisal of its pharmacodynamic and pharmacokinetic properties, and therapeutic efficacy. Drugs 35: 244–285

Tolman E L, Partridge R 1975 Multiple sites of interaction between prostaglandins and nonsteroidal anti-inflammatory agents. Prostaglandins 9: 349–359

Tonkin A L, Wing L M H 1988 Interactions of nonsteroidal anti-inflammatory drugs. In: Brooks P M (ed) Bailliere's Clinical Rheumatology. Anti-rheumatic drugs, vol 2/No 2. Bailliere Tindall, London, pp 455–483

Ventafridda V, Tamburini M, Caraceni A, de Conno F, Naldi F 1987 A validation study of the WHO method for cancer pain relief. Cancer 59: 851–856

Waldum H L, Hamre T, Kleveland P M et al 1992 Can NSAIDs cause acute biliary pain with cholestasis? Journal of Clinical Gastroenterology 14: 328–330

Warshaw A L, Carey R W, Robinson D R 1981 Control of fever associated with visceral cancers by indomethacin. Surgery 89: 414–416

Wong V, Daly M, Boon A, Heatley V 1993 Paracetamol and acute biliary pain with cholestasis. Lancet 342: 869

CHAPTER 12 | Nonopioids II

In this chapter, the adverse effects of aspirin and other nonsteroidal anti-inflammatory drugs (NSAIDs) are considered. Adverse drug reactions can be classified as (Rawlins & Thompson 1977):

- *type A* ('augmented') = predictable, dose dependent
- *type B* ('bizarre') = unpredictable, not dose dependent.

NSAIDs manifest both types. Apart from platelet dysfunction, gastro-duodenal injury, hepatotoxicity and salt and water retention, the adverse effects of NSAIDs fall into type B.

HYPERSENSITIVITY

Although most people tolerate aspirin and other NSAIDs well, some manifest allergic reactions (i.e. mediated through an immunological mechanism such as specific antibodies or sensitized T-lymphocytes). In others, aspirin may precipitate or exacerbate urticaria or asthma by a nonimmunological mechanism ('pseudo-allergy'), probably as the result of a chemical imbalance at cellular level induced by cyclo-oxygenase inhibition (Szczeklik 1986).

Anaphylaxis

Anaphylaxis is characterized by the following symptoms and signs which develop *within seconds or minutes* of taking aspirin:

- flushing
- palpitations
- weakness
- dizziness
- tingling of the extremities

BOX 12.A
TREATMENT OF ANAPHYLACTIC SHOCK (Szczeklik 1986, BNF 1993)

IM adrenaline 500 µg–1 mg (i.e. 0.5–1 ml adrenaline 1 in 1000)

Repeat every 10 minutes until pulse and blood pressure satisfactory

If patient is unconscious, double the dose

IV chlorpheniramine 10 mg is a useful adjunct

IV corticosteroids are only of secondary value because their impact is not immediate

Even so, they should be given to severely affected patients to prevent further deterioration

---

- urticaria
- angio-oedema
- agitation.

Asthma occurs in $< 10\%$; hypotension, pallor and other manifestations of shock are also uncommon (Szczeklik 1986). Patients with systemic lupus erythematosus or with aspirin induced asthma are at greater risk of anaphylaxis, although only a minority of patients developing anaphylaxis has a history of asthma or chronic rhinitis.

Anaphylaxis is specific to a given drug or chemically related class of drugs. Thus in one study, patients sensitive to dipyrone (metamizole) and its congener aminopyrine (aminophenazone) were not affected by aspirin or other NSAIDs (Szczeklik 1986). Anaphylaxis requires prompt treatment with adrenaline (Box 12.A).

Aspirin induced asthma

About 4% of adult asthmatics give a history of aspirin induced asthma (Szczeklik 1986). The frequency is much higher if spirometry is used for diagnosis, possibly as high as 20%. Most people with aspirin induced asthma, give a negative history of chronic asthma. It is rare in children. It is 50% more common in women than men (Box 12.B). Aspirin induced asthma

---

BOX 12.B
IDENTIKIT DESCRIPTION OF ASPIRIN INDUCED ASTHMA (Szczeklik 1986)

Beginning in the 20s or 30s, the patient develops intermittent and profuse watery rhinorrhoea (vasomotor rhinitis). This leads in time to chronic nasal congestion and nasal polyps.

Asthma develops subsequently within an hour of taking aspirin. It is associated with conjunctival irritation and flushing.

Since most patients have taken aspirin in the past without any problems, the reaction is unexpected and initially is often not attributed to the drug.

Table 12.1   NSAID induced asthma

Precipitate attacks of asthma	Well tolerated (cause no bronchoconstriction)
Aspirin	Choline salicylate Sodium salicylate
Amidopyrine Diclofenac Diflunisal Fenamic acids Fenoprofen Indomethacin Ketoprofen Naproxen Phenylbutazone Piroxicam Sulindac Sulphinpyrazone Tiaprofenic acid Tolmetin	Azapropazone Benzydamine Chloroquine Paracetamol[a]

[a] When beginning therapy, give half a tablet of paracetamol and observe 2–3 h for symptoms, which occur in no more than 5% of patients.

is dangerous. A single tablet of aspirin or other NSAID can precipitate severe bronchospasm, shock, coma and respiratory arrest (Virchow 1976).

In a few patients oculonasal symptoms occur without bronchospasm. Once developed, aspirin intolerance is generally permanent. Repeated challenges with aspirin are therefore positive, although variable in response. Desensitization can be undertaken. Most patients, however, use alternative drugs (Table 12.1).

Tartrazine, a yellow azo dye used for colouring foods, drinks, drugs and cosmetics, induces bronchoconstriction in some aspirin/NSAID sensitive subjects (Szczeklik et al 1977, Settipane 1983).

Aspirin induced asthma is related to cyclo-oxygenase inhibition. Aspirin sensitive subjects possibly differ from other people with asthma by depending more on the bronchodilating activity of PGE_2 than on the beta-adrenergic system. Aspirin inhibits the production of PGE_2 with the result that more arachidonic acid is available as a substrate for leukotriene production. Leukotrienes C_4 and D_4 are known to be potent bronchoconstrictors and mucus secretagogues. Other unidentified bronchoconstrictors could also be involved (Capron et al 1985).

Aspirin improved asthma

Cases of asthma improved by aspirin, indomethacin, dipyrone, aminopyrine and mefenamic acid have been reported (Szczeklik 1986). Aspirin in a single dose of 300–1200 mg produces bronchodilation accompanied by the relief of asthma for up to 24 h. The syndrome affects less than 1% of adult asthmatics.

Asthmatics who benefit from aspirin are not readily distinguishable from those in whom aspirin provokes bronchoconstriction. The striking difference between the two syndromes is their response to analgesics. Thus, the same drugs which precipitate bronchoconstriction in some patients produce bronchodilatation in others. Because all the active drugs are cyclo-oxygenase inhibitors, it is likely that the relief of asthma is the result of the removal from the respiratory tract of a product of arachidonic acid metabolism. This could be thromboxane A_2, prostaglandin F_2 or prostaglandin D_2.

HAEMATOLOGICAL EFFECTS

Daily doses of aspirin 80 mg inhibit platelet aggregation and prolong bleeding time in healthy individuals (Herd et al 1987). These effects stem from inhibition of platelet cyclo-oxygenase and hence thromboxane production. As a result platelet adhesiveness is reduced. Because aspirin irreversibly inhibits cyclo-oxygenase by acetylation, this effect persists until the acetylated platelets are replaced by new platelets which have not been exposed to aspirin. About 10% of the platelet population is replaced each day.

In contrast, nonacetylated salicylates have no effect on platelet function in normal therapeutic doses (Estes & Kaplan 1980, Green et al 1981, Danesh et al 1987). Other NSAIDs inhibit platelet cyclo-oxygenase but, unlike aspirin, the effect is reversible when treatment is stopped (Ikeda 1977, Stevens et al 1985; Table 12.2).

Thus, to avoid excessive bleeding at surgery, aspirin should be stopped one week before the operation, whereas other NSAIDs need be stopped only long enough to allow their excretion. For example, ibuprofen needs to be stopped only 12–24 h before operation.

Protein bound NSAIDs can also affect coagulation by displacing warfarin and other coumarin anticoagulants. It is clinically relevant, however, only with phenylbutazone (not now generally used) and salicylates in toxic concentrations.

GASTRODUODENAL INJURY

It is estimated that every year in the UK there are 30 000 serious gastro-intestinal events (i.e. haemorrhage or perforation) associated with NSAID use (Beardon et al 1989). It is accepted that these events have a mortality rate of about 10%, i.e. there are some 3000 NSAID related deaths each

Table 12.2 NSAIDs and platelet function

Drug	Effect on platelet cyclo-oxygenase
Aspirin	Irreversible inhibition by acetylation
Nonacetylated salicylates (diflunisal $\leqslant$ 500 mg b.i.d.)	No effect
Other NSAIDs	Reversible inhibition

BOX 12.C
TERMINOLOGY OF NSAID GASTROPATHY

Endoscopy
Erythema may be diffuse or patchy; latter may be linear or macular

Erosion = loss of mucosal surface with a white, yellowish or haemorrhagic base with margin of erythema; does not penetrate muscularis mucosae; ranges in diameter from 1 mm to several cm

Ulcer = lesion which penetrates muscularis mucosae into the submucosa or muscularis propria; ranges in diameter from 2 mm to many cm — usually > 0.5 cm

Adaptation = the process by which visible gastric mucosal injury lessens, and may resolve entirely, despite the continued administration of a noxious substance such as a NSAID (Graham 1988)

Histology
Acute gastritis = damage to or loss of surface epithelial cells, haemorrhage, congestion and oedema; often focal in nature; common after acute drug damage

Chronic gastritis = infiltration by inflammatory cells; diffuse; subdivided into chronic superficial gastritis, chronic atrophic gastritis and gastric atrophy

---

year. This accounts for 80% of those dying from ulcer complications (Cockel 1987). Others have suggested that the figure for NSAID related deaths, is higher, i.e. > 4000/year (Armstrong & Blower 1987). NSAIDs, therefore, are probably the most toxic drugs used in pain relief and palliative care. This is not always appreciated.

All NSAIDs injure gastric mucosa (Box 12.C). Anyone who takes two 300 mg tablets of aspirin with a glass of water will suffer some gastric bleeding (Ivey 1991). Anyone who continues to take aspirin over a 24 h period will develop gastric erosions, and 50% will develop duodenal ones as well. The following figures relate to patients with rheumatoid arthritis taking aspirin or other NSAID for 3 months or more (Ivey 1991):

- gastric erosions　　　　= 40%
- gastric ulceration　　　= 20%
- iron deficiency anaemia　= 10%
- duodenal ulcer　　　　= 5%

NSAID induced acute erosions and chronic peptic ulceration are distinct phenomena (McCarthy 1989, Soll et al 1991; Table 12.3). NSAID and nonNSAID peptic ulcers are also distinct (Table 12.4).

The gastric mucosa prevents the stomach from being digested by its own acid-peptic contents. The most important part of the mucosa is the epithelial surface membrane (Ivey 1986). Because the membrane comprises lipid and protein, water soluble molecules are restricted in their passage through it. Fat soluble compounds cross the membrane by dissolving in the lipid. In the stomach, the pH is about 2.5 and 90% of aspirin is nonionized and lipid soluble. In the gastric mucosa, however, the pH is about 7 and ionisation occurs. This results in a concentration gradient of nonionized aspirin

Table 12.3 NSAID induced gastric erosions and ulcers

Erosions	Ulcers
Rare with nonacetylated salicylates and prodrugs	Occur with all NSAIDs and all routes of administration
Symptoms absent	Up to 50% symptomatic
Shallow, no scarring	Deep, with scarring
Onset immediate (15 min)	Onset delayed (weeks or months)
Generally short lasting	Often long lasting
Lessen with adaptation	Occur despite adaptation
Caused mainly by topical injury	Caused mainly by systemic effects
Incidence decreased by enteric coated tablets	Enteric coating not of benefit
Usually multiple	Often solitary
Diffuse	Mainly distal stomach
Usually associated with mucosal haemorrhages	Mucosal haemorrhages usually absent
Correlated with antiplatelet activity	Correlated with inhibitory effect on mucin synthesis

Table 12.4 NSAID and nonNSAID peptic ulcer disease

Feature	NSAID	NonNSAID
Site	Antrum Prepylorus	Duodenum
Causal associations	NSAID	Nonerosive gastritis Helicobacter pylori
Risk groups	Older Women	Younger Men
Treatment	Cytoprotection	Acid suppression

across the mucosal surface with a high intracellular ionized aspirin concentration — which causes mucosal injury. The mucosa then becomes abnormally permeable to water soluble compounds and ions. Bleeding may subsequently occur, not because of the aspirin but because of secondary acid induced injury (Davenport 1964). In addition, histamine release within the damaged mucosa causes vasodilatation and exacerbates any bleeding tendency.

Gastric mucosal protaglandins (PGs) have a cytoprotective role. Because of reduced PG synthesis, aspirin will damage the gastric mucosa more readily. Reduction of gastric mucosal PGs, however, is not the key mechanism underlying aspirin induced injury. Buffered aspirin (pH 7) and IV aspirin also reduce gastric mucosal PG content but do not produce mucosal injury. Even in the absence of hydrochloric acid, aspirin can damage the gastric mucosa as a result of a high intracellular concentration. A solution of two 300 mg aspirin tablets has a pH of about 2.5.

A topical irritant effect has been observed in the mouth within 30 min of placing an aspirin tablet between the gum and the cheek (Roth 1963). Biopsy showed acute superficial necrosis of the epithelium. Similar changes can occur in the rectum with an aspirin suppository.

There may be an ischaemic component to NSAID ulceration (Wallace

& Granger 1992). PGs accelerate gastric ulcer healing by increasing gastric mucosal blood flow (Sato et al 1987). Long term NSAID administration may selectively inhibit blood flow in the mucosa of the gastric antrum (Ohtsuka 1992).

The relative infrequency of melaena or haematemesis after aspirin ingestion probably relates to several factors. For example, the random localization of an aspirin particle in the proximity of a blood vessel may determine whether aspirin causes a major haemorrhage. The likelihood of a tablet fragment getting trapped in a mucosal fold, and permitting prolonged topical action, depends partly on the disintegration time and dissolution rate of the preparation used and partly on whether the tablet is taken on an empty or a full stomach. Alcohol and/or smoking also have a bearing.

Adaptation

Gastric mucosal adaptation has been documented in animals (St John et al 1973, Eastwood & Quimby 1982) and in volunteers (O'Laughlin et al 1981, Graham et al 1983, Graham 1988, Shorrock et al 1990). For example, in a study of indomethacin 150 mg/day, endoscopy was performed after 24 h, 7 days and 28 days (Shorrock et al 1990). Acute gastroduodenal injury was maximal at 24 h. Resolution was not universal, however, and 2/14 volunteers developed ulcers. Adaptation is less evident in volunteers with higher doses of aspirin (Graham 1988).

The mechanism of adaptation in these studies is unknown. The effect is probably the result of several interrelated factors, including increased cellular regeneration (Graham 1988). Different mechanisms could be involved in acute and chronic injury. Healing of acute erosions (commonly seen in volunteer studies) may be independent of PG related mechanisms.

The relevance of volunteer studies to chronic NSAID use is debatable. Certainly, in a group of elderly patients with rheumatoid arthritis, there was no evidence of gastric adaptation after 2 weeks (Metzger et al 1976). The prevalence of gastric mucosal damage (up to 60%; Silvoso et al 1979, Larkai et al 1987) and ulceration (10–30%; Graham et al 1988, Graham 1989, Graham 1990, Shield et al 1990, Soll et al 1991) seen in endoscopic studies of arthritic patients taking NSAIDs long term suggests that adaptation is not taking place to any significant extent in these patients.

The constant rate of hospitalization for ulcer complications over 4 years with long term aspirin also suggests that mucosal adaptation is not occurring (Kurata & Abbey 1990). In rheumatoid arthritis 70% of ulcers had not healed after 3 months when aspirin was continued (Roth 1988). These data suggest that the higher doses of NSAIDs used in arthritis are often above the level where adaptation is able to prevent visible injury (Graham 1989).

In patients taking a NSAID long term, mucosal proliferation at the edge of a NSAID associated ulcer (which is important for ulcer healing) is reduced (Levi et al 1990, Soll et al 1991). NSAID injury is dose related (Agrawal 1991, Griffin et al 1991, Colin Jones et al 1992, Lanza et al 1992) and multiple NSAID therapy is associated with increased injury (Agrawal 1991).

Management

A number of therapeutic manoeuvres can reduce NSAID associated gastro-duodenal injury (Box 12.D). Gastric injury is reduced if aspirin is taken with sufficient antacid. Buffered aspirin preparations, however, do not all contain enough antacid for this purpose (Lanza et al 1980). For long term therapy, aspirin is best given enteric coated.

A prospective survey of the use of an H_2 receptor antagonist in patients with NSAID peptic ulcers suggests that such drugs are of value (Table 12.5).

BOX 12.D
PREVENTION OF NSAID ASSOCIATED GASTROPATHY

Use smallest dose necessary

Combine aspirin with sodium bicarbonate (short term)

Use enteric coated aspirin

Use NSAID with better record, e.g. ibuprofen (available without prescription for this reason)

Use a NSAID which is only poorly absorbed in the stomach, e.g. diclofenac, diflunisal, ibuprofen

Combine administration with misoprostol

Table 12.5   Controlled trials of H_2-receptor antagonists in the healing of NSAID associated ulcers and injury: NSAID was continued in all studies unless stated

n	Type of injury	Duration (weeks)	Comparator	Result	Author
Cimetidine					
27	Ulcers (GD)	6	Placebo	NS	Davies et al 1986
104	Erosions	8	Placebo	NS	Roth et al 1987
18	Ulcers (G)	8	Placebo	NS	O'Laughlin et al 1982
626	Ulcers	4	Placebo	Cimetidine daily NS Cimetidine b.i.d. p = 0.01	Wallin et al 1988
70	Ulcers (G)	6	Placebo + antacid	p < 0.001	Loiudice et al 1981
72	Ulcers (GD)	4	Bismuth	NS	Bianchi Porro et al 1987
26	Erosions	6	Sucralfate	NS	Shepherd et al 1989
Ranitidine					
48	Erosions	4	Placebo	p < 0.05	Bianchi Porro et al 1987
46	Erosions	4	Placebo	p < 0.05	Simon et al 1988
24	Erosions	24	Placebo	NS	Swift et al 1989
149	Ulcers (GD)	4	Placebo (NSAID stopped)	NS	Tildesley et al 1993
65	Ulcers (GD)	9	Sucralfate	Equivalent	Manniche et al 1987
68	Ulcers (G)	4	Omeprazole	Omeprazole p = 0.02	Walan et al 1989

G = gastric; D = duodenal; NS = not significant at 0.05 probability level.
Based on Fenn & Robinson 1991

Table 12.6   Healing of NSAID associated peptic ulcers by an H_2-receptor antagonist

Time (weeks)	% Healing (stomach)		% Healing (duodenum)	
	Stop NSAID	Continue NSAID	Stop NSAID	Continue NSAID
4	71	54	74	57
8	95	63	100	84
12	100	79	100	92

From Lancaster-Smith et al 1991

It is not known, however, what the rate of healing would have been with a placebo. Controlled trials indicate that:

- cimetidine and ranitidine *prevent* NSAID associated duodenal ulcers (Table 12.6)
- cimetidine and ranitidine do *not* prevent NSAID associated gastric ulcers (Table 12.6)
- ranitidine but not cimetidine facilitates *healing* of NSAID associated ulcers (Table 12.7).

On the other hand, misoprostol, a synthetic analogue of PGE_1, both *prevents* NSAID associated gastric and duodenal ulcers and enhances ulcer *healing* (Fenn & Robinson 1991, Bardhan et al 1993). Recommended doses are:

- for prevention: 200 µg b.i.d.–q.i.d. (depending on dose of NSAID)
- for healing: 200 µg q.i.d. or 400 µg b.i.d.

In one study in patients with arthritis the cumulative incidence of gastric ulcer during 1 year on both misoprostol and a NSAID was 13%, compared with 29% in patients taking a NSAID alone ($p < 0.05$; Elliott et al 1990). The development of large gastric erosions was also reduced significantly in the misoprostol group.

Misoprostol is equal but not superior to H_2-receptor antagonists in healing nonNSAID peptic ulcers (Nicholson 1985, Rachmilewitz et al 1986, Simjee et al 1987). In this situation, relief of symptoms is not as rapid as with H_2-receptor antagonists (Watkinson et al 1988).

HEPATOTOXICITY

Acute abdominal pain and cholestasis 24–48 h after taking therapeutic doses of paracetamol, aspirin or naproxen have been reported in three women (Waldum et al 1992, Wong et al 1993). Hepatocellular injury is also occasionally seen with NSAIDs (Prescott 1986). Indeed, several NSAIDs have been withdrawn because of hepatotoxicity (benoxaprofen, fenclofenac, ibufenac).

About 50% of patients given aspirin regularly in anti-inflammatory doses develop mild dose dependent reversible liver damage as evidenced by an increase in plasma aminotransferase concentration (Table 12.8). Liver damage is occasionally severe and may be complicated by disseminated intravascular coagulation and encephalopathy.

Table 12.7 Controlled trials of H_2-receptor antagonists in the prevention of NSAID associated gastroduodenal injury

n	Volunteer or patient	Duration (weeks)	Gastric injury	Duodenal injury	Author
Ranitidine					
43	V	3d	$p < 0.01$	$p < 0.05$	Berkowitz et al 1986
246	P	4	NS	NA	Bianchi Porro et al 1987
263	P	4/8	NS	$p = 0.024$ ulcers NS erosions	Ehsanullah et al 1988
144	P	4/8	NS	$p < 0.01$	Robinson et al 1989
110	P	1	NS	NS	Stalnikowicz et al 1989
16	V	1	NS	$p = 0.004$	Oddsson et al 1990
40	P	2	$p = 0.002$	$p = 0.002$	Yanagawa et al 1990
72	P	2/4/8	$p < 0.01$	NS	Yanagawa et al 1991
421	P	8	Inferior to misoprostol ($p = 0.03$)	= misoprostol	Raskin et al 1991
28	V	2	$p < 0.05$	$p < 0.05$	Muller & Simon 1992
Cimetidine					
8	V	1d	NS	NA	Hogan et al 1986
50	V	1	Inferior to enprostil ($p = 0.05$)	$p = 0.05$ (v placebo)	Stiel et al 1986
26	P	40	NS	NA	Roth et al 1987
30	V	1d	$p < 0.001$	NA	Kimmey et al 1988
30	V	1	NS	$p < 0.05$	Lanza et al 1988
90	V	1	Inferior to misoprostol ($p = 0.006$)	$p = 0.004$ (v placebo)	Lanza et al 1988
92	P	1	NS	$p < 0.01$	Stalnikowicz et al 1988
17	V	1	NS erosions	NS erosions	Aabakken et al 1989
80	V	1	NS erosions/ulcers	NS erosions/ulcers	Lanza et al 1990
223	P	12	$p < 0.05$	$p < 0.05$	Wallin et al 1990

V = volunteer, P = patient, NA = not assessed, NS = not statistically significant. p value indicates statistical superiority over placebo or comparative agent.
Based on Fenn & Robinson 1991

Table 12.8 Incidence of salicylate induced hepatic injury

Diagnosis	Incidence (%)
Normal subjects and patients with nonrheumatic disease	0–30
Juvenile rheumatoid arthritis[a]	25–70
Adult rheumatoid arthritis	20
Systemic lupus erythematosus[a]	50
Rheumatic fever	50–70

[a] Active disease has higher incidence and greater severity of injury than quiescent disease.
From Zimmerman 1981

Reye's syndrome in children and young adults is considered generally to be related to aspirin. This is characterized by:

- mild influenza-like prodromal illness
- impaired liver function

- hypoglycaemia
- acidosis
- encephalopathy.

In some ways, Reye's syndrome resembles subacute salicylate intoxication, although aspirin cannot be implicated in all cases (Prescott 1986). Even so, aspirin is no longer prescribed for children under 12 years old and breast feeding mothers.

NEPHROPATHY

NSAIDs affect renal function. By increasing sodium and fluid retention, they cause oedema, hypertension, hypokalaemia and, even, congestive cardiac failure. A general property of NSAIDs, therefore, is to reduce the effect of diuretics and antihypertensives. Various other NSAID induced renal effects are seen occasionally (Clive & Stoff 1984, Anonymous 1986):

- acute renal failure
- acute on chronic renal failure
- acute interstitial nephritis and nephrotic syndrome
- chronic interstitial nephritis and papillary necrosis
- hyperkalaemia
- hyponatraemia.

Patients at risk of acute renal failure are those in whom there is true or functional intravascular hypovolaemia (Clive & Stoff 1984):

- diuretics
- haemorrhage
- surgery
- congestive cardiac failure
- cirrhosis
- nephrotic syndrome.

Underlying renal disease and old age are probably additional concurrent risk factors. The kidneys are normally protected from the generalized vasoconstriction produced by activation of the catecholamine and renin-angiotensin systems in response to true or functional hypovolaemia. Prostacyclin, a powerful vasodilator, is produced in the kidneys and safeguards renal blood flow (Fig. 12.1). Renal blood flow and glomerular filtration rate are critically dependent on prostacyclin production in patients with impaired renal function (Ciabattoni et al 1984). Sulindac does not affect renal production of prostacyclin or PGE_2 (Fig. 12.2) and does not affect renal function. It can be used safely in patients with renal dysfunction. Chronic renal failure and interstitial nephritis with nephrotic syndrome have been reported following the use of topical, benzydamine and piroxicam respectively (O'Callaghan et al 1994).

With interstitial nephritis, cyclo-oxygenase inhibition probably leads to an excess of pro-inflammatory leukotrienes which cause renal damage. These

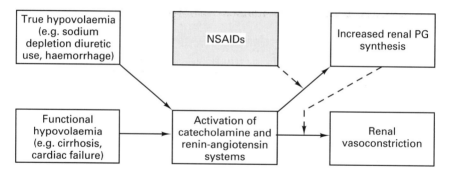

Fig. 12.1 Pathophysiology of NSAID mediated renal failure. Dotted arrows = inhibitory effects. (Reproduced with permission from Clive & Stoff 1985.)

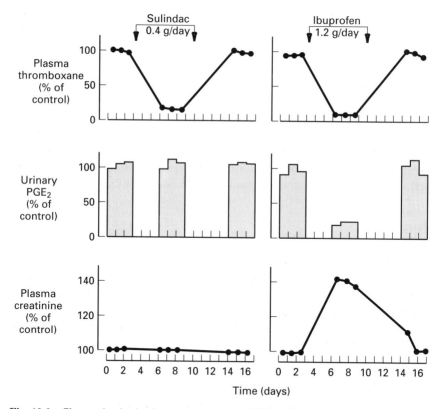

Fig. 12.2 Changes in platelet thromboxane B_2, renal PGs and plasma creatinine in two groups of 10 patients with chronic glomerulonephritis treated with sulindac and ibuprofen. (Reproduced with permission from Ciabattoni et al 1984.)

syndromes have been reported with several NSAIDs. They are, however, sporadic and unpredictable, and manifest days or months after starting treatment (Table 12.9). Eosinophilia, eosinophiluria, fever and gross proteinuria are present in the acute form.

Misoprostol protects renal blood flow in patients with cirrhosis and

Table 12.9   NSAIDs and interstitial nephritis

Drug	Acute interstitial nephritis and nephrotic syndrome	Chronic interstitial nephritis and papillary necrosis
Ibuprofen	0	+
Indomethacin	+	+
Mefenamic acid	+	+
Naproxen	+	+
Fenoprofen	+	0
Tolmetin	+	0

ascites who are taking NSAIDs (Antillon et al 1990). Misoprostol did not affect renal function in patients with rheumatoid arthritis and some renal impairment who were taking NSAIDs long term (Boers et al 1991). Thus, although misoprostol prevents acute (functional) renal impairment, it cannot reverse chronic injury (Weir et al 1989, Wilkie et al 1992).

SKIN REACTIONS

Urticaria and angio-oedema

A few people react to aspirin by developing urticaria (i.e. weals and swellings). In addition, up to 40% of patients with chronic urticaria develop an obvious increase in symptoms if they take aspirin during a phase of active urticaria (Szczeklik 1986). There are several different causal types of urticaria. Aspirin exacerbates:

- idiopathic urticaria
- delayed pressure urticaria
- cholinergic urticaria.

It does *not* exacerbate cold urticaria (Doeglas 1983). Aspirin can also convert a mild allergic response to another allergen into a life threatening one. People with urticaria should avoid aspirin in any form, and also drug additives and colourants such as benzoates and tartrazine because there is cross reactivity in up to 50% (Szczeklik 1986).

Photosensitivity

The cutaneous photosensitivity seen with some NSAIDs is elicited by a phototoxic mechanism. The response occurs within minutes of exposure to ultraviolet (UV) light and comprises:

- pruritus
- burning
- erythema
- weals.

This reaction differs from the delayed response ('exaggerated sunburn') seen with tetracyclines and psoralens. Most NSAIDs which cause phototoxicity are propionic acid derivatives (Kochevar 1989):

- benoxaprofen (withdrawn)
- carprofen
- ketoprofen
- naproxen
- nabumetone
- tiaprofenic acid.

Piroxicam, which is not a propionic acid derivative, also causes photo-sensitivity, but not for several days after commencing treatment (Kaidbey & Mitchell 1989). This cannot be reproduced in volunteers or animals (Kochevar 1989). The mechanism is probably allergic rather than phototoxic.
  Photosensitivity has *not* been reported with:

- aspirin
- ibuprofen
- indomethacin.

Considering the widespread use of naproxen, for example, photosensitivity must be uncommon. An incidence of 0.3% has been suggested (Kaidbey & Mitchell 1989). Characteristics of the drugs which cause photosensitivity include:

- ability to absorb UV radiation of wavelength > 310 nm
- photoreactivity
- photo-instability
- adequate concentration in skin.

When the above criteria are met, injury to the skin occurs. There may also be mast cell degranulation with histamine release (Kochevar 1989). Ibuprofen, while sharing the property of photo-instability with other propionic acid derivatives, does not absorb UV radiation of the right wavelength. In contrast, indomethacin absorbs UV radiation of the right wavelength but is not photoreactive. Indeed, indomethacin can be used topically as a sunscreen (Kochevar 1989).

Other skin reactions

Other skin reactions to NSAIDs include (Szczeklik 1986):

- fixed eruptions
- toxic epidermal necrosis
- erythema multiforme and Stevens-Johnson syndrome
- purpura (aspirin, phenylbutazone)
- lichen planus-like eruptions (aminophenazone).

REFERENCES

Aabakken L, Larsen S, Osnes M 1989 Cimetidine tablets or suspension for the prevention of gastrointestinal mucosal lesions caused by nonsteroidal anti-inflammatory drugs. Scandinavian Journal of Rheumatology 18: 369–375

Agrawal N 1991 Risk factors for gastrointestinal ulcers caused by NSAIDs. Journal of Family Practice 32: 619–624

Anonymous 1986 Nonsteroidal anti-inflammatory drugs and the kidney. British Medical Journal 294: 1621–1622

Antillon M, Cominelli F, Lo S, Moran M et al 1990 Effects of oral prostaglandins on indomethacin-induced renal failure in patients with cirrhosis and ascites. Journal of Rheumatology (Suppl 20) 17: 46–49

Armstrong C P, Blower A L 1987 Nonsteroidal anti-inflammatory drugs and life threatening complications of peptic ulceration. Gut 28: 527–532

Bardhan K D, Bjarnason I, Scott D L et al 1993 The prevention and healing of acute NSAID-associated gastroduodenal mucosal damage by misoprostol. British Journal of Rheumatology 32: 990–995

Beardon P H G, Brown S V, McDevitt D G 1989 Gastrointestinal events in patients prescribed non-steroidal anti-inflammatory drugs: a controlled study using record linkage in Tayside. Quarterly Journal of Medicine 71: 497–505

Berkowitz J M, Adler S N, Sharp J T, Warner C W 1986 Reduction of aspirin induced gastroduodenal mucosal damage with ranitidine. Journal of Clinical Gastroenterology 8 (3): 377–380

Bianchi Porro G, Pace F, Caruso I 1987 Why are nonsteroidal anti-inflammatory drugs important in peptic ulceration? Alimentary Pharmacology and Therapeutics 1: 540S–547S

Boers M, Dijkmans B A C, Breedveld F C et al 1991 No effect of misoprostol on renal function of rheumatoid patients treated with diclofenac. British Journal of Rheumatology 30: 56–59

British National Formulary 1993 A Joint Publication of the British Medical Association and the Royal Pharmaceutical Society of Great Britain, London, No 26 (September 1993) pp 131–132

Capron A, Ameisen J C, Joseph M, Auriault C, Tonnel A B, Caen J 1985 New functions for platelets and their pathological implications. International Archives of Allergy and Applied Immunology 77: 107–114

Ciabattoni G, Cinotti G A, Pierucci A et al 1984 Effects of sulindac and ibuprofen in patients with chronic glomerular disease. New England Journal of Medicine 310: 279–283

Clive D M, Stoff J S 1984 Renal syndromes associated with nonsteroidal anti-inflammatory drugs. New England Journal of Medicine 310: 563–572

Clive D M, Stoff J S 1985 Nonsteroidal anti-inflammatory drugs and the kidney. Medical Times 113 (4): 29–34

Cockel R 1987 NSAIDs: should every prescription carry a government health warning? Gut 28: 515–518

Colin Jones D, Langman M, Lawson D et al 1992 Risk associated with treatment by individual nonsteroidal anti-inflammatory drugs. Gut suppl 33 (2): T191

Danesh B J Z, Saniabadi A R, Russell R I, Lowe G D O 1987 Therapeutic potential of choline magnesium trisalicylate as an alternative to aspirin for patients with bleeding tendencies. Scottish Medical Journal 32: 167–168

Davenport H W 1964 Gastric mucosal injury by fatty and acetylsalicylic acids. Gastroenterology 46: 245–250

Davies J, Collins A J, Dixon A J 1986 The influence of cimetidine on peptic ulcer in patients with arthritis taking anti-inflammatory drugs. British Journal of Rheumatology 25: 54–58

Doeglas H M G 1983 Chronic urticaria: intolerance for aspirin and food additives and relationship to atopy. British Journal of Dermatology 108: 108

Eastwood G L, Quimby G F 1982 Effect of chronic aspirin ingestion on epithelial proliferation in rat fundus, antrum, and duodenum. Gastroenterology 82: 852–856

Ehsanullah R S B, Page M C, Tildesley G, Wood J R 1988 Prevention of gastroduodenal damage induced by nonsteroidal anti-inflammatory drugs: controlled trial of ranitidine. British Medical Journal 297: 1017–1021

Elliott S L, Yeomans N D, Buchanan R R C et al 1990 Longterm effects of misoprostol on gastropathy induced by nonsteroidal anti-inflammatory drugs (NSAIDs). Clinical and Experimental Rheumatology 8 (Suppl 4):58

Estes D, Kaplan K 1980 Lack of platelet effect with aspirin analog. Arthritis and Rheumatism 23: 1303–1307

Fenn G C, Robinson G C 1991 Misoprostol: a logical therapeutic approach to gastroduodenal mucosal injury induced by nonsteroidal anti-inflammatory drugs. Journal of Clinical Pharmacy and Therapies 16: 385–409

Graham D Y 1988 Gastric adaptation: studies in humans during continuous aspirin administration. Gastroenterology 95: 327–333

Graham D Y 1989 Prevention of gastroduodenal injury induced by chronic nonsteroidal anti-inflammatory drug therapy. Gastroenterology 96: 675–681

Graham D Y 1990 The relationship between nonsteroidal anti-inflammatory drug use and peptic ulcer disease. Gastro-enterology Clinics of North America 19(1): 171–182

Graham D Y, Smith J L, Dobbs S M 1983 Gastric adaptation occurs with aspirin administration in man. Digestive Diseases and Sciences 28: 1–6

Graham D Y, Agrawal N N, Roth S H 1988 Prevention of NSAID-induced gastric ulcer with misoprostol: multicentre double-blind, placebo-controlled trial. Lancet 2: 1277–1280

Green D, Davies R O, Holmes G I et al 1981 Effects of diflunisal on platelet function and faecal blood loss. Clinical Pharmacology and Therapeutics 30: 378–384

Griffin M R, Piper J M, Daugherty J R et al 1991 Nonsteroidal anti-inflammatory drug use and increased risk of peptic ulcer disease in elderly persons. Annals of Internal Medicine 114: 257–263

Herd C M, Rodgers S E, Lloyd J V, Bochner F, Duncan E M, Tunbridge L J 1987 A dose-ranging study of the antiplatelet effect of enteric coated aspirin in man. Australian and New Zealand Journal of Medicine 17: 195–200

Hogan D L, Thomas F J, Isenberg J I 1986 A single dose of cimetidine prevents aspirin-induced gastric damage in man. Digestive Diseases and Sciences 31 (10): 4815

Ikeda Y 1977 The effect of ibuprofen on platelet function in vivo. Keio Journal of Medicine 26: 213–222

Ivey K J 1986 Gastrointestinal intolerance and bleeding with non-narcotic analgesics. Drugs 32 (suppl 4): 71–89

Ivey K J 1991 Pathophysiology of NSAID induced gastroduodenal damage: epidemiology and mechanisms of action of therapeutic agents. Alimentary Pharmacology and Therapeutics 5 (suppl 1): 91–98

Kaidbey K H, Mitchell F N 1989 Photosensitizing potential of certain nonsteroidal anti-inflammatory agents. Archives of Dermatology 125: 783–786

Kimmey M B, Silversten F E 1988 Role of H_2 receptor blockers in the prevention of gastric injury resulting from nonsteroidal anti-inflammatory agents. American Journal of Medicine 84 (2A): 49–52

Kochevar I E 1989 Phototoxicity of nonsteroidal anti-inflammatory drugs. Archives of Dermatology 125: 824–826

Kurata J H, Abbey D E 1990 The effect of chronic aspirin use on duodenal and gastric ulcer hospitalizations. Journal of Clinical Gastroenterology 12: 260–266

Lancaster-Smith M J, Jaderberg M E, Jackson D A 1991 Ranitidine in the treatment of nonsteroidal anti-inflammatory drug associated gastric and duodenal ulcers. Gut 32: 252–255

Lanza F L, Roger G L, Nelson R S 1980 Endoscopic evaluation of the effects of aspirin, buffered aspirin and enteric-coated aspirin in gastric and duodenal mucosa. New England Journal of Medicine 303: 136–138

Lanza F L, Aspinall R L, Swabb E A, Davis R E, Rack M F, Rubin A 1988 Double-blind, placebo-controlled, endoscopic comparison of the mucosal protective effects of misoprostol versus cimetidine on tolmetin-induced mucosal injury to the stomach and duodenum. Gastroenterology 95: 289–294

Lanza F L, Graham D Y, Davies R E, Rack M F 1990 Endoscopic comparison of cimetidine and sucralfate for prevention of naproxen-induced acute gastroduodenal injury. Digestive Diseases and Sciences 35 (12): 1494–1499

Lanza F L, Roger G L, Rack M L 1992 NSAID induced gastric ulceration is dose related. Gastroenterology 102 (4): A109

Larkai E N, Lacey Smith J, Lidskmy M D, Graham D Y 1987 Gastroduodenal mucosa and dyspeptic symptoms in arthritic patients during chronic nonsteroidal anti-inflammatory drug use. American Journal of Gastroenterology 82: 1153–1158

Levi S, Goodlad R A, Lee C Y et al 1990 Inhibitory effect of nonsteroidal anti-inflammatory drugs on mucosal cell proliferation associated with gastric ulcer healing. Lancet 336: 840–843

Loiudice T A, Saleem T, Lang J A 1981 Cimetidine in the treatment of gastric ulcer induced by steroidal and nonsteroidal anti-inflammatory drugs. American Journal of Gastroenterology 75: 104–110

McCarthy D M 1989 Nonsteroidal anti-inflammatory drug induced ulcers: management by traditional therapies. Gastroenterology 96: 662–674

Manniche C, Malchow-Moller A, Andersen J R 1987 Randomized study of the influence of nonsteroidal anti-inflammatory drugs on the treatment of peptide ulcer in patients with rheumatic disease. Gut 28: 226–229

Metzger W H, McAddam L, Bluestone R, Guth P H 1976 Acute gastric mucosal injury during continuous or interrupted aspirin ingestion in humans. American Journal of Digestive Diseases 21: 963–968

Muller P, Simon B 1992 Schutzwirkung von ranitidin in magen and duodenum gegenuber piroxicam. Arzneim-Forsch/Drug Research 42: 1492–1494

Nicholson P A 1985 A multicenter international controlled comparison of two dosage regimes of misoprostol and cimetidine in the treatment of duodenal ulcer in outpatients. Digestive Diseases and Sciences 30 (suppl): 171S–177S

O'Callaghan C A, Andrews P A, Ogg C S 1994 Renal disease and use of topical NSAIDs. British Medical Journal 308: 110–111

Oddsson E, Gudjonsson H, Thjodleifsson B 1990 Protective effect of omeprazole or ranitidine against naproxen induced damage to the human gastroduodenal mucosa. World Congress of Gastroenterology, Sydney FP22

Ohtsuka E 1992 Upper gastrointestinal endoscopic findings and gastric mucosal blood flow in patients with rheumatoid arthritis. Fukuoka Igaku Zasshi 83 (2): 62–71

O'Laughlin J C, Hofteizer J W, Ivey K J 1981 Effect of aspirin on the human stomach in normals; endoscopic comparison of damage produced one hour, 24 hours and 2 weeks after administration. Scandinavian Journal of Gastroenterology 16 (suppl 67): 211–214

O'Laughlin J C, Silvoso G K, Ivey K J 1982 Resistance to medical therapy of gastric ulcers in rheumatic disease patients taking aspirin. Digestive Diseases and Sciences 27 (11): 976–980

Prescott L F 1986 Effects of non-narcotic analgesics on the liver. Drugs 32 (suppl 4): 129–147

Rachmilewitz D, Chapman J W, Nicholson P A 1986 A multicenter international controlled comparison of two dosage regimes of misoprostol and cimetidine in the treatment of gastric ulcer in outpatients. Digestive Diseases and Sciences 31 (Suppl): 75S–80S

Raskin J, White R, Jaszewski R 1991 Double-blind comparative study of the efficacy and safety of misoprostol and ranitidine in the prevention of NSAID-induced gastric ulcers and upper GI symptoms: preliminary findings. Digestion 49 (suppl 1): 50–51

Rawlins M D, Thompson J W 1977 Pathogenesis of adverse drug reactions. In: Davis D M (ed) Textbook of adverse drug reactions. Oxford University Press, Oxford, pp 11–34

Robinson M G, Griffin J W, Bowers J et al 1989 Effect of ranitidine on gastroduodenal damage induced by nonsteroidal anti-inflammatory drugs. Digestive Diseases and Sciences 34: 424–428

Roth J L A 1963 Report of symposium on salicylates. Gastroenterology 44: 389–391

Roth S H 1988 Nonsteroidal anti-inflammatory drugs: gastropathy, death and medical practice. Annals of Internal Medicine 109: 353–354

Roth S H 1992 Prophylaxis against nonsteroidal induced upper gastrointestinal side effects. Annals of Rheumatoid Diseases 51: 1412

Roth S H, Bennett R E, Mitchell C S 1987 Cimetidine therapy in nonsteroidal anti-inflammatory drug gastropathy. Double-blind by term evaluation. Archives of Internal Medicine 147: 1798–1801

St John D J B, Yeomans N D, McDermott F T, de Boer W G R M 1973 Adaptation of the gastric mucosa to repeated administration of aspirin in the rat. American Journal of Digestive Diseases 18: 881–886

Sato N, Kawano S, Fukada M, Kamada T 1987 The effects of a PGE_1 analogue misoprostol on gastric mucosal blood volume index and haemoglobin oxygenation in humans. Journal of Gastroenterology and Hepatology 2: 499–505

Settipane G A 1983 Aspirin and allergic diseases: a review. American Journal of Medicine 74: 102–107

Shepherd H A, Fine D, Hillier K et al 1989 Effect of sucralfate and cimetidine on rheumatoid patients with active gastroduodenal lesions who are taking nonsteroidal anti-inflammatory drugs. American Journal of Medicine 86 (6A): 49–54

Shield M J, Fenn G C, Kiff P, Stead H, Geis S 1990 Do differential rates of NSAID-associated gastroduodenal damage exist? British Journal of Rheumatology 29 (suppl 1): 5

Shorrock C J, Prescott R J, Rees W D W 1990 The effects of indomethacin on gastroduodenal morphology and mucosal pH gradient in the healthy human subject. Gastroenterology 99: 334–339

Silvoso G R, Ivey K J, Butt J H et al 1979 Incidence of gastric lesions in patients with rheumatic disease on chronic aspirin therapy. Annals of Internal Medicine 91 (4): 517–520

Simjee A E, Spitaels J M, Pettengell K E, Manion G L 1987 A comparative study of misoprostol and ranitidine in the healing of duodenal ulcers: a double-blind controlled trial. South African Medical Journal 72: 15–17

Simon B, Damman H G, Leucht U, Muller P 1988 Ranitidine in the therapy of NSAID-induced gastroduodenal lesions. Scandinavian Journal of Gastroenterology 23 (154): 18–21

Soll A H, Weinstein W M, Kurata J, McCarthy D 1991 Nonsteroidal anti-inflammatory drugs and peptic ulcer disease. Annals of Internal Medicine 114: 307–319

Stalnikowicz R, Pollak D, Eliakim A 1988 Cimetidine decreases indomethacin induced duodenal mucosal damage in patients with acute musculoskeletal disorders. Gut 29: 1578–1582

Stalnikowicz R, Goldin E, Fich et al 1989 Indomethacin-induced gastroduodenal damage is not affected by co-treatment with ranitidine. Journal of Clinical Gastroenterology 1: 178–182

Steven M M, Small M, Pinkerton L, Madhok R, Sturrock R D, Forbes C D 1985 Non-steroidal anti-inflammatory drugs in haemophilic arthritis. Haemostasis 15: 204–209

Stiel D, Ellard K T, Hills L J, Brooks P M 1986 Protective effect of enprostil against aspirin-induced gastroduodenal mucosal injury in man. Comparison with cimetidine and sucralfate. American Journal of Medicine 81 (Suppl 2A): 54–58

Swift G L, Heneghan M, Williams G T et al 1989 Effect of ranitidine on gastroduodenal mucosal damage in patients on longterm nonsteroidal anti-inflammatory drugs. Digestion 44: 86–94

Szczeklik A 1986 Analgesics, allergy and asthma. Drugs 32 (suppl 4) 148–163

Szczeklik A, Gryglewski R J, Czerniawska-Mysik G 1977 Clinical patterns of hypersensitivity to nonsteroidal anti-inflammatory drugs and their pathogenesis. Journal of Allergy and Clinical Immunology 60: 276–284

Tildesley G, Ehsanullah R S B, Wood J R 1993 Ranitidine in the treatment of gastric and duodenal ulcers associated with nonsteroidal anti-inflammatory drugs. British Journal of Rheumatology 32: 474–478

Virchow C 1976 Analgetika-intoleranz bei asthmatikern (Analgetika-Asthma-Syndrom). Praxis und Klinik der Pneumologie 30: 642–692

Walan A, Bader J-P, Classen M, Lamers C B H W, Piper D W, Rutgersson K, Eriksson S 1989 Effect of omeprazole and ranitidine on ulcer healing and relapse rates in patients with benign gastric ulcer. New England Journal of Medicine 320: 69–75

Waldum H L, Hamre T, Kleveland P M et al 1992 Can NSAIDs cause acute biliary pain with cholestasis? Journal of Clinical Gastroenterology 14: 328–330

Wallace J L, Granger D N 1992 Pathogenesis of NSAID gastropathy: are neutrophils the culprits? Trends Pharmacology Science f13: 129–130

Wallin M D, Frank W O, Fox M J et al 1988 The effects of cimetidine drug on the healing of nonsteroidal anti-inflammatory drug-induced gastroduodenal damage while continuing NSAID therapy. American Journal of Gastroenterology 83 (9): 1076

Wallin B A, Grier C E, Fox M J, McCafferty J P, Wetherington J D, Palmer R H 1990 Prevention of NSAID-induced ulcers with cimetidine: results of a double blind placebo controlled trial. Gastroenterology 98 (5) part 2: A146

Watkinson G, Hopkins A, Akbar F A 1988 The therapeutic efficacy of misoprostol in peptic ulcer disease. Postgraduate Medical Journal 64 (Suppl 1): 60–73

Weir M R, Klassen D K, Hall P S, Schubert C 1989 Misoprostol minimizes indomethacin-induced renal dysfunction in healthy women. American Society of Nephrology, 22nd Annual meeting

Wilkie M E, Davies G R, Marsh F P, Rampton D S 1992 Effects of indomethacin and misoprostol on renal function in healthy volunteers. Clinical Nephrology 38: 334–337

Wong V, Daly M, Boon A, Heatley V 1993 Paracetamol and acute biliary pain with cholestasis. Lancet 342: 869

Yanagawa A, Endo T, Nakagawa T, Mizushima Y 1990 Prophylactic efficacy of ranitidine against gastroduodenal mucosal damage from nonsteroidal anti-inflammatory drugs: a randomized placebo-controlled study. Round Table Series 21: 97–103

Yanagawa A, Mizushima Y, Endoh T, Kobayashi K, Sugihara M 1991 Prophylactic efficacy of the H_2-blocker ranitidine against gastroduodenal lesions caused by nonsteroidal anti-inflammatory drugs (NSAIDs): controlled trial study. Japanese Journal of Rheumatology 3: 275–287

Zimmerman H J 1981 Effects of aspirin and acetaminophen on the liver. Archives of Internal Medicine 141: 333–342

Weak opioids

NOMENCLATURE

In the Revised Method for Relief of Cancer Pain (WHO 1994), step 2 analgesics are described as 'opioids for mild to moderate pain' rather than 'weak opioids'. This change is associated with an increased number of drugs in step 2. Three of the six listed step 2 analgesics, however, are regarded as 'strong opioids' by many people (Table 13.1). This difference of opinion emphasizes that, in certain respects, the division between 'weak' and 'strong' opioids is arbitrary.

One characteristic of weak opioids such as dihydrocodeine and dextropropoxyphene is that oral codeine, rather than IM morphine, is used as the reference drug for comparison. This is not the case with newer drugs, however, which are available in both oral and parenteral forms.

Classification on the basis of Controlled/Scheduled Drug regulations provides a pragmatic solution; opioids which are not restricted by narcotic control laws can be classed as 'weak opioids' and the rest as 'strong'. Even on this basis, however, there are exceptions — ethoheptazine and pentazocine

Table 13.1 Step 2 opioids

Author's list	WHO revised list
Codeine	Codeine
Dihydrocodeine	Dihydrocodeine
Dextropropoxyphene	Dextropropoxyphene
Ethoheptazine	Standard opium
Meptazinol	Oxycodone[b]
Tramadol[a]	Buprenorphine[b]
Pentazocine	

[a] Tramadol is not yet available in the UK or the USA but is marketed in many countries.
[b] Regarded as step 3 analgesics in this book.

are both Controlled/Scheduled Drugs but, when given by mouth, are both best described as weak opioids. In fact, when originally marketed, both were not Controlled Drugs; they were subsequently reclassified because of abuse by addicts.

By injection, all the weak opioids can provide analgesia equivalent or nearly equivalent to morphine 10 mg. In clinical practice, however, codeine, dihydrocodeine, dextropropoxyphene and ethoheptazine are not used par-enterally. Pentazocine, meptazinol and tramadol are available in both oral and parenteral forms.

COMBINATION (COMPOUND) PREPARATIONS

As nonopioids and weak opioids have different mechanisms of action, there is no fundamental pharmacological objection to the use of compound tablets. Combined use has been shown to produce an additive effect (Houde et al 1966). In the UK, however, the amount of codeine and dihydrocodeine in many compound tablets is generally much less than would be given if used alone (Table 13.2).

One study of compound analgesic tablets in cancer patients indicated that dextropropoxyphene and ethoheptazine are ineffectual when given by mouth in conjunction with aspirin (Fig. 13.1). Other studies, however, do not support this negative result (see p. 241). The following points should be noted:

- single dose analgesic studies do not always predict the performance of a drug when taken repeatedly
- drugs which are slowly absorbed will show up less well in single dose studies
- drugs with a prolonged plasma halflife cumulate when given repeatedly, which tends to enhance efficacy
- in this study, all preparations were given in standardized (double-blind) blue gelatin capsules, and no information was offered concerning the bio-availability or the absorption characteristics of the drugs when given in this way
- the end point (percentage of patients achieving 50% relief) is perhaps not the best for cancer pain patients.

Table 13.2   Some weak opioid compound preparations in the UK

Preparation	Weak opioid	Nonopioid
Co-codaprin	Codeine 8 mg	Aspirin 400 mg
Co-codamol	Codeine 8 mg	Paracetamol 500 mg
Solpadol, Tylex	Codeine 30 mg	Paracetamol 500 mg
Co-dydramol	Dihydrocodeine 10 mg	Paracetamol 500 mg
Remedeine	Dihydrocodeine 20 mg	Paracetamol 500 mg
Remedeine forte	Dihydrocodeine 30 mg	Paracetamol 500 mg
Co-proxamol	Dextropropoxyphene hydrochloride 32.5 mg	Paracetamol 325 mg

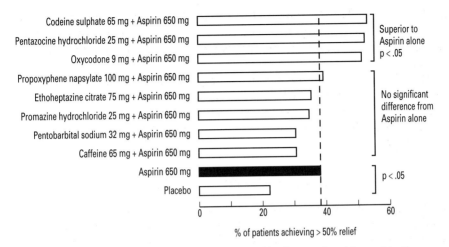

Fig. 13.1 Comparative analgesic effect of placebo, aspirin alone, and aspirin combinations as indicated by the percentage of patients achieving more than 50% relief of pain. (Reproduced with permission from Moertel et al 1974.)

CEILING EFFECT

Weak opioids are often said to have a 'ceiling' effect for analgesia. This is an oversimplification. Whereas mixed agonist-antagonists such as pentazocine have a true ceiling effect, the maximum effective dose of weak opioid agonists is arbitrary. At higher doses there are progressively more adverse effects, notably nausea and vomiting, which outweigh any extra analgesic effect.

The amount of dextropropoxyphene and ethoheptazine in compound tablets was chosen so that only a small minority of patients would experience nausea and vomiting with two tablets. This adds a further constraint; the upper dose is limited by the number of tablets which a patient will accept — possibly only two or three of any preparation.

There is little to choose between the weak opioids in terms of efficacy (Table 13.3). Codeine and dihydrocodeine are more constipating. For this

Table 13.3 Weak opioids

Drug	Bio-availability (%)	Time to maximum concentration (h)	Plasma halflife (h)	Duration of analgesia (h)[a]	Potency ratio with codeine
Codeine	40 (12–84)	–	2.5	4–5	1
Dextropropoxyphene	40	–	12–15	6–8	7/8[b]
Dihydrocodeine	20	1.6–1.8	2.5–3	3–4	4/3
Ethoheptazine	–	1	–	5–7	1/5–1/3
Meptazinol	<10	0.5–2	3.5–5[c]	3–4	2/5[d]
Pentazocine	20	1	3	2–3	(1)[d]
Tramadol	70	2	6	4–6	(2)[d]

[a] When used in usual doses for mild to moderate pain.
[b] Multiple doses; single dose = 1/2–2/3.
[c] Multiple doses in elderly; single dose = 2 h.
[d] Estimated on basis of potency ratio with morphine.

reason, co-proxamol is preferred at most palliative care units in the UK (Table 13.2). Meptazinol is not widely used and tramadol is not presently available. The following general rules should be observed:

- a weak opioid should be *added to*, not substituted for, a nonopioid
- if a weak opioid is inadequate when given regularly change to something definitely stronger (i.e. morphine)
- do not 'kangaroo' from weak opioid to weak opioid.

CODEINE

■ DRUG PORTRAIT

Codeine (methylmorphine) occurs naturally in opium. It is about 1/12 as potent as morphine. Codeine is the parent weak opioid and is used to relieve mild to moderate pain. It is well absorbed after administration by mouth. The major metabolite is codeine-6-glucuronide. Codeine exerts its analgesic effect mainly through partial biotransformation to morphine.

There is a linear dose-response curve in doses up to 360 mg IM; higher doses have not been examined. Oral bio-availability varies considerably with a mean of 40%. The plasma halflife is about 2.5 h. The maximum plasma concentration is higher after multiple doses than after a single dose. Duration of effect is comparable to morphine. Usual oral doses are 30–60 mg q4h–q6h; higher doses can be given. Codeine is also used as an antitussive and an antidiarrhoeal.

The plasma halflife of codeine varies in different studies from 2.5–4.5 h (Persson et al 1992). The lower figure is probably more reliable. Single dose studies indicate that parenterally codeine is less than 1/12 as potent as morphine (Lasagna & Beecher 1954) and between 1/3 and 1/4 as potent by mouth (Eddy et al 1968). If this were true of repeated administration, it would mean that codeine 60 mg is as potent as morphine 15–20 mg PO. This is not so; the majority of patients with poor relief from weak opioids or compound preparations obtain good relief from morphine 10 mg q4h.

In a recent study using high performance liquid chromatography (HPLC), oral bio-availability varied extensively, ranging between 12 and 84% with a mean of 40% (Persson et al 1992). These figures are similar to those for morphine, and suggest that the codeine:morphine potency ratio is probably the same for both parenteral and oral administration, i.e. about 1/12.

In a single dose study in patients with terminal cancer, it was not possible to distinguish between 32 mg of codeine and 650 mg of aspirin, although both were better than a placebo (Houde et al 1966). When taken together, an additive effect was noted, lending support to the common practice of combining aspirin with codeine (Fig. 13.2).

No clinical trial has distinguished between codeine 15 mg PO and placebo, and not all have with codeine 30 mg. However, codeine 20 mg and ibuprofen 400 mg show an additive effect (Fig. 13.3). Further, the analgesic effect after

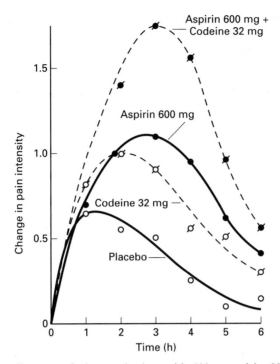

Fig. 13.2   Time-effect curves for lactose placebo, aspirin 600 mg, codeine 32 mg and a combination of aspirin 600 mg and codeine 32 mg. Changes in pain intensity are plotted against time in hours. Treatments were administered in a randomized order on a complete crossover basis to 11 patients with pain due to cancer. Nine of the patients repeated the crossover twice. (Reproduced with permission from Houde et al 1966.)

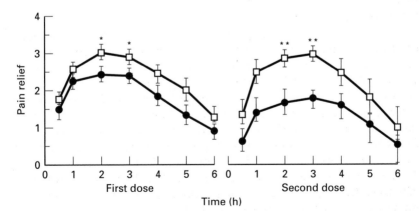

Fig. 13.3   Mean pain relief scores against time for the first and second doses. □ = combination of ibuprofen 400 mg and codeine phosphate 25.6 mg; ● = ibuprofen 400 mg. * = $p < 0.05$; ** = $p < 0.02$, Wilcoxon matched-pairs signed-ranks test. (Reproduced with permission from McQuay et al 1989.)

the second dose is significantly greater than after the first (McQuay et al 1989). This fits with the observation that the maximum plasma concentration of codeine is higher after multiple doses than after a single dose (Chen et al 1991). The only currently available compound preparation in the UK of codeine and ibuprofen is a m/r tablet containing codeine 20 mg and ibuprofen 300 mg (Codafen Continus). Price apart, the very low content of both drugs in this preparation means that it has no real place in cancer pain management.

Biotransformation of codeine to morphine

Codeine is eliminated primarily by glucuronidation to codeine-6-glucuronide (Fig. 13.4). Minor metabolic pathways are O-demethylation to morphine and N-demethylation to norcodeine, each accounting for about 10% of the dose (Adler et al 1955). Whereas both morphine-6-glucuronide and normorphine are known to be active metabolites of morphine, comparable information is not available for the corresponding codeine metabolites. For many years, however, it has been suggested that the analgesic effect of codeine may be mediated via morphine itself (Sanfilippo 1948). Although not without its critics (Quiding et al 1986), this view is supported by experiments which show that, even though 1/12 as potent as morphine, the affinity of codeine for the mu opioid receptor is 3000 times less than that of morphine (Pert & Snyder 1973).

It is now known that some people are slow metabolizers of debrisoquine because they lack a necessary gene (Heim & Meyer 1990). This drug is used to test the CYP2D6 metabolic pathway (alias P450 II D6 or sparteine oxygenase pathway). Many drugs, including tricyclic antidepressants, are metabolized by this pathway and toxic drug plasma concentrations are likely to occur in enzyme deficient people. In these same people, codeine is not converted to morphine (Sindrup et al 1991), and the analgesic effect of codeine is minimal (Desmeules et al 1991). Likewise, pretreatment with quinidine (an inhibitor of the same enzyme system), also markedly impairs the analgesic effect of codeine (Sindrup et al 1992). These data imply that

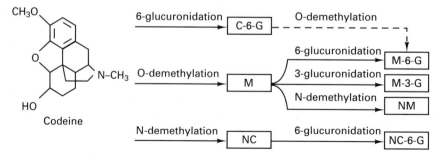

Fig. 13.4 Pattern of codeine metabolism in humans. C-6-G = codeine-6-glucuronide; M = morphine; NC = norcodeine; M-6-G = morphine-6-glucuronide; M-3-G = morphine-3-glucuronide; NM = normorphine; NC-6-G = norcodeine-6-glucuronide. (Reproduced with permission from Sindrup et al 1991.)

the 5–10% of the population who cannot produce morphine from codeine will get little or no analgesic effect from codeine.

Although this conclusion has been challenged, it surely means that people who say they do not obtain relief with codeine should be believed. Methods to determine if a person is genetically deficient in this respect have been developed and can identify more than 95% of affected people (Heim & Meyer 1990).

Animal studies have shown that brain slices and brain microsomes can convert codeine to morphine (Chen et al 1990). The same is likely to be true for humans. Thus, even if plasma morphine concentrations after systemic codeine are below the minimal effective concentration, it is still possible that codeine analgesia may be mediated by morphine produced in the CNS.

DIHYDROCODEINE

■ DRUG PORTRAIT

Dihydrocodeine is a semisynthetic weak opioid agonist with a potency about 1/3 greater than codeine. Its plasma halflife is 2.5–3 h and it is metabolized along the same pathways as codeine. Duration of useful effect is consistently less than morphine. Usual doses are 30–60 mg q4h–q6h; higher doses can be given. M/r dihydrocodeine tablets are available in many countries but not in the USA.

Dihydrocodeine was introduced in Germany as an antitussive about 70 years ago. Interest in its analgesic potential is more recent, dating back some 40 years. Although it has been claimed to be twice as potent as codeine, some trials have reported it to be less potent (Seed 1958). Usually, the effect has been equal or slightly greater, on average by about one third. It is suggested that the optimal parenteral dose is 30 mg (Eddy et al 1956). At 60 mg IM pain relief is increased only slightly and morphine-like adverse effects become more evident. By mouth, if an oral to parenteral potency ratio of 1:3 is assumed, the optimal dose limit will be of the order of 90–120 mg. At all dose levels studied, the duration of relief is shorter with dihydrocodeine than with morphine (Beecher et al 1957).

Presystemic metabolism, presumably in the gut wall and liver reduces the oral bio-availability of dihydrocodeine to 20%. The metabolism of dihydrocodeine has not been fully established. Assuming that it undergoes similar biotransformation to codeine, its major metabolites would be (Rowell et al 1983):

- dihydrocodeine-6-glucuronide (as the major metabolite)
- dihydromorphine and glucuronide metabolites
- N-de-alkylcodeine and glucuronide metabolites.

Life threatening respiratory failure peaked 36–48 h after an overdose of dihydrocodeine in a patient with renal failure (Redfern 1983). This suggests that dihydrocodeine-6-glucuronide could be an active agent. Metabolic acidosis could have reduced tissue penetration and resulted in higher plasma concentrations (Barnes et al 1985), but the prolonged effect is difficult to explain in these terms alone.

Dihydrocodeine 30–60 mg has been compared with ibuprofen 400 mg q.i.d. as needed for 6 days in postdental extraction pain (McQuay et al 1993). About half the patients receiving dihydrocodeine were withdrawn from the study on the first postoperative day because of adverse effects (nausea, vomiting, drowsiness) and/or inadequate relief, compared with 6/44 patients receiving ibuprofen. This trial demonstrates, once again, that a nonsteroidal anti-inflammatory drug (NSAID) may well be a better analgesic (i.e. more relief, less adverse effects) than an opioid for moderately severe pain.

There are few controlled trials of oral dihydrocodeine with other oral opioids. A 60 mg dose of dihydrocodeine is probably equivalent to about 6 mg of morphine sulphate. As with codeine, a starting dose of morphine 10 mg q4h is indicated for patients obtaining inadequate relief with dihydrocodeine 60 mg. In a few, the dose may need to be increased rapidly to 20 mg.

In a study of 95 healthy volunteers who took dihydrocodeine 30 mg on three consecutive mornings after breakfast, compared with placebo taken in the same way a week later, nausea and dizziness occurred significantly more often in the 41 females than in the 54 male participants. The results also suggested that dihydrocodeine may be more constipating in men than in women ($p = 0.064$) (Palmer et al 1966). Whether these differences hold true for codeine or morphine is not known.

M/r tablets contain dihydrocodeine 60 mg, 90 mg and 120 mg equivalent to m/r morphine 6 mg, 9 mg and 12 mg respectively. In practice m/r dihydrocodeine is prescribed mainly for patients with chronic nonmalignant pain, e.g. low back pain.

DEXTROPROPOXYPHENE

■ DRUG PORTRAIT

Dextropropoxyphene is a synthetic analgesic structurally related to methadone. It is a weak opioid agonist and is readily absorbed from the gastro-intestinal tract over 2–3 h. Single doses are approximately 1/2–2/3 as potent as codeine; multiple doses about 7/8 as potent. Dextropropoxyphene injections are not available; they are painful and have a toxic effect on soft tissues and veins.

Dextropropoxyphene is N-demethylated in the liver to yield norpropoxyphene which has substantially less central depressant effect. Dextropropoxyphene has a plasma halflife of 12–15 h, whereas that of norpropoxyphene is 30–36 h. The latter is slowly excreted in the urine. The usual dose of dextropropoxyphene hydrochloride is 65 mg q6h; this is equivalent to dextropropoxyphene napsylate 100 mg. Higher doses can be given.

Single dose studies of dextropropoxyphene indicate that it is definitely less potent than codeine as an analgesic (Beaver 1966). However, it has a much longer plasma halflife and cumulates when taken regularly (Waife et al 1975). When given q6h, the plasma concentration increases progressively and reaches a steady state after 2–3 days (McLeod 1972). A potency ratio of 7/8 or more is a reasonable estimate for multiple doses (Beaver 1984). Its laevorotatory isomer, levopropoxyphene, is not an analgesic, but is marketed in the USA as a cough suppressant (Novrad).

In the UK, dextropropoxyphene is generally prescribed in combination with paracetamol (32.5 mg + 325 mg; co-proxamol). It is also available alone in a tablet containing dextropropoxyphene napsylate 100 mg. In the USA it is used more commonly alone than in combination.

In the 1970s there was much controversy about the efficacy of dextropropoxyphene because of equivocal results in single dose studies (Miller et al 1970). However, the dose-response curves obtained in a study of postoperative and fracture pain, show unequivocally that dextropropoxyphene is an active and efficacious opioid analgesic (Fig. 13.5). It is not possible to have a dose-response curve of this nature with an inactive substance. The study also suggested that dextropropoxyphene may be more bio-available when administered as the napsylate salt rather than the hydrochloride.

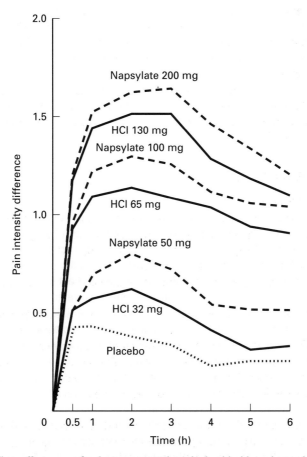

Fig. 13.5 Time-effect curves for dextropropoxyphene hydrochloride and napsylate. (Reproduced with permission from Beaver 1984; adapted from Sunshine et al 1971.)

Co-proxamol is generally a well tolerated preparation. In a few patients, both young and old, it causes unacceptable central effects, notably, muzziness, lightheadedness, dysphoria and/or confusional symptoms. There is no way of predicting such patients. As with other opioids, constipation is a common adverse effect, although usually not as troublesome as with codeine and dihydrocodeine. Occasional patients will experience nausea and/or vomiting. Thus, as with all opioid analgesics, when prescribed dextropropoxyphene, the patient should be advised who to contact and how in the event of unacceptable adverse effects.

Drug interactions

An important drug interaction has been reported in three patients (Dam & Christiansen 1977). They were also taking carbamazepine and complained of headache, dizziness, ataxia, nausea and tiredness. Combined use resulted in an increase of the plasma concentration of carbamazepine which accounted for the symptoms. Dextropropoxyphene is thought to inhibit the oxidation of carbamazepine (Dam & Christiansen 1977).

It has also been reported that, when taken regularly, dextropropoxyphene may interfere with coumarin anticoagulants. Up to 150 mg of dextropropoxyphene a day once or twice a week is safe, but the regular ingestion of 200 mg or more may require a reduction in the dose of the oral anticoagulant (Standing Advisory Committee 1982). As paracetamol may also increase thrombotest times, anticoagulated patients commencing co-proxamol should be closely monitored and the dose of anticoagulant reduced if necessary.

ETHOHEPTAZINE

■ DRUG PORTRAIT

Ethoheptazine is structurally related to pethidine/meperidine but is less potent. It is about 1/4 as potent as codeine. It is readily absorbed from the gastrointestinal tract and peak plasma concentration is reached in 1 h. The plasma halflife is not known. It is extensively metabolized in the liver and the metabolites excreted in the urine. The duration of useful effect is 5–7 h. The usual dose is ethoheptazine *citrate* 150 mg q6h–q8h (equivalent to ethoheptazine base 100 mg). Higher doses can be given. In the UK, ethoheptazine is available only in a compound tablet containing ethoheptazine citrate 75 mg, meprobamate 150 mg and aspirin 250 mg. It is not available within the National Health Service in the UK and is a Controlled Drug.

Ethoheptazine may be thought of as weak pethidine. Its basic structure comprises a heterocyclic ring of seven members, whereas pethidine, a piperidine, has six. Ethoheptazine is about 1/3 as potent as pethidine (Gleesman & Seifter 1956). Its plasma halflife is not known. By injection, it is longer acting than both pethidine and morphine, with most patients requesting it at intervals of 5–7 h (Grossman et al 1956). When first introduced, concern was expressed about cumulative CNS toxicity after days or weeks of regular administration. This took the form of nervousness, headache, dizziness, 'visual symptoms' and syncope (Golbey et al 1955). Subsequently it was decided that these had been caused by an impurity in the original batch of medication. In contrast to pethidine, ethoheptazine does not (Seifter et al 1954):

- cause lethargy in rats
- produce morphine-like excitement in cats
- depress respiration until very high doses are administered.

Ethoheptazine has been used in doses of up to 500 mg q4h in patients with various acute and chronic pains (Grossman et al 1956). Two thirds of those who received 250 mg q4h experienced adverse effects. Some patients developed toxic reactions after 1–3 weeks. However, two patients received 500 mg q4h without toxicity. When the dose was reduced to 75 mg any adverse effects were predominantly gastric, i.e. nausea, vomiting and epigastric discomfort.

As a result of this study (Grossman et al 1956), 50 mg of ethoheptazine base (75 mg of ethoheptazine citrate) has been adopted as the standard quantity per tablet. This gives a dose of 100 mg (citrate 150 mg) in two tablets. It would seem, however, that there may be occasions when a higher dose could be safely used. The single dose study referred to already (Moertel et al 1974) almost certainly employed a suboptimal dose of ethoheptazine (Cass et al 1958). Further, an analgesic with a relatively long duration of action is likely to have a relatively long plasma halflife. This means that, with regular administration, the plasma concentration will rise substantially over several days, and result in progressively more relief.

In the doses commonly used, ethoheptazine is as effective as codeine but, on a mg for mg basis, is only 1/3–1/5 as potent. Ethoheptazine is less constipating and causes less nausea. Drowsiness is unusual (Grossman et al 1956). This makes ethoheptazine a more attractive drug than codeine in situations in which one wishes to avoid adverse alimentary and CNS effects.

Equagesic is the only commonly used preparation containing ethoheptazine in the UK and the USA. It also contains aspirin and meprobamate. Aspirin may itself cause gastritis, whereas meprobamate (a mild anxiolytic and muscle relaxant) may cause drowsiness. This is usually transient, and clears after 2–3 days. Occasionally, patients are hypersensitive to meprobamate and experience malaise or a skin rash after a few doses.

MEPTAZINOL

■ DRUG PORTRAIT

Meptazinol is a synthetic centrally acting analgesic. It has both opioid and nonopioid properties. It is a partial mu_1 opioid agonist with central cholinergic properties (Green 1983, Spiegel & Pasternak 1984). It precipitates abstinence phenonema in animals dependent on morphine. The analgesic effect of meptazinol is antagonized by naloxone and by drugs with central anticholinergic properties, e.g. atropine and hyoscine (Bensreti et al 1983). Parenterally meptazinol is as potent as pethidine. Because of extensive hepatic first pass metabolism, oral bio-availability is less than 10%. Peak plasma concentrations are reached in 0.5–2 h.

Meptazinol is extensively metabolized mainly to a glucuronide; less than 5% of unchanged drug is recovered in the urine. Plasma halflife is about 2 h. Multiple doses in the elderly extend the plasma halflife from 3.5 h to 5 h, though the peak plasma concentration is not significantly increased. Meptazinol is available for PO, IM and IV use. It is shorter acting than morphine and injections of 75–100 mg may need to be given q2h. The recommended oral dose is twice that of the injection, although this provides only 20% as much drug systemically. Meptazinol is therefore a weak opioid when used by mouth. The usual oral dose is 200 mg q3h–q4h; higher doses can be given.

Radioligand binding studies show that meptazinol has only low affinity for opioid receptors (Spiegel & Pasternak 1984, Pasternak et al 1985). In contrast, high affinity sites for meptazinol have been identified in the cerebral cortex and the spinal cord of rats in areas that are distinct from those with high density opioid receptors (Green 1983). This binding is not affected by morphine, buprenorphine or naloxone. Unlike opioid receptors, meptazinol binding sites lack stereospecificity. In animals, meptazinol has also been shown to increase noradrenaline content in the brain stem and hypothalamus, and to increase serotonin content in the brain stem (Kmieciak-Kolada & Herman 1988).

Postoperatively, meptazinol 100 mg IM is as effective as papaveretum 20 mg IM (Moyes et al 1979). It is, however, shorter acting; the duration of useful effect being less than 3 h in many patients. Like pethidine, meptazinol does not effect pupil diameter. It has remarkably little effect on respiration, nor does it cause constipation (Holmes & Ward 1985). Meptazinol precipitates withdrawal phenomena in animals, including primates, and reverses respiratory depression induced by morphine (Stephens et al 1978). In complete contrast to morphine and pentazocine, however, meptazinol potentiates the electrically induced twitch of an isolated guinea pig ileum (Stephens et al 1978). Similarly, in other morphine sensitive tissues such as the mouse and the rat vas deferens, meptazinol has effects opposite to those of morphine and pentazocine.

The analgesic effect of meptazinol is almost completely reversed by naloxone, although higher doses are required than are necessary for other opioid agonists. The analgesic effect of meptazinol in mice is also antagonized by low doses of centrally acting anticholinergic drugs such as hyoscine (Green 1983).

Meptazinol delays paracetamol absorption to a greater extent than morphine (Fig. 13.6), and will presumably delay the absorption of other drugs given concurrently.

TRAMADOL

■ DRUG PORTRAIT

Tramadol is a synthetic centrally acting analgesic. It has both opioid and

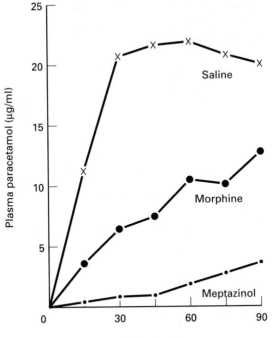

Fig. 13.6 Mean plasma paracetamol concentrations after saline, morphine and meptazinol. (Reproduced with permission from Nimmo et al 1986.)

nonopioid properties (Raffa et al 1992, Lee et al 1993). The latter are related to stimulation of neuronal serotonin release and inhibition of presynaptic re-uptake of noradrenaline and serotonin. Tramadol is readily absorbed from the gastro-intestinal tract and has an oral bio-availability of about 70%. Parenterally it is 1/10 as potent as morphine. Tramadol is converted in the liver to O-desmethyltramadol which is itself an active substance, two to four times more potent than tramadol. Further biotransformation results in inactive metabolites which are excreted by the kidneys. Tramadol has a plasma halflife of 6 h. Duration of analgesic effect is 4–6 h depending on the dose given and the intensity of pain. Usual oral doses are 50–100 mg q4h–q6h; higher doses can be given.

The opioid properties of tramadol relate to mu, delta and kappa opioid receptor agonism, with a 20-fold preference for the mu receptor ((+)enantiomer). The nonopioid properties are related to stimulation of serotonin release ((+)enantiomer) and inhibition of presynaptic re-uptake of noradrenaline and serotonin ((–)enantiomer). As noted in Chapter 3, noradrenaline and serotonin are neurotransmitters for the descending inhibitory pathways which modulate nociception.

The actions of tramadol are best demonstrated by observing the impact of an alpha$_2$-adrenergic antagonist, yohimbine, on the antinociceptive effect

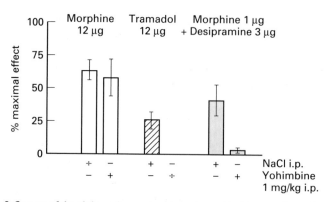

Fig. 13.7 Influence of the alpha$_2$-adrenergic antagonist, yohimbine, on the analgesic effect of morphine, tramadol and the combination of subthreshold doses of morphine and desipramine. i.p. = intraperitoneally. (Reproduced with permission from Driessen et al 1990.)

of morphine, morphine and desipramine (a selective noradrenaline re-uptake inhibitor) and tramadol (Fig. 13.7). Yohimbine has no impact on morphine analgesia but antagonizes the effect of tramadol and also the combined effect of morphine and desipramine (given at doses which are ineffective when given alone). An analogous effect can be shown by blocking serotonin receptors with ritanserin. Naloxone only partially reverses the analgesic effect of tramadol (Raffa et al 1992). A comparison of receptor site affinities and mono-amine re-uptake inhibition illustrates the unique combination of properties which underlie the action of tramadol (Table 13.4 & 13.5). A synergistic interaction is necessary to explain its analgesic effect.

Table 13.4 Opioid receptor affinities: K_i (uM) values[a]

	Mu	Delta	Kappa
Morphine	0.0003	0.09	0.6
Dextropropoxyphene	0.03	0.38	1.2
Codeine	0.2	5	6
Tramadol	2	58	43

[a] The lower the K_i value, the greater the receptor affinity.
From Raffa et al 1992

Table 13.5 Inhibition of mono-amine uptake: K_i (uM) values[a]

	Noradrenaline	Serotonin
Imipramine	0.0066	0.021
Tramadol	0.78	0.99
Dextropropoxyphene	} IA[b]	IA
Codeine		
Morphine		

[a] The lower the K_i value, the greater the receptor affinity.
[b] IA = inactive at 10 uM.
From Raffa et al 1992

The principal metabolite of tramadol, mono-O-desmethyltramadol, is also pharmacologically active. It has a higher affinity for opioid receptors than tramadol itself. The quantity produced in man is small, however, and its contribution to analgesia is probably also small. Parenterally, tramadol and pethidine are equipotent, about 1/10 as potent as morphine (Vickers et al 1992).

Tramadol is used extensively in many countries, although it is not yet licensed as an analgesic in the UK or the USA. Tramadol can be administered PO, PR, SC, IM and IV. It has been used for IV patient controlled analgesia (PCA) postoperatively (Chrubasik et al 1992). An open study of the use of tramadol in cancer pain has been published (Grond et al 1992). Despite very good oral bio-availability (about 70%), some centres use the same potency ratio with morphine (1/10) when changing between oral preparations as when changing between parenteral ones (Zech D 1993 Personal Communication). A double-blind trial of morphine and tramadol in cancer patients concluded, however, that the oral potency ratio is approximately 1/4 (Wilder-Smith et al 1994).

Tramadol is usually administered in doses of 50–100 mg q4h–q6h. Experience with higher doses is limited. 200 mg is a typical *daily* dose for moderate pain. Tramadol is as effective as codeine when used as a cough suppressant (Szekely & Vickers 1992). Tramadol causes much less constipation and respiratory depression than equi-analgesic doses of other opioids (Houmes et al 1992, Vickers et al 1992). Its dependence liability is also considerably less (Preston et al 1991), and it is not a Controlled Drug.

PENTAZOCINE

■ DRUG PORTRAIT

Pentazocine is a synthetic centrally acting analgesic. It is the N-allyl derivative of phenazocine and a partial mu and kappa agonist, and delta antagonist (Hill 1992). Pentazocine 30–60 mg IM is as effective as morphine 10 mg IM (Hoskin & Hanks 1991). It is shorter acting than morphine, analgesia lasting up to 3 h. A ceiling effect is observed with parenteral doses above 100 mg. Usual oral doses are 25–100 mg q3h–q4h. Because of its short duration of action and its ability to cause psychotomimetic effects, pentazocine is not recommended for cancer pain management.

Pentazocine was the first mixed agonist-antagonist opioid to be introduced for clinical use (Houde 1979, Martin 1979). Originally, it was regarded as a mu antagonist, kappa agonist. Consequently, it was stated that pentazocine should not be administered with or after morphine. A *synergistic* effect between morphine and pentazocine, however, has been noted (Levine & Gordon 1988). Thus, although neither pentazocine 15 mg IV nor morphine 2 mg IV produced significant analgesia on their own, in combination they produced significantly greater analgesia than either pentazocine *30 mg* or morphine *4 mg* alone. The analgesia produced was comparable to that obtained with morphine 16 mg (Levine & Gordon 1988). The analgesia produced by a combination of pentazocine 30 mg and morphine 4 mg, however, was not significantly greater than that obtained with the lower doses. This indicates that there is a limit to the synergy between the two preparations.

In certain circumstances, however, pentazocine does reverse the analgesic effect of morphine. Whereas in opioid naive patients morphine 8 mg IM and pentazocine 40 mg and 80 mg IM show additive effects, in opioid tolerant patients pentazocine 10 mg, 20 mg and 40 mg caused a progressive reduction in the effect of morphine (Houde et al 1972, Houde 1974). In addition, pentazocine has been used postoperatively in elderly patients to reverse the respiratory depression induced by fentanyl administered during surgery while, at the same time, maintaining analgesia (Rifat 1972).

Like most opioids, pentazocine increases the tone of the sphincter of Oddi and raises the pressure within the pancreatic and biliary ducts (Staritz et al 1985).

By mouth, pentazocine is a weak opioid. In cancer patients, pentazocine 50 mg is less potent than two tablets of co-codaprin or co-proxamol (Robbie & Samarasinghe 1973). Further, considering there are safer alternatives, the proportion of patients experiencing psychotomimetic effects is unacceptably high. In hospital patients who received parenteral pentazocine for acute pain, the incidence was 7–10% (Woods et al 1974). The incidence in patients with terminal cancer is almost certainly higher because of concurrence with other factors which also can cause such symptoms. Although these effects tend to be dose related, they have occurred after even small doses by mouth. Psychotomimetic effects occur occasionally with all opioid analgesics, including morphine, but probably in no more than 1–2% of patients.

The ability of pentazocine in some situations to reverse morphine analgesia could cause problems. Patients are sometimes in possession of several different opioid containing preparations — one of which could contain pentazocine. Thus, to avoid antagonism resulting from concurrent use, pentazocine is best not used at all in the management of cancer pain.

ANTIDIARRHOEALS

Opioids affect the gastro-intestinal tract in various ways (Box 13.A). Increased absorption of electrolytes and water from the intestinal lumen and a prolonged intestinal transit time account for the antidiarrhoeal effect of opioids. The prolonged transit time results from increased segmentation of the circular muscle coat and diminished peristalsis. This effect is mediated by a specific opioid receptor in the intestinal wall which causes the release of serotonin (5HT). This in turn acts through both cholinergic and non-cholinergic pathways. Effects are dose related and, in animal models, are inhibited by naloxone, 5HT antagonists and the belladonna alkaloids. Clinically, however, the belladonna alkaloids do not relieve constipation in patients receiving opioids. This may be partly because of the relative doses used. More likely, it reflects the fact that atropine and hyoscine (and other

> **BOX 13.A**
> **OPIOIDS AND THE GASTRO-INTESTINAL TRACT** (Krueger 1937, Beubler 1983)
>
> **Actions**
> Increase sphincter tone:
>
> - Oddi
> - ileocaecal
> - anal
>
> Increase segmentation (ring contractions):
>
> - pyloric antrum
> - small intestine
> - colon
>
> Increase electrolyte and water absorption:
>
> - small intestine
> - large intestine
>
> Impair defaecation reflex:
>
> - rectum less sensitive to distension
> - increased internal anal sphincter tone
>
> **Effects**
> Delay gastric emptying:
>
> - epigastric fullness
> - flatulence
> - anorexia
> - nausea
> - vomiting
>
> Infrequent defaecation }
> Hard faeces   }   constipation

anticholinergic drugs) have a diffuse antimotility effect on the intestinal musculature. This means that such drugs not only reduce segmentation but also diminish peristalsis. Codeine and morphine are often used as anti-diarrhoeals. Diphenoxylate and loperamide, however, are opioid agonists used solely as antidiarrhoeals.

Diphenoxylate

■ DRUG PORTRAIT

Diphenoxylate is an opioid agonist derived from pethidine but devoid of analgesic activity. Like codeine and morphine, it interacts both centrally and peripherally with opioid receptors. It can therefore cause typical adverse opioid effects, although with recommended doses the incidence of such effects is low. Diphenoxylate is well absorbed by mouth. Peak plasma levels occur within 3 h of administration. Difenoxin is the major metabolite. This also has antimotility properties. The combined plasma halflife of the two substances is 6 h. The duration of useful effect is 6–8 h. The initial recommended dose is diphenoxylate 10 mg, followed by 5 mg q6h. Less frequent administration may be satisfactory, depending on individual needs and response. Diphenoxylate is available only with atropine (co-phenotrope). This contains the two substances in a ratio of 100:1, i.e. diphenoxylate 2.5 mg with atropine 25 μg.

Loperamide

■ DRUG PORTRAIT

Loperamide is a peripherally acting opioid agonist derived from butyramide. It is chemically related to both haloperidol and pethidine. Loperamide differs from codeine, morphine and diphenoxylate in that it has no central opioid activity at normal oral therapeutic doses. It is poorly absorbed by mouth. Peak plasma levels occur within 4 h of administration, and the plasma halflife is 7–15 h. Excretion is mainly in the faeces; 40% of an oral dose is excreted unchanged by this route in 8 days. 10% is excreted in the urine either unchanged or conjugated with glucuronic acid. Biliary elimination is an important route of excretion in rats but this has not so far been studied in man. The initial recommended dose for acute diarrhoea is 4 mg, followed by 2 mg with each loose motion, up to 16 mg/day. When used chronically, individual needs vary widely, from 2 mg once a day to 4 mg q.i.d.. Higher doses can be used.

Loperamide is about three times more potent than diphenoxylate and 50 times more potent than codeine (Schuermans et al 1974). It is also longer acting, and may need to be given only once or twice a day. The following regimens are approximately equivalent in terms of antidiarrhoeal effect:

loperamide	2 mg b.i.d.
diphenoxylate	2.5 mg (as co-phenotrope) q.i.d
codeine phosphate	60 mg t.i.d.–q.i.d.

Tablet or capsule size obviously imposes an artificial restraint. This makes it impossible to give regimens of exact equivalence. All three agents are also available in liquid (syrup) forms. In the UK, kaolin and morphine mixture BPC is a useful alternative.

Loperamide should be regarded as the opioid of choice for the non-specific treatment of diarrhoea in patients who do not require analgesic or antitussive medication. This is because, with loperamide, the dissociation of opioid gastro-intestinal effects from opioid CNS effects is almost complete. When small amounts only are needed, codeine 30 mg b.i.d.–t.i.d. may be preferable as it is cheaper.

Loperamide is devoid of central activity even at doses four times higher than the constipating dose (Schuermans et al 1974). When it is injected IV, however, opioid CNS effects have been described (Niemegeers et al 1979). It has no abuse potential. Loperamide is well tolerated by patients and adverse effects are rare in doses up to 10 mg/day. Adverse effects include fatigue in 2% and abdominal colic in 6% (Palmer et al 1980).

Studies of loperamide demonstrate a specific antisecretory effect (Burleigh 1991). In the rat jejunum, loperamide inhibits the secretion of water and sodium and chloride ions induced by cholera toxin. Loperamide also inhibits jejunal secretion induced by prostaglandins and bile salts. It has no effect on the osmotic secretion induced by intraluminal hypertonic mannitol (Sandhu et al 1983). This indicates that the antisecretory effect is mediated by specific transport mechanisms, and is not merely a passive diffusional process. Loperamide may have a specific action on the anal sphincter (Read et al 1982). This could be of value in patients with diarrhoea complicated by faecal incontinence.

REFERENCES

Adler T K, Fujimoto J M, Way E L, Baker E M 1955 The metabolic fate of codeine in man. Journal of Pharmacology and Experimental Therapeutics 114: 251–262

Barnes J N, Williams A J, Tomson M J F, Toseland P A, Goodwin F J 1985 Dihydrocodeine in renal failure: further evidence for an important role of the kidney in the handling of opioid drugs. British Medical Journal 290: 740–742

Beaver W T 1966 Mild analgesics: a review of their clinical pharmacology (Part II). American Journal of Medical Science 251: 576–599

Beaver W T 1984 Analgesic efficacy of dextropropoxyphene and dextropropoxyphene-containing combinations: a review. Human Toxicology 3: 191s–220s

Beecher H K, Gravenstein J S, Pederson D P, Smith G M 1957 Analgesic effect and side effect liability of dihydrocodeine, codeine and morphine in man. Federal Proceedings 16: 281

Bensreti M M, Golley S, Gonzalez J P et al 1983 Selective and combined antagonism of the biphasic antinociceptive activity of meptazinol using opiate and cholinergic antagonists. British Journal of Pharmacology 80: 559

Beubler E 1983 Opiates and intestinal transport: in vivo studies. In: Turnberg L A (ed) Intestinal secretion. Smith, Kline & French Laboratories, Hertfordshire, pp 53–55

Burleigh D E 1991 Loperamide but not morphine has antisecretory effects in human colon in vitro. European Journal of Pharmacology 202: 277–280

Cass L J, Frederick W S, Batholomey A F 1958 Methods in evaluating ethoheptazine and ethoheptazine combined with aspirin. Journal of the American Medical Association 166: 1829–1833

Chen Z R, Irvine R J, Bochner F, Somogyi A A 1990 Morphine formation from codeine in rat brain: a possible mechanism of codeine analgesia. Life Sciences 46: 1067–1074

Chen Z R, Somogyi A A, Reynolds G, Bochner F 1991 Disposition and metabolism of codeine after single and chronic doses in one poor and seven extensive metabolisers. British Journal of Clinical Pharmacology 31: 381–390

Chrubasik J, Buzina M, Schulte-Monting J, Atanassoff P, Alon E 1992 Intravenous tramadol for post-operative pain: comparison of intermittent dose regimens with and without maintenance infusion. European Journal of Anaesthesiology 9: 23–28

Dam M, Christiansen J 1977 Interaction of propoxyphene with carbamazepine. Lancet ii: 509

Desmeules J, Gascon M-P, Dayer P, Magistris M 1991 Impact of environmental and genetic factors on codeine analgesia. European Journal of Clinical Pharmacology 41: 23–26

Driessen B, Schlutz H, Reimann W 1990 Evidence for a non-opioid component in the analgesic action of tramadol. Naunyn Schmiedeberg's Archives of Pharmacology 341: R104

Eddy N B, Halden H, Braenden O J 1956 Synthetic substances with morphine-like effect: relationship between analgesic action and addiction liability, with discussion of chemical structure of addiction – producing substances. Bulletin of World Health Organisation 14: 353–402, 835–836

Eddy N B, Friebel H, Hahn K-J, Hallbach H 1968 Codeine and its alternatives for pain and cough relief. 1. Bulletin of World Health Organization 38: 673–741

Gleesman J M, Seifter J 1956 The analgesic activity of some phenylhexamethylenimine derivatives. Journal of Pharmacology and Experimental Therapeutics 116: 23–24

Golbey M, Gittinger W C, Batterman R C 1955 Analgesic potency of parenterally administered azocycloheptane derivatives in man. Federation Proceedings 14: 344

Green D 1983 Current concepts concerning the mode of action of meptazinol as an analgesic. Postgraduate Medical Journal 59 (suppl 1): 9–12

Grond S, Zech D, Lynch J, Schug S, Lehmann K A 1992 Tramadol: a weak opioid for relief of cancer pain. The Pain Clinic 5: 241–247

Grossman A J, Golbey M, Gittinger W C, Batterman R C 1956 Clinical effectiveness and safety of a new series of analgesic compounds. Journal of the American Gerontology Society 4: 187–192

Heim M, Meyer U A 1990 Genotyping of poor metabolisers of debrisoquine by allelo-specific PCR amplication. Lancet 336: 529–532

Hill R G 1992 Multiple opioid receptors and their ligands. Frontiers of Pain 4: 1–4

Holmes B, Ward A 1985 Meptazinol: a review of its pharmacodynamic and pharmacokinetic properties and therapeutic efficacy. Drugs 30: 285–312

Hoskin P J, Hanks G W 1991 Opioid agonist-antagonist drugs in acute and chronic pain states. Drugs 41: 326–344

Houde R W 1974 The use and misuse of narcotics in the treatment of chronic pain. In: Bonica J J (ed) Advances in neurology, vol 4. Raven Press, New York, pp 527–536

Houde R W 1979 Analgesic effectiveness of the narcotic agonist-antagonists. British Journal of Clinical Pharmacology 7: 297s–308s

Houde R W, Wallenstein S L, Beaver W T 1966 Evaluation of analgesics in patients with cancer pain. In: Lasagna L (ed) Clinical pharmacology. Section 6 of International encyclopedia of pharmacology and therapeutics. Pergamon, Oxford, pp 59–97

Houde R W, Wallenstein S L, Rogers A 1972 Analgesic studies program of the Sloan-Kettering Institute for Cancer Research. In: Report of the 34th Annual Scientific Meeting, Committee on problems of drug dependence. National Academy of Sciences, Washington DC, pp 151–172

Houmes R J M, Voets M A, Verkaaik A, Erdmann W and Lachmann B 1992 Efficacy and safety of tramadol versus morphine for moderate and severe postoperative pain with special regard to respiratory depression. Anesthesia Analgesia 74: 510–514

Kmieciak-Kolada K, Herman Z S 1988 Influence of meptazinol on levels of biogenicamines in discrete brain areas of rat. Acta Poloniae Pharmaceutica 45: 276–279

Krueger H 1937 The action of morphine on the digestive tract. Physiology Reviews 17: 618–645

Lasagna L, Beecher K H 1954 The analgesic effectiveness of codeine and meperidine (Demerol). Journal of Pharmacology and Experimental Therapeutics 112: 306–311

Lee C R, McTavish D, Sorkin E M 1993 Tramadol: a preliminary review of its pharmacodynamic and pharmacokinetic properties, and therapeutic potential in acute and chronic pain states. Drugs 46: 313–340

Levine J D, Gordon N C 1988 Synergism between the analgesic actions of morphine and pentazocine. Pain 33: 369–372

McLeod D C 1972 Propoxyphenes – drug evaluation data. Drug Intelligence and Clinical Pharmacy 6: 143–144

McQuay H J, Carroll D, Watts P G, Juniper R P, Moore R A 1989 Codeine 20 mg increases pain relief from ibuprofen 400 mg after third molar surgery. A repeat-dosing comparison of ibuprofen and an ibuprofen-codeine combination. Pain 37: 7–13

McQuay H J, Carroll D, Guest P G, Robson S, Wiffen P J, Juniper R P 1993 A multiple dose comparison of ibuprofen and dihydrocodeine after third molar surgery. British Journal of Oral and Maxillofacial Surgery 31: 95–100

Martin W R 1979 History and development of mixed opioid agonists, partial agonists and antagonists. British Journal of Clinical Pharmacology 7: 273s–279s

Miller R R, Ferrigold A, Paxinos J 1970 Propoxyphene hydrochloride. Journal of the American Medical Association 213: 996–1006

Moertel C G, Ahmann D L, Taylor W F, Schwartau N 1974 Relief of pain by oral medications. Journal of the American Medical Association 229: 55–59

Moyes D G, Miller M T, Aldridge N J 1979 A comparison between meptazinol and omnopon in the relief of postoperative pain. SA Medical Journal 55: 865–866

Niemegeers C J E, McGuire J L, Heykants J J P, Janssen P A J 1979 Dissociation between opiate-like and antidiarrhoeal activities of antidiarrhoeal drugs. Journal of Pharmacology and Experimental Therapeutics 210: 327–333

Nimmo W S, Todd J G, Vogel J 1986 Effect of meptazinol on drug absorption and gastric emptying. European Journal of Anaesthesiology 3: 295–298

Owen M, Hills L J 1980 How safe is dextropropoxyphene? Medical Journal of Australia 1: 617–618

Palmer R W, Eade O E, O'Shea P J, Cuthbert M F 1966 Incidence of unwanted effects of dihydrocodeine bitartrate in health volunteers. Lancet ii: 620–621

Palmer K R, Corbett C L, Holdsworth C D 1980 Double-blind cross-over study comparing loperamide, codeine and diphenoxylate in the treatment of chronic diarrhoea. Gastroenterology 79: 1272–1275

Pasternak G W, Adler B A, Rodriguez J 1985 Characterization of the opioid receptor binding and animal pharmacology of meptazinol. Postgraduate Medical Journal 61 (suppl 2): 5–12

Persson K , Hammarlund-Udenaes M, Mortimer O, Rane A 1992 The postoperative pharmacokinetics of codeine. European Journal of Clinical Pharmacology 42: 663–666

Pert C B, Snyder S H 1973 Properties of opiate-receptor binding in rat brain. Proceedings of the National Academy of Sciences 70: 2243–2247

Preston K L, Jasinski D R, Testa M 1991 Abuse potential and pharmacological comparison of tramadol and morphine. Drug and Alcohol Dependence 27: 7–18

Quiding H, Anderson P, Bondesson U, Boreus L O, Hynning P-A 1986 Plasma concentrations of codeine and its metabolite, morphine, after single and repeated oral administration. European Journal of Clinical Pharmacology 30: 673–677

Raffa R B, Friderichs E, Reimann W, Shank R P, Codd E E, Vaught J L 1992 Opioid and nonopioid components independently contribute to the mechanism of action of tramadol, an 'atypical' opioid analgesic. Journal of Pharmacology and Experimental Therapeutics 260: 275–285

Read M, Read N W, Barber D C 1982 Effects of loperamide on anal sphincter function in patients complaining of chronic diarrhoea with faecal incontinence and urgency. Digestive Diseases and Sciences 27: 807–813

Redfern N 1983 Dihydrocodeine overdose treated with naloxone infusion. British Medical Journal 287: 751–752

Rifat K 1972 Pentazocine in sequential analgesic anaesthesia. British Journal of Anaesthesia 44: 175–182

Robbie D S, Samarasinghe J 1973 Comparison of aspirin-codeine and paracetamol-dextropropoxyphene compound tablets with pentazocine in relief of cancer pain. Journal of International Medical Research 1: 246–252

Rowell F J, Seymour R A, Rawlins M D 1983 Pharmacokinetics of intravenous and oral dihydrocodeine and its acid metabolites. European Journal of Clinical Pharmacology 25: 419–424

Sandhu B K, Milla P J, Harries J T 1983 Mechanisms of action of loperamide. Scandinavian Journal of Gastroenterology 18 (suppl 84): 85–92

Sanfilippo G 1948 Contributo sperimentala all'ipotesi della smetilazione della codeina nell' organismo. I. Influence della dose sull' assuefazione alla codeina. II. Assuefazione alla codeina attenuata con somministrazione prolungata di morfina. Bolletino Societa Italiana di Biologia Spermimentale 24: 723–726

Schuermans V, Van Lommel R, Dom J, Brugmans J 1974 Loperamide (R18553), a novel type of antidiarrhoeal agent. Part 6: clinical pharmacology. Placebo-controlled comparison of the constipating activity and safety of loperamide, diphenoxylate and codeine in normal volunteers. Arzneimittel-Forschung 24: 1653–1657

Seed J C, Wallenstein S L, Houde R W, Belville J W 1958 A comparison of the analgesic and respiratory effects of dihydrocodeine and morphine in man. Archives of International Pharmacodynamics 116: 293–339

Seifter J, Eckfield D K, Letchack I, Gore E M, Glassman J M 1954 Pharmacological properties of some azocycloheptane analgesics. Federation Proceedings 13: 403

Sindrup S H, Brosen K, Bjerring P et al 1991 Codeine increases pain thresholds to copper vapor laser stimuli in extensive but not poor metabolizers of sparteine. Clinical Pharmacology and Therapeutics 49: 686–693

Sindrup S H, Arendt-Nielsen L, Brosen K et al 1992 The effect of quinidine on the analgesic effect of codeine. European Journal of Clinical Pharmacology 42: 587–592

Spiegel K, Pasternak G W 1984 Meptazinol: a novel mu_1 selective opioid analgesic. Journal of Pharmacology and Experimental Therapeutics 228: 414–419

Standing Advisory Committee for Haematology of the Royal College of Pathologists 1982. Drug interaction with coumarin derivative anticoagulants. British Medical Journal 285: 274–275

Staritz M, Poralla T, Manns M, Ewe K, Meyer zum Buschenfelde K-H 1985 Pentazocine hampers bile flow. Lancet i: 573–574

Stephens R J, Waterfall J F, Franklin R A 1978 A review of the biological properties and metabolic disposition of the new analgesic agent, meptazinol. General Pharmacology 9: 73–78

Sunshine A, Laska E, Slafta J, Fleischman E 1971 A comparative analgesia study of propoxyphene hydrochloride, propoxyphene napsylate, and placebo. Toxicology Applied Pharmacology 19: 512–518

Szekely S M and Vickers M D 1992 A comparison of the effects of codeine and tramadol on laryngeal reactivity. European Journal of Anaesthesiology 9: 111–120

Vickers M D, O'Flaherty D, Szekely S M, Read M, Yoshizumi J 1992 Tramadol: pain relief by an opioid without depression of respiration. Anaesthesia 47: 291–296

Waife S O, Gruber C M, Rodder B E, Nash J F 1975 Problems and solutions to single-dose testing of analgesics: comparison of propoxyphene, codeine and fenoprofen. International Journal of Clinical Pharmacology 12: 301–304.

Wilder-Smith C H, Schimke J, Osterwalder B, Senn H-J 1994 Oral tramadol and morphine for strong cancer-related pain. Annals of Oncology 5: 141–146

Woods A J J, Moir D C, Campbell C et al 1974 Medicines evaluation and monitoring group: central nervous system effects of pentazocine. British Medical Journal 1: 305–307

World Health Organization 1994 Revised Method for Relief of Cancer Pain and other symptoms management. WHO, Geneva [In Press]

Strong opioids I

This chapter focuses on morphine and closely related drugs such as diamorphine and papaveretum. Other strong opioids are discussed in Chapter 15. More details about the use of morphine are given in Chapters 16–20.

MORPHINE

Morphine is the strong opioid of choice for cancer pain (WHO 1986). It is important, however, to have a second strong opioid available for the small minority of patients who cannot tolerate morphine.

■ DRUG PORTRAIT

Morphine is the main pharmacologically active constituent of opium. It is a strong analgesic and is used primarily in severe nociceptive pain. Its effects are mediated by specific opioid receptors, mainly within the CNS. Peripherally its main action is on smooth muscle. It is readily absorbed by all routes of administration. When given regularly, the oral to SC potency ratio is about 1/2; oral to IV about 1/3. The plasma halflife of an oral dose is 2–2.5 h; that of a parenteral dose about 1.5 h. The main site of metabolism is the liver where morphine is converted principally to morphine-3-glucuronide (inactive) and morphine-6-glucuronide (active). Cumulation of these metabolites occurs in renal failure. The duration of useful analgesia is 3–6 h.

Morphine-3-glucuronide (M3G) and morphine-6-glucuronide (M6G) are the major metabolites of morphine in man (Sawe et al 1981, McQuay et al 1990). M6G binds to opioid receptors whereas M3G does not. In rats, M6G is 45 times more potent than morphine intracerebrally, and about 4 times more potent subcutaneously (Shimomura et al 1971). Comparable results have been obtained in mice (Francis et al 1992). An analgesic effect has been shown in humans (Osborne et al 1988, Morley et al 1992). M6G may also have greater emetic potency (Thompson et al 1992).

Prolonged respiratory depression has been reported in man in association with negligible plasma concentrations of morphine but with very high concentrations of M3G and M6G (Osborne et al 1986). M6G contributes substantially to the analgesic effect of morphine, in both single and repeated doses.

Glucuronides are normally highly polar hydrophilic compounds which are unable to cross the blood-brain barrier. Morphine salts, such as the sulphate and hydrochloride, are also hydrophilic in contrast to morphine itself. M6G and M3G are, however, far more lipophilic than expected (Carrupt et al 1991). They exist in equilibrium between extended and folded forms. The extended form is (as expected) highly hydrophilic, whereas the folded form is almost as lipophilic as morphine itself. This form may well predominate in biological membranes, thereby facilitating movement into the CNS (Hand et al 1987). It is known, however, that the brain itself is able to metabolize M3G and M6G (Sandouk et al 1991).

Renal function

> 'Of all the lessons which were hammered into me during my hospital career, none was more persistently driven home than the fact that it is extremely dangerous to administer morphia in kidney disease' (Toogood 1898).

This quotation appeared in the British Medical Journal almost 100 years ago. In patients with severely impaired renal function, morphine and its active congeners have an increased and prolonged effect (McQuay & Moore 1984, Barnes et al 1985, Osborne et al 1993). A series of case reports confirm this observation (Mostert et al 1971, Don et al 1975, Barnes & Goodwin 1983, Redfern 1983, Stiefel & Morant 1991).

■ CASE HISTORY
A 70 year-old man underwent emergency surgery for peritonitis and subsequently developed severe acute renal failure. He received 415 mg of papaveretum (strong opium) over 3 days. Respiratory depression requiring ventilation persisted for 3 days after treatment with papaveretum was stopped. Table 14.1 shows the concentrations of morphine, M3G and M6G (Osborne et al 1986).

Cumulation of M6G provides an explanation for this phenomenon (Table 14.2). The metabolism of morphine itself is unimpaired in renal failure, even in anephric patients (Aitkenhead et al 1984, Sawe et al 1985a, Woolner et al 1986, Wolff et al 1988, Portenoy et al 1991).

Hepatic function

Evidence favours the liver as the principal site of morphine metabolism in man (Sawe et al 1985b, Hasselstrom et al 1986). As in other species,

Table 14.1   Concentrations of morphine, M3G and M6G in a patient with renal failure given papaveretum

Time after opioid was stopped (h)	Respiratory depression	Morphine (nmol/l)	M3G[a] (nmol/l)	M6G[b] (nmol/l)
40	Yes	39	10220	2342
62	Yes	< 10	9230	2026
117	Yes	< 10	9720	1562
135	Yes	< 10	7670	1350
161	Yes	< 10	5040	1023
185	Yes	< 10	4940	872

[a] In this patient, plasma halflife of M3G = 136 h.
[b] In this patient, plasma halflife of M6G = 103 h.
From Osborne et al 1986

Table 14.2   Oral morphine: influences on morphine and metabolite plasma concentrations

Factor	Effect
Age > 70 years Plasma creatinine > 150 mmol/l	M3G & M6G increased
Male	Morphine & M6G decreased
Ranitidine	Morphine increased
Elevated plasma creatinine + concurrent ranitidine	M6G increased
Elevated plasma creatinine + concurrent tricyclic antidepressants	M3G increased

From McQuay et al 1990

metabolism also occurs in other organs (Mazoit et al 1984) notably the CNS (McQuay 1986, Wahlstrom et al 1988, Sandouk et al 1991). Glucuronidation is rarely impaired in hepatic failure (Patwardhan et al 1981, Hasselstrom et al 1986). This reflects clinical experience; morphine is well tolerated in most patients with impairment of hepatic function (Laidlaw et al 1961, Regnard & Twycross 1984).

In a group of eight jaundiced cirrhotic patients with prolonged prothrombin times, however, the plasma halflife of morphine was found to be significantly longer than in six noncirrhotics; nearly 3.5 h compared with < 2 h (Mazoit et al 1987). In such patients, morphine should probably be given less often, i.e. q6h–q8h.

Morphine induced pain

Occasionally, at very high IV and high intrathecal (IT) doses, additional morphine exacerbates pain (Stillman et al 1987, De Conno et al 1991, Sjogren et al 1993). Examples of this phenomenon have already been given in Chapter 4 (see p. 74). One report tells of a patient with metastatic pelvic and back pain whose pain was exacerbated by IT morphine 60 mg daily (Morley et al 1992). CSF analysis showed a very high concentration of M3G but no M6G. When the patient was given IT injections of M6G 1 mg, there was complete pain relief for 7 h on each occasion.

Morphine induced pain, therefore, may be the result of abnormal morphine metabolism, i.e. production of M3G but no M6G. It has also been suggested that M3G antagonizes the effects of both morphine and M6G (Smith et al 1990, Gong et al 1992). Normally, however, M3G does not bind to opioid receptors. But, perhaps in the absence of M6G and at very high concentrations, receptor binding might occur. M3G may also be a nonspecific CNS stimulant.

■ CASE HISTORY

A 49 year-old male with advanced lung cancer had had chest pain on the right side since the onset of disease. Treatment was started with oral methadone and diclofenac. Because of poor relief, it was decided to try IT morphine. A bolus test dose of morphine 1 mg was administered with only slight pain relief. A second injection with morphine 3 mg was given and 75% pain relief was recorded. This was reproduced on three different days and lasted about 15 h. The patient was offered an implanted IT system.

The infusion was started with morphine 5 mg/day. Over 2 months, the dose was increased to 30 mg/day because of incomplete pain relief. During the third month, the pain became much worse and the dose was increased to 80 mg/day without any effect (Fig. 14.1). Computed tomography (CT) revealed marked local progression of the disease but excluded cerebral metastases.

The patient complained of an increased and unusual kind of pain and developed multifocal myoclonus particularly in the legs. Pain and allodynia were present in the lumbosacral and lower thoracic dermatomes. This was completely different from the cancer related thoracic pain.

The morphine infusion was reduced. After lowering the dose to 50 mg/day and prescribing diazepam, the allodynia and myoclonus remitted (Fig. 14.1).

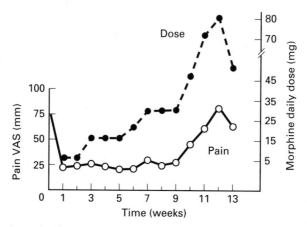

Fig. 14.1   The figure depicts pain intensity on a VAS and the daily dose of morphine administered by continuous infusion IT. Data refer to the last day of the each week. (Reproduced with permission from De Conno 1991.)

The patient became very drowsy, and died of a pulmonary haemorrhage one week later (De Conno et al 1991).

Oral to parenteral potency ratio of morphine

In the USA, it is still often stated that the oral to parenteral potency ratio of morphine is 1:6. This view is based on the results of a single dose study in postoperative cancer patients (Houde et al 1965). The bio-availability of orally administered morphine varies, however, between 15 and 64%, with a mean of 38% (Sawe et al 1981). Using IV patient controlled analgesia (PCA), it has been shown that approximately three times as much oral morphine is needed to match the previously satisfactory parenteral dose, i.e. the *oral to IV* potency ratio is 1:3 (Kalso & Vainio 1990), reflecting the earlier bio-availability study. Bio-availability by SC injection, however, is only about 80% (Hanna M 1992 Personal Communication). This means that the *oral to SC* potency ratio should be regarded as 1:2 (Consensus Statement 1994).

The discrepancy between a ratio of 1:6 with single doses for acute pain and 1:3 or 1:2 with repeated doses for chronic pain has led to much confusion (Kaiko 1986). It has been suggested that the reason for the discrepancy could relate to a greater contribution by M6G to the analgesic effect of repeatedly administered oral morphine (Hanks 1991, Portenoy et al 1992). Because of hepatic first pass metabolism, the plasma M6G to morphine ratio is significantly higher after regular oral administration of morphine than with IV or SC infusion (Table 14.3). There is no published data, however, which shows that the M6G to morphine ratio is higher after multiple oral doses than after a single oral dose.

Enterohepatic recirculation of morphine is a possible alternative explanation. It has been shown in rats (Walsh & Levine 1975, Dahlstrom & Paalzow 1978) but not in man. The phenomenon of greater efficacy with repeat oral doses has been noted with codeine, a prodrug of morphine (McQuay et al 1988). Alternatively, the original clinical trial could have produced a 'rogue' result. The results of trials with m/r morphine postoperatively suggests that this may well be the case.

Table 14.3 Mean plasma concentrations and ratios of morphine and metabolites during chronic administration of morphine

Dose (mg/24 h)	n	Concentration (mmol/l)			Ratio		
		Morphine	M3G	M6G	M6G: Morphine	M3G: Morphine	M6G: M3G
IV 60 (48–72)	5	0.04	0.19	0.05	0.88	4.4	0.34
SC 142 (60–300)	5	0.18	1.1	0.3	1.03	3.5	0.28
PO 302 (30–800)	5	0.03	0.44	0.19	7.22[a]	13.6[a]	0.59

[a] Significant differences from the groups treated SC and IV ($p < 0.05$).
From Janicki et al 1991

Table 14.4 Pain relief with morphine after abdominal hysterectomy

	Placebo			Morphine		
		10 mg IM	m/r 30 mg	m/r 60 mg	m/r 90 mg	m/r 120 mg
Number of patients	38	41	21	21	19	6
Peak pain relief	1.5	2.8[a]	2.0	2.7[a]	2.6[a]	3.2[b]
Pain relief at 6 h	0.2	0.7	1.1	1.5[c]	2.0[c]	2.8[d]
Total pain relief	3.7	9.6	9.8	15.5[a]	18.7[c]	25.2
Adverse drug reactions (%)	45	61	48	71	64	100

m/r = modified-release tablets. Letters indicate results significantly different from: (a) placebo; (b) placebo and m/r 30 mg; (c) placebo, 10 mg IM and m/r 30 mg; (d) placebo, 10 mg IM, and m/r 30 mg and 60 mg.
From Kaiko et al 1990

Oral morphine for postoperative pain

Controlled trials of oral morphine postoperatively have been mainly restricted to m/r morphine tablets. Results have been variable (Kaiko 1986). Relief is better if m/r morphine is given *pre-operatively* (see p. 46). In a study which examined dose-response relationships, total pain relief was the same with morphine 10 mg IM and m/r morphine 30 mg (Table 14.4). One patient developed serious respiratory depression with m/r morphine 120 mg which resulted in this dose being abandoned (Kaiko et al 1990).

Age and morphine requirements

Children

In neonates of 1–4 days of age, the plasma halflife for morphine is significantly longer than in older infants (nearly 7 h compared with about 4 h), and renal clearance is less than half (Lynn & Slattery 1987). This is reflected in a considerably lower M3G/morphine plasma concentration ratio compared with older children, 7 v. 24 (Choonara et al 1992).

In 19 neonates who were mechanically ventilated because of respiratory distress and who received morphine, the plasma halflife was even longer, almost 10 h $\pm$ 3 h (Chay et al 1992). In infants over 1 month, morphine clearance reaches or surpasses adult levels. Children are, therefore, no more sensitive to respiratory depression than adults.

Adults

It is known that elderly patients require less morphine than younger patients. The oral morphine requirements of a group of patients over 60 years were about half those of a group of younger patients (Forman et al 1992). The smaller doses correlated with decreased creatinine clearance. Nausea and constipation were more frequent in the older group despite smaller doses.

A difference has also been demonstrated in 80 volunteers aged 26–30 years

Table 14.5   Pharmacokinetic data for morphine in volunteers

	IV	Oral solution	M/r tablets
Area under curve			
Young (n = 80)	97	26	28
Elderly (n = 9)	139[a]	62[a]	43[a]
Bio-availability (%)			
Young	100	36	35
Elderly	100	48	45

[a] Significantly different from young group (p < 0.05).
From Baillie et al 1989

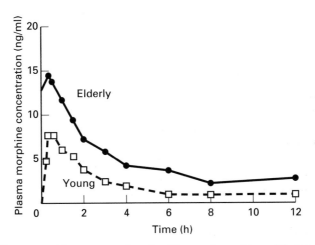

Fig. 14.2   Plasma morphine concentration after 10 mg oral morphine sulphate solution in young and old volunteers (mean ± SEM). (Reproduced with permission from Baillie et al 1989.)

and nine aged 68–90 years for IV morphine, oral morphine solution and m/r morphine tablets (Table 14.5, Fig. 14.2). The increased oral bio-availability in the elderly is compatible with decreased first pass hepatic metabolism.

A review of nearly 1400 patients with advanced cancer demonstrated yet again that morphine requirements reduce with age (Fig. 14.3). In addition, an association was noted between primary site and dose of morphine (Table 14.6). The high opioid needs of patients with pelvic cancers may relate to the common association with lumbosacral plexopathy — a cancer pain syndrome which is generally difficult to relieve with primary analgesics alone.

DIAMORPHINE

■ DRUG PORTRAIT

Diamorphine (di-acetylmorphine, heroin) is a semisynthetic derivative of morphine which is used mainly as a strong opioid analgesic, principally in the UK. Diamorphine, however, is a prodrug without intrinsic activity of its own. In vivo or in solution, it is rapidly de-acetylated to mono-acetylmorphine and then more slowly to morphine itself (Barrett et al 1992). It is well absorbed by

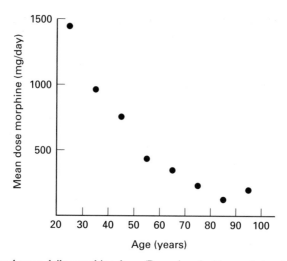

Fig. 14.3   Age and mean daily morphine dose. (Reproduced with permission from Rees 1990.)

Table 14.6   Hierarchy of morphine requirements

Cancers	Dose (mg q4h)	Mean dose (mg/24 h)
Brain, gall bladder	10	60
Larynx, oesophagus, caecum, stomach, vulva	30	180
Unknown, colon, prostate, lung, ovary, bladder	40	240
Melanoma, pancreas, kidney, breast	60	360
Dual cancers, nonHodgkins lymphoma	75	480
Mouth, thyroid, sarcoma, rectum, uncommon cancers	90	540
Uterus, myeloma	105	630
Cervix	130	780

From Rees 1990

all routes of administration. Because of greater lipophilicity, diamorphine and mono-acetylmorphine cross the blood-brain barrier more readily than morphine. This accounts for the observed potency difference between parenteral diamorphine and morphine. IM diamorphine is more than twice as potent as morphine. By mouth, however, the two opioids are almost equipotent. The duration of useful analgesia is 3–6 h.

Di-acetylmorphine was first prepared in 1874 at St. Mary's Hospital, London (Wright 1874). Initially it was largely ignored by the medical profession but 20 years later interest rapidly developed as a result of animal experiments conducted in Germany. Commercial production was started in 1898 by the Bayer Company who marketed the drug under the trade name of heroin. It was used initially in various respiratory conditions, for example, dyspnoea, pharyngitis, laryngitis, bronchitis, asthma and pulmonary tuberculosis. Later, hay fever, colds, coughs, pertussis and pneumonia were added to the advertisers' list of indications. It was also recommended, in the

USA, as a remedy for morphine dependence. Unfortunately, this only served to introduce diamorphine to the addict population and resulted in increasing abuse.

Its reputation as an analgesic developed later. By then, its use in so many respiratory conditions was falling into disfavour. Eventually, because of the increasing number of addicts, its medicinal use was banned in the USA in 1924. Since then all but a few countries have fallen into line with what subsequently became the policy of the League of Nations and, later, the United Nations. Diamorphine, however, is still widely used in the UK.

Diamorphine is a classical prodrug. It does not bind to opioid receptors, and is devoid of analgesic activity itself (Inturrisi et al 1983, Inturrisi et al 1984). It is metabolized into analgesically active 6-mono-acetylmorphine, morphine and M6G (Fig. 14.4). In terms of analgesic efficacy and effect on mood, diamorphine has no clinical advantage over morphine by oral or IM routes (Twycross 1977, Beaver et al 1981, Kaiko et al 1981, Inturrisi et al 1984).

Diamorphine IM has a slightly faster onset of action than morphine IM (Reichle et al 1962, Dundee et al 1966). This probably relates to the greater lipid solubility of diamorphine, permitting more rapid absorption from the site of injection. On the other hand, morphine acts more quickly IV (Morrison et al 1991). The explanation for this apparent paradox probably lies in differences in plasma protein binding (diamorphine 40%, morphine 20%) and the need for diamorphine to be converted into an active metabolite.

The use of diamorphine in the UK as the *parenteral* strong opioid of choice has caused some doctors elsewhere to believe that diamorphine is better than morphine (Tattersall 1981, Katz et al 1984, Levine et al 1986, Sellers 1986, McCarthy Montagne 1993). It is not (Twycross 1977, Lipman 1993). There is, therefore, no pharmacological justification for seeking to introduce diamorphine for medicinal use on the grounds that it is better than morphine. If a pain is opioid responsive it will respond equally well to both morphine and diamorphine. If the pain is opioid resistant it will respond equally badly.

The major advantage of diamorphine over morphine is that, when injections are necessary, the high solubility of diamorphine means that large doses can be given in a small volume (Tables 14.7, 14.8). This advantage is irrelevant if hydromorphone is available as in the USA and Canada. Hydromorphone is more potent than diamorphine and almost as soluble.

Morphine/diamorphine potency ratio

Diamorphine IM is two to two and a half times more potent than morphine IM (Reichle et al 1962, Beaver et al 1981, Kaiko et al 1981). If diamorphine is only a prodrug, this is perhaps surprising. The following points provide an explanation:

- diamorphine is a prodrug for mono-acetylmorphine as well as morphine

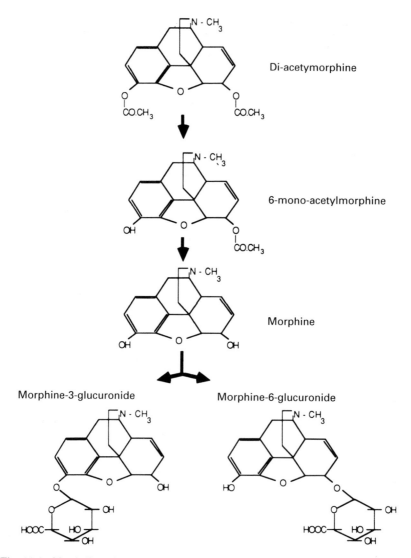

Fig. 14.4 Metabolic pathway of diamorpine (di-acetylmorphine) and morphine. 6-mono-acetylmorphine, morphine and morphine-6-glucuronide bind to opioid receptors; di-acetylmorphine and morphine-3-glucuronide do not.

- mono-acetylmorphine may well be more potent than morphine (Wright & Barbour 1935)
- by injection, hepatic first pass metabolism is circumvented and more mono-acetylmorphine will be available
- diamorphine is highly lipophilic and crosses the blood-brain barrier more readily than morphine.

There is still controversy about the potency ratio of oral diamorphine and morphine. A controlled trial suggested that the potency ratio is about 1.5:1 (Twycross 1977). In practice, however, many centres convert patients from

Table 14.7 Solubility of morphine and selected opioids

Preparation	Amount of water needed to dissolve 1 g at 25°C (ml)
Morphine	5000
Morphine hydrochloride	24
Morphine sulphate	21
Morphine tartrate	10
Morphine acetate	2.5
Diamorphine hydrochloride	1.6
Hydromorphone	3
Oxymorphone	4

1 g of diamorphine hydrochloride dissolved in 1.6 ml has a volume of 2.4 ml (Hanks & Hoskin 1987).

Table 14.8 Volume of injection of equi-analgesic doses of diamorphine hydrochloride and morphine sulphate[a]

Doses of drug (mg)		Approximate volume of injection (ml)		
Diamorphine[b] hydrochloride	Morphine sulphate	Diamorphine[b] freeze-dried	Morphine 15 mg/ml[c]	30 mg/ml[d]
5	12.5	0.1	1	0.5
10	25	0.1	2	1
20	50	0.1	4	2
30	75	0.1	5	2.5
60	150	0.2	10	5
100	250	0.3	17	8.5
500	1250	1.2	84	42

[a] Using a potency ratio of 2.5:1 (Beaver et al 1981). If the potency ratio is taken to be 2:1 (Kaiko et al 1981), the volumes given should be reduced by 1/5.
[b] Every 100 mg of added opioid salt will increase the volume by about 0.1 ml (Jones et al 1985).
[c] Maximum strength generally available in USA; some centres manufacture 50 mg/ml (Edgar & Hatheway 1990).
[d] Maximum strength available in UK.

diamorphine q4h to m/r morphine q12h using a 1:1 ratio. The following points provide an explanation:

- in the trial in question, the figure of 1.5:1 was a convenient approximation, i.e. the real figure might be 1:4 or 1:3
- in the male patients, the figure was nearer 1.25:1; the figure of 1.5:1 related to females
- if, in fact the real potency ratio is only 1.3 or 1.2, this may be irrelevant given the tendency to 'round up' the dose of m/r morphine (e.g. 100 mg rather than 95 mg)
- it is also possible that m/r morphine is more 'efficient' than q4h medication because of a smoothing out of the peaks and troughs of more frequent drug administration.

Thus, although the potency ratio of oral diamorphine and morphine has been shown to be greater than one, it may well be possible to ignore this when converting from diamorphine q4h PO to m/r morphine q12h. The '1–2–3' rule (diamorphine 1 mg SC = diamorphine 2 mg PO or morphine 3 mg PO) used when converting either oral morphine or oral diamorphine to SC diamorphine need not be used when changing between oral preparations.

THE BROMPTON COCKTAIL

The Brompton cocktail is now part of medical history. It was a mixture of morphine and cocaine in a vehicle of alcohol, syrup and chloroform water. For several decades it was the standard way in the UK of administering oral morphine to relieve pain or respiratory distress in patients with terminal disease.

The first record of the combined use of morphine and cocaine appeared in the British Medical Journal about 100 years ago (Snow 1896). Because of the cost, the use of cocaine was discontinued the next year at the insistence of the hospital's Board of Governors (Snow 1897). Some 30 years later, it was re-introduced by Roberts at the Brompton Chest Hospital, who used a morphine and cocaine elixir as a postthoracotomy analgesic (Kerrane 1975).

At other hospitals, similar elixirs were used in advanced malignant or terminal respiratory disease. These were known by various names:

- mistura pro moribundo
- mistura pro euthanasia
- mistura euphoriens.

It was not until 1952, when the Brompton Hospital produced its own supplement to the British National Formulary, that the composition of a morphine and cocaine elixir appeared in print. In this it was called 'Haustus E' and contained:

> morphine hydrochloride 1/4 grain (15 mg)
> cocaine hydrochloride 1/6 grain (10 mg)
> alcohol 90% 30 minims (2 ml)
> syrup 60 minims (4 ml)
> chloroform water to 1/2 fl oz (15 ml).

This was a modification of the earlier formulation which contained gin and honey instead of alcohol and syrup. It appeared subsequently in Martindale's Extra Pharmacopoeia (1958) together with three variant formulations.

In the 1960s and 1970s, diamorphine was commonly used in the UK instead of morphine as the analgesic component in such elixirs, and was by then generally known as the Brompton Cocktail. A controlled trial demonstrated, however, that apart from a small difference in potency, the efficacy and adverse effects of oral diamorphine and morphine are identical (Twycross 1977). Since then the use of oral preparations of diamorphine has steadily declined.

There was a tendency to endow the Brompton Cocktail with mystical properties and to regard it as the panacea for terminal cancer pain. It did, however, contain four substances all of which could cause adverse effects, including an unpleasant taste in the mouth and a burning sensation in the throat. Sometimes these effects resulted in noncompliance by the patient.

The Brompton Cocktail fell into disrepute principally as a result of two controlled trials which failed to show any benefit from the addition of alcohol and cocaine (Melzack et al 1979, Twycross 1979).

SCHLESSINGER'S SOLUTION

Schlessinger's solution is also historical. It was used in the USA, and comprises:

morphine sulphate 1 g
ethylmorphine 2 g
hyoscine hydrobromide 12 mg
distilled water to 50 ml.

One ml contains 20 mg of morphine sulphate. Ethylmorphine is comparable to codeine (methylmorphine). Sometimes morphine sulphate was substituted for ethylmorphine making the solution considerably more potent.

Schlessinger's solution is very bitter and each dose (1, 2, 3 ml, etc.) was diluted with juice or water before administration. With a 1 ml dose, the amount of hyoscine is relatively small (240 µg), although this is sufficient to cause anticholinergic effects in some patients. With larger doses, there will be a much greater likelihood of dry mouth, urinary retention, disorientation and delirium. Schlessinger's solution clearly offers no advantage over a simple solution of morphine sulphate. It has a number of disadvantages and its use cannot be recommended.

NEPENTHE

At one time nepenthe was a standardized alcoholic tincture of opium (Martindale 1972). Some years ago, it was reformulated (Martindale 1977). *Nepenthe oral solution* still contains the equivalent of anhydrous morphine 0.84% but only 0.05% of this derives from opium tincture; the rest is morphine (Table 14.9). This is equivalent to almost 1.2% morphine sulphate. Nepenthe is usually diluted and given as a 10% solution. Thus, 10 ml of 10% nepenthe contains the equivalent of approximately 12 mg of morphine sulphate. Stronger solutions can also be prepared. Because nepenthe has no advantage over morphine sulphate, its use cannot be recommended.

Table 14.9   The changing face of nepenthe

Source	Description
Martindale: The Extra Pharmacopoeia, 26th Edition 1972	A liquid preparation of opium with added morphine containing the equivalent of 0.84% anhydrous morphine.
Martindale: The Extra Pharmacopoeia, 27th Edition 1977	Oral solution. Contains anhydrous morphine 0.84% (0.05% from papaveretum and 0.79% from morphine hydrochloride).

Nepenthe is often prescribed with aspirin. It is not always appreciated that the aspirin must be dispensed separately, and two 300 mg dispersible aspirin tablets added at the time of administration. If the aspirin is dissolved in nepenthe by the pharmacy, hydrolysis occurs with the formation of the less potent salicylic acid. Patients supplied with such a mixture have observed that 'the new medicine is not so good as the first lot'. Reverting to separately prescribed nepenthe and aspirin resolves this problem.

OPIUM

Opium contains a variable mixture of about 25 alkaloids, including morphine 9–17%, noscapine 2–9%, codeine 0.3–4%, and smaller proportions of thebaine, narceine, papaverine and hydrocotarnine. Pharmaceutical opium powder is standardized to contain some 10% of morphine by weight. In some countries concentrated opium (papaveretum) is available. This contains 50% morphine together with the other opium alkaloids (see below).

The weight of morphine in these preparations denotes the content of morphine base. In other circumstances, morphine content refers to the weight of morphine salt (sulphate, hydrochloride, etc.). To allow a better comparison with morphine sulphate, it is necessary to adjust the morphine content of opium upwards. Thus, 100 mg of opium is equivalent to 10 mg of morphine base, which is approximately equivalent to 13 mg of morphine sulphate.

Powdered opium is used in opium and belladonna suppositories (B & O Supprette, USA). Two strengths are available containing either 30 mg of powdered opium and 16.2 mg of belladonna extract (approximately equivalent to 0.2 mg of atropine or hyoscine) or 60 mg with 15 mg. The belladonna is said to counteract the ureteric spasm and increased gastro-intestinal muscle tone produced by morphine. This claim has not been objectively evaluated.

Some palliative care services in the USA use these suppositories for rectal tenesmoid pain, particularly if associated with rectal colic and/or spasm of the pelvic floor. Generally, however, ordinary morphine sulphate suppositories should be used if rectal administration is indicated.

PAPAVERETUM

A number of preparations containing concentrated opium are available in both the UK and the USA:

- papaveretum tablets 10 mg (Omnopon UK)
- papaveretum injections 20 mg/l ml (Omnopon UK, Pantopon USA)
- papaveretum 10 mg and aspirin 500 mg tablets (Aspav UK).

There is no place for papaveretum injections; morphine or diamorphine should be used instead. The aspirin and papaveretum tablets are of interest for two reasons:

- although the tablets are large, they are effervescent and relatively easy to take

- they do not come under the Controlled Drugs regulations in the UK.

Each tablet contains papaveretum 10 mg, equivalent to anhydrous morphine 5 mg. As each tablet weighs over 2.5 g, the anhydrous morphine equivalent content is less than 0.2%. This is the cut off point below which morphine preparations are exempt from the Controlled Drugs regulations. A tablet containing the same quantity of papaveretum but weighing less would not be. There are no other advantages to be gained by its use. The disadvantages are those common to fixed drug combinations. Accordingly, the use of these tablets is not recommended.

The aspirin and opium (A & O) tablets available in parts of India contain powdered opium, not papaveretum. The opium content (30 mg) is only 10% morphine base, equivalent to some 4 mg of morphine sulphate.

MORPHINE INTOLERANCE

From time to time a patient experiences intolerable adverse effects with morphine (Table 14.10). In some patients, reducing the dose of morphine and/or initiating appropriate corrective measures resolves the problem or reduces it to an acceptable level. If the patient has severe pain, however, reducing the dose of morphine may not be feasible.

Table 14.10   Morphine intolerance

Type	Description	Initial action	Comment
Gastric stasis	Epigastric fullness flatulence, anorexia persistent nausea	Metoclopramide 10–20 mg q4h	If intolerance persists, change to an alternative opioid
Sedation	Intolerable sedation and delirium	Reduce dose of morphine; consider trial of dexamphetamine 5 mg daily–b.i.d.	Sedation may be caused by other factors (see p. 322); stimulant only rarely indicated
Psychotomimesis	Notably dysphoria and hallucinations	Haloperidol 3–5 mg nocte	
Vestibular stimulation	Incapacitating movement induced nausea and vomiting	Cyclizine 50–100 mg q4h–q6h; meclozine 25 mg q8h–q12h (USA); promethazine theoclate 25–50 mg q6h–q8h	Rare; try alternative opioid or methotrimeprazine/ levomepromazine
Histamine release			
Cutaneous	Pruritus	Oral antihistamine	If intolerance does not settle in a few days, prescribe an alternative opioid
Bronchial	Bronchoconstriction → dyspnoea	IV/IM antihistamine (e.g. chlorpheniramine 5–10 mg) + bronchodilator	Very rare; change to a chemically distinct opioid immediately
Morphine induced pain	Morphine causes increased pain and allodynia	Change to alternative strong opioid (e.g. fentanyl, methadone)	A rare syndrome in patients receiving high dose IV or IT morphine (see p. 257)

The only common form of intolerance is vomiting caused by morphine induced delayed gastric emptying. This usually responds to a prokinetic agent, e.g. metoclopramide, cisapride (Rowbotham et al 1988, McNeil et al 1990).

In a few patients, it becomes clear that the situation is not improving and it is necessary to change to another strong opioid (Kalso & Vainio 1990, Galer et al 1992).

■ CASE HISTORY

A 48 year-old woman with advanced breast cancer vomited intermittently when taking morphine 30 mg q4h. Haloperidol 5 mg nocte and cyclizine 50 mg q4h helped much of the time but it was necessary to limit food intake. Metoclopramide 10 mg q4h did not help. Changing to phenazocine 5 mg q4h maintained pain relief and the intermittent attacks of nausea and vomiting cleared up. She looked better and began to eat well.

■ CASE HISTORY

A 54 year-old man with prostatic cancer complained of pruritus when morphine 10 mg q4h was prescribed. This cleared within 24 h of changing to levorphanol 1.5–3 mg q4h.

A few patients who remain psychologically averse to taking morphine in any form also require an alternative opioid. A series of five morphine intolerant patients has been reported (Table 14.11), including the two case histories below.

■ CASE HISTORY

A 57 year-old woman with recurrent ovarian cancer reported a severe deep abdominal pain associated with a small area of intense allodynia. The dose of oral morphine was increased progressively to 180 mg/day but she developed intolerable sedation with little pain relief. She was empirically changed to oral levorphanol, and the dose was gradually increased to 48 mg/day. At this dose, she had complete relief from the deep pain with only minimal sedation and no other adverse effects. The allodynia was unchanged (Galer et al 1992).

■ CASE HISTORY

A 52 year-old man with squamous cell cancer of the pharynx developed progressive head, neck and chest pain from an enlarging tumour mass. The pain responded to radiotherapy but then recurred. Oral morphine was prescribed. At 270 mg/day, the pain was eased but the patient experienced hallucinations and sedation. Levorphanol was substituted for morphine at a dose about one quarter of the equi-analgesic morphine dose. Pain relief was better but still inadequate. Severe nausea, vomiting and sedation precluded further dose increases. Levorphanol was discontinued and a trial of oral methadone was initiated. With 20 mg q6h, the patient had almost complete relief of pain and no adverse effects (Galer et al 1992).

Table 14.11 Selective intolerance to opioids

Patient Sex	Age	Diagnosis	Morpine (mg/day)	Effects	Alternative opioid (mg/day)	EDDM[a]	Effects (mg/day)
F	21	Osteoblastoma	230 IV	Pain Hallucinations Dizziness Nausea	Hydromorphone 96 IV	580 IV	Pain relief 90%; no adverse effects
F	57	Ovarian cancer	180 PO	Pain Allodynia Severe sedation	Levorphanol 48	240 PO	Deep pain relief; allodynia unchanged; sedation minimal; same dose 2 *years* later
F	75	Bronchogenic cancer (brachial plexopathy)[b]	216 IV	Pain Sedation Confusion	Methadone 60 PO	60–80 IV	Pain relief 'substantial'; complete after 5 days
			Hydromorphone Levorphanol	} Same outcome			
M	52	Pharyngeal cancer	270 PO	Pain Hallucination Sedation	Methadone 80 PO	240–320 PO	Pain relief <100%; no adverse effects; maintained till death 3 months later
			Levorphanol	Pain relief better } Sedation Severe vomiting			
F	46	Posttraumatic paraplegia[b]	300 PO	Pain relief slight Severe sedation Anxiety	Methadone 60 PO	180–240 PO	Pain relief > 60%; minimal sedation; no anxiety; no change *1 year* later

[a] EDDM = equivalent daily dose of morphine.
[b] Neuropathic pain.
From Galer et al 1992

In each case, an opioid was identified which provided a satisfactory balance between pain relief and adverse effects. Two of the patients had neuropathic pain syndromes which were poorly responsive to morphine but which responded to methadone in considerably lower equivalent doses.

Differential opioid receptor affinity probably accounts for the variability in response. Levorphanol, for example, has greater affinity for delta receptors (Moulin et al 1988). Genetic factors may also be involved (Galer et al 1992). For example, mouse strains exist which differ in their sensitivity to morphine by more than 100 times (Vaught et al 1988). It is also known that tolerance develops independently at each receptor subtype (Ling et al 1989, Sosnowski & Yaksh 1990, Foley 1991).

The mechanism of the pain may also be important in determining the pattern of responses produced by different opioids. In animals, the analgesic efficacy of a delta receptor agonist and a kappa agonist varied according to the type of nociceptive stimulus, whether cutaneous thermal or visceral chemical (Schmauss & Yaksh 1983). Pharmacokinetic factors may also be contributory. For example, there is variability in the amount of M6G which is produced by patients receiving morphine (Osborne et al 1990, Portenoy et al 1991, Morley et al 1993).

Poor pain relief and intolerable adverse effects (agitation, delirium and myoclonus) have also been reported with rapidly achieved very high dose hydromorphone (65–200 mg/h by IV infusion; MacDonald et al 1993). The adverse effects cleared when morphine was substituted on a one to one basis, i.e. much less than the normally accepted equivalent analgesic dose. At more typical lower oral doses, hydromorphone and morphine are interchanged using a potency ratio of five or six. It seems, however, that this does not hold true at very high doses. Presumably, hydromorphone and morphine do not share the same affinity for all opioid receptor subtypes and, in consequence, cross-tolerance is incomplete. Hallucinations with hydromorphone have also been reported (Bruera et al 1992). These resolved on changing to morphine or diamorphine.

■ CASE HISTORY

A 32 year-old woman with advanced cancer of the ovary was admitted for pain relief. In hospital, increasing doses of hydromorphone were required to relieve pain. She ultimately received an IV infusion of hydromorphone 65 mg/h. The pain remained poorly relieved and she developed an agitated delirium and myoclonus.

Liver function tests were slightly raised but renal function was normal. The patient was changed to morphine 75 mg/h by IV infusion (23% of the equivalent dose of hydromorphone). Within 24 h the myoclonus and agitation cleared. The patient was drowsy but painfree. Two days later it was decided that the patient was oversedated and the morphine infusion was decreased to 50 mg/h. The pain remained relieved and the patient was more alert.

The concept of incomplete cross-tolerance is not new. It has been recommended for some years that when changing to an alternative opioid, the dose of the second drug should be half to two thirds of the anticipated normal equivalent dose (McGivney & Crooks 1984, Foley 1985). This advice is relevant only at high doses. With oral medication at more typical doses, the 'correct' equivalent dose should be used when changing from one strong opioid to another.

REFERENCES

Aitkenhead A R, Vater M, Achola K, Cooper C M S, Smith G 1984 Pharmacokinetics of single dose IV morphine in normal volunteers and patients with end-stage renal failure. British Journal of Anaesthesia 56: 813–819

Baillie S P, Bateman D N, Coates P E, Woodhouse K W 1989 Age and the pharmacokinetics of morphine. Age and Ageing 18: 258–262

Barnes J N, Goodwin F J 1983 Dihydrocodeine narcosis in renal failure. British Medical Journal 286: 438–439

Barnes J N, Williams A J, Tomson M J, Toseland P A, Goodwin F J 1985 Dihydrocodeine in renal failure: further evidence for an important role in the kidney in the handling of opioid drugs. British Medical Journal 290: 740–742

Barrett D A, Dyssegaard A L P, Shaw N 1992 The effect of temperature and pH on the deacetylation of diamorphine in aqueous solution and in human plasma. Journal of Pharmacy and Pharmacology 44: 606–608

Beaver W T, Schein P S, Hext M 1981 Comparison of the analgesic effect of intramuscular heroin and morphine in patients with cancer pain. Clinical Pharmacology and Therapeutics 29: 232

Bruera E, Schoeller T, Montejo G 1992 Organic hallucinosis in patients receiving high doses of opiates for cancer pain. Pain 48: 397–399

Carrupt P-A, Testa B, Bechalany A, El Tayar N, Descas P, Perrissoud D 1991 Morphine 6-glucuronide and morphine 3-glucuronide as molecular chameleons with unexpected lipophilicity. Journal of Medicinal Chemistry 34 1272–1275

Chay P C W, Duffy B J, Walker J S 1992 Pharmacokinetic-pharmacodynamic relationships of morphine in neonates. Clinical Pharmacology and Therapeutics 51: 334–342

Choonara I, Lawrence A, Michalkiewicz A, Bowhay A, Ratcliffe J 1992 Morphine metabolism in neonates and infants. British Journal of Clinical Pharmacology 34: 434–437

Consensus Statement 1993 Use of morphine for cancer pain. European Association for Palliative Care

Dahlstrom B E, Paalzow L K 1978 Pharmacokinetic interpretation of the enterohepatic recirculation and first-pass elimination of morphine in the rat. Journal of Pharmacokinetics and Biopharmaceutics 6: 505–519

De Conno F, Caraceni A, Martini C, Spoldi E, Salvetti M, Ventafridda V 1991 Hyperalgesia and myoclonus with intrathecal infusion of high-dose morphine. Pain 47: 337–339

Don H F, Dieppa R A, Taylor P 1975 Narcotic analgesics in anuric patients. Anesthesiology 42: 745–747

Dundee J W, Loan W B, Clarke S J 1966 Studies of drugs given before anaesthesia XI: diamorphine (heroin) and morphine. British Journal of Anaesthesia 38: 610–619

Edgar S P, Hatheway G J 1990 Concentrated morphine sulfate injection. American Journal of Hospital Pharmacy 47: 1529

Foley K M 1985 The treatment of cancer pain. New England Journal of Medicine 313: 84–95

Foley K M 1991 Clinical tolerance. In: Basbaum A, Besson J-M (eds) Towards a new pharmacotherapy of pain. John Wiley, New York, pp 181–203

Forman B, Portenoy R K, Yanagihara R H, Hunt W C, Kush R, Shepard K 1992 Elderly cancer patients with pain: response to oral morphine (MS) dose, pain and toxicity. Journal of the American Geriatric Society 40 (10): SA26

Francis B, Gout R, Monsarrat B, Cros J, Zajac J-M 1992 Further evidence that morphine-6B-glucuronide is a more potent opioid agonist than morphine. Journal of Pharmacology and Experimental Therapeutics 262: 25–31

Galer B S, Coyle N, Pasternak G W, Portenoy R K 1992 Individual variability in the response to different opioids: report of five cases. Pain 49: 87–91

Gong Q-L, Hedner J, Bjorkman R, Hedner T 1992 Morphine 3-glucuronide may functionally antagonize morphine-6-glucuronide induced antinociception and ventilatory depression in the rat. Pain 48: 249–255

Hand C W, Blunnie W P, Claffey L P, McShane A J, McQuay H J, Moore R A 1987 Potential analgesic contribution from morphine-6-glucuronide in CSF. Lancet ii: 1207–1208

Hanks G W 1991 Morphine pharmacokinetics and analgesia after oral administration. Postgraduate Medical Journal 67 (suppl 2): S60–S63

Hanks G W, Hoskin P 1987 Opioid analgesics in the management of pain in patients with cancer: a review. Palliative Medicine 1: 1–25

Hasselstrom J, Eriksson L S, Persson A, Rane A, Svensson J, Sawe J 1986 Morphine metabolism in patients with liver cirrhosis, Acta Pharmacologica et Toxicologica (suppl V): abstract 101

Houde R W, Wallenstein S L, Beaver W T 1965 Clinical measurement of pain. In: de Stevens G (ed) Analgesics. Academic Press, New York, pp 75–122

Inturrisi C E, Schultz M, Shin S, Umans J G, Angel L, Simon E J 1983 Evidence from opiate binding studies that heroin acts through its metabolites. Life Sciences 33: 773–776

Inturrisi C E, Max M B, Foley K M, Schultz M, Shin S U, Houde R W 1984 The pharmacokinetics of heroin in patients with chronic pain. New England Journal of Medicine 310: 1213–1217

Janicki P K, Erskine W A R, James M F M 1991 The route of prolonged morphine administration affects the pattern of its metabolites in the urine of chronically treated patients. European Journal of Clinical Chemistry and Clinical Biochemistry 29: 391–393

Jones V, Murphy A, Hanks G W 1985 Solubility of diamorphine. Pharmaceutical Journal 235: 426

Kaiko R F 1986 Discussion. In: Foley K, Inturrisi C E (eds) Advances in pain research and therapy, vol 8, Raven Press. New York, pp 235–237

Kaiko R F, Wallenstein S L, Rogers A G, Grabinski P Y, Houde R W 1981 Analgesic and mood effects of heroin and morphine in cancer patients with postoperative pain. New England Journal of Medicine 304: 1501–1505

Kaiko R F, Van Wagoner J, Brown J et al 1990 Controlled-release oral morphine (MS contin tablets, MSC) in postoperative pain. European Journal of Pharmacology 183: 147–148

Kalso E, Vainio A 1990 Morphine and oxycodone in the management of cancer pain. Clinical Pharmacology and Therapeutics 47: 639–646

Katz M D, Fritz W L, Lor E 1984 Heroin: should it be legalized for the treatment of cancer pain? Arizona Medicine 51: 602–603

Kerrane T A 1975 The Brompton Cocktail. Nursing Mirror 140: 59

Laidlaw J, Read A E, Sherlock S 1961 Morphine tolerance in hepatic cirrhosis. Gastroenterology 40: 389–396

Levine M N, Sackett D L, Bush H 1986 Heroin versus morphine for cancer pain? Archives of Internal Medicine 146: 353–356

Ling G S F, Paul D, Simantov R, Pasternak G W 1989 Differential development of acute tolerance to analgesia, respiratory depression, gastrointestinal transit and hormone release in a morphine model. Life Science 45: 1627–1636

Lipman A G 1993 The argument against therapeutic use of heroin in pain management. American Journal of Hospital Pharmacy 50: 996–998

Lynn A M, Slattery J T 1987 Morphine pharmacokinetics in early infancy. Anesthesiology 66: 136–139

McCarthy R L, Montagne M 1993 The argument for therapeutic use of heroin in pain management. American Journal of Hospital Pharmacy 50: 992–996

MacDonald N, Der L, Allan S, Champion P 1993 Opioid hyperexcitability: the application of alternate opioid therapy. Pain 53: 353–355

McGivney W T, Crooks G M 1984 The care of patients with severe chronic pain in terminal illness. Journal of the American Medical Association 251: 1182–1188

McNeill M J, Ho E T, Kenny G N C 1990 Effect of IV metoclopramide on gastric emptying after opioid premedication. British Journal of Anaesthesia 64: 450–452

McQuay H J 1986 Opiate metabolism and excretion. In: Levy J, Budd K (eds) Opioids: use and abuse. Royal Society of Medicine Services, London, pp 27–34

McQuay H J, Moore R A 1984 Be aware of renal function when prescribing morphine. Lancet ii: 284–285

McQuay H J, Carroll D, Watts P G, Juniper R P, Moore R A 1988 Codeine increases pain relief from ibuprofen after third molar surgery. Pain 37: 7–13

McQuay H J, Carroll D, Faura C C, Gavaghan D J, Hand C W, Moore R A 1990 Oral morphine in cancer pain: influences on morphine and metabolite concentration. Clinical Pharmacology and Therapeutics 48: 236–244

Martindale 1958 The Extra Pharmacopoeia, 24th edn. The Pharmaceutical Press, London, p 911

Martindale 1972 The Extra Pharmacopoeia, 26th edn. The Pharmaceutical Press, London, p 1128

Martindale 1977 The Extra Pharmacopoeia, 27th edn. The Pharmaceutical Press, London, p 973

Mazoit J-X, Sandouk P, Roche A 1984 Extrahepatic metabolism of morphine occurs in humans. Anaesthesiology 69: A456

Mazoit J-X, Sandouk P, Zetlaoui P, Scherrman J-M 1987 Pharmacokinetics of unchanged morphine in normal and cirrhotic subjects. Anesthesia and Analgesia 66: 293–298

Melzack R, Mount B M, Gordon J M 1979 The Brompton mixture versus morphine solution given orally: effects on pain. Canadian Medical Association Journal 120: 435–439

Morley J S, Miles J B, Wells J C, Bowsher D 1992 Paradoxical pain. Lancet 340: 1045

Morley J S, Watt J W G, Wells J C, Miles J B, Finnegan M J, Leng G 1993 Methadone in pain uncontrolled by morphine. Lancet 342: 1243

Morrison L M, Payne M, Drummond G B 1991 Comparison of speed of onset of analgesic effect of diamorphine and morphine. British Journal of Anaesthesia 66: 656–659

Mostert J W, Evers J L, Hobika G H, Moore R H, Ambrus J L 1971 Cardiorespiratory effects of anaesthesia with morphine or fentanyl in chronic renal failure and cerebral toxicity after morphine. British Journal of Anaesthesia 43: 1053–1060

Moulin D E, Ling G S F, Pasternak G W 1988 Unidirectional analgesic cross-tolerance between morphine and levorphanol in the rat. Pain 33: 233–239

Osborne R J, Joel S P, Slevin M L 1986 Morphine intoxication in renal failure: the role of morphine-6-glucuronide. British Medical Journal 292: 1548–1549

Osborne R, Joel S, Trew D, Slevin D 1988 Analgesic activity of morphine-6-glucuronide. Lancet i: 828

Osborne R, Joel S, Trew D, Slevin M 1990 Morphine and metabolite behavior after different routes of morphine administration: demonstration of the importance of the active metabolite morphine-6-glucuronide. Clinical Pharmacology and Therapeutics 47: 12–19

Osborne R, Joel S, Grebenik K, Trew D, Slevin M 1993 The pharmacokinetics of morphine and morphine glucuronides in kidney failure. Clinical Pharmacology and Therapeutics 54: 158–167

Patwardhan R V, Johnson R F, Hoyumpa A et al 1981 Normal metabolism of morphine in cirrhosis. Gastroenterology 81: 1006–1011

Portenoy R K, Foley K M, Stulman J et al 1991 Plasma morphine and morphine-6-glucuronide during chronic morphine therapy for cancer pain: plasma profiles, steady-state concentrations and the consequences of renal failure. Pain 47: 13–19

Portenoy R K, Moulin D E, Rogers A, Inturrisi C E, Foley K M 1992 Intravenous infusion of opioids for cancer pain: clinical review and guidelines for use. Cancer Treatment Reports 70: 575–581

Redfern N 1983 Dihydrocodeine overdose treated with naloxone infusion. British Medical Journal 287: 751–752

Rees W D 1990 Opioid needs of terminal care patients: variations with age and primary site. Clinical Oncology 2: 79–83

Regnard C F B, Twycross R G 1984 Metabolism of narcotics. British Medical Journal 288: 860

Reichle C W, Smith G M, Gravenstein J S, Macris S G, Beecher H K 1962 Comparative analgesic potency of heroin and morphine in postoperative patients. Journal of Pharmacology 136: 43–46

Rowbotham D J, Bamber P A, Nimmo W S 1988 Comparison of the effect of cisapride and metoclopramide on morphine-induced delay in gastric emptying. British Journal of Clinical Pharmacology 26: 741–746

Sandouk P, Serrie A, Scherrmann J M, Langlade A, Bourre J M 1991 Presence of morphine metabolites in human cerebrospinal fluid after intracerebroventricular administration of morphine. European Journal of Drug Metabolism and Pharmacology 16 (suppl 3): 166–171

Sawe J, Dahlstrom B, Paalzow L, Rane A 1981 Morphine kinetics in cancer patients. Clinical Pharmacology and Therapeutics 30: 629–635

Sawe J, Svensson J O, Odar-Cederlof I 1985a Kinetics of morphine in patients with renal failure. Lancet ii: 211

Sawe J, Kager L, Svensson J O, Rane A 1985b Oral morphine in cancer patients: in vivo kinetics and in vitro hepatic glucuronidation. British Journal of Clinical Pharmacology 19: 495–501

Schmauss C, Yaksh T L 1983 In vivo studies on spinal opiate receptor systems mediating antinociception. II. Pharmacological profiles suggesting a differential association of mu, delta and kappa receptors with visceral, chemical and cutaneous stimuli in the rat. Journal of Pharmacology and Experimental Therapeutics 228: 1–2

Sellers E M 1986 Therapeutic use of heroin: the scientist's role in social policy development. Clinical and Investigative Medicine 9: 139–140

Shimomura K, Kamata O, Ueki S 1971 Analgesic effect of morphine glucuronides. Tohoku Journal of Experimental Medicine 105: 45–52

Sjogren P, Jonsson T, Jensen N-H, Drenck N-E, Jensen T S 1993 Hyperalgesia and myoclonus in terminal cancer patients treated with continuous intravenous morphine. Pain 55: 93–97

Smith M T, Watt J A, Cramond T 1990 Morphine-3-glucuronide — a potent antagonist of morphine analgesia. Life Sciences 47: 579–585

Snow H 1896 Opium and cocaine in the treatment of cancerous disease. British Medical Journal 2: 718–719

Snow H 1897 The opium-cocaine treatment of malignant disease. British Medical Journal 1: 1019–1020

Sosnowski M, Yaksh T L 1990 Differential cross-tolerance between intrathecal morphine and sufentanil in the rat. Anesthesiology 73: 1141–1147

Stiefel H, Morant R 1991 Morphine intoxication during acute reversible renal insufficiency. Journal of Palliative Care 7 (4): 45–47

Stillman M J, Moulin D E, Foley K M 1987 Paradoxical pain following high-dose spinal morphine. Pain (suppl 4): S389

Tattersall M H N 1981 Pain: heroin versus morphine. Medical Journal of Australia 1: 492

Thompson P I, Bingham S, Andrews P L R, Patel N, Joel S P, Slevin M L 1992 Morphine 6-glucuronide: a metabolite of morphine with greater emetic potency than morphine in the ferret. British Journal of Pharmacology 106: 3–8

Toogood F S 1898 The use of morphia in cardiac disease. Lancet ii: 1393–1394

Twycross R G 1977 Choice of strong analgesic in terminal cancer: diamorphine or morphine? Pain 3: 93–104

Twycross R G 1979 Effect of cocaine in the Brompton Cocktail. In: Bonica J J, Liebeskind J C, Albe-Fessard D G (eds) Advances in Pain Research and Therapy vol 3. Raven Press, New York, pp 927–932

Vaught J L, Mathiasen J R, Raffa R B 1988 Examination of the involvement of supraspinal and spinal mu and delta opioid receptors in analgesia using the mu receptor deficient CXBK mouse. Journal of Pharmacology and Experimental Therapeutics 245: 13–16

Wahlstrom A, Winblad B, Bixo M, Rane A 1988 Human brain metabolism of morphine and naloxone. Pain 35: 121–127

Walsh C T, Levine R R 1975 Studies of the enterohepatic circulation of morphine in the rat. Journal of Pharmacology and Experimental Therapeutics 195: 303–310

Wolff J, Bigler D, Christensen C B, Rasmussen S N, Andersen H B, Tonnesen K H 1988 Influence of renal function on the elimination of morphine and morphine glucuronides. European Journal of Clinical Pharmacology 34: 353–357

Woolner D F, Winter D, Frendin T J, Begg E J, Lynn K L, Wright G J 1986 Renal failure does not impair the metabolism of morphine. British Journal of Clinical Pharmacology 22: 55–59

World Health Organization 1986 Cancer Pain Relief. World Health Organization, Geneva

Wright C R A 1874 On the action of organic acids and their anhydrides on the natural alkaloids. Journal of the Chemical Society 12 (NS): 1031–1042

Wright C I, Barbour F A 1935 The respiratory effects of morphine, codeine and related substances. Journal of Pharmacology and Experimental Therapeutics 54: 25–33

CHAPTER 15 | Strong opioids II

ALTERNATIVE STRONG OPIOIDS

Morphine-like drugs are classified in a number of ways (see Chapter 10). The most basic classification relates to potency-efficacy and divides opioids into weak and strong. An alternative classification is based on the agonist and antagonist actions of each opioid at the different receptor subtypes. A third way is by chemical structure (Box 15.A).

If a patient appears to have persistent intolerance to morphine, an alternative opioid should be used. Theoretically, the choice of a chemically distinct opioid would seem best. A change from morphine to oxycodone, however, may be sufficient in some instances (Kalso & Vainio 1990). Choice also depends on the dose of morphine to be substituted and the age of the patient (Table 15.1). With an elderly patient, levorphanol and methadone would generally not be good choices because of the greater danger of cumulation.

The following strong opioids will not be discussed in this chapter:

- anileridine (available in Canada)
- bezitramide (available in the Netherlands)
- ketobemidone (available in Scandinavia)
- trimeperidine (available in Russia and CIS).

Dipipanone, dextromoramide and phenazocine are included because of their availability in the UK. Methadone and pethidine (meperidine) are given more coverage because they are relatively cheap, widely available and, on a global basis, extensively used. Methadone is a useful alternative to morphine but is more difficult to use because of its long plasma halflife. In contrast, however, the use of pethidine should be discouraged (see p. 286).

When changing from one strong opioid to another it is important to give

---

BOX 15.A
CLASSIFICATION OF OPIOIDS ACCORDING TO CHEMICAL STRUCTURE

Opium
Standardized opium
Papaveretum ('strong opium')

Naturally occurring (opium alkaloids)
Codeine
Morphine } extracted from opium

Semisynthetic (formerly called opiates)
Dihydrocodeine
Oxycodone
Diamorphine
Hydromorphone } obtained by relatively simple structural
Oxymorphone   modifications of codeine, morphine or thebaine
Nalbuphine
Buprenorphine

Synthetic
Morphinans
   butorphanol
   levorphanol

Benzomorphans
   pentazocine
   phenazocine

Piperidines
   pethidine (meperidine)   synthetic compounds with structural
   anileridine   resemblance to the whole or to
   ketobemidone   a part of the morphine molecule
   fentånyl
   sufentanil

Diphenylpropylamines
   dextropropoxyphene
   dipipanone
   dextromoramide
   methadone

---

an adequate dose (Table 15.1). The following factors should also be taken into account:

- speed of onset and duration of action
- receptor site affinity
- adverse effects
- drug interactions.

Table 15.1   Opioids by mouth: approximate equivalence to oral morphine sulphate[a]

Analgesic	Proprietary name	Potency ratio with morphine sulphate	Duration of action (h)[b]
Codeine		1/12[c]	3–5
Pethidine/meperidine	Demerol (USA)	1/8[c]	2–3
Tramadol	Tramal	1/4	4–5
Dipipanone	in Diconal (UK)	1/2	3–5
Papaveretum	Omnopon (UK), Pantopon (USA)	2/3[d]	3–5
Oxycodone	in Percodan, Percocet, Tylox (USA)	4/3[e]	5–6
Dextromoramide	Palfium (UK)	[2][f]	2–3
Methadone	Physeptone (UK), Dolophine (USA)	[3–4][g]	6–12
Levorphanol	Dromoran (UK), Levo-dromoran (USA)	5[c]	6–8
Phenazocine	Narphen (UK)	5[h]	6–8
Hydromorphone	Dilaudid (USA)	5–6[c]	3–5
Buprenorphine	Temgesic	60[i]	6–8

[a] Multiply dose of opioid by its potency ratio to determine the equivalent dose of morphine sulphate.
[b] Dependent in part on severity of pain and on dose; often longer lasting in very elderly and those with renal dysfunction.
[c] Determined parenterally but seems to hold true clinically for oral route as well.
[d] Papaveretum (strong opium) is standardized to contain 50% morphine base; potency ratio expressed in relation to morphine sulphate.
[e] Oxycodone is 3/4 as potent as morphine by injection but, because of greater oral bioavailability, it is more potent by mouth (Kalso & Vainio 1990).
[f] Dextromoramide: a single 5 mg dose is equivalent to morphine 15 mg in terms of peak effect but is shorter acting; overall potency ratio adjusted accordingly.
[g] Methadone: a single 5 mg dose is equivalent to morphine 7.5 mg. Has a long plasma halflife which leads to cumulation when given repeatedly; overall potency ratio adjusted accordingly (Inturrisi & Verebely 1972).
[h] Unpublished observations (Twycross 1973).
[i] Must be taken *sublingually*; potency diminished if swallowed (Zenz et al 1985). In the USA, buprenorphine is currently available only as an injection.

Speed of onset and duration of action

There is little to choose between different opioids in terms of speed of onset of action. Most begin to take effect about 20–30 min after oral administration. If a rapid onset of action is needed, the IV route should be used.

Absorption after IM injection is influenced by the blood supply of the muscle. Uptake from gluteal muscles is slower in females than in males, and uptake from the deltoid is faster than uptake from gluteal muscles (Kaiko 1986). Rapid onset is not crucial for patients receiving regular medication.

A longer duration of action permits fewer doses to be given. Opioids with a longer duration of action than morphine include:

- oxycodone (marginally)
- phenazocine
- levorphanol
- buprenorphine
- methadone.

Table 15.2   Disease induced alterations in opioid pharmacokinetics

Opioid	Effect	Reference
	Cirrhosis	
Dextropropoxyphene		Giacomini et al 1980
Pentazocine	Increased bio-availability and decreased clearance = cumulation	Neal et al 1979
Pethidine		Klotz et al 1974
		Pond et al 1981
	Renal failure	
Dihydrocodeine	Decreased clearance = cumulation	Barnes et al 1985
Dextropropoxyphene	Increased norpropoxyphene (toxic metabolite) = cumulation	Gibson et al 1980
Pethidine	Increased norpethidine (toxic metabolite) = cumulation	Szeto et al 1977
Morphine	Increased morphine-6-glucuronide (active metabolite) = cumulation	Sawe et al 1985
		Osborne et al 1986
		Osborne et al 1993

With the availability of m/r morphine, however, there is little reason for choosing an alternative opioid because of a longer duration of action. Hepatic and renal dysfunction alter the metabolism and excretion of some opioids (Table 15.2).

Receptor site affinity

All opioids do not bind equally to all opioid receptors (Table 15.3). For example, pentazocine and butorphanol are:

- mu, kappa and sigma agonists
- delta antagonists.

Table 15.3   Receptor selectivity of opioid analgesics

Drug	Receptor type		
	Mu	Kappa	Delta
Morphine	A	a	a
Buprenorphine	pA	Ant	A
Butorphanol	pA	A	Ant
Fentanyl	A	a	a
Levorphanol	A	x	A
Methadone	A	x	A
Nalbuphine	Ant	pA	ant
Oxymorphone	A	a	a
Pentazocine	pA	A	ant
Pethidine	a	–	–
Naloxone	Ant	Ant	Ant

A = strong agonist; a = weak agonist; Ant = strong antagonist; ant = weak antagonist;
pA = partial agonist; x = negligible activity, – = no activity.
Sources: Hill 1992, Corbett et al 1993

In contrast, morphine is a mu, kappa and delta agonist with negligible sigma activity. Opioids with conflicting receptor affinities are best not administered concurrently. Partial agonists, by definition, have a ceiling to their analgesic effect.

Adverse effects

For the clinically important adverse effects of constipation and nausea there are no comparative data from chronic studies to suggest that any of the alternatives is consistently preferable to morphine.

Postoperatively, pethidine causes significantly more nausea and vomiting than morphine (Morrison et al 1968), and oxycodone significantly less (Kantor et al 1981). In cancer patients, however, oxycodone may have a greater propensity to cause sweating. On the other hand, it has been substituted satisfactorily in patients who hallucinated with morphine (Kalso & Vainio 1990).

Dysphoria

Activity at the sigma receptor is associated with psychotomimetic effects (Box 15.B). Dextromethorphan (an opioid cough sedative) and its metabolite dextrorphan and levorphanol all manifest phencyclidine-like activity at the NMDA receptor (Church et al 1988, Bonuccelli et al 1992). Dextrorphan is 5–7 times more potent than the other two opioids. This probably explains the psychosis occasionally seen in abusers of dextromethorphan (Benylin DM, Canada; Walker & Yatham 1993).

The use of opioids which produce a higher incidence of psychotomimetic effects than codeine or morphine without any specific advantage is difficult to justify. The mixed agonist-antagonists *nalbuphine, butorphanol,* and *pentazocine* all come into this category (Houde 1986, Wallenstein et al 1986).

Toxic metabolite

This is a potential problem with *pethidine.* Its chief metabolite, norpethidine, causes CNS excitation, i.e. agitation, tremor, myoclonus and convulsions (Szeto et al 1977).

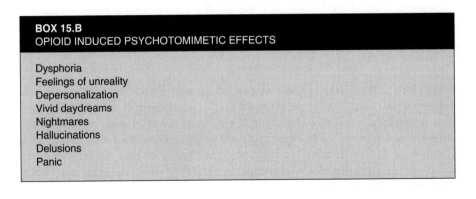

BOX 15.B
OPIOID INDUCED PSYCHOTOMIMETIC EFFECTS

Dysphoria
Feelings of unreality
Depersonalization
Vivid daydreams
Nightmares
Hallucinations
Delusions
Panic

Table 15.4   Drug induced alterations in opioid pharmacology

Opioid	Interaction	Result	Reference
Any opioid	Alcohol or other CNS depressants, beta-adrenergic blockers (?)	} Increased CNS depression	Davis & Hatoum 1979
Pethidine	Mono-amine oxidase inhibitors	Serotonergic crisis	Rogers & Thornton 1969
	Chlorpromazine Phenobarbitone Phenytoin	} Increased metabolism to norpethidine	Stambaugh & Wainer 1981 Stambaugh et al 1977 Pond & Kretschzmar 1981
Morphine	Amitriptyline Clomipramine	} Increased bio-availability	Ventafridda et al 1987 Ventafridda et al 1987
Methadone	Cimetidine	Slower metabolism	Sorkin & Ugawa 1983
	Phenytoin Rifampicin	} Increased metabolism	Tong et al 1981 Kreek et al 1976

Drug interactions

Because of the possibility of an additive sedative effect, care needs to be taken when strong opioids and psychotropic drugs are used concurrently. In addition, several specific interactions occur between opioids and other drugs (Table 15.4). Cimetidine, for example, inhibits the metabolism of methadone. This may lead to increasing drowsiness or even coma (Sorkin & Ugawa 1983). On the other hand, rifampicin speeds up methadone metabolism and may precipitate opioid withdrawal symptoms (Kreek et al 1976).

SEMISYNTHETIC OPIOIDS

Buprenorphine

■ DRUG PORTRAIT

Buprenorphine is a derivative of the opium alkaloid, thebaine. It is a partial mu agonist, kappa antagonist and delta agonist. Because of extensive first pass metabolism, buprenorphine is not given PO. Buprenorphine is well absorbed SL, but onset of action is relatively slow (about 30 min). Peak effects occur after 3 h (morphine = 1 h). The plasma halflife is about 3 h. The duration of useful effect is some 6–9 h (morphine = 3–5 h). The dose-response curve for subjective effects is bell-shaped, and doses of 1.2 mg produce less effect than 0.6 mg (Heel et al 1979). Morphine-like effects are maximal at a dose of about 1 mg SC.

Buprenorphine is used at some centres as an alternative to morphine in the lower part of morphine's dose range (Box 15.C; Atkinson et al 1990). Because it is a partial mu agonist buprenorphine can never be a total substitute for morphine. Opinions differ, however, as to the presence or the height of a therapeutic ceiling. It has been suggested that it may be effective only in doses up to about 5 mg in 24 h (Zenz et al 1985). This view has been vigorously challenged (Budd 1990).

> **BOX 15.C**
> **GUIDE TO THE USE OF BUPRENORPHINE**
>
> An alternative to oral morphine in the low to middle part of morphine's dose range.
>
> In low doses, buprenorphine and morphine are additive in their effects; at high doses, antagonism by buprenorphine may occur.
>
> Buprenorphine is available as a SL tablet; ingestion reduces bio-availability.
>
> Needs to be given only q8h; to give more often is to make life unnecessarily harder for a hard-pressed patient.
>
> With daily doses of over 3 mg, patients may prefer to take fewer tablets more often, i.e. q6h.
>
> Analgesic ceiling at a daily dose of 3–5 mg; this is equivalent to 180–300 mg of morphine.
>
> Buprenorphine is *not* an alternative to codeine or dextropropoxyphene. Like morphine, it should be used when a weak opioid has failed.
>
> Assuming previous regular use of codeine or dextropropoxyphene, patients should commence on 200 µg q8h with the advice that:
>
> > 'If it is not more effective than your previous tablets take a further 200 µg after 1 h, and 400 µg q8h after that'.
>
> When changing to morphine, multiply total daily dose of buprenorphine by 60. If pain previously poorly relieved, multiply by 100.
>
> Adverse effects need to be monitored as with morphine: nausea, vomiting, constipation, drowsiness.
>
> There is never a need to prescribe both buprenorphine and morphine. Use one or the other; then unintended antagonism cannot occur.

Most patients are satisfactorily controlled on a q8h regimen. Subjective and physiological effects are generally similar to morphine, including drowsiness when used postoperatively or during the first few days of chronic use. There are two important differences:

- vomiting is more common after SL than after IM administration
- naloxone does not reverse the effects of buprenorphine when used in standard doses of 400–800 µg IV.

Buprenorphine is almost as potent SL as by injection; 400 µg SL is equivalent to 300 µg IM. Buprenorphine by injection is 30–40 times more potent than morphine, and longer lasting. Compared with oral morphine, SL buprenorphine is some 60 times more potent. Thus, when changing from an *unsatisfactory* buprenorphine regimen to morphine, the total daily dose of buprenorphine should be multiplied by 100 and converted into a convenient q4h or q12h regimen.

In a long term open study, 70 patients with chronic pain (two thirds with cancer) received buprenorphine SL (Adriaensen et al 1981). The total daily dose ranged from 400 µg to 4 mg. While 10% experienced little or no benefit, over half reported good or complete relief. Most patients (number unspecified), however, withdrew from the study because of adverse effects.

Unlike most opioids, buprenorphine does not increase pressure within the biliary and pancreatic ducts (Staritz et al 1985). Buprenorphine is less constipating than morphine. Patients with advanced cancer, however, usually need a laxative when buprenorphine is given regularly. Animal studies confirm that buprenorphine slows intestinal transit (Anonymous 1979).

One man who took an overdose of 40 buprenorphine 400 µg tablets recovered uneventfully after 24 h without respiratory depression (Heel et al 1979). The only symptoms referable to buprenorphine were vomiting and drowsiness. Serious respiratory depression is unlikely to occur in clinical practice. If serious respiratory depression occurred as a result of self-poisoning, the use of very large doses of naloxone (up to 16 mg) would probably be necessary, and assisted ventilation considered. The manufacturers recommend the use of doxapram, a respiratory stimulant, by injection or infusion.

In a study specifically aimed at assessing dependence liability, it was shown that tolerance can be induced by increasing the dose. When medication was stopped suddenly after receiving 8 mg/day for 2 weeks, withdrawal symptoms typical of opioid physical dependence occurred but not until day 14. Buprenorphine is generally considered to have a low abuse potential and is not a Controlled Drug in countries where it is available.

Hydromorphone

Hydromorphone is an analogue of morphine with similar pharmacokinetic and pharmacodynamic properties. It is 5–6 times more potent than morphine (Vallner et al 1981). Oral bio-availability is similar or better than morphine. Published mean figures range from 37–62% (Babul & Darke 1992). As with morphine, there is wide interpatient variation. The main metabolite is hydromorphone-3-glucuronide. Hydromorphone-6-glucuronide is also formed but whether this has a comparable effect to M6G is not known (Babul & Darke 1992). Two other minor metabolites, dihydro-isomorphine and dihydromorphine, are pharmacologically active. By the spinal route in opioid naive subjects, hydromorphone causes much less pruritus than morphine, 11% v. 44% (Chaplan et al 1992).

Hydromorphone is widely used in the USA. It is available in oral solid (1, 2, 3, 4 mg tablets), oral liquid, rectal (3 mg suppository) and parenteral forms. It is well absorbed following oral administration. Hydromorphone injection is also available in a highly concentrated form (10 mg/ml) for parenteral use when a high dose, low volume injection is needed. It is anticipated that a range of hydromorphone preparations will become available in the UK during 1994. Hydromorphone provides useful analgesia for about 4–5 h.

Oxycodone

Oxycodone is an analogue of morphine with similar pharmacokinetic and pharmacodynamic properties. Parenterally it is about 3/4 as potent as morphine (Kalso & Vainio 1990). Oral bio-availability is about 2/3, compared with 1/3 for morphine. By mouth, therefore, oxycodone is more potent than morphine (Table 15.1). It is available in several countries. For many years in the USA its use was largely limited to several popular compound tablet or capsule formulations with either aspirin (Percodan) or paracetamol/acetaminophen (Percocet, Tylox). The potential toxicity of the nonopioid component restricted the amount of oxycodone which could be taken. Oxycodone alone is now recognized as a useful alternative strong opioid (Glare & Walsh 1993, Poyhia et al 1993). It has a plasma halflife of about 5 h, i.e. twice that of morphine (Poyhia et al 1992). It is given every 4–5 h, but possibly could be given less frequently.

Oxymorphone

Oxymorphone is an analogue of morphine with similar properties. By SC injection, it is 10 times more potent than morphine (Dundee et al 1974). Oxymorphone is available in the USA as a 5 mg suppository. Oxymorphone PR is much less potent; 5 mg is equivalent to morphine 10 mg PO/PR.

MORPHINANS

Butorphanol

Butorphanol is structurally related to pentazocine and to levorphanol. It is a mixed agonist-antagonist (Table 15.3) and has a similar pharmacological profile to pentazocine (see p. 247) but is considerably more potent. Butorphanol neither precipitates nor suppresses abstinence in morphine dependent subjects. Naloxone precipitates a moderately severe withdrawal syndrome.

Postoperatively, butorphanol is 5–8 times more potent than morphine. In cancer patients, a potency ratio of 4:1 has been observed (Heel et al 1978). It is about 20 times more potent than pentazocine (Lewis 1980). The plasma halflife is 2.5–3.5 h and the duration of effect after IM injection is 3–4 h (Heel et al 1978).

Butorphanol is metabolized primarily to the inactive hydroxybutorphanol which is mostly excreted in the urine, and some in the bile. It acts promptly and the main adverse effect is drowsiness. A high incidence of psychotomimetic effects has been reported in cancer patients; 6/18 after 18 mg PO and 6/32 after 2 mg IM (Heel et al 1978). It is available for parenteral use in solutions 1 mg/ml and 2 mg/ml. Butorphanol is not a Controlled Drug. It is no longer available in the UK.

Levorphanol

Levorphanol is available in both the UK and the USA. In animal studies, levorphanol shows high affinity for mu, kappa and delta receptors, whereas morphine is relatively selective for mu receptors (Moulin et al 1988). Thus, levorphanol infusions in rats result in tolerance to both morphine and levorphanol whereas morphine infusions produce tolerance to morphine alone. The fact that levorphanol is more broad spectrum than morphine probably explains why it is of benefit in some morphine intolerant patients (see p. 269).

Levorphanol causes less nausea and vomiting than morphine and usually provides relief for 6 h. The longer duration of action relates in part to lipid solubility and cumulation of the drug in body fat. Levorphanol has a plasma halflife of 12–16 h. As with methadone, this may result in unacceptable sedation in the elderly.

BENZOMORPHANS

Phenazocine

Phenazocine is sometimes used in the UK in cancer patients who are intolerant of morphine. It is available as a 5 mg tablet, equivalent to 20–25 mg of morphine sulphate by mouth (Twycross R G 1973 Unpublished Observations). One tablet q4h may therefore be excessive. The tablets can, however, be halved and need not be taken as often as morphine. For example, 2.5 mg q.i.d. is approximately equivalent to 10 mg morphine q4h. Although not manufactured specifically for SL use, the tablets dissolve readily in the mouth. Phenazocine appears to be equipotent by SL and PO routes.

PIPERIDINES

Fentanyl

Fentanyl is a short acting synthetic opioid used extensively as a perioperative analgesic. A transdermal preparation is also available (Supplement 1992, Portenoy et al 1993). Transdermal patches (TTS-fentanyl) are supplied in 25, 50, 75 and 100 µg/h strengths, and are intended to last for 72 h (Shaw & Chandrasekaran 1985). Peak plasma concentrations of fentanyl are achieved after 12–24 h and a depot remains in the skin for 24 h after the patch is removed.

The patches are much more expensive than oral morphine and they do not permit rapid dose titration because of the slow onset of activity after application and delayed cessation of activity after removal (Duthie et al 1988). There is inter-patient variation in the amount of drug delivered to the skin. The unintended application of a pad over a fentanyl patch has resulted in a systemic overdose (Rose et al 1993). Some patients obtain relief for only 48 h rather than the intended 72 h.

Fentanyl patches are useful for patients whose opioid dose is constant and who cannot or will not take oral medication regularly. Because of the slow onset of maximum analgesic effect, rescue medication may be necessary during the first 24 h. A conversion table for oral morphine to fentanyl is available (Table 15.5).

Pethidine

■ DRUG PORTRAIT

Pethidine (meperidine) is a synthetic opioid analgesic. Its effects are generally similar to those of morphine, despite substantial structural differences. It also

Table 15.5   Converting oral morphine sulphate to TTS-fentanyl[a]

Oral morphine (mg q4h)	Oral morphine (mg/day)	TTS-fentanyl delivery rate (μg/h)
≤ 22	≤ 134	25
23–37	135–224	50
38–52	225–314	75
53–67	315–404	100
68–82	405–494	125
83–97	495–584	150

[a] Recommendations supplied by Jansen UK. A potency ratio of morphine 10 mg IM/q4h to fentanyl 100 μg/h transdermally was used to derive this conversion table.

has anticholinergic effects. Its central effects are mediated via CNS morphine receptors; peripherally it acts directly on smooth muscle. It is absorbed from all routes of administration, and is about 1/3 as potent by mouth as by SC or IM injection. Peak plasma concentrations occur 1–2 h after ingestion. Absorption from the alimentary canal is more variable than with morphine, making it a less reliable oral analgesic. The plasma halflife is about 3–4 h.

Pethidine is hydrolyzed to pethidinic acid which, in turn, is partially conjugated. It is also N-demethylated to norpethidine which may then be hydrolyzed to norpethidinic acid and conjugated. Norpethidine is a CNS stimulant and causes agitation, tremor, multifocal myoclonus and convulsions. This limits the amount of pethidine which can safely be given on a regular basis. About one third of administered pethidine can be accounted for in the urine as N-demethylated derivatives. Little is excreted unchanged, but more if the urine is acid. Pethidine is about 1/8 as potent as morphine. Despite a longer plasma halflife, pethidine is generally shorter acting than morphine, useful analgesia lasting only 2–4 h.

Pethidine differs from morphine in a number of ways (Box 15.D). Like

BOX 15.D
PETHIDINE DIFFERS FROM MORPHINE

Shorter duration of action
Ceiling effect because of toxic metabolite
Not antitussive
Less constipating
Less smooth muscle spasm (e.g. biliary tract, sphincter of Oddi)
More vomiting
Anticholinergic effects
Pupils not constricted
Metabolism → norpethidine; causes tremors, multifocal myoclonus, agitation, convulsions
Interactions with:

- phenobarbitone   } increase production of norpethidine
- chlorpromazine   }
- mono-amine oxidase inhibitors (see Box 15.E)

morphine it can cause sedation and respiratory depression. Physical dependence develops with repeated regular use over several weeks. Compared with morphine, withdrawal symptoms:

- develop more rapidly
- are generally not so intense
- are shorter in duration.

For acute severe pain, pethidine 100–150 mg IM or 50–100 mg IV may be given as needed q2h–q3h. The solution for injection is irritant and should not be given SC. For severe cancer pain, 100–300 mg PO q2h–q3h may be necessary.

Pethidine can substitute for morphine up to about morphine 30 mg PO q4h. Unfortunately, pethidine is often prescribed with little regard for its pharmacodynamics. Attention must be paid to analgesic equivalence and duration of action (Table 15.1). A q6h order condemns most patients to pain for much of the day.

It is generally difficult to persuade a patient to take more than pethidine 200 mg q3h because of the number of tablets this means. Further, the incidence of adverse CNS effects increases considerably at doses above this level. Pethidine is not, therefore, a complete alternative to morphine.

Pethidine is commonly used for obstetric analgesia because of its short duration of action. It is often used in preference to morphine to relieve biliary colic because it causes less biliary tract spasm (Gaensler et al 1948). Pethidine is not an antitussive.

Renal failure

Pethidine should not be given to patients with impaired renal function because of the likelihood of irritability, myoclonus and convulsions caused by cumulation of norpethidine (Szeto et al 1977). Phenobarbitone and chlorpromazine enhance the production of norpethidine (Stambaugh et al 1977, Stambaugh & Wainer 1981).

■ CASE HISTORY

A 42 year-old man with osteogenic sarcoma received pethidine 150 mg IM q2h–q3h. Plasma biochemistry indicated mild renal insufficiency. He became agitated and confused, and had two grand mal fits. By then, he had received a total of 63 doses of pethidine. After the second fit, drug assay showed a plasma norpethidine/pethidine ratio of almost 5:1. Pethidine was discontinued and levorphanol and phenytoin were started. The fits did not recur (Szeto et al 1977).

■ CASE HISTORY

A 25 year-old woman with chronic renal failure received pethidine 75 mg IM q3h for deep painful leg ulcers. After 2 weeks she became very irritable and had multifocal myoclonus. She had a plasma norpethidine/pethidine ratio of over 6:1 Pethidine was discontinued and morphine started. The irritability and myoclonus subsided over the next two days (Szeto et al 1977).

Mono-amine oxidase inhibitors

Pethidine is totally contra-indicated in patients receiving a mono-amine oxidase inhibitor (MAOI). The administration of pethidine to a patient receiving a MAOI can cause a severe, and sometimes fatal reaction (Shee 1960). Three MAOIs are available in the UK:

- phenelzine (Nardil)
- isocarboxazid (Marplan)
- tranylcypromine (Parnate).

■ CASE HISTORY

A 38 year-old woman had been treated with phenelzine for a fortnight when she developed a severe headache; for this she was given pethidine 100 mg IM, without untoward effects. A month later, while on a slightly larger dose of phenelzine, she had another severe headache and was again given pethidine 100 mg IM. Within 20 min she was incoherent, excitable and was making wild movements. Her blood pressure at the time was 260/120 mm Hg (normally 120/80). On admission to hospital she was disorientated, had macabre hallucinations, tunnel vision and could not walk. For 36 h she was semicomatose but had occasional moments of lucidity. Over 3 days she gradually recovered without treatment (Taylor 1962).

Typically, the reaction is seen within minutes of the administration of pethidine (Box 15.E). It was originally suggested that it was caused by a reduction in the rate of metabolism of pethidine by the liver (London & Milne 1962). The immediacy of the reaction, however, rules out this explanation. Animal studies indicate that the reaction is precipitated by an increased concentration of cerebral serotonin (Rogers & Thornton 1969). A critical level of serotonin in the brain is necessary before the drug interaction occurs. Animal studies suggest a figure of some 60% above control values (Rogers & Thornton 1969). This would explain why the woman described above reacted normally after pethidine on one occasion, but abnormally on the second occasion when taking a higher dose of MAOI.

This drug interaction has not been reported with other strong opioids.

BOX 15.E
INTERACTION BETWEEN PETHIDINE AND MAOIs (Anonymous 1967)

Within minutes of administration of pethidine injection:

- restless, possibly violent
- multifocal myoclonus
- sweating
- cyanosis
- hypertension
- increased tendon reflexes
- extensor plantar responses
- Cheyne-Stokes respirations

Thus, there was no problem with morphine in a patient who subsequently had a serious reaction to pethidine (Shee 1960). On the other hand, pretreatment of mice with a MAOI potentiates the toxicity of morphine, pentazocine and phenazocine as well as pethidine (Clark et al 1972). This effect, however, is probably related to inhibition of opioid metabolism and, at worst, would only result in excessive sedation with these drugs (Cocks & Passmore-Rowe 1962).

Overdosage

Because norpethidine (plasma halflife = 15 h) causes excitation, overdosage with pethidine tends to present a picture of mixed CNS depression and excitation. When pethidine is given parenterally, the rate of absorption exceeds the rate of norpethidine formation, and the result is primarily one of CNS depression. Orally, the rate of absorption does not exceed the capacity of the liver to convert pethidine to norpethidine. Hence the ratio of norpethidine to pethidine increases and results in both stupor and convulsions.

Naloxone does not prevent or stop norpethidine induced convulsions. Thus, if convulsions occur before or after the correction of the respiratory depression with naloxone, IV midazolam or diazepam should be given.

DIPHENYLPROPYLAMINES

Dipipanone

Dipipanone is a synthetic opioid available in the UK as a compound tablet containing dipipanone 10 mg and cyclizine 30 mg (Diconal). It is 1/2 as potent as morphine. There is no advantage in its use unless an antihistamine anti-emetic is also indicated. Even so, in patients taking more than two tablets, the anticholinergic and sedative effects of cyclizine tend to be troublesome, particularly dry mouth and blurring of vision, together with drowsiness. Dipipanone is used less often than in the past.

Dextromoramide

Dextromoramide is a synthetic opioid available in the UK as 5 mg and 10 mg tablets. It is rapidly absorbed with peak plasma concentrations occurring in many patients after 1 h, sometimes less (Pagani et al 1989). Some patients show a biphasic elimination pattern, others monophasic. In the latter, the plasma halflife ranges from 1.5–4.7 h. In the former, the halflife for the first phase is 0.4–1.6 h and 6–22 h for the terminal phase (Pagani et al 1989). Hepatic first pass metabolism is probably less than with many other opioids.

In terms of peak effect, dextromoramide is three times more potent than morphine. As with methadone, however, the plasma halflife of dextromoramide appears not to correlate closely with the duration of analgesic effect. Although several reports state 4–6 h (Kolodny 1960, Flavell-Matts 1962, Kay 1973), the general opinion among palliative care doctors is that the usual duration of action is only about 2–3 h (Wilkes 1974, Lamerton 1979, Judd et al 1981).

When used more widely in the past, the 'failed dextromoramide' patient was a recurring phenomenon. Typically, such a patient had severe pain and was taking 10–20 mg q4h. Good relief of pain was obtained but only for about 2 h. This resulted in a vicious 'on-off' effect which often led to overwhelming pain.

Dextromoramide is still used at some centres in the UK as a 'top up' analgesic before a painful procedure, such as changing an adherent dressing. It should not be used to provide 'round the clock' analgesia.

Methadone

■ DRUG PORTRAIT

Methadone is a synthetic opioid analgesic. Its effects are generally similar to those of morphine despite substantial structural differences. Its central effects are mediated via CNS opioid receptors; peripherally it acts directly on smooth muscle. Methadone is a racemic mixture. L-methadone is responsible for almost all the analgesic effect, whereas D-methadone is a useful anti-tussive. Methadone is a basic and lipophilic drug which is absorbed well from all routes of administration. Mean oral bio-availability is about 80%. There is a high volume of distribution with only about 1% of the drug in the blood. Methadone accumulates in tissues when given repeatedly, which creates an extensive reservoir (Robinson & Williams 1971). Protein binding (principally to a glycoprotein) is 60–90% (Eap et al 1990). This is double that of morphine. Both volume of distribution and protein binding contribute to the long plasma halflife. This varies considerably from under 10 h to 75 h (Sawe 1986). The halflife is longer in older than in younger patients. Acidifying the urine results in a shorter halflife (20 h) and raising the pH with sodium bicarbonate a longer halflife (> 40 h; Nilsson et al 1982a). Renal and liver disease do not affect methadone clearance (Kreek et al 1980, Novick et al 1981). In single doses methadone PO is about 1/2 as potent as IM (Beaver et al 1967), and IM a single dose of methadone is marginally more potent than morphine. With repeated doses, methadone is several times more potent.

Methadone is metabolized chiefly in the liver to several metabolites (Fainsinger et al 1993). About half of the drug and its metabolites are excreted by the intestines, and half by the kidneys (Inturrisi & Verebely 1972). It is generally longer acting than morphine. With chronic administration, useful analgesia lasts 6–12 h.

Like morphine, methadone has no obvious ceiling effect. It is used at some centres as the strong analgesic of choice (Bertler et al 1980, Fainsinger et al 1993). Methadone has a high mean oral bio-availability of about 80% ranging from 40% to almost 100% (Meresaar et al 1981, Nilsson et al 1982b). It differs from morphine in several ways (Box 15.F). Its very long halflife is the most important difference. The relationship between plasma concen-

---

BOX 15.F
METHADONE DIFFERS FROM MORPHINE

No active metabolite
Long halflife
Cumulation when given regularly
Longer duration of action
Faeces a major route of excretion
Renal failure does not alter pharmacodynamics
Nonlinear relationship between plasma concentration and analgesia
SC injection more likely to cause local reaction

---

tration and analgesia is not straightforward (Sawe et al 1981). With a single dose, analgesia is maximal after 1–2 h, whereas peak plasma levels occur after 4–6 h. By 6 h pain relief has fallen to 25% or less, even though the plasma concentration is still near maximal (Berkowitz 1976). Clearly, the plasma concentrations do not reflect the concentration at the receptors (Sawe 1986). In contrast, miosis correlates closely with plasma levels.

Uses and contra-indications

Methadone can be used as an alternative to morphine for the relief of acute or persistent pain, or as an antitussive. Some centres change to methadone from morphine if only a poor response has been obtained in cases of nociceptive pain (Morley et al 1993). Methadone is also useful in cases of morphine intolerance (see p. 269). Because of its longer halflife, there is the greater likelihood of cumulative toxicity (Twycross 1977). Methadone is best not used in patients who:

- are elderly or demented
- are delirious (confused)
- have raised intracranial pressure
- are in respiratory, hepatic or renal failure.

Close supervision is needed until a patient's response to methadone has been fully evaluated. The plasma concentration may not reach a steady state for 2–3 weeks. Particular care should be taken when psychotropic drugs are administered concurrently.

■ CASE HISTORY

A 78 year-old woman with lung cancer was given methadone 3 mg PO q6h for persistent chest pain. Instead of this, she took 12 mg PO q6h. 12 days later she was admitted to hospital unresponsive with shallow slow respirations (3/min). Liver and kidney function was essentially normal. With naloxone 800 μg IV she became alert and oriented with a respiratory rate of 16/min. Over the next 24 h she became comatose on several occasions and each time was given naloxone 400 μg IV. She was discharged after 3 days (Ettinger et al 1979).

■ CASE HISTORY

A 59 year-old woman with lung cancer complained of severe pain and a rash on the right buttock, caused by herpes zoster. She was prescribed methadone 10 mg PO q4h–q6h. After three doses she became weak and unable to move from her bed. When admitted to hospital she was very drowsy and cyanosed. Liver and kidney function was essentially normal. Naloxone 400 μg IV was administered. Respiratory rate and level of consciousness improved. Further doses of naloxone were required over the next 8 h. Further opioids were withheld and the patient was discharged after 8 days (Ettinger et al 1979).

Methadone is well absorbed rectally; doses of up to 600 mg/suppository have been used. In comparison with parenteral morphine or hydromorphone, the cost of methadone suppositories is about one tenth (Bruera et al 1992). This makes it an attractive option for use in economically poorer countries. Rectal methadone carries the same risk of toxic cumulation.

Methadone can also be given by the buccal or SL routes. One third of the content of 1 ml of a methadone solution was absorbed in 10 min (Weinberg et al 1988). If the pH of the mouth was raised to 8.5, the absorption increased to three quarters.

Interactions

Methadone can be displaced from its protein binding by high concentrations of propranolol, phenothiazines and tricyclic antidepressants (Abramson 1982). This interaction is probably not relevant with normal doses of these drugs. A number of important interactions between methadone and other drugs, however, have been reported. Rifampicin, an antibiotic, speeds up methadone metabolism and has occasionally precipitated withdrawal symptoms (Kreek et al 1976). Cimetidine inhibits the metabolism of methadone; this may lead to drowsiness or even coma (Sorkin & Ugawa 1983).

■ CASE HISTORY

A 76 year-old man with disseminated lung cancer was prescribed methadone solution 5 mg PO t.i.d. On day 6, cimetidine 300 mg q.i.d. was started. He was comfortable on this regimen, with occasional SC morphine injections. On day 12, the patient was found unresponsive with small reactive pupils; respirations were 2/min and pulse 54. Naloxone 400 μg IV was administered. The patient immediately became alert and oriented, with respirations 20/min. More IV naloxone was needed 6 h later. Methadone, morphine and cimetidine were discontinued and a cimetidine-methadone interaction suspected. All opioids were withheld for 24 h after which methadone 2.5 mg PO t.i.d. was restarted. The patient remained comfortable and painfree. Cimetidine was replaced by aluminium hydroxide. The patient was discharged painfree some weeks later (Sorkin & Ugawa 1983).

Treatment regimens

Methadone is not recommended for acute severe pain. In advanced cancer, the starting dose will depend on the patient's previous medication. Various regimens are currently used.

Children Methadone has been used in children from the age of 1 year with various forms of malignant disease for periods of more than 3 months (Martinson et al 1978). Most were on a q6h or q8h regimen, with three q12h. Doses ranged from 2.5–40 mg (median 10 mg). Two thirds also received hydroxyzine (see p. 408). No information was provided about reasons for choice of timing. The children had good pain relief and were not excessively drowsy.

Adults Several schedules have been recommended with adults:

- *q4h–q6h*: stems from a single dose study (Beaver et al 1976) and from an atypical trial of IV methadone given by PCA over 6 days (Grochow et al 1989, Gourlay et al 1990). With such a regimen, there must be provision for dose reduction to prevent toxic cumulation (Twycross 1977). Generally, a long term regimen of q4h should not be used
- *reducing frequency*: q6h for 3 days followed by q8h (Ventafridda et al 1986)
- *ad libitum*: patients with severe pain are advised to take a fixed dose of 10 mg when needed. After 5–7 days, the amount of methadone taken over the previous 2–3 days is noted and the patient advised to convert to a regular q8h–q12h regimen.

Using a reducing frequency regimen in 27 randomly allocated patients, it was shown that the dose of methadone remained stable over the first 2 weeks of therapy, whereas in a second group of patients the dose of morphine increased by 63% (Fig. 15.1). The residual pain scores were the same in both groups (Ventafridda et al 1986).

At another centre, where 14 patients used an ad libitum approach, the total dose of methadone in the first 24 h ranged between 30–100 mg (Jakobsson et al 1980). After 1 week, the mean daily dose had fallen to 22 mg. Intervals between doses were initially 3–7 h but subsequently increased to about 10 h. Plasma concentrations of methadone increased sevenfold over 5 days. Most patients had complete or almost complete pain relief; some experienced mild drowsiness. One patient discontinued medication because of vomiting.

As with morphine, there are wide variations in dose requirements. In over 100 patients treated for up to 2 years, the daily doses ranged from 20–880 mg (Breivik & Rennemo 1982).

MU ANTAGONISTS

A pure antagonist is a substance which has a high degree of affinity for a receptor site but no intrinsic activity. Two compounds fit this description, naloxone and naltrexone. Naloxone is available commercially and is the

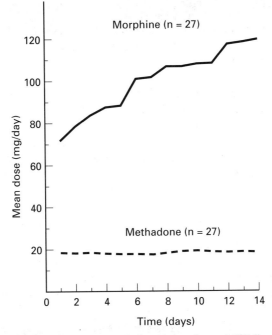

Fig. 15.1 Morphine and methadone doses during 14 days (mean ± SD) linear regression analysis: morphine p < 0.001; methadone p < 0.6. (Reproduced with permission from Ventafridda et al 1986.)

standard opioid antagonist in clinical use. Naltrexone is available in the USA. It is an oral opioid antagonist used in postdetoxification programmes (Kleber et al 1980). In contrast, nalorphine and nalbuphine are both mixed kappa agonists-mu antagonists.

Nalorphine

Nalorphine was used to antagonize morphine induced respiratory depression before the introduction of naloxone. Nalorphine has the following characteristics:

- it is as potent as morphine (Lasagna & Beecher 1954)
- it causes disturbing psychotomimetic adverse effects in most patients
- when given after morphine, nalorphine reverses the effects of morphine
- above a certain dose, nalorphine is less antagonistic to morphine (Houde & Wallenstein 1956)
- its capacity for producing physical dependence is much less than morphine
- in physically dependent animals and humans, the withdrawal syndrome associated with the use of nalorphine differs in certain respects from that seen with morphine.

Now that naloxone is generally available, nalorphine is no longer used.

BOX 15.G
WITHDRAWAL PHENOMENA IN MORPHINE DEPENDENT SUBJECTS

Mild
Yawning
Lacrimation
Rhinorrhoea   } develop after 8–16 h
Perspiration
Irritability

Moderate
Dilated pupils
Gooseflesh   } develop after 24–36 h
Tremor
Anorexia

Severe
Vomiting
Diarrhoea
Weight loss
Myoclonus
Cramps

Prolonged
Insomnia
Restlessness
Hyperpnoea
Blood pressure elevated
Pyrexia

Maximum after 2 or 3 days
Duration up to 2 weeks

Nalbuphine

Nalbuphine is chemically closely related to naloxone and to oxymorphone. It is slightly more potent than morphine. The duration of action is 3–6 h (Lewis 1980). Nalbuphine can be given SC, IM and IV. It is available in ampoules containing 10 mg/ml.

Abruptly stopping nalbuphine after prolonged use causes opioid withdrawal symptoms. Nalbuphine is 1/4 as potent as nalorphine in precipitating withdrawal symptoms in morphine dependent subjects (Box 15.G), but *suppresses* withdrawal symptoms in subjects dependent on only small doses of morphine. This paradoxical effect stems from differences in affinity for the opioid receptor subtypes. Nalbuphine reverses pruritus caused by epidural morphine in opioid naive subjects without reversing analgesia (Cohen et al 1992). It is not a Controlled Drug.

Naloxone

■ DRUG PORTRAIT

Naloxone is a potent opioid antagonist. It has a high affinity for morphine receptor sites and reverses the effect of opioid analgesics by displacement. The degree of displacement is dose related. Partial antagonism may be obtained by using small doses. Activity after oral administration is low; it is only 1/15 as potent by mouth as by injection. IV naloxone acts within 1 or 2 min, and has a plasma halflife of about 20 min. It is rapidly metabolized by the liver, primarily by conjugation with glucuronic acid. The conjugate is excreted by the kidneys. Naloxone is best given IV but, if not practical, may be given IM or SC. After IV injection, antagonism lasts for between 15 and 90 min.

Naloxone has no opioid effect; it is a pure antagonist. Tolerance does not develop during clinical use and, if abruptly withdrawn after repeated administration, no abstinence phenomena occur. Overdosage has not been reported. A single IV dose of 24 mg caused only slight drowsiness (Jasinski et al 1967). On the other hand, life threatening cardiac complications have occurred after doses as small as 100–400 µg) (see p. 298).

The most important clinical property of naloxone is reversal of opioid induced respiratory depression. It also antagonizes the sedative, analgesic and miotic effects of systemically administered opioid analgesics. In contrast to the nalorphine, a mixed agonist-antagonist, it does not increase respiratory depression should the diagnosis of opioid intoxication be wrong. It does not cause psychotomimetic effects.

Naloxone is not effective against respiratory depression caused by non-opioids such as barbiturates. It reverses the respiratory depression caused either by an overdose of an opioid (including codeine and dextropropoxyphene) or by an exaggerated response to conventional doses. It also counteracts the opioid effects of pentazocine and other mixed agonist-antagonists. Antagonism of buprenorphine is less complete because of its high receptor affinity.

Although naloxone is a pure opioid antagonist, it can cause other effects in certain circumstances. These actions of naloxone can be grouped into several categories:

- relief of poststroke pain
- correction of hyperendorphinism
- miscellaneous uses
- sporadic adverse effects.

Poststroke pain

This neuropathic pain syndrome has been reported after ischaemic injury to several sites in the brain causing partial de-afferentation of the lemniscal-thalamic-parietal pathway (Anonymous 1992). Pain relief has been achieved by repeated high doses of naloxone (Budd 1985, Ray & Tai 1988). The results of a controlled trial with doses up to 8 mg IV were disappointing, however (Bainton et al 1992).

Naloxone can inhibit evoked nociceptive activity in the rat thalamus (Jurna 1988). *Lower* doses of naloxone consistently caused inhibition, whereas higher doses sometimes inhibited and sometimes enhanced nociceptive activity. Whether these findings have implications for the treatment of poststroke pain is not known.

Correction of hyperendorphinism

Naloxone in doses of 800–1200 µg corrects congenital insensitivity to pain (Willer et al 1978). This suggests that this syndrome is related to a permanent hyperactivity of the body's endogenous opioid systems. Naloxone was also of benefit in a case of acquired insensitivity to pain associated with generalized hypothalamic dysfunction (Dunger et al 1980).

Benefit with naloxone has also been shown in patients with chronic idiopathic constipation (Kreek et al 1983). The effect was considered peripheral (i.e. intestinal) rather than central because of the response to both oral and IV naloxone. The results support the hypothesis that an excess of endogenous opioids is responsible for this condition.

Miscellaneous uses

Naloxone has been used in various conditions with variable response. For example, in septic shock, over half the patients showed an increase in systolic blood pressure of nearly 50% within minutes of naloxone 400–1200 µg IV (Peters et al 1981). In patients receiving morphine, naloxone reverses morphine induced peripheral vasodilatation (Cohen & Coffman 1980).

Naloxone has also been used to reverse ischaemic central neurological deficits (Baskin & Hosobuchi 1981, Bousigue et al 1982). Benefit occurred without any change in systemic blood pressure.

Naltrexone, an alternative opioid antagonist, has been used successfully in some patients with bulimia (Jonas & Gold 1986).

Sporadic adverse effects

The large doses used in poststroke pain and in the correction of massive opioid overdose indicate that naloxone has a wide margin of safety. On the other hand, a series of reports (Pallasch & Gill 1981, Cuss et al 1984, Partridge & Ward 1986) indicates that naloxone occasionally causes:

- severe hypertension
- pulmonary oedema
- tachycardia
- cardiac arrest.

Some have been in patients with identifiable pre-existing cardiac abnormalities (e.g. cardiomyopathy) or after open heart surgery. Doses as small as 100–400 µg of naloxone have been implicated (Pallasch & Gill 1981). It has been suggested that the mechanism of these sporadic events is related to the centrally mediated catecholamine responses to opioid reversal (Smith & Pinnock 1985).

Naloxone reversal of respiratory depression after spinal opioids

Naloxone 400 µg IV/SC reverses respiratory depression secondary to spinal opioids without significantly reversing analgesia (Scott & Fischer 1982, Korbon et al 1985). This claim, however, has been challenged (Gowan et al 1988). In a double-blind controlled trial, naloxone was administered in three different IV dose schedules over 20 h to patients who had received epidural morphine 6–7 mg before thoracotomy. Naloxone produced a 'trend towards decreased analgesia' as measured by:

- analgesic requirements
- intervals between analgesic doses
- VAS scores.

Surprisingly, an infusion of naloxone of about 30 µg/h had the same impact as one of 300 µg/h. In a second randomized controlled trial, however, a prophylactic IV infusion of naloxone 166 µg/h for 12 h in women undergoing caesarean section, did not reduce the analgesic effect of epidural morphine 4 mg given immediately postoperatively (Thind et al 1986).

The effect of naloxone will, of course, vary according to clinical circumstances. In the initial reports, the patients had respiratory depression whereas, in the clinical trials, it was given prophylactically.

Naloxone and the relief of opioid induced constipation

Oral naloxone may have a place in the management of constipation induced by opioids (Sykes 1991, Culpepper-Morgan et al 1992). In one study, 4/5 patients receiving naloxone q4h at 20–40% of their oral morphine dose experienced a strong laxative effect, whereas none of 12 patients obtained a response with a naloxone dose of 10% or less (Sykes 1991). The severity of response in 3 patients was undesirable, and possibly represented an opioid withdrawal reaction limited to the gastro-intestinal tract. The 20% dose of naloxone may therefore be excessive, particulary for patients receiving higher doses of morphine. Prolonged administration of the 10% dose of naloxone might be effective.

Naloxone in palliative care

The effect of IV naloxone lasts for 15–90 min and depends on the dose and the duration of action of the previously administered opioid and the interval since administration. A dose in excess of that needed to reverse depressed respiratory function will reverse sedation and analgesia. It may also cause sweating and tachycardia. If the patient is opioid dependent, naloxone precipitates withdrawal phenomena (Box 15.G). It is important, therefore, not to give too much. The amount needed to improve respiratory function is usually not more than 100–200 µg. A standard ampoule (400 µg) is usually excessive. In addition to pain and agitation, the patient may experience generalized allodynia and hyperaesthesia making further IV injections painful and difficult. If naloxone is required, a butterfly cannula should be inserted and naloxone 100 µg IV injected every 2–3 min.

OPIOID OVERDOSAGE

Adults

In adult self-poisoning with opioid analgesics, the overdose is considerably greater and the usual initial dose of naloxone is 400 µg. Larger doses can be given. The manufacturer's Data Sheet states that the initial dose may be as much as 2 mg. Doses can be repeated every 2 or 3 min. If no improvement is observed after 10 mg, the diagnosis of opioid induced respiratory depression should be questioned.

As most opioids act for longer than naloxone, respiratory depression may recur, especially with methadone and dextropropoxyphene. It can be prevented by a continuous IV infusion (Bradberry & Raebel 1981). Alternatively, repeated IV or IM injections can be administered as needed every 1 or 2 h. Observation for up to 48 h may be necessary, particularly if the amount or nature of the opioid administered is unknown.

Buprenorphine overdose is reversed by naloxone, but larger amounts of naloxone are required (Table 15.6). In the case of buprenorphine overdosage, the initial dose of naloxone should be at least 4 mg (10 × 400 µg ampoules). Subsequent doses of between 4 and 8 mg should be given, depending on the initial response. If necessary, doxapram, a respiratory stimulant, should also be used. A bolus of 100 mg IV should be followed by an infusion of 200 mg/h (3 mg/kg body weight). The rate may be increased up to 1 g/h (Dundee et al 1974).

Children

The usual initial dose of naloxone for children is 5–10 µg/kg body weight. This dose may be repeated at 2 or 3 min intervals in accordance with the adult administration guidelines. Continuous IV naloxone infusion has been recommended for use in children (Gourlay & Coulthard 1983, Lewis et al 1984).

Table 15.6   Initial naloxone dose for opioid overdosage

	IV dose
Iatrogenic respiratory depression	100 µg
Self-poisoning with opioid	400 µg
Self-poisoning with buprenorphine	4 mg

REFERENCES

Abramson F P 1982 Methadone plasma protein binding: alterations in cancer and displacement from alpha 1-acid glycoprotein. Clinical Pharmacology and Therapeutics 32: 652–658

Adriaensen H, Mattelaere B, Varmeenen H 1981 A long-term open assessment of sublingual buprenorphine in patients suffering from chronic pain. Pain suppl 1: 838

Anonymous 1967 Analgesics and monoamine oxidase inhibitors. British Medical Journal ii: 284

Anonymous 1979 Buprenorphine injection (Temgesic). Drug and Therapeutics Bulletin 17: 17–19

Anonymous 1992 More on central poststroke pain: treatment with naloxone. Topics in Pain Management 8: 3–4

Atkinson R E, Schofield P, Mellor P 1990 The efficacy in sequential use of buprenorphine and morphine in advanced cancer pain. In: Doyle D (ed) Opioids in the treatment of cancer pain. Royal Society of Medicine Services, London, pp 81–87

Babul N, Darke A C 1992 Putative role of hydromorphone metabolites in myoclonus. Pain 51: 260–261

Bainton T, Fox M, Bowsher D, Wells C 1992 A double-blind trial of naloxone in central poststroke pain. Pain 48: 159–162

Barnes J N, Williams A J, Tomson M J, Toseland P A, Goodwin F J 1985 Dihydrocodeine in renal failure: further evidence for an important role in the kidney in the handling of opioid drugs. British Medical Journal 290: 740–742

Baskin D S, Hosobuchi Y 1981 Naloxone reversal of ischaemic neurological deficits in man. Lancet ii: 272–275

Beaver W T, Wallenstein S L, Houde R W, Rogers A 1967 A clinical comparison of the analgesic effects of methadone and morphine administered intramuscularly and of orally and parenterally administered methadone. Clinical Pharmacology and Therapeutics 8: 415–426

Berkowitz B A 1976 The relationship of pharmacokinetics to pharmacological activity; morphine, methadone and naloxone. Clinical Pharmacokinetics 1: 219–230

Bertler A, Erelius N, Elwin C E 1980 Coordinated activity at a university hospital of analgesic treatment in terminal care. Presented at Symposium on Narcotic Analgesics. Stockholm,

Bonuccelli U, Del Dotto P, Piccini P, Behge F, Corsini G U, Muratorio A 1992 Dextromethorphan and Parkinsonism. Lancet 340: 53

Bousigue J-Y, Giraud L, Fournie D, Tremoulet M 1982 Naloxone reversal of neurological deficit. Lancet ii: 618–619

Bradberry J C, Raebel M A 1981 Continuous infusion of naloxone in the treatment of narcotic overdose. Drug Intelligence and Clinical Pharmacy 15: 945–950

Breivik H, Rennemo F 1982 Clinical evaluation of combined treatment with methadone and psychotropic drugs in cancer patients. Acta Anaesthesiologica Scandinavica 26 (suppl 74): 135–140

Bruera E, Schoeller T, Fainsinger R, Kastelan C 1992 Custom made suppositories of methadone for severe cancer pain. Journal of Pain and Symptom Management 7: 372–374

Budd K 1985 The use of the opiate antagonist, naloxone, in the treatment of intractable pain. Neuropeptides 5: 419–422

Budd K 1990 Experience with partial agonists in the treatment of cancer pain. In: Opioids in the treatment of cancer pain. Royal Society of Medicine Services, London, pp 51–55

Chaplan S R, Duncan S R, Brodsky J B, Brose W G 1992 Morphine and hydromorphone epidural analgesia. Anesthesiology 77: 1090–1094

Church J, Jones M G, Davies S N, Lodge D 1988 Antitussive agents as N-methylaspartate antagonists: further studies. Canadian Journal of Physiology and Pharmacology 67: 561–567

Clark B, Thompson J W, Widdrington G 1972 Analysis of the inhibition of pethidine N-demethylation by monoamine oxidase inhibitors and some other drugs with special reference to drug interactions in man. British Journal of Pharmacology 44: 89–99

Cocks D P, Passmore-Rowe A 1962 Dangers of monoamine oxidase inhibitors. British Medical Journal ii: 1545–1546

Cohen R A, Coffman J D 1980 Naloxone reversal of morphine-induced peripheral vasodilatation. Clinical Pharmacology and Therapeutics 28: 541–544

Cohen S E, Ratner E F, Kreitzman T R, Archer J H, Mignano L R 1992 Nalbuphine is better than naloxone for treatment of side effects after epidural morphine. Anesthesia and Analgesia 75: 747–752

Corbett A D, Paterson S J, Kosterlitz H W 1993 Selectivity of ligands for opioid receptors. In Herz A (ed) Opioids I Springer Verlag, London, pp 657–672

Culpepper-Morgan J A, Inturrisi C E, Portenoy R K et al 1992 Treatment of opioid-induced constipation with oral naloxone: a pilot study. Clinical Pharmacology and Therapeutics 52: 90–95

Cuss F M, Colaco C B, Baron J H 1984 Cardiac arrest after reversal of effects of opiates with naloxone. British Medical Journal 288: 363–364

Davis W M, Hatoum N S 1979 Lethal synergism between morphine or other narcotic analgesics and propranolol. Toxicology 14: 141–151

Dundee J W, Gray R C, Gupta P R 1974 Doxapram in the treatment of acute drug poisoning. Anaesthesia 29: 710–714

Dunger D B, Leonard J V, Wolff O H, Preece M A 1980 Effect of naloxone in a previously undescribed hypothalamic syndrome. Lancet i: 1277–1281

Duthie D J R, Rowbotham D J, Wyld R, Henderson P D, Nimmo W S 1988 Plasma fentanyl concentrations during transdermal delivery of fentanyl to surgical patients. British Journal of Anaesthesia 60: 614–618

Eap C B, Cuendet C, Baumann P 1990 Binding of D-methadone, L-methadone and DL-methadone to proteins in plasma of healthy volunteers: role of variants of X1-acid glycoprotein. Clinical Pharmacology and Therapeutics 47: 338–346

Ettinger D S, Vitale P J, Trump D L 1979 Important clinical pharmacological considerations in the use of methadone in cancer patients. Cancer Treatment Reports 63: 457–459

Fainsinger R, Schoeller T, Bruera E 1993 Methadone in the management of cancer pain: a review. Pain 52: 137–147

Flavell-Matts S G 1962 Dextromoramide analgesia in the acute general medical patient. Practitioner 188: 524–526

Gaensler E A, McGowan J M, Henderson F F 1948 A comparative study of the action of demerol and opium alkaloids in relation to biliary spasm. Surgery 23: 211–220

Giacomini K M, Giacomini J C, Gibson T P, Levy G 1980 Propoxyphene and norpropoxyphene plasma concentrations after oral propoxyphene in cirrhotic patients with and without surgically constructed portacaval shunt. Clinical Pharmacology and Therapeutics 30: 183–188

Gibson T P, Giacomini K M, Briggs W A, Whitman W, Levy G 1980 Propoxyphene and norpropoxyphene plasma concentrations in the anephric patient. Clinical Pharmacology and Therapeutics 27: 665–670

Glare P A, Walsh T D 1993 Dose-ranging study of oxycodone for chronic pain in advanced cancer. Journal of Clinical Oncology 11: 973–978

Gourlay G K, Coulthard K 1983 The role of naloxone infusions in the treatment of overdoses of long halflife narcotic agonists: application to nor-methadone. British Journal of Clinical Pharmacology 15: 269–272

Gourlay G K, Plummer S L, Cherry D A, Cousins M J 1990 Does intravenous methadone provide longer lasting analgesia than intravenous morphine? Pain 42: 383–384

Gowan J D, Hurtig J B, Fraser R A, Torbicki E, Kitts J 1988 Naloxone infusion after prophylactic epidural morphine: effects on incidence of postoperative side-effects and quality of analgesia. Canadian Journal of Anaesthesia 35: 143–148

Grochow L, Sheidler V, Grossman S, Green L, Enterline J 1989 Does intravenous methadone provide longer lasting analgesia than intravenous morphine? A randomized, double-blind study. Pain 38: 151–157

Heel R C, Brogden R N, Speight T M, Avery G S 1978 Butorphanol: a review of its pharmacological properties and therapeutic efficacy. Drugs 16: 473–505

Heel R C, Brogden R N, Speight T M, Avery G S 1979 Buprenorphine: a review of its pharmacological properties and therapeutic efficacy. Drugs 17: 81–110

Hill R G 1992 Multiple opioid receptors and their ligands. Frontiers of Pain 4: 1–4

Houde R W 1986 Discussion. In: Foley K M, Inturrisi C E (eds) Advances in pain research and therapy, vol 8. Raven Press, New York, pp 261–263

Houde R W, Wallenstein S L 1956 Federation Proceedings 15: 440

Inturrisi C E, Verebely K 1972 The levels of methadone in the plasma in methadone maintenance. Clinical Pharmacology and Therapeutics 13: 633–637

Jakobsson P A, Ginman C, Hanson J, et al 1980 Clinical evaluation of methadone treatment in cancer pain. Presented at Symposium on Narcotic Analgesics. Stockholm

Jasinski D R, Martin W R, Haertzen C A 1967 The human pharmacology and abuse potential of N-allyl-noroxymorphone (naloxone). Journal of Pharmacology and Experimental Therapeutics 157: 420–426

Jonas J M, Gold M S 1986 Naltrexone reverses bulimic symptoms. Lancet i: 807

Judd A T, Tempest S M, Clarke I M C 1981 The anaesthetist and the pain clinic; dextromoramide analgesia. British Medical Journal 282: 75–76

Jurna I 1988 Dose-dependent inhibition by naloxone of nociceptive activity evoked in the rat thalamus. Pain 35: 349–354

Kaiko R F 1986 Discussion. In: Foley K, Inturrisi C E (eds) Advances in pain research and therapy, vol 8, Raven Press. New York, pp 235–237

Kalso E, Vainio A 1990 Morphine and oxycodone in the management of cancer pain. Clinical Pharmacology and Therapeutics 47: 639–646

Kantor T G, Hopper M, Laska E 1981 Adverse effects of commonly ordered oral narcotics. Journal of Clinical Pharmacology 21: 1–8

Kay B 1973 A study of strong oral analgesics; the relief of postoperative pain using dextromoramide, pentazocine and bezitramide. British Journal of Anaesthesia 45: 623–628

Kleber H D, Gold M S, Riodan C E 1980 The use of clonidine in detoxification from opiates. Bulletin on Narcotics 32: 1–10

Klotz U, McHorse T S, Wilkinson G R, Schenker S 1974 The effect of cirrhosis on the disposition and elimination of meperidine in man. Clinical Pharmacology and Therapeutics 16: 667–675

Kolodny A L 1960 Dextromoramide (Palfium) a new synthetic analgesic for relief of acute and chronic pain. Antibiotic Medicine and Clinical Therapy 7: 695–701

Korbon G A, James D J, Verlander J M et al 1985 Intramuscular naloxone reverses the side effects of epidural morphine while preserving analgesia. Regional Anesthesia 10: 16–20

Kreek H J, Garfield J W, Gutjahr C L, Giusti L M 1976 Rifampin-induced methadone withdrawal. New England Journal of Medicine 294: 1104–1106

Kreek M J, Schecter A J, Gutjahr C L, Hecht M 1980 Methadone use in patients with chronic renal disease. Drug Alcohol Dependence 5: 197–205

Kreek M-J, Schaefer R A, Hahn E F, Fishman J 1983 Naloxone, a specific opioid antagonist, reverses chronic idiopathic constipation. Lancet i: 261–262

Lamerton R C 1979 Cancer patients dying at home. The last 24 hours. Practitioner 223: 813–817

Lasagna L, Beecher H K 1954 The analgesic effectiveness of codeine and meperidine (Demerol). Journal of Pharmacology and Experimental Therapeutics 112: 306–311

Lewis J R 1980 Evaluation of new analgesics. Butorphanol and nalbuphine. Journal of the American Medical Association 243: 1465–1467

Lewis J M, Klein-Schwartz W, Benson B E, Oderda G M, Takai S 1984 Continuous naloxone infusion in pediatric narcotic overdose. American Journal of Diseases of Children 138: 944–946

London D R, Milne M D 1962 Dangers of monoamine oxidase inhibitors. British Medical Journal ii: 1752

Martinson I M, Armstrong G D, Geis D P et al 1978 Home care for children dying of cancer. Paediatrics 62: 106–113

Meresaar U, Nilsson M I, Holmstrand J, Anggard E 1981 Single dose pharmacokinetics and bioavailability of methadone in man studied with a stable isotope method. European Journal of Clinical Pharmacology 20: 473–478

Morley J S, Watt J W G, Wells J C, Miles J B, Finnegan M J, Leng G 1993 Methadone in pain uncontrolled by morphine. Lancet 342: 1243

Morrison J D, Hill G B, Dundee J W 1968 Studies of drugs given before anaesthesia XV: evaluation of the method of study after 10,000 observations. British Journal of Anaesthesia 40: 890–900

Moulin D E, Ling G S F, Pasternak G W 1988 Unidirectional analgesic cross-tolerance between morphine and levorphanol in the rat. Pain 33: 233–239

Neal E A, Meffin P J, Gregory P B, Blaschke T F 1979 Enhanced bioavailability and decreased clearance of analgesics in patients with cirrhosis. Gastroenterology 77: 96–102

Nilsson M I, Meresaar U, Anggard E 1982a Clinical pharmacokinetics of methadone. Acta Anaesthesiologica Scandinavica suppl 74: 66–69

Nilsson M I, Anggard E, Holmstrand H, Gunne L M 1982b Pharmacokinetics of methadone during maintenance treatment: adaptive changes during the induction phase. European Journal of Clinical Pharmacology 22: 343–349

Novick D M, Kreek M J, Fanizza A M, Yancovitz S R, Gelb A M, Stenger R J 1981 Methadone disposition in patients with chronic liver disease. Clinical Pharmacology and Therapeutics 30: 353–362

Osborne R J, Joel S P, Slevin M L 1986 Morphine intoxication in renal failure: the role of morphine-6-glucuronide. British Medical Journal 292: 1548–1549

Osborne R, Joel S, Grebenik K, Trew D, Slevin M 1993 The pharmacokinetics of morphine and morphine glucuronides in kidney failure. Clinical Pharmacology and Therapeutics 54: 158–167

Pagani I, Barzaghi N, Crema F, Perucca E, Ego D, Rovei V 1989 Pharmacokinetics of dextromoramide in surgical patients. Fundamental and Clinical Pharmacology 3: 27–35

Pallasch T J, Gill C J 1981 Naloxone associated morbidity and mortality. Oral Surgery 52: 602–603

Partridge B L, Ward C F 1986 Pulmonary oedema following low-dose naloxone administration. Anesthesiology 65: 709–710

Peters W P, Johnson M W, Friedman P A, Mitch W E 1981 Pressor effect of naloxone in septic shock. Lancet i: 529–532

Pond S M, Kretschzmar K M 1981 Effect of phenytoin on meperidine clearance and normeperidine formation. Clinical Pharmacology and Therapeutics 30: 680–686

Pond S M, Tong T, Benowitz N L, Jacob P, Rigod J 1981 Presystemic metabolism of meperidine to normeperidine in normal and cirrhotic subjects. Clinical Pharmacology and Therapeutics 30: 183–188

Portenoy R K, Southam M A, Gupta S K et al 1993 Transdermal fentanyl for cancer pain: repeated dose pharmacokinetics. Anesthesiology 78: 36–43

Poyhia R, Seppala T, Olkkola K T, Kalso E 1992 The pharmacokinetics and metabolism of oxycodone after intramuscular and oral administration to healthy subjects. British Journal of Clinical Pharmacology 33: 617–621

Poyhia R, Vainio A, Kalso E 1993 Oxycodone: an alternative to morphine for cancer pain. A review. Journal of Pain and Symptom Management 8: 63–67

Ray D A A, Tai Y M A 1988 Infusions of naloxone in thalamic pain. British Medical Journal 296: 969–970

Robinson A E, Williams F M 1971 The distribution of methadone in man. Journal of Pharmacy and Pharmacology 23: 353–358

Rogers K J, Thornton J A 1969 the interaction between monoamine oxidase inhibitors and narcotic analgesics in mice. British Journal of Pharmacology 36: 470–480

Rose P G, Macfee M S, Boswell M V 1993 Fentanyl transdermal system overdoses secondary to cutaneous hyperthermia. Anesthesia and Analgesia 77: 390–391

Sawe J 1986 High-dose morphine and methadone in cancer patients: clinical pharmacokinetic consideration of oral treatment. Clinical Pharmacology 11: 87–106

Sawe J, Hansen J, Ginman C et al 1981 Patient-controlled dose regimen of methadone for chronic cancer pain. British Medical Journal 282: 771–773

Sawe J, Kager L, Svensson J O, Rane A 1985 Oral morphine in cancer patients: in vivo kinetics and in vitro hepatic glucuronidation. British Journal of Clinical Pharmacology 19: 495–501

Scott P V, Fischer H B J 1982 Intraspinal opiates and itching: a new reflex? British Medical Journal 284: 1015–1016

Shaw J E, Chandrasekaran S K 1985 Transdermal therapeutic systems. In: Prescott L F, Nimmo W E (eds) Drug absorption. Proceedings of the International Conference on Drug Absorption, ADIS Press, Edinburgh, pp 186–193

Shee J C 1960 Dangerous potentiation of pethidine by iproniazid, and its treatment. British Medical Journal ii: 507

Smith G, Pinnock C 1985 Editorial: naloxone – paradox or panacea? British Journal of Anaesthesia 57: 547–549

Sorkin E M, Ugawa C S 1983 Cimetidine potentiation of narcotic action. Drug Intelligence and Clinical Pharmacy 17: 60–61

Stambaugh J E, Wainer I W 1981 Drug interaction: meperidine and chlorpromazine, a toxic combination. Journal of Clinical Pharmacology 21: 140–146

Stambaugh J E, Wainer I W, Hemphill D M, Schwartz I 1977 A potentially toxic drug interaction between pethidine (meperidine) and phenobarbitone. Lancet 1: 398–399

Staritz M, Poralla T, Manns M, Ewe K, Meyer zum Buschenfelde K-H 1985 Pentazocine hampers bile flow. Lancet i: 573–574

Supplement 1992 The role of the fentanyl series for pain management: novel delivery systems. Journal of Pain and Symptom Management 7 (Suppl 3): S1–S62

Sykes N P 1991 Oral naloxone in opioid-associated constipation. Lancet 337: 1475

Szeto H H, Inturrisi C E, Houde R et al 1977 Accumulation of normeperidine an active metabolite of meperidine in patients with renal failure or cancer. Annals of Internal Medicine 86: 738–741

Taylor D C 1962 Alarming reaction to pethidine in patients on phenelzine. Lancet ii: 401–402

Thind G S, Wells J C D, Wilkes R G 1986 The effects of continuous intravenous naloxone on epidural morphine analgesia. Anesthesia 41: 582–585

Tong T G, Pond S M, Kreek M J, Jaffery N F, Benowitz N L 1981 Phenytoin-induced methadone withdrawal. Annals of Internal Medicine 94: 349–351

Twycross R G 1977 A comparison of diamorphine with cocaine and methadone. British Journal of Clinical Pharmacology 4: 691–693

Vallner J, Stewaqrt J, Kotzan J, Kirsten E, Hongberg I 1981 Pharmacokinetics and bioavailability of hydromorphone following intravenous and oral administration to human subjects. Journal of Clinical Pharmacology 21: 152–156

Ventafridda V, Ripamonti C, Bianchi M, Sbanotto A, De Conno F 1986 A randomized study on oral administration of morphine and methadone in the treatment of cancer pain. Journal of Pain and Symptom Management 1: 203–207

Ventafridda V, Ripamonti C, De Conno F, Bianchi M, Pazzuconi F, Panerai A E 1987 Antidepressants increase bioavailability of morphine in cancer patients (letter). Lancet i: 1204

Walker J, Yatham L N 1993 Benylin (dextromethorphan) abuse and mania. British Medical Journal 306: 896

Wallenstein S L, Rogers A G, Kaiko R F, Houde R W 1986 Nalbuphine: clinical analgesic studies. In: Foley K M, Inturrisi C E (eds) Advances in pain research and therapy, vol 8. Raven Press, New York, pp 247–252

Weinberg D S, Inturrisi C E, Reidenberg B et al 1988 Sublingual administration of selected opioid analgesics. Clinical Pharmacology and Therapeutics 44: 335–342

Wilkes E 1974 Some problems in cancer management. Proceedings of the Royal Society of Medicine 67: 1001–1005

Willer J C, Dehen H, Boureau F, Cambier J 1978 Congenital insensitivity to pain and naloxone. Lancet ii: 739

Zenz M, Piepenbrock S, Tryba M, Glocke M, Everlien M, Klauke W 1985 Kontrollierte studie mit buprenorphine. Deutsche Medizinische Woschensechrict 110: 448–453

Oral morphine

'Morphine exists to be given, not merely to be withheld'.

The mode of action of morphine is discussed in Chapter 10 and its general pharmacology in Chapter 14. This chapter deals specifically with the practical aspects of the use of morphine by mouth in the relief of cancer pain.

In advanced cancer, morphine is used principally to relieve pain and/or dyspnoea. It also has a place in the management of cough and diarrhoea. When used to relieve severe acute pain, the route of administration is normally parenteral. In cancer, however, the oral route is preferred because it enhances the patient's independence, is noninvasive, and costs less.

ORAL PREPARATIONS

The choice lies between solutions or tablets of morphine sulphate/hydrochloride and m/r preparations (Table 16.1). The molecular weights of morphine sulphate or hydrochloride are similar and they may be regarded as interchangeable. Morphine solution and ordinary tablets are administered q4h; m/r preparations q12h. Proprietary preparations of both formulations are available. Some pharmacies, however, still produce their own morphine solutions.

The following have been shown to be equally efficacious and to have identical adverse effects profiles:

- morphine solution q4h and m/r tablets q12h (Hanks et al 1987, Arkinstall et al 1989, Walsh et al 1992)
- morphine tablets q4h and m/r tablets q12h (Deschamps et al 1992)
- m/r tablets q12h and m/r suspension q12h (Boureau et al 1992).

M/r preparations are not necessarily identical (Bloomfield et al 1993). A new m/r morphine capsule is being marketed in 1994 in several countries. Its

Table 16.1   Proprietary oral preparations of morphine sulphate (UK)

Formulation	Content	
Tablet	10 mg	
	20 mg	
Oral solution	10 mg/5 ml	
	30 mg/5 ml	} unit dose vials
	100 mg/5 ml	
	2 mg/ml[a]	
	20 mg/ml[b]	} bottles
M/r tablets	10 mg	
	15 mg	
	30 mg	
	60 mg	
	100 mg	
	200 mg	
M/r powder[c]	20 mg	
	30 mg	
	60 mg	
	100 mg	
	200 mg	

[a] Because content of morphine base is less than 2% (i.e. 2 g/l), this preparation is *not* a Controlled Drug in the UK.
[b] Coloured red to facilitate use of calibrated dropper.
[c] Given in water as a suspension. Weight for weight is several times more expensive than m/r tablets.

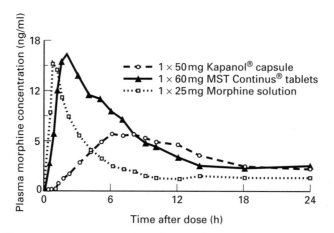

Fig. 16.1   Plasma morphine concentrations after a single dose of morphine solution and two m/r preparations. (Reproduced with permission from West & Maccarrone 1993.)

pharmacokinetic profile is clearly more attractive than that of MST-Continus (Figs. 16.1, 16.2). The absence of an early peak with the new preparation may reduce:

- adverse effects in some patients
- breakthrough pain towards the end of each 12 h dose interval.

At some centres m/r tablets are considered the formulation of choice, while

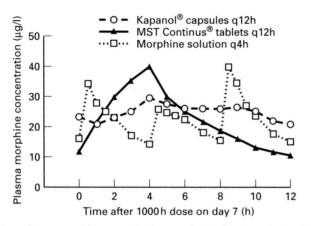

Fig. 16.2   Mean plasma morphine concentrations on day 7 of treatment with either morphine solution or one of two m/r morphine preparations. Total number of patients = 24. (Reproduced with permission from Gourlay et al 1993.)

at others morphine solutions or ordinary tablets are preferred. The convenience of a b.i.d. regimen compared with q4h makes m/r tablets an attractive option, particularly for those at home.

In economically poorer countries, the cost of m/r tablets is likely to limit their use. The cost of m/r morphine suspensions is even greater. On the other hand, if the professional time used to administer morphine to inpatients is taken into account, the cost differential is reduced. In one study, it took 9 min to administer m/r morphine b.i.d. compared with 24 min for morphine solution q4h (Goughnour & Arkinstall 1991).

Initial dose titration with morphine solution or ordinary tablets is recommended (Hanks 1989). At Sobell House, inpatients who have been stabilized on aqueous morphine q4h are transferred to m/r morphine q12h as part of the preparation for going home. At some centres, however, m/r tablets are used throughout.

The change from one preparation to the other is straightforward. Either at 1000 h or 2200 h the m/r morphine tablets can be introduced, and continued on a b.i.d. 'after breakfast and bedtime' schedule. There is no need for a loading dose of morphine solution or ordinary tablets to be given (Hoskin et al 1989).

Provided a patient can swallow liquids or tablets and is not vomiting repeatedly, morphine can and should be given by mouth; injections are not necessary. Any other limitation to the use of oral morphine will be shared also by parenteral morphine. In other words:

- if a pain is opioid responsive, oral morphine will give relief
- if the pain is opioid resistant, morphine will not give relief even if administered parenterally.

This general statement is *not* true, however, in relation to spinal morphine which may well be superior to SC or IV morphine in patients with seemingly morphine resistant pain (see p. 365).

CHOICE OF STARTING DOSE

The initial dose of morphine sulphate depends mainly on the patient's previous medication. Age and general condition are also important. For patients who have been taking a weak opioid, a starting dose of 10 mg is generally appropriate. If step 2 (weak opioid) is omitted, a 5 mg dose is usually more appropriate.

In the frail elderly patient, or patients with respiratory or hepatic failure, it is often prudent to start on a dose which is likely to be suboptimal. This prevents distress in both patient and family, and noncompliance, should the patient on a higher dose become very drowsy, dizzy or confused.

It is sometimes stated that it is best to start on a 'high' dose and then, when the pain is relieved, reduce to a lower maintenance level. Such an approach cannot be recommended although, in some patients, the liberal use of 'as needed' extra doses may speed up the initial dose titration. The analgesic effect of morphine is *not* an 'all or none' phenomenon. With rare exceptions, it is possible to choose a starting dose that is at least as effective as the previous medication, and usually more so.

Changing from an alternative strong opioid

For those who have been receiving an alternative strong opioid, it is necessary to determine as closely as possible what the patient has been taking over a 24 h period and convert to 'morphine sulphate equivalents' (Table 16.2, Box 16.A). For a patient on very high doses, however, a dose of about half to two thirds the theoretical equivalent is generally advisable (see p. 272). This is because of incomplete cross-tolerance (McGivney & Crooks 1984, Foley 1985).

Equivalency tables are only approximate. Unless the patient has been taking a mixed agonist-antagonist such as pentazocine, the previous medication can be used for 'topping up' over the first few days until the correct dose of morphine is determined. This prevents the patient becoming disillusioned and even more anxious should the chosen starting dose of morphine be too low.

Because of the gross difference in plasma halflives, it is difficult to give equivalent doses for morphine and methadone. On the other hand, methadone is a useful alternative strong opioid. This means that it is unlikely that there will be a need to change to morphine because of unrelieved pain. The only common reason for wishing to change is excessive drowsiness and confusional symptoms resulting from cumulation. In this circumstance, prescribing morphine sulphate initially in a ratio of 1:1 would be appropriate.

One other drug conversion may be difficult, namely, from dextromoramide. Patients with severe pain often take dextromoramide q2h–q3h and occasionally more often. Here there is a psychological problem. If you have been taking medication q2h–q3h and obtaining a fair measure of relief, it may be difficult to accept that anything can and will last 4 h. Further, dextromoramide has a rapid onset of action. Thus, if a patient has been taking his medication partly 'as needed', he may experience worsening pain

Table 16.2 Opioids by mouth: approximate equivalence to oral morphine sulphate[a]

Analgesic	Proprietary name	Potency ratio with morphine sulphate	Duration of action (h)[b]
Codeine		1/12[c]	3–5
Pethidine/meperidine	Demerol (USA)	1/8[c]	2–3
Tramadol	Tramal	1/4	4–5
Dipipanone	in Diconal (UK)	1/2	3–5
Papaveretum	Omnopon (UK), Pantopon (USA)	2/3[d]	3–5
Oxycodone	in Percodan, Percocet, Tylox (USA)	4/3[e]	5–6
Dextromoramide	Palfium (UK)	[2][f]	2–3
Methadone	Physeptone (UK), Dolophine (USA)	[3–4][g]	6–12
Levorphanol	Dromoran (UK), Levo-dromoran (USA)	5[c]	6–8
Phenazocine	Narphen (UK)	5[h]	6–8
Hydromorphone	Dilaudid (USA)	5–6[c]	3–5
Buprenorphine	Temgesic	60[i]	6–8

[a] Multiply dose of opioid by its potency ratio to determine the equivalent dose of morphine sulphate (Box 16.A).

[b] Dependent in part on severity of pain and on dose; often longer lasting in very elderly and those with renal dysfunction.

[c] Determined in parenteral study but clinically seems to hold true for oral route as well.

[d] Papaveretum (strong opium) is standardized to contain 50% morphine base; potency ratio expressed in relation to morphine sulphate.

[e] Oxycodone is 3/4 as potent as morphine by injection but, because of greater oral bio-availability, it is more potent by mouth (Kalso & Vainio 1990)

[f] Dextromoramide: a single 5 mg dose is equivalent to morphine 15 mg in terms of peak effect but is shorter acting; overall potency ratio adjusted accordingly.

[g] Methadone: a single 5 mg dose is equivalent to morphine 7.5 mg. Has a long plasma halflife which leads to cumulation when given repeatedly; overall potency ratio adjusted accordingly (Inturrisi & Verebely 1972).

[h] Unpublished observations (Twycross 1973).

[i] Must be taken *sublingually*; potency diminished if swallowed (Zenz et al 1985). In the USA, buprenorphine is currently available only as an injection.

BOX 16.A
CONVERTING TO MORPHINE FROM AN ALTERNATIVE OPIOID

Add up the total dose in milligrams of the alternative strong opioid taken in an average 24 h period.

Multiply this by the potency of the strong opioid in question (see Table 16.2). This is the *total daily dose of morphine* that will give comparable relief.

If the patient has been in pain despite the use of the alternative strong opioid, the total daily dose of morphine should be increased by about 50%.

If using morphine solution or ordinary morphine tablets, divide this by *six* and 'round up' to the nearest convenient 5 mg or 10 mg. This is the correct starting dose of morphine q4h. This may be 60 mg or even more.

If using m/r morphine, divide by *two* and 'round up' to the nearest convenient twice a day dose. This may be as much as 200 mg.

after the first dose of morphine, even if theoretically adequate, because of slower absorption. For someone with severe pain, this could devastate morale. When changing from dextromoramide, therefore, the starting dose of morphine should err on the side of generosity (Table 16.2). In addition, both at home and in hospital, the patient should be allowed initially to keep some dextromoramide tablets to use for breakthrough pain.

ADJUSTMENT OF DOSE

The patient and family should be advised that the starting dose may not relieve the pain completely:

'If the morphine is less effective than your old medication, 'top up' with a dose of the old and increase the next dose of morphine solution from 5 ml to 8 ml.' *or*

'If the morphine is less effective than your old medication, take another dose after 2 h and increase the next regular dose from 5 ml to 8 ml.' *or*

'If your pain is not 90% relieved by this time tomorrow, increase the dose of morphine solution from 5 ml to 8 ml.'

There is less room for manoeuvre with tablets; a patient on morphine 10 mg would have to double the dose to 20 mg. In addition, the following general advice should be given:

'If you are unhappy about anything concerning the new medication, contact me at. . . (name and telephone number of doctor or nurse).' *or*

'I (or nurse) will be in touch later today/tomorrow to review progress.' *or*

'Would you phone me tomorrow at. . . to let me know how things are going?'

Further, if an unknown team member is scheduled to be on duty, give the patient the name of the person available and a few words of introduction and reassurance:

'Dr X/Nurse Y is on call tonight. We work closely together, and I will tell him/her about you before I go off duty.'

During the first few days, it is often necessary to adjust the dose of morphine. It should be exceptional, therefore, for a patient not to be visited on the second day of treatment by either a doctor or nurse familiar with the use of oral morphine.

The patient and family usually have many questions they want to ask about the regular use of morphine, for example 'Will I become addicted?' Professional time must be made for such discussion.

Personal professional support is necessary to encourage the patient and family during the period of initial adverse effects. Also, only the trained professional can recognize when the dose of morphine should be reduced temporarily or when morphine intolerance cannot be circumvented. *It is negligent to prescribe morphine and not to arrange close supervision by somebody familiar with its use* (Box 16.B).

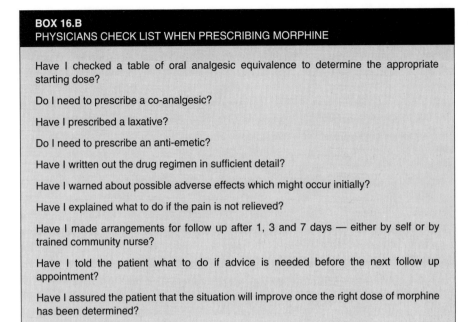

BOX 16.B
PHYSICIANS CHECK LIST WHEN PRESCRIBING MORPHINE

Have I checked a table of oral analgesic equivalence to determine the appropriate starting dose?

Do I need to prescribe a co-analgesic?

Have I prescribed a laxative?

Do I need to prescribe an anti-emetic?

Have I written out the drug regimen in sufficient detail?

Have I warned about possible adverse effects which might occur initially?

Have I explained what to do if the pain is not relieved?

Have I made arrangements for follow up after 1, 3 and 7 days — either by self or by trained community nurse?

Have I told the patient what to do if advice is needed before the next follow up appointment?

Have I assured the patient that the situation will improve once the right dose of morphine has been determined?

Most patients obtain relief with morphine sulphate in doses of between 10 and 30 mg q4h (Fig. 16.3). If previously they have been taking an alternative strong opioid, such as hydromorphone, levorphanol, methadone or phenazocine, the effective analgesic dose may be considerably higher. If the pain is not much relieved after one or two increments of 100% (low starting dose) or 50% (high starting dose) it is possible that the patient has

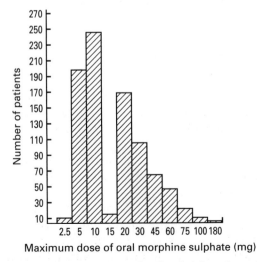

Fig. 16.3   Histogram of maximum q4h doses of orally administered morphine sulphate in 955 patients at St. Christopher's Hospice (1978–79). Median dose = 10 mg. 75 includes 80 and 90 mg; 100 includes 110 and 120 mg.

> **BOX 16.C**
> **REASONS FOR INCOMPLETE RELIEF WITH MORPHINE IN A PATIENT RECEIVING MORPHINE REGULARLY ON AN APPROPRIATE TIME SCHEDULE**
>
> Need to prescribe NSAID or paracetamol
>
> Need to increase the dose of morphine
>
> Pain precipitated by activity
>
> Unresolved anger, anxiety, fear (see Chapter 2)
>
> Poor compliance because living alone, forgetfulness, etc.
>
> Difficulty in swallowing medication, with loss through drooling and spluttering (see Chapter 18)
>
> Vomiting shortly after taking oral morphine (see Chapter 18)
>
> Inability to increase the dose further because of intolerable adverse effects (see Chapters 15, 18, 19)
>
> Failure to use an appropriate secondary analgesic (see Chapters 21–23)
>
> Failure to use appropriate nondrug measures (see Chapters 24–26)
>
> Patient has morphine resistant pain (see Chapters 19, 21–26)

an opioid resistant pain. In this circumstance, the use of alternative measures should be considered (Box 16.C).

A poor response may also indicate that there is a higher than average psychological component to the pain. This will demand:

- more time
- more psychotherapeutic support
- possibly the prescription of an anxiolytic or an antidepressant.

DOSE INCREMENTS

At lower doses, increments are generally greater in percentage terms than when adjusting a higher dose:

$5 \text{ mg} \rightarrow 10 \text{ mg} = 100\%$ increase

$\left. \begin{array}{l} 10 \text{ mg} \rightarrow 15 \text{ mg} \\ 20 \text{ mg} \rightarrow 30 \text{ mg} \\ 40 \text{ mg} \rightarrow 60 \text{ mg} \end{array} \right\} = 50\%$ increase

$\left. \begin{array}{l} 30 \text{ mg} \rightarrow 40 \text{ mg} \\ 60 \text{ mg} \rightarrow 80 \text{ mg} \end{array} \right\} = 33\%$ increase

Occasionally, satisfactory pain relief may be achieved by increasing from, say, 60 mg to 70 mg. Such a small increment is not recommended, however, because experience indicates that it does not often have a significant impact. In general, the following are convenient steps:

$5 \rightarrow 10 \rightarrow 15 \rightarrow 20 \rightarrow 30 \rightarrow 40 \rightarrow 60 \rightarrow 90/100 \rightarrow 120/160 \rightarrow 200/240 \rightarrow 300/400$ mg.

A change from $20 \rightarrow 25$ mg or $40 \rightarrow 50$ mg is definitely *not* recommended. Each adjustment takes time and, if there is little benefit, time and confidence are lost.

NIGHT TIME

When a patient is receiving morphine q4h it is generally possible to manage without an 0200 h dose. If a patient does not normally wake in the night to micturate, a double dose may be given at bedtime (Fig. 16.4). A retrospective survey of the time of death of 365 patients who died either in a palliative care unit (213) or the associated general hospital (152) confirmed that, in patients who received a double dose of morphine at bedtime, there were no excess deaths during the night hours (Table 16.3).

If a regular dose is needed in the middle of the night, patients taking morphine solution at home should be advised to prepare it in advance. This can be done at bedtime and left in an easily accessible place by the bed. Then, when the patient wakes, it is not necessary to measure an exact amount of morphine solution, it simply has to be taken. Further, if the patient wakes again later, he does not have to wonder if he has had the 0200 h dose; if the medicine cup is empty — he has.

EXTRA DOSES OF MORPHINE

Patients should be instructed to take an extra dose of morphine solution

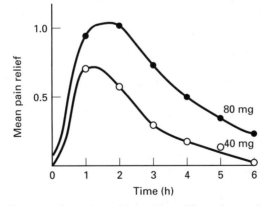

Fig. 16.4   Time-effect curves for oral morphine sulphate. Those shown relate to the approximate mean upper and lower doses investigated in 25 cancer patients who received a series of single doses in random order. After 40 mg, a mean pain relief score of 0.5 or more is achieved for 2 h; after 80 mg for 4 h. This explains why a double dose of morphine sulphate at night usually obviates the need for an 0200 h dose. The increased potential for drowsiness with the higher dose helps ensure a good night's rest. (Reproduced with permission from Houde et al 1965.)

Table 16.3 The influence of age, opioids, hypnotics and dyspnoea on the time of death

Group	n	Day (0600–2159 h)	Night (2200–0559 h)	Chi-squared and probability
Noncancer	152	122 (80)[a]	30 (20)[a]	11.53
Cancer	213	136 (64)	77 (36)	p = 0.0007
Cancer patients				
Male	83	51 (61)	32 (39)	0.34
Female	130	85 (65)	45 (35)	p = 0.56
Age 75+	53	32 (60)	21 (40)	0.13
Age < 75	160	101 (63)	59 (37)	p = 0.72
On opioids	194	123 (63)	71 (37)	0.01
Not on opioids	17	11 (65)	6 (35)	p = 0.92
Low opioid dose	92	59 (64)	33 (36)	0.01
High opioid dose	101	64 (63)	37 (37)	p = 0.91
Single 2200 h dose	87	51 (59)	36 (41)	1.19
Increased 2200 h dose	50	34 (68)	16 (32)	p = 0.28
Opioid and hypnotic	149	96 (64)	53 (36)	0.07
Opioid, no hypnotic	45	28 (62)	17 (38)	p = 0.78
Dyspnoea, on opioids	14	12 (86)	2 (14)	3.24
No dyspnoea, on opioids	180	111 (62)	69 (38)	p = 0.07

[a] Numbers in parenthesis = percentage of deaths.
From Regnard & Badger 1987

or ordinary tablets if they experience troublesome breakthrough pain. Because an immediate effect is necessary, m/r tablets are not ideal in this situation. The extra dose is normally the same as the q4h dose, or roughly one third of the q12h dose of m/r tablets.

If the pain occurs less than 1 h before a scheduled dose, taking the next dose early may suffice. If this results in a progressive movement towards a q3h regimen, however, it means that the regular dose is insufficient. Thus if breakthrough pain is experienced between most or all regular doses, it almost certainly means that the regular dose needs to be increased.

Most extra doses of morphine are required between 1000 h and 0200 h (Bruera et al 1992). Possible reasons for the diurnal variation include:

- increased daytime mobility
- fatigue
- lack of distraction
- decreased perception of pain at night
- circadian variation in the pharmacokinetics of opioids
- circadian variation in the sensitivity of opioid receptors.

EXCEPTIONS TO 'EVERY FOUR HOURS'

There are times when it is appropriate to prescribe ordinary morphine sulphate tablets or solutions other than q4h:

- *renal failure* — because of cumulation of morphine-6-glucuronide (M6G) (plasma halflife ⩽ 7.5 h), morphine may need to be given only q8h

- *initiation of treatment in the very elderly, particularly at home* — the potential for adverse effects is obviously greater in an elderly frail patient. It may be wise to start with a test bedtime dose and review the next morning. Depending on how the patient has fared, one can continue with the same regimen (using a weak opioid during the day) or carefully introduce two or three daytime doses linked to meal times for convenience
- *the very elderly* — the duration of action of morphine increases progressively with age (Kaiko 1980). Thus, in a frail patient of over 80 years of age, a q6h regimen may well be adequate
- *night pain only*
- *evening and night pain only* — a few patients fall into these categories and either bedtime only or 1800 h and bedtime is appropriate. Some patients have pain which is made worse by lying down, particularly if for an extended period of time. Indeed, occasionally a patient taking regular morphine needs a relatively higher 2200 h dose, i.e. *three times* the daytime q4h morphine dose or *one and a half times* the morning m/r morphine dose
- *occasional attacks of severe pain* — some patients may obtain relief from a weak opioid but fear a return of their previously intolerable pain. They are re-assured by having a small supply of morphine 'in reserve'. The quantity need be only 200 ml but, if going on holiday, 500 ml may be more re-assuring
- *fast metabolizers* — rarely, a patient repeatedly experiences a return of pain before the next dose despite several dose increments. Increasing the dose further seems merely to increase the adverse drug effects. The right course is for the patient to revert to the former, smaller dose and to take it more often, i.e. q3h or, if m/r, q8h.

A q3h regimen is, however, more inconvenient. It is important, therefore, to be sure that increasing the regular dose will not bridge the gap before adopting the lower dose and greater frequency option. In practice, the number who require morphine q3h is very small — much less than 1%.

ADVERSE EFFECTS

Most patients experience adverse effects with morphine (Box 16.D). The most common is constipation, followed by nausea and vomiting.

Constipation

Morphine affects gut motility and function in a number of ways (Box 16.E). Constipation is the norm. A laxative should be prescribed, therefore, when a patient is prescribed morphine, unless there is a definite reason for not doing so, e.g. steatorrhoea or an ileostomy (Twycross & Harcourt 1991). Although patients generally need more laxative when the dose of morphine is increased, higher doses of morphine are relatively less constipating than lower ones (Sykes 1991).

Experience at many centres indicates that a combination of a contact laxative (peristaltic stimulant) and a surface-wetting agent (faecal softener)

BOX 16.D
ADVERSE EFFECTS OF MORPHINE THERAPY

Initial
Nausea and vomiting
Drowsiness
Delirium:
- muddled thinking
- disorientation
Unsteadiness

Continuing
Constipation
Nausea and vomiting
Inactivity drowsiness
Dry mouth

Occasional
Urinary retention
Sweating
Myoclonus

---

achieves the best results, e.g. standardized senna (up to 75 mg a day) and docusate (up to 600 mg a day). Combination preparations reduce the number of tablets/capsules the patient has to swallow (e.g. co-danthrusate (UK) and casanthranol-docusate (USA)). The median number of co-danthrusate capsules prescribed at Sobell House for patients on morphine is four, i.e. danthron 300 mg (Box 16.F).

When first seen, some patients have been on an opioid analgesic for several weeks and may already be severely constipated or even impacted (Glare & Lickiss 1992). Abdominal examination alone may demonstrate that the colon is full of faeces as far back as the caecum. If this is so, inpatient treatment is probably going to be necessary to sort it out. More than one third of inpatients with terminal cancer continue to need rectal measures (suppositories, enemas or manual evacuations) in addition to oral laxatives (Twycross & Lack 1986).

As noted on page 299, oral naloxone has been used to treat morphine induced constipation (Sykes 1991, Culpepper-Morgan et al 1992). The routine use of naloxone in this way is not yet a practical proposition.

Nausea and vomiting

If the patient vomits after taking morphine, the morphine will not be absorbed, the patient remains in pain, and confidence in the new medicine is lost. To avoid this, some doctors use an anti-emetic routinely when morphine is prescribed. While this is probably good advice for the inexperienced prescriber, once a doctor and the team feel confident in the use of oral morphine, a more discriminatory approach is possible.

BOX 16.E
OPIOIDS AND THE GASTRO-INTESTINAL TRACT (Krueger 1937, Beubler 1983)

Actions
Increase sphincter tone:

- Oddi
- ileocaecal
- anal

Increase segmentation:

- pyloric antrum
- small intestine
- colon

Increase electrolyte and water absorption:

- small intestine
- large intestine

Impair defaecation reflex:

- rectum less sensitive to distension
- increased internal anal sphincter tone

Effects
Delay gastric emptying:

- epigastric fullness
- flatulence
- anorexia
- nausea
- vomiting

Infrequent defaecation
Hard faeces
} constipation

The following patients should be prescribed an anti-emetic prophylactically:

- those who are already troubled by nausea and vomiting
- those who are vomiting as a result of the use of codeine or other weak opioid
- those who have vomited with opioids in the past.

The following patients need *not* be prescribed an anti-emetic prophylactically:

- those with no current nausea and vomiting
- those taking a weak or alternative strong analgesic regularly without nausea or vomiting.

One third of all patients prescribed morphine never need an anti-emetic.

The choice of anti-emetic depends on whether or not morphine is the main or only cause of vomiting (Table 16.4). Haloperidol and fluphenazine are

---

BOX 16.F
GUIDELINES FOR MANAGEMENT OF OPIOID INDUCED CONSTIPATION

Ask about the patient's usual bowel habit and use of laxatives.

Do a rectal examination if you suspect faecal impaction or if there is diarrhoea and/or faecal incontinence (to exclude impaction with overflow).

Record bowel motions each day in a 'Bowel Book'.

Encourage fluids generally, fruit juice, fruit and bran.

Prescribe prophylactically co-danthrusate (UK) 1 capsule at bedtime or casanthranol 30 mg with docusate 100 mg (Peri-Colace USA) 1 capsule twice a day.

If already constipated, prescribe co-danthrusate 2 capsules at bedtime or casanthranol-docusate 2 capsules b.i.d.

Adjust every few days according to results, up to 3 capsules q.i.d.

If necessary, 'uncork' with the help of bisacodyl 10 mg suppository + glycerine suppository.

If suppositories are ineffective, administer a phosphate enema followed by a soap enema if no result.

If the maximum dose of co-danthrusate or casanthranol-docusate is ineffective, reduce by half and add an osmotic laxative ('small bowel flusher'), e.g. lactulose 20 ml b.i.d.

If co-danthrusate or casanthranol-docusate causes abdominal cramps, divide daily dose or change to a small bowel flusher, e.g. lactulose syrup 20–40 ml once daily to t.i.d.

Lactulose may be preferable in patients with a history of irritable bowel syndrome (spastic colon) or of cramps with other contact laxatives ('peristaltic stimulants'), e.g. senna.

Sometimes it is appropriate to optimize a patient's existing bowel regimen, rather than change automatically to co-danthrusate or cansanthranol-docusate.

Table 16.4   Choice of anti-emetic

Cause		Anti-emetic	Usual doses
Drugs Biochemical	}	Haloperidol Fluphenazine Prochlorperazine	1–3 mg nocte–b.i.d. 0.5–2 mg b.i.d. 5 mg t.i.d.
Bowel obstruction (functional, partial)		Metoclopramide Domperidone	10 mg q4h–q8h 10 mg q4h–q8h
Bowel obstruction (marked or complete) Raised intracranial pressure	}	Cyclizine Promethazine Meclozine (USA)	50 mg t.i.d.–q.i.d. 25–50 mg t.i.d.–q.i.d. 25 mg b.i.d.–t.i.d.

equally good choices for nausea and vomiting induced by morphine. They should be used in preference to prochlorperazine which is more likely to cause drowsiness. In the UK, apart from depot injections for use in psychotic patients, fluphenazine is available only as 1 mg and 2.5 mg tablets. This limits its usefulness as an anti-emetic. It is, however, a broad spectrum anti-emetic and will therefore sometimes be of more benefit than haloperidol which is limited in its impact to the chemoreceptor trigger zone (Peroutka & Snyder 1982).

Although stimulation of the chemoreceptor trigger zone in the brain stem is the most common cause of morphine induced vomiting, morphine can precipitate vomiting by other mechanisms:

- delayed gastric emptying
- secondary to constipation
- vestibular disturbance (rare).

Vomiting secondary to delayed gastric emptying is a problem in some 5–10% of patients prescribed oral morphine. It is reminiscent of pyloric stenosis. The use of a prokinetic agent (e.g. metoclopramide or domperidone 10 mg q4h) normally permits the continued use of morphine. In patients given morphine 10 mg IM as surgical premedication, metoclopramide 10 mg IM did not reverse the delayed gastric emptying, whereas 10 mg IV did (McNeill et al 1990). This suggests that there is a dose-response curve for metoclopramide. Clearly, if 10 mg PO is ineffectual, a higher dose should be considered. Cisapride is more effective than metoclopramide (Rowbotham et al 1988) but is more expensive. The normal dose is 10 mg t.i.d.

Vomiting with morphine is sometimes only an initial adverse effect. If an anti-emetic was prescribed prophylactically, and not to control pre-existing nausea and vomiting, it is good practice to stop it after the patient has been on a steady dose of morphine for 1 week. If necessary, the anti-emetic can be restarted.

'Opioid bowel syndrome'

Occasionally a patient will develop a functional obstruction (paralytic ileus) with morphine or other strong opioid (Bruera et al 1987). The concurrent use of an anticholinergic drug may be the precipitating factor. When this is the case, stopping the drug and prescribing oral metoclopramide may be enough to reverse the ileus. If the patient does not respond to an oral prokinetic drug and a stimulant laxative, however, morphine/diamorphine and metoclopramide 60 mg/24 h should be given by SC infusion. After a few days, when the obstructive picture has resolved, it is usually possible to revert to oral medication (Bruera et al 1987).

Drowsiness

Like nausea and vomiting, drowsiness may be troublesome during the first few days, as well as subsequently if an upward dose adjustment is made. Patients should be warned about initial drowsiness and encouraged to persevere in the knowledge that it will almost certainly lessen. Occasionally, in a very old frail patient, it is necessary to reduce the dose of morphine and then increase it again more slowly, every 2–3 days, until adequate relief is obtained.

Occasionally, a patient will go on feeling very drowsy and drugged

---

BOX 16.G
CHECKLIST FOR EXCESSIVE DROWSINESS IN PATIENTS RECEIVING ORAL MORPHINE

General Factors

Is the patient still recuperating from prolonged fatigue?
Is the patient more ill than I thought?

- renal failure
- hypercalaemia
- hyponatraemia
- hyperglycaemia
- hepatic failure
- cerebral metastases
- septicaemia
- cardiac failure
- hypotension

Drug Factors

Is the patient completely painfree?

- if yes, reduce the dose and review both drowsiness and pain relief.

Is the patient on a psychotropic drug, notably a long acting benzodiazepine (e.g. flurazepam, diazepam, nitrazepam) or a phenothiazine (e.g. chlorpromazine)? Is it necessary?

- if not, stop it
- if yes, can the dose be reduced?

If the patient is taking a phenothiazine anti-emetic, can it be changed to haloperidol or metoclopramide?

(Box 16.G). It is important to distinguish between persistent drowsiness and inactivity or boredom drowsiness. Most patients receiving morphine 'catnap' with ease. This means that they will fall asleep if sitting quietly and alone. As many of these patients have little stamina, they need more rest and sleep than when healthy. Provided that they are easily roused and can converse readily when joined by family or friends, continuing inactivity drowsiness should be seen as a bonus. Indeed, many patients find that it helps to pass what otherwise might be a long and exhausting day.

If stamina is not limited, the patient will be able to live an active life because any continuing drowsiness will be related to physical inactivity. Objective testing has shown that Continuous Reaction Time, a neuropsychological test, is significantly affected in patients receiving opioids compared with patients receiving only nonopioids (Banning et al 1992). The correlation between outcome of a Continuous Reaction Time test and ability to handle complex situations in everyday life, however, has not been established. In another study using a battery of tests (tapping speed, arithmetic, reverse digits, serial memory), patients who had had an increase in dose of morphine of at least 30% within the previous 3 days were found to have impairment of cognitive function (Bruera et al 1989). On the other hand, patients on a stable dose of morphine had no impairment of cognitive function, confirming that tolerance develops to these effects.

Patients with renal failure are particularly likely to become drowsy because of cumulation of M6G. This necessitates a reduction in dose of morphine. As already noted, moderate hepatic insufficiency does *not* affect the metabolism of morphine (Patwardhan et al 1981, Hasselstrom et al 1986) and morphine is well tolerated in patients up to the point of hepatic encephalopathy (Laidlaw et al 1961).

The use of cerebral stimulants is discussed in Chapter 21.

Delirium

Delirium (confusion) may occur, particularly in the elderly, who are more sensitive to the effects of morphine. It may be necessary, therefore, to titrate the dose of morphine more slowly in these patients. It is best to warn those over 70 years of age that they may become muddled at times during the first few days, but to persevere.

Delirium may also be precipitated by the concurrent use of psychotropic drugs. If symptoms of delirium persist, a reduction in psychotropic medication should be considered (Box 16.G).

Unsteadiness

This may occur as a result of orthostatic (postural) hypotension, particularly in the elderly. Patients over 70 years of age should be warned about the possibility. Sometimes because of this and for confusional symptoms, it is necessary to reduce the dose for 3–4 days before carefully increasing it again if the pain is still not fully relieved.

Dry mouth

In a prospective survey of patients admitted during a period of 8 weeks to a cancer hospital, patients were evaluated for dry mouth (Table 16.5). Patients

Table 16.5   Evaluation of dryness of mouth during previous 24 h in 199 cancer patients

Analgesic group	n	Dryness of mouth			
		Normal	Slightly dry	Moderately dry	Extremely dry
Concurrent treatment expected to cause dry mouth					
Morphine	35	10 (29)	3 (9)	9 (26)	13 (37)
Nonopioid, weak opioid, or no analgesic	37	18 (49)	6 (16)	7 (19)	6 (16)
No concurrent treatment or treatment not expected to cause dry mouth					
Morphine	32	8 (25)	5 (16)	14 (44)	5 (16)
Nonopioid, weak opioid, or no analgesic	95	61 (64)	11 (12)	21 (22)	2 (2)

Numbers in parenthesis = percentages.
From White et al 1989

who had nondrug reasons for dry mouth were excluded (e.g. radiotherapy or surgery to the head and neck). A highly significant association was found between the use of morphine and dryness of the mouth (White et al 1989). Even when the contribution of concurrent medication was taken into account, patients receiving morphine were nearly four times more likely to have a dry mouth of any severity compared with patients taking weak opioids, nonopioids or no analgesic.

Urinary symptoms

Morphine has an effect on the muscle of the urinary tract. Experimentally, in animals, urinary retention occurs with all species even with analgesic doses of morphine. In man, morphine contracts the vesical sphincter making it more difficult to pass urine. It also increases the tone of the detrusor muscle, which may give rise to urinary urgency. As the central depressant effect of morphine makes the patient less attentive to impulses from the bladder, the overall effect is a tendency to urinary retention (Weinstock 1971).

Respiratory depression

Respiratory depression is not generally of clinical importance (see p. 335). Morphine 10 mg IM raises the pCO_2 by about 5 mm Hg (Weinstock 1971). This is the same as the usual nocturnal elevation of pCO_2 which occurs in the general population. In patients with raised intracranial pressure, however, elevation of the pCO_2 results in a reflex increase in cerebral vasodilatation with a resultant increase in intracranial pressure which may exacerbate or precipitate headache.

Morphine should, therefore, be used with more care in patients with chronic obstructive airways disease (COAD), limited respiratory reserve and raised intracranial pressure. On the other hand, these conditions are not contra-indications to the use of oral morphine in the terminally ill. In patients distressed by tachypnoea at rest, the prescription of morphine 5–10 mg q4h may reduce the respiratory rate from 30–40/min down to 20–25/min. This makes the patient feel better and able to do more (see Chapter 20).

Myoclonus

Several reports speak of myoclonus (twitching) with morphine therapy. Some are dubious because of polypharmacy, including drugs with anticholinergic effects (Potter et al 1989). Other cases are unequivocal. In most instances the patient has been receiving a very high dose of morphine. Morphine-3-glucuronide (M3G) has been implicated (Sjogren et al 1993). If it is not possible to reduce the dose of morphine, an anticonvulsant benzodiazepine such as clonazepam should be given (Eisele et al 1992).

■ CASE HISTORY
An 87 year-old woman with a 6 year history of breast cancer and multiple bone

metastases had been treated with tamoxifen, medroxyprogesterone acetate and local radiotherapy. Bone pain was fully relieved by m/r ketoprofen 200 mg daily. M/r morphine 10 mg b.i.d., then 20 mg b.i.d., was prescribed for increasing chest wall and breast pain with good effect. She also took frusemide and lactulose.

Two weeks after starting oral morphine she began to develop episodic myoclonic jerking. Each spasm started abruptly and lasted several seconds. They became more frequent and prolonged. Neurological examination was unremarkable. Plasma urea, electrolytes and calcium concentrations were normal, as were an electro-encephalogram (EEG) and CT scan. Withdrawing m/r morphine lessened but did not stop the myoclonus. Increasing pain necessitated restarting morphine. The addition of clonazepam 1 mg nocte stopped the myoclonus (Shorvon 1984), which did not recur even though the dose of morphine rose to 180 mg/24 h (Boyd & Quigley 1992).

Pruritus

Pruritus (itching) is a rare complication of morphine therapy, associated with intradermal histamine release. A patient developed pruritus when receiving morphine, hydromorphone and methadone (Rogers 1991). Levorphanol caused nausea and vomiting, and pethidine caused marked irritability. With oxymorphone 0.5 mg IV q3h, however, there was good pain relief and no pruritus.

Histamine release is dose related and lower doses of morphine might not cause pruritus in a susceptible person. Morphine induced histamine release is not inhibited by naloxone (Hermens et al 1985). There are no reports of oxycodone, oxymorphone and fentanyl causing pruritus.

DRUG INTERACTIONS

Polypharmacy — the use of several drugs concurrently — is often necessary in patients with advanced cancer. Provided the physician is aware of the potential for interactions and the patient is reviewed after each drug innovation, it is unlikely that anything will go dangerously wrong.

Psychotropic drugs

The sedative and respiratory depressant effects of morphine tend to be potentiated and prolonged by psychotropic drugs (e.g. phenothiazine, benzodiazepines, antidepressants) and alcohol. It is generally wise, therefore, to prescribe relatively small doses of psychotropic drugs initially. Morphine will also potentiate the hypotensive effect of these drugs.

Beta-blockers

The cardiac effects of adrenergic beta-blockers (e.g. propranolol, atenolol) may be enhanced by morphine (Davis & Hatoum 1981).

Cimetidine

High parenteral doses of morphine produce significant cardiovascular effects that are attributable to histamine release. In a study of morphine anaesthesia in which 1 mg of morphine/kg body weight was administered to 40 patients scheduled for elective coronary artery bypass surgery, it was shown that significant haemodynamic protection can be obtained by the use of histamine antagonists. Diphenhydramine and cimetidine together are superior to either drug given alone (Philbin et al 1981). Although of interest, these observations are probably irrelevant in the care of the patient with advanced cancer.

More important are reports that cimetidine impairs the elimination of morphine, and causes greater toxicity. In rats the plasma halflife of morphine was increased from 2 h to nearly 4 h following pretreatment with cimetidine for 3 days (Mojaverian et al 1982a). In a comparable study in seven healthy male volunteers aged 28–30 years, however, cimetidine had no effect on the pharmacokinetics of morphine (Mojaverian et al 1982b). A report of an apparent morphine-cimetidine interaction in a patient on haemodialysis probably related to cumulation of M6G (Fine & Churchill 1981).

INSTRUCTIONS TO PATIENTS AND FAMILIES

Patients need to know they are receiving morphine. It should be presented as the next logical step in their pain management. It can be pointed out that, broadly speaking, there are only two basic analgesics, namely aspirin and morphine. Their previous medication can be explained in these terms, either as 'weak morphine'; (if a weak opioid agonist) or 'a synthetic or artificial morphine' (if an alternative strong opioid). Morphine is, however, a negative emotive word. As with other negative words (e.g. 'cancer' and 'dying') a qualifying adjective or phrase does much to soften an initial negative impact:

> 'What we need to do is to get you sorted out with the help of good old-fashioned morphine.' *or*

> 'The best medicine for you is liquid morphine.'

The patient will ask or wonder about addiction and tolerance and, at some stage, these concerns have to be addressed (see Chapter 17).

A medication chart for the patient to work from is necessary. Adequate follow up for patients at home is essential.

MORPHINE ON GENERAL WARDS

In wards with 4-hourly medicine rounds, the administration of morphine q4h should present few problems. Most wards, however, have only four drug rounds a day, at approximately 0700, 1300, 1700 and 2200 h. These are commonly styled 0600, 1200/1400, 1800 and 2200 h. Further, in some countries, the usual hospital method of charting drug administration does not clearly indicate at what time a regular drug is actually given. Special provision may need to be made to enable a patient to receive morphine q4h.

A further difficulty is that the interval between the first drug round (0700) and the last (2200) is less than 16 hours. In practice, it is not uncommon to see a series of entries such as:

0725, 1125, 1550, 2130
0725, 1125, 1525, 1925, 2350

In the first, it proved impossible to give the third dose on time and the fourth has been delayed partly for convenience and partly to 'help the patient have a better night'. In the second example, the day staff have coped in an exemplary fashion with a highly individual drug regimen — until bedtime:

'Here is your night sedative Mr. Smith. You cannot have your morphine yet, that is not due yet. We'll bring that later. . .'

The patient either fails to get to sleep because of unrelieved pain (or worry about the possibility) or complains bitterly when woken from a deep sleep by a nurse an hour or so later. In both instances, the comfort (and sleep) of the patient is put in jeopardy by a pharisaical attitude to the concept of 'q4h'.

The following should be borne in mind:

- it is important to make the q4h regimen as easy to adhere to as possible
- the day may well be less than 16 h both at home and in hospital
- it is necessary, therefore, to catch up at some stages in the day. Generally, catching up is best done at 1000 h. If 'time slippage' occurs by mistake or inevitably later in the day, catching up should be repeated at 2200 h. This may mean that the interval between the 0600 (on waking dose) and the 1000 h dose is less than 4 h, occasionally less than 3 h, and similarly between the 1800 h and bedtime doses. It is necessary, therefore, to advise nursing staff specifically on this point
- when catching up is practised, it is much easier for the nursing staff to administer q4h medication. In fact, the only administration additional to the routine drug rounds is likely to be 1000 h. This is a time when the maximum number of nurses are available, and when the book keeping associated with the use of a Controlled Drug is most easy to complete
- such a regimen, namely, on waking, 1000, 1400, 1800, bedtime ($\pm$ middle of night), reflects outpatient recommendations. This makes the transition from hospital to home easier as the patient already knows the benefit of the regimen he is recommended to continue
- it helps the nursing staff considerably if, on the medicine chart, the 'official' times of administration are included appropriately by the prescribing doctor (0200, 0600, 1000, 1400, 1800, 2200 h). This requires the use of two lines on charts which have only four boxes per drug for the nurse's signature (Fig. 16.5)
- it is necessary to check daily to ensure that doses have not been omitted through oversight or through the cumulative effect of time slippage
- most patients given a double dose at bedtime will sleep painfree beyond

MEDICINE SHEET

MONTH May 1982   DATE

DATE	DETAILS OF DRUG ADMINISTRATION	Time to be given	Signature of Prescribing Doctor	5 / 6	7 / 8		
5/5/82	MORPHINE (10 mg in 10 ml) P.O.	0200					
		0600					
	to take 10 ml 4 hourly	1000	*Morris*				
		1400					
		1800					
	● and 20 ml nocte	● 2200					
5/5/82	MORPHINE (10 mg in 10 ml) P.O.						
	to take 10 ml 2 hourly PRN		*Morris*				
5/5/82	HALOPERIDOL 1.5 mg tab. P.O.						
	nocte	2200	*Morris*				
5/5/82	DORBANEX SYRUP 10 ml P.O.						
	nocte	2200	*Morris*				

Fig. 16.5 A suggested way of writing up a q4h regimen on a medication chart which permits only four entries a day.

0200 h. The nursing staff should be advised to delay the middle of the night dose until about 0300 h if the patient is sleeping soundly. On the other hand, if the patient wakes regularly at 0100 h to micturate or because of pain, the 0200 h dose should be given earlier
- provision should be made for additional 'as needed' morphine, in the event of breakthrough pain. Instructions must be clear: the use of 'as needed' morphine does not mean that the next dose of regular morphine is omitted or delayed
- if 'as needed' morphine is taken several times a day, it is probably an indication that the regular dose should be increased.

MORPHINE AND DRIVING

Most patients requiring treatment with morphine are not fit to drive on account of their general poor state of health. From time to time, however, a patient asks, 'And can I drive, doctor?' This may be when morphine is first started. Alternatively, the patient may have improved since starting morphine so that he begins to think about taking up some of his former activities, including driving. The following points must be borne in mind:

- driving or being in charge of a vehicle when under the influence of a drug is an offence in all countries and states

- in the UK, conviction carries an automatic penalty of disqualification from driving for 6 months
- it is the driver's responsibility to know when he is unable to drive safely
- without guidance from his doctor he may not realize the danger until too late.

Broadly speaking, drivers can be classified as *vocational, professional,* and *occasional* (Raffee 1978). Vocational drivers are those who drive all or most of their working day in heavy goods vehicles (HGV). Professional drivers include taxi drivers and commercial travellers. In the absence of formal testing to show that attention and reaction time are unimpaired, vocational drivers must be advised not to drive HGV, and taxi drivers similarly. But what of the patient who drives 20–30 miles to work each day? Or of the retired person who just wants to go 1–2 miles to the shops?

Over the past 25 years, a significant number of my patients have driven while taking regular oral morphine. To date there have been no accidents. The advice they are given is summarized in Box 16.H.

There is a legal requirement on every driver, as soon as he becomes aware of it, to report to the Licensing Centre any disability likely to make him now or in the future a danger when driving. Applicants for driving licences are also required to report such disabilities. Temporary disabilities unlikely to exceed 3 months are excluded. The obligation to notify the Licensing Authority falls on the patient, but he can only do this if his doctor advises him that he has a disability that is likely to affect his driving.

If the Licensing Centre becomes aware that a person holding a licence or applying for a licence has a disability it may require him to authorize his doctor to supply information about his disability to the Medical Adviser at the Centre. If he refuses he may be required to undergo medical examination by a nominated doctor or doctors. In some districts of the USA, there are

---

BOX 16.H
ADVICE TO PATIENTS TAKING MORPHINE ABOUT DRIVING

The medicines you are taking do *not* necessarily disqualify you from driving. The speed of your reactions and general alertness may, however, be affected.

You should take the following precautions, particularly if you have not driven for some weeks because of your illness:

- do not drive in the dark or when conditions are bad
- do not drink alcohol, however little, during the day
- check your fitness to drive in the following way:
  - choose a quiet time of the day, when the light is good
  - choose an area where there are a number of quiet roads
  - take a companion (spouse, partner, friend)
  - drive for 10–15 minutes on quiet roads
  - if both you and your companion are happy with your alertness, concentration, reactions and general ability, then it is all right to drive for short distances
- do not exhaust yourself by long journeys.

driving evaluation centres. A test at one of these will provide an objective evaluation of a person's capability to drive.

In the UK, any doctor in doubt about the advice he should give his patient can discuss the matter with the Medical Advisory Branch at the Driver and Vehicle Licensing Centre at Swansea (0792 42731). This is an answering service and the doctor leaves his name and telephone number. After these details have been checked, the doctor is telephoned back. There may be occasions when the doctor considers it necessary to take the initiative and notify the Licensing Centre of a patient's disability and its effect on his driving. Each case is a matter for the individual doctor's discretion.

CONCLUSION

Morphine by mouth is a versatile, reliable and safe drug. It is the strong analgesic of choice for cancer patients with severe pain. It is not, however, the panacea. Many factors will influence morphine requirements. In most patients, it is necessary to use a co-analgesic and other forms of adjuvant medication, and also nondrug measures.

REFERENCES

Arkinstall W W, Goughnour B R, White J A, Stewart J H 1989 Control of severe pain with sustained-release morphine tablets v. oral morphine solution. Canadian Medical Association Journal 140: 653–661
Banning A, Sjogren P, Kaiser F 1992 Reaction time in cancer patients receiving peripherally acting analgesics alone or in combination with opioids. Acta Anaesthesiologica Scandinavica 36: 480–482
Beubler E 1983 Opiates and intestinal transport in vivo studies. In: Turnberg L A (ed) Intestinal secretion. Smith, Kline and French Laboratories, Herefordshire, pp 53–55
Bloomfield S S, Cissell G B, Mitchell J et al 1993 Analgesic efficacy and potency of two oral controlled-release morphine preparations. Clinical Pharmacology and Therapeutics 53: 469–478
Boureau F, Saudubray F, d'Arnoux C et al 1992 A comparative study of controlled-release morphine (CRM) suspension and CRM tablets in chronic cancer pain. Journal of Pain and Symptom Management 7: 393–399
Boyd K, Quigley C 1992 Morphine-induced myoclonus. Palliative Medicine 6: 167
Bruera E, Brenneis C, Michaud M, MacDonald N 1987 Continuous SC infusion of metoclopramide for treatment of narcotic bowel syndrome. Cancer Treatment Reports 71: 1121–1122
Bruera E, Macmillan K, Hanson J, MacDonald R N 1989 The cognitive effects of the administration of narcotic analgesics in patients with cancer pain. Pain 39: 13–16
Bruera E, Macmillan K, Kuehn N, Miller M J 1992 Circadian distribution of extra doses of narcotic analgesics in patients with cancer pain: a preliminary report. Pain 49: 311–314
Culpepper-Morgan J A, Inturrisi C E, Portenoy R K et al 1992 The treatment of opioid-induced constipation with oral naloxone: a pilot study. Clinical Pharmacology and Therapeutics 52: 90–95
Davis W M, Hatoum N S 1981 Possible toxic interaction of propranolol and narcotic analgesics. Drug Intelligence and Clinical Pharmacy 15: 290–291
Deschamps M, Band P R, Hislop T G, Rusthoven J, Iscoe N, Warr D 1992 The evaluation of analgesic effects in cancer patients as exemplified by a double-blind, crossover study of immediate-release versus controlled-release morphine. Journal of Pain and Symptom Management 7: 384–392
Eisele J H, Grigsby E J, Dea G 1992 Clonazepam treatment of myoclonic contractions associated with high-dose opioids: case report. Pain 49: 231–232

Fine A, Churchill D N 1981 Potentially lethal interaction of cimetidine and morphine. Canadian Medical Association Journal 124: 1434–1436

Foley K M 1985 The treatment of cancer pain. New England Journal of Medicine 313: 84–95

Glare P, Lickiss J N 1992 Unrecognized constipation in patients with advanced cancer: a recipe for therapeutic disaster. Journal of Pain and Symptom Management 7: 369–371

Goughnour B R, Arkinstall W W 1991 Potential cost-avoidance with oral extended-release morphine sulfate tablets versus morphine sulfate solution. American Journal of Hospital Pharmacy 48: 101–104

Gourlay G K, Plummer J I, Cherry D A, Onley M M, Fugere F 1993 A comparison of Kapanol (a new sustained-release morphine formulation), MST Continus and morphine solution in cancer patients: pharmacokinetic aspects. Presented at the VIIth World Congress on Pain.

Hanks G W 1989 Controlled release morphine (MST Contin) in advanced cancer: the European experience. Cancer 63: 2378–2382

Hanks G W, Twycross R G, Bliss J M 1987 Controlled release morphine tablets: a double-blind trial in patients with advanced cancer. Anaesthesia 42: 840–844

Hasselstrom J, Eriksson L S, Persson A, Rane A, Svensson J, Sawe J 1986 Morphine metabolism in patients with liver cirrhosis, Acta Pharmacologica et Toxicologica (suppl V): abstract 101

Hermens J M, Ebertz J M, Hanifin J M, Hirshman C A 1985 Comparison of histamine release in human skin mast cells induced by morphine, fentanyl, and oxymorphone. Anesthesiology 62: 124–129

Hoskin P J, Poulain P, Hanks G W 1989 Controlled-release morphine in cancer pain: is a loading dose required when the formulation is changed? Anaesthesia 44: 897–901

Houde R W, Wallenstein S L, Beaver W T 1965 Clinical measurement of pain. In: de Stevens G (ed) Analgetics. Academic Press, New York, pp 75–122

Inturrisi C E, Verebely K 1972 The levels of methadone in the plasma in methadone maintenance. Clinical Pharmacology and Therapeutics 13: 633–637

Kaiko R F 1980 Age and morphine analgesia in cancer patients with postoperative pain. Clinical Pharmacology and Therapeutics. 28: 823–826

Kalso E, Vainio A 1990 Morphine and oxycodone in the management of cancer pain. Clinical Pharmacology and Therapeutics 47: 639–646

Krueger H 1937 The action of morphine on the digestive tract. Physiological Review 17: 618–645

Laidlaw J, Read A E, Sherlock S 1961 Morphine tolerance in hepatic cirrhosis. Gastroenterology 40: 389–396

McGivney W T, Crooks G M 1984 The care of patients with severe chronic pain in terminal illness. Journal of the American Medical Association 251: 1182–1188

McNeill M J, Ho E T, Kenny G N C 1990 Effect of IV metoclopramide on gastric emptying after opioid premedication. British Journal of Anaesthesia 64: 450–452

Mojaverian P, Swanson B N, Vlasses P, Ferguson R K 1982a Cimetidine impairs elimination of morphine in rats. Federation Proceedings 41: 1337

Mojaverian P, Fedder I L, Vlasses P H, et al 1982b Cimetidine does not alter morphine disposition in man. British Journal of Clinical Pharmacology 14: 809–813

Patwardhan R V, Johnson R F, Hoyumpa A et al 1981 Normal metabolism of morphine in cirrhosis. Gastroenterology 81: 1006–1011

Peroutka S J, Snyder S H 1982 Antiemetics: neurotransmitter receptor binding predicts therapeutic actions. Lancet i: 658–659

Philbin D M, Moss J, Atkins C W et al 1981 The use of H1 and H2 histamine antagonists with morphine anaesthesia: a double study. Anesthesiology 55: 292–296

Potter J M, Reid D B, Shaw R J et al 1989 Myoclonus associated with treatment with high doses of morphine: the role of supplemental drugs. British Medical Journal 299: 150–153

Raffee A (ed) 1978 Medical Aspects of Fitness to Drive. Medical Commission on Accident Prevention, London

Regnard C, Badger C 1987 Opioids, sleep and the time of death. Palliative Medicine 1: 107–110

Rogers A G 1991 Considering histamine release in prescribing opioid analgesics. Journal of Pain and Symptom Management 6: 44–45

Rowbotham D J, Bamber P A, Nimmo W S 1988 Comparison of the effect of cisapride and metoclopramide on morphine-induced delay in gastric emptying. British Journal of Clinical Pharmacology 26: 741–746

Shorvon S D 1984 Neurology seminar: epilepsy update. Hospital Update 10: 541–546

Sjogren P, Jonsson T, Jensen N-H, Drenck N-E, Jensen T S 1993 Hyperalgesia and myoclonus in terminal cancer patients treated with continuous intravenous morphine. Pain 55: 93–97

Sykes N P 1991 Oral naloxone in opioid-associated constipation. Lancet 337: 1475
Twycross R G, Lack S A 1986 Control of alimentary symptoms in far-advanced cancer. Churchill Livingstone, Edinburgh, pp 368
Twycross R G, Harcourt J M V 1991 Use of laxatives at a palliative care centre. Palliative Medicine 5: 27–33
Walsh T D, MacDonald N, Bruera E, Shepard K V, Michaud M, Zanes R 1992 A controlled study of sustained-release morphine sulfate tablets in chronic pain from advanced cancer. American Journal of Clinical Oncology (CCT) 15: 268–272
Weinstock M 1971 Site of action of opioid analgesic drugs in peripheral tissues. In: Clouet D (ed) Narcotic drugs. Biochemical pharmacology. Plenum Press, New York, pp 394–407
West R J, Maccarrone C 1993 Single dose pharmacokinetics of a new oral sustained-release morphine formulation, Kapanol capsules. Presented at the VIIth World Congress on Pain.
White I D, Hoskin P J, Hanks G W, Bliss J M 1989 Morphine and dryness of the mouth. British Medical Journal 298: 1222–1223
Zenz M, Piepenbrock S, Tryba M, Glocke M, Everlien M, Klauke W 1985 Kontrollierte studie mit buprenorphine. Deutsche Medizinische Woschensechrict 110: 448–453

Misunder-standings about morphine

MORPHINE CONSUMPTION

In 1980, the world-wide medicinal use of morphine was 2300 kg. A decade later this had risen to over 7200 kg. As already noted, the use of morphine still varies greatly between countries. Thus, in 1990, about 80% of all medicinal morphine was used in only 10 countries (Fig. 17.1). The remainder was used in 133 other countries containing most of the world's population. These countries generally registered little change in morphine consumption throughout the decade. In addition, over 60 countries reported no morphine consumption at all.

It is encouraging to note, however, that the largest percentage increases occurred in countries with historically low per capita consumption. Thus, from 1984 to 1990 the use of morphine increased dramatically in (Joranson 1992; figures rounded):

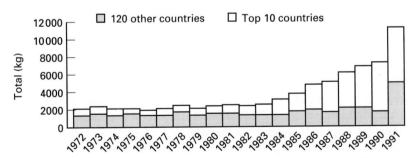

Fig. 17.1 World consumption of morphine 1972–1990. Figure prepared by the University of Wisconsin Pain Research Group, 1992. Top 10 countries: Australia, Canada, Denmark, Iceland, Ireland, New Zealand, Norway, Sweden, UK, USA. (Reproduced with permission from Joranson 1992.)

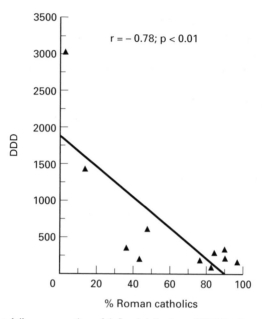

Fig. 17.2   Average daily consumption of defined daily doses (DDD) of morphine per million inhabitants 1986–90 related to percentage of Roman Catholic people in 11 European countries. (Reproduced with permission from Banos & Bosch 1993.)

Germany (900%)
France (700%)
Israel (700%)
Finland (700%)
Norway (600%)
Spain (500%)
Austria (400%)
Japan (300%).

In addition, morphine is now available for the first time in Mexico, Vietnam and India.

In Europe, an association has been noted between low morphine consumption and Roman Catholicism (Fig. 17.2). Inordinate concern about impaired cognition and hastening death, together with a tendency to glorify suffering, may be responsible for this.

MISUNDERSTANDINGS CAUSE MISMANAGEMENT

There is a widespread tendency to overstate the potential for harm with morphine and related drugs. This stems from several deeply held false beliefs. As noted in Chapter 1, collectively these cause 'opiophobia' in drug regulatory authorities. In the general public, opiophobia is associated with a pathological fear of death which often leads to an unethical conspiracy of silence between the health care professionals and the patient's family:

'[In Italy] a large proportion of patients do not receive precise information about the nature of their illness. Relatives often ask the physician not to tell the patient about the severity of the disease, especially in cancer cases . . . False clinical documents are even compiled on occasions to conceal the fact that the patient has cancer. In some cases it is a source of relief after the patient dies for the relatives to be able to say "He/she died without knowing it was cancer". In this sort of atmosphere it is obviously difficult to prescribe morphine, which is associated in the minds of relatives and patients with the end of all hope' (Garattini 1993).

MISUNDERSTANDINGS QUANTIFIED

A survey of nearly 250 doctors in part of Minnesota showed that misunderstandings are still common in a country with a relatively liberal attitude towards medicinal opioids (Table 17.1). Comparable attitudes have been noted in medical students (Weissman & Dahl 1990). If representative of the USA, the results are disturbing. They emphasize once more the need for better education at all levels of the medical profession.

'MORPHINE IS DANGEROUS BECAUSE IT DEPRESSES RESPIRATION'

The respiratory depressant effect of opioids has been demonstrated in volunteer studies (Rigg 1978). Respiratory depression is also a risk postoperatively; patients generally receive a standard dose of morphine which, for some, will be excessive. Postoperative and cancer patients, however, are not comparable. Unlike postoperative patients, cancer patients with pain:

- have usually been receiving a weak opioid for sometime (i.e. are not opioid naive)
- take medication by mouth (slower absorption, lower peak concentration)
- titrate the dose upwards step by step (less likelihood of an excessive dose being given).

Table 17.1   Misunderstandings about morphine in a group of 150 doctors

Item	% Misunderstanding
Tolerance and pain relief	51
Tolerance and adverse effects	39
Adjuvant drugs	29
Parenteral drugs for severe pain	27
Addiction	20
Inevitable pain	19
Morphine ceiling dose	17
Physical dependence	16
'As needed' administration	11
Morphine efficacy	10
Respiratory depression	7
Poor prognosis	4

From Elliott & Elliott 1992

Postoperative respiratory depression is caused by both pulmonary (atelectasis) and drug related factors (Brismar et al 1985, Heneghan & Jones 1985, Jones & Jordan 1987). Opioid doses larger than those needed for pain relief will increase any depression. In cancer patients, however, when the dose of morphine is titrated against the patient's pain, clinically important respiratory depression does not occur. This is because *pain itself is a physiological antagonist to the central depressant effects of morphine.*

A review of the time of death of cancer patients showed that a double dose of morphine at bedtime caused no excess mortality during the night (Regnard & Badger 1987). There is, therefore, a broad margin of safety.

Further, in 20 cancer patients of median age 59 years who were taking more than morphine 100 mg/24 h PO, the respiratory rates were all ≥ 12/min at rest (Walsh 1984). Twelve of the patients had a history of chronic bronchitis and 8 had cancer of the bronchus. All p_aCO_2 values except one were within the normal range (i.e. <45 mm Hg); 12 were hypoxic but only one severely so ($pO_2 = 48$ mm Hg). If p_aCO_2 is used as the index of ventilatory failure, this seems to be neither common nor severe in cancer patients treated with oral morphine. Given the frequency of respiratory tract disease in this group of patients, some degree of hypoxia might be expected.

Respiratory depression does occur, however, if the underlying pain is suddenly removed and the dose of morphine is not reduced. A 76 year-old man with a pleural mesothelioma needed oral morphine 90 mg q4h to relieve severe chest pain (Hanks et al 1981). Several hours after a successful nerve block with intrathecal chlorocresol, the patient became drowsy, confused and cyanosed with a respiratory rate of 3–4/min. He required naloxone on two occasions to correct this. There is need for caution, therefore, if the level of pain is suddenly altered as a result of nondrug measures particularly in those with limited respiratory reserve.

If a patient's pain is treated successfully by neurolytic or neurosurgical technique, the dose of morphine should be immediately reduced to 25% of the previously used analgesic dose. If the nerve block is totally successful, it will be possible to phase out the rest of the morphine over the next 1 or 2 weeks. If only partly successful, however, it may be necessary to increase the dose again to 50–60% of the original dose, or even more.

Respiratory depression may occur with spinal opioids. This is more likely in opioid naive patients (Writer et al 1985). In advanced cancer, because patients have invariably already been receiving opioids PO/SC regularly, serious respiratory depression is very rare. Morphine, therefore, is a safe drug for cancer pain management.

'MORPHINE ONLY ALTERS A PATIENT'S RESPONSE TO HIS PAIN'

It has been stated that opioids do not relieve a patient's pain but simply change the psychological reaction to it. In other words, the patient is still aware of the pain but its quality is less distressing. Sometimes this may be so, but in opioid responsive pain the goal of treatment is total relief from pain. This is possible if the analgesic is given prophylactically in a dose adjusted to individual need.

The danger of believing that morphine only alters a patient's response to pain is that the doctor may well not titrate the dose properly, and the patient will be left unnecessarily with residual pain. With pains that are morphine resistant, however, the patient continues to complain of pain and continues to be distressed by it.

'MORPHINE INDUCES EUPHORIA'

It is often stated that the use of morphine induces a state of euphoria. This is not so. Euphoria is rarely seen in cancer patients receiving morphine. Patients with unrelieved pain are understandably dysphoric. Relief of pain with morphine or other opioid results in a return to a more normal mood; this is not euphoria.

The belief that opioids commonly cause euphoria derives partly from the writings and experiences of literary figures, such as de Quincy and Coleridge, and to the unqualified transfer of the results of studies on drug addicts to nonaddicts. Evidence from volunteer studies and clinical experience both indicate that this belief is unfounded (Smith & Beecher 1962). In advanced cancer, morphine and other opioids do not cause euphoria.

Indeed, data collected in the 1970s indicated that the longer a patient received oral diamorphine the greater the likelihood of depression (Twycross & Wald 1976). A similar association between morphine and depression, however, has not been noted at Sobell House. This suggests that the cause of the depression was probably related to the then routine concomitant prescription of a phenothiazine or to other factors.

'MORPHINE IS ADDICTIVE'

Until 30 years ago, the word 'addiction' was used to describe the nonmedical use of socially unacceptable drugs (cannabis, cocaine, heroin) and 'habituation' was used for socially acceptable ones (alcohol, caffeine, nicotine). When this distinction was recognized to be scientifically dubious, the word 'dependence' was adopted to encompass both habituation and addiction. The WHO has defined addiction as:

> 'A state, psychic and sometimes also physical, resulting from the interactions between a living organism and a drug, characterized by behavioural and other responses that always include a compulsion to take the drug on a continuous or periodic basis in order to experience its psychic effects, and sometimes to avoid the discomfort of its absence. Tolerance may or may not be present' (WHO 1969).

This definition approximates closely to the popular conception of addiction as a compulsion or overpowering drive to take the drug in order to experience psychological effects.

The fear of causing psychological dependence is still a major cause for not prescribing strong opioids in cancer patients with pain (Hill 1987).

Published data indicate, however, that this fear is unfounded. For example, among nearly 12 000 hospital patients who received strong opioids, there were only four reasonably well documented cases of addiction in patients who had no history of drug abuse (Porter & Jick 1980). The dependence was considered major in only one instance, which suggests that the medical use of strong opioids rarely leads to addiction.

Studies of chronically ill patients have shown that abuse of nonopioid analgesics or combinations of weak opioids and nonopioids is more common than abuse of strong opioids (Maruta et al 1979, Tennant & Rawson 1982, Tennant & Uelman 1983). In patients with pain of nonmalignant origin, studies indicate that long term opioid use is not associated with psychological dependence (Taub 1982, Portenoy & Foley 1986). This suggests that drug use alone is not the major determinant in the development of psychological dependence. Support for this view comes from studies of USA military personnel addicted to strong opioids in Vietnam (Robins et al 1974). In this group, drug abuse was strongly dependent on factors such as:

- personality
- social environment
- availability of money.

From time to time, a patient may be encountered who is thought to be addicted because he is demanding an injection every two or three hours. Typically such a patient has a long history of poor pain relief and for several weeks has been receiving repeated ('q4h as needed') but inadequate opioid injections. With regular oral medication and when the pain has been relieved, however, the clock watching and demanding behaviour stops. This situation has been called 'pseudo-addiction' (Weissman & Haddox 1989). It is not true psychological dependence because the patient is not demanding an opioid in order to experience its psychological effects but to obtain relief from pain for one or two hours.

PAIN MANAGEMENT IN AN ADDICT OR EX-ADDICT

More difficult to deal with is the rare patient, usually young, who was a 'street addict' before becoming ill. Usually one of two errors will be made. On the one hand his pain is discounted by the professional staff and requests for strong opioids resisted ('After all he is an addict'). On the other hand the patient is treated as a nonaddict patient and allowed to escalate his opioid intake far beyond reasonable estimates of what is likely to be necessary to relieve the pain. This is one situation in which the patient's statements about what hurts must be carefully balanced by the judgement of an experienced and compassionate doctor (Box 17.A).

Addicts are able to extract about two thirds of the morphine content from m/r tablets (Bloor & Smalldridge 1990). The following case history is from a substance abuse unit in the UK:

■ CASE HISTORY
A 26 year-old woman had a long history of IV diamorphine abuse. She had

> **BOX 17.A**
> **GUIDELINES FOR USING MORPHINE IN PAST OR PRESENT 'STREET ADDICTS'**
>
> Most palliative care staff are unaccustomed to dealing with opioid dependent patients. Outside advice can be very helpful in achieving a successful synthesis between standard palliative care methods and those of drug dependency units.
>
> The patient should be under the care of an experienced doctor who can make a reasonable estimate of the patient's opioid requirements given the extent of the disease.
>
> The patient should be under the care of an experienced palliative care nurse who can identify nonverbal signs of pain and who can advise less experienced members of the nursing team.
>
> Opioids should be prescribed by one doctor only.
>
> Change the patient from parenteral to oral or rectal opioids as soon as confidence has been established. This immediately breaks the association with the street ritual of injecting drugs, and establishes a new link between drugs and pain relief.
>
> The doctor should make an explicit 'contract' about what he is prepared to do and what not:
>
> > 'I am prepared to increase your oral morphine at bedtime because this will stop you waking in pain in the night'.
>
> > 'I will give you an extra supply of oral morphine when you go home for the day on Saturday because the extra activity may exacerbate your pain'.
>
> > 'I will not give you morphine injections to take home because they are not necessary for pain relief, and because of the difficulties you have had in the past'.
>
> A clear statement must be in the nursing plan about what to do if the patient requests morphine for breakthrough pain.

been free of drugs for 1 year when inoperable cancer of the cervix was diagnosed. She was prescribed m/r morphine tablets 60 mg t.i.d. for abdominal pain. Although the tumour responded to radiotherapy, her use of m/r morphine sulphate tablets increased to 240 mg a day. She started extracting morphine from the tablets and injected it IV up to 12 times a day (Bloor & Smalldridge 1990).

'TOLERANCE TO MORPHINE DEVELOPS RAPIDLY'

In the past, predictions about dose escalation were made on the basis of animal and volunteer studies. The subjects were not in pain and the emphasis was on inducing tolerance and physical dependence as rapidly as possible by using maximum tolerated doses rather than by administering the drugs in doses and at intervals comparable to a clinical regimen. Although such studies may be useful in predicting abuse liability, they are irrelevant to clinical practice.

To allow predictions to be made on the basis of clinical experience, the notes of 500 patients admitted consecutively to St. Christopher's Hospice were reviewed (Twycross 1974). A total of 205 patients received diamorphine regularly for at least 1 week. By grouping the patients according to survival

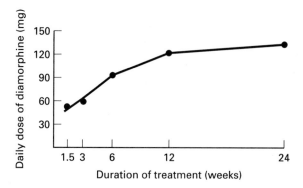

Fig. 17.3   205 patients admitted consecutively with advanced cancer were grouped according to survival following the start of treatment with diamorphine; group median final daily dose of diamorphine is shown plotted against group median duration of treatment. (Reproduced with permission from Twycross 1974.)

after commencing diamorphine, it was shown that the longer the duration of treatment the slower the rate of rise in dose (Fig. 17.3).

In a second review, 115 patients who had received diamorphine regularly for at least 12 weeks were selected from approximately 3000 patients admitted over 7 years (Twycross & Wald 1976). Visual analysis of graphs of diamorphine use over time indicated that there was an initial phase when the dose was increased several times within 1 or 2 weeks, followed by a prolonged phase when the dose was increased less often or not at all (Fig. 17.4). It was also clearly shown that the longer a patient survived after prescription of diamorphine, the greater the likelihood of a reduction in dose.

Dose reductions were made on a trial and error basis in patients who had improved generally over a number of weeks and who had had no recent episodes of breakthrough pain. Reductions were also made after successful intrathecal nerve blocks in five patients and after chemotherapy or irradiation in several others. Nine of the 115 patients stopped receiving diamorphine. Three never required any more. The other six did, however, when severe pain recurred — two after about 3 weeks and four after more than 4 months.

In summary, the data showed that the longer the duration of treatment with diamorphine:

- the slower the rate of rise in dose
- the longer the periods without a dose increase
- the greater the likelihood of a dose reduction
- the greater the likelihood of stopping medication altogether.

The pattern when prescribing morphine is identical.

A more recent study of nearly 1000 patients with advanced cancer who received regular opioids produced similar results. Only 5% of patients required an average daily increase of more than 10% of the previous dose; 81% were said to have a stable dose pattern; and 14% discontinued opioids (Brescia et al 1992).

Thus, when used within the context of continuing comprehensive bio-

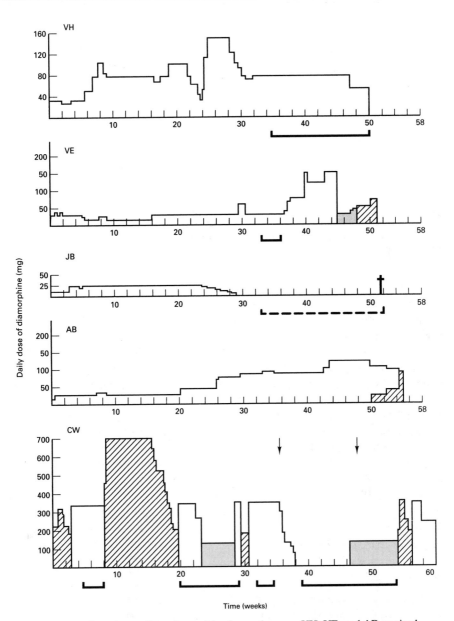

Fig. 17.4   Dose-time charts of 5 patients with advanced cancer. VH, VE, and AB received diamorphine up to the time of death; CW was still alive at the time of the report. (Reproduced with permission from Twycross & Wald 1976.)

psychosocial care, morphine and other strong opioids can be used for long periods in cancer patients without concern about tolerance. Further, although physical dependence may develop after several weeks of continuous treatment, this does not prevent a downward adjustment of dose should the pain be relieved by nondrug measures (e.g. radiotherapy or neurolytic block).

With the exception of constipation and miosis, tolerance to the adverse effects of morphine develops more readily than tolerance to analgesia (Bruera et al 1989, Ling et al 1989). Should tolerance develop, an upward adjustment of dose is all that is necessary to regain pain relief. The main reason for increasing the dose is not tolerance, however, but progression of the disease (Twycross 1974, Kanner & Foley 1981, Brescia et al 1992, Collin et al 1993).

Tolerance does occur in other contexts. Street addicts develop tolerance, and may need increasing doses to obtain the same effect. They use opioids in the absence of pain. Acute tolerance in the absence of pain has also been shown in animals (Colpaert et al 1980).

Various drugs administered concurrently with morphine have been observed to attenuate the development of *induced* tolerance in animals, e.g. cocaine (Misra et al 1989). The relevance of such studies to clinical practice is uncertain. Several studies in man about attenuation or reversal of tolerance to opioids need careful evaluation because the word tolerance is not always used consistently and often no control data are available (Hosobuchi et al 1980).

'IF A CANCER PATIENT IS GIVEN MORPHINE, HE IS GOING TO DIE SOON'

Many patients prescribed morphine are near to death and remain near to death. These will die soon. On the other hand, data on file indicate that one third of patients survive more than 4 weeks and 10% for more than 3 months (Fig. 17.5). These figures are underestimates because the duration of treatment was measured only from the first inpatient admission to Sobell House. Many had been taking morphine for several weeks before this.

Whether the patient dies in a short time depends on when morphine is

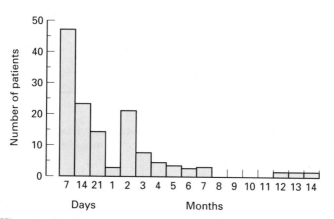

Fig. 17.5 Histogram showing survival after commencing treatment with morphine sulphate in 129 patients admitted to Sobell House in 1978. As some patients received morphine for several weeks before referral to Sobell House, the data understates the survival in these patients. Median duration of treatment = 13 days; 33% of patients survived for more than 4 weeks; 12% for more than 3 months.

started. Circumstantial evidence suggests, however, that the correct use of morphine *prolongs* the life of a cancer patient because of:

- freedom from pain
- improved rest and sleep
- increased appetite and strength
- increased physical activity.

On the other hand, giving morphine to a patient totally exhausted by pain and insomnia, particularly if elderly, may lead to pneumonia consequent upon a combination of somnolence and cough suppression. If used earlier, however, when the need first arises, the risk is negligible.

It has recently been suggested that this 'misunderstanding' may reflect reality in the Netherlands:

> 'Dutch doctors frequently use morphine in doses higher than necessary for effective pain treatment. 82% of Dutch doctors agree with this practice and 16.3% of all deaths (more than 20 000 people annually) in the Netherlands are probably due to increased opioid dosage with the intention of hastening death (Van der Mass 1991). Because morphine is so often used for this purpose many patients and doctors refrain from prescribing it or are initiating therapy very late. One study revealed that 30% of patients actually decreased the dose or discontinued opioid drugs immediately after discharge (Dorrepaal 1989)' (Zylicz 1993).

'IF A PATIENT HAS MORPHINE AT HOME, IT WILL GET STOLEN'

The diversion of medicinal opioids for illicit use by other people is a concern of Governments and law enforcement agencies. The experience in Sweden should do much to allay this fear. There, the medicinal use of morphine and methadone increased 17 times between 1975 and 1982 because of an increasing use of oral strong opioids to relieve cancer pain (Agenas et al 1982). There was, however, no associated increase in illicit drug use or diversion of strong opioids to established addicts. The same experience has been noted in Wisconsin, USA. (Joranson D 1991 Personal Communication).

In one country, however, a few doctors have been conned into prescribing m/r morphine tablets to 'patients' claiming to have chronic pain for which they need strong opioids. This is clearly a problem but is distinct from the theft of morphine from cancer patients.

It is extremely rare for a patient's supply of morphine to be misappropriated by another person. A patient who was short of money sold his 'Brompton Mixture' to a group of addicts who found it cheaper and longer lasting in its effects than street heroin (Fischbeck et al 1980). In another case, a family member misappropriated a patient's medication for personal use.

'PATIENTS WILL USE MORPHINE TO COMMIT SUICIDE'

I know of no cases of self-poisoning by a cancer patient in which the agent used was morphine. Further, the incidence of suicide in cancer patients is only about twice that of the general population (Breitbart 1992).

'A KIND OF LIVING DEATH'

As already noted, many doctors and nurses have a very negative attitude towards morphine. The use of the word 'estupefaciente' to describe opioids in Southern European countries re-inforces such attitudes (Alloza 1993). One doctor wrote:

> 'What about the inoperable cancer patient who may not die for months or a year, and yet who is suffering agonies from chronic pain? . . . Is a doctor then justified in prescribing such drugs when he knows full well he will be sentencing his patient to a kind of living death?' (Bunyard 1971).

Although they might not express it so succinctly, globally many doctors share the view of the doctor who said:

> 'I try to postpone giving morphia until the very end and am best pleased if the first dose of morphia is also the last' (Anonymous 1972).

These views stem from ignorance about the appropriate use of morphine in cancer patients. Indeed, the patients who are truly sentenced to 'a kind of living death' are the ones who are *not* prescribed an adequate analgesic regimen. One such man had been bedridden because of pain for 2 months. His wife then found him crawling around the living room on his hands and knees searching for the gun which she had hidden to prevent him shooting himself. The subsequent use of morphine enabled this patient to start living again. The same is true for many others, as a visit to any palliative care unit will demonstrate.

■ CASE HISTORY

A 30 year-old Swedish woman was found to have cancer of the ovaries in early 1985. Although her doctors could not say how long she would live, they used the WHO 3-step ladder without hesitation. The woman progressed from aspirin and paracetamol to codeine. When this was no longer effective, she was prescribed morphine. The dose was increased gradually to 6 g/day. The woman functioned well on her medication and was in no way a 'zombie'. Until her death in November 1989 she led a full life without the debilitating effects of constant pain. She continued working, running aerobics classes, and maintained an active social diary (Anonymous 1990).

'CANCER PATIENTS EXPERIENCE A FINAL CRESCENDO OF PAIN'

There are many studies of symptoms in dying patients (Twycross & Lichter 1993). Those which often require attention during the last 48 hours include:

- pain
- dyspnoea
- restlessness
- agitation.

In one survey, 26% of patients at the end of life had unendurable pain which necessitated heavy sedation (Ventafridda et al 1990). This raises the question as to whether a final crescendo of pain is a common feature in patients dying from cancer.

A longitudinal study of over 400 cancer patients receiving regular diamorphine for one or more weeks showed that the median final dose was lower than the median maximum dose (Twycross 1974). A second study spanned the last week of life in 100 terminally ill cancer patients (Scott et al 1992). In these the mean daily dose of morphine increased from 211 to 213 mg. In a third study of the final 48 hours of 200 cancer patients (both inpatient and home care), the doses in those receiving a strong opioid were (Lichter & Hunt 1990):

- decreased in 13%
- unchanged in 43%
- increased in 44%.

In the latter, a single upward dose adjustment ± adjuvant medication proved sufficient in two thirds. In the rest, further adjustments or other treatment were necessary to relieve the pain. Relief was not complete in about 10%, but persisting severe pain occurred in only 1%.

None of these surveys from palliative care units supports the idea of a final crescendo of pain. Thus, if pain relief has previously been good and psychosocial aspects of care addressed, pain is unlikely to be a problem at the very end of life (Lombard & Oliver 1989, McIllmurray & Warren 1989, Saunders 1989). Pain relief in the last days of a patient's life is, in essence, a continuation of what is already being done.

New problems may emerge, however, and re-evaluation is necessary if the patient appears to be in pain. Sometimes specific measures are of greater benefit than a 'blanket' increase in the dose of morphine and/or other medication. For example:

- a painful bedsore may be helped by the application of benzydamine cream or a local anaesthetic gel (Jepson 1992)
- a distended bladder can be relieved by catheterization
- a loaded rectum can be emptied by manual removal.

Patients may be disturbed by pain even when unconscious. They may also be physically dependent on opioids and withdrawal restlessness will occur if analgesic medication is stopped suddenly when they can no longer swallow. Analgesics, therefore, must be given by an alternative route, i.e. SL, PR, SC.

In the terminal phase, patients may have pain on movement. They may show signs of discomfort even when apparently deeply unconscious, and may moan or cry out when moved. Such 'disturbance pain' may be due to muscle and joint stiffness as a result of prolonged immobility (Saunders 1989). A muscle relaxant such as diazepam or midazolam is often helpful.

Signs of discomfort may also be a form of 'alarm response' to being disturbed and may be particularly evident in the blind, the deaf, and the confused. In addition, dying patients may call out to check whether someone is with them or when they are aware that they are unattended (Livesley 1985). These cries may be misinterpreted as pain and be a source of concern to family and carers.

Disturbance pain is minimized by keeping the patient informed of intended interventions, by describing any procedure that is to be undertaken, and by gentle slow handling. At some centres, activity related pain is managed by administration of a short acting strong opioid (e.g. dextromoramide) for major disturbances such as sponging.

REFERENCES

Agenas I, Gustafsson L, Rane A, Sawe 1982 Analgetikaterapi for cancerpatienter. Lakartidningen 79: 287–289
Alloza J-L 1993 Opiophobia and cancer pain. Lancet 341: 1474–1475
Anonymous 1972 in Postal Symposium No. 1: Management of Terminal Illness. Smith & Nephew Pharmaceuticals, p 29
Anonymous 1990 Readers digest covers cancer pain issue. Cancer Pain Update 18: 3
Banos J-E, Bosch F 1993 Opiophobia and cancer pain. Lancet 341: 1474
Bloor R N, Smalldridge N J F 1990 Intravenous use of slow release morphine sulphate tablets. British Medical Journal 300: 640–641
Breitbart W 1992 Suicide. In: Holland J C, Rowland J H (eds) Handbook of psychooncology. Oxford University Press, Oxford, pp 291–299
Brescia F J, Portenoy R K, Ryan M, Krasnoff L, Gray G 1992 Pain, opioid use, and survival in hospitalized patients with advanced cancer. Journal of Clinical Oncology 10: 149–155
Brismar B, Hedenstierna G, Lundquist H, Strandberg A, Svensson L, Tokics L 1985 Pulmonary densities during anesthesia with muscular relaxation: a proposal of atelectasis. Anesthesiology 62: 422–428
Bruera E, Macmillan K, Hanson J, MacDonald R N 1989 The cognitive effects of the administration of narcotic analgesics in patients with cancer pain. Pain 39: 13–16
Bunyard P 1971 Intractable pain — how treatable is it? World Medicine Dec 1: 17
Collin E, Poulain P, Gauvain-Piquard A, Petit G, Pichard-Leandri E 1993 IS disease progression the major factor in morphine 'tolerance' in cancer pain treatment. Pain 55: 319–326
Colpaert F C, Niemegeers C J E, Janssen P A J, Maroli A N 1980 The effects of prior fentanyl administration and of pain on fentanyl analgesia: tolerance to and enhancement of narcotic analgesia. Journal of Pharmacology and Experimental Therapeutics 213: 418–426
Dorrepaal K L 1989 Pijn bij patienten met kanker (thesis). Amsterdam University, Amsterdam (Krips Repro)
Elliott T E, Elliott B A 1992 Physician attitudes and beliefs about use of morphine for cancer pain. Journal of Pain and Symptom Management 7: 141–148
Fischbeck K H, Mata M, D'Aquisto, Caronna J J 1980 Brompton mixture taken intravenously by a heroin addict. Western Journal of Medicine 133: 80
Garattini S 1993 Pain relief: narcotic drug use for severe pain. Lancet 341: 1061–1062
Hanks G W, Twycross R G, Lloyd J W 1981 Unexpected complication of successful nerve block. Anaesthesia 36: 37–39
Heneghan C P H, Jones J G 1985 Pulmonary gas exchange and diaphragmatic position. British Journal of Anaesthetics 57: 1161–1166
Hill S C 1987 Painful prescriptions. Journal of the American Medical Association 257: 2081
Hosobuchi Y, Lamb S, Bascom D 1980 Tryptophan loading may reverse tolerance to opiate analgesics in humans: a preliminary report. Pain 9: 161–169
Jepson B A 1992 Relieving the pain of pressure sores. Lancet 339: 503–504
Jones J G, Jordan C 1987 Postoperative analgesia and respiratory complications. Hospital Update 13: 115–124
Joranson D E 1992 Progress and issues in opioid availability. IASP Newsletter July/August: 9–10
Kanner R, Foley K M 1981 Patterns of narcotic drug use in cancer pain clinic. Annals of New York Academy of Sciences 362: 162–172
Lichter I, Hunt E 1990 The last 48 hours of life. Journal of Palliative Care 6: 7–15
Ling G S F, Paul D, Simantov R, Pasternak G W 1989 Differential development of acute

tolerance to analgesia, respiratory depression, gastrointestinal transit and hormone release in a morphine infusion model. Life Sciences 45: 1627–1636

Livesley B 1985 The management of the dying patient. In: Pathy M S J (ed) Principles and practice of geriatric medicine. John Wiley, London, pp 1287–1295

Lombard D J, Oliver D J 1989 The use of opioid analgesics in the last 24 hours of life of patients with advanced cancer. Palliative Medicine 3: 27–29

McIllmurray M B, Warren M R 1989 Evaluation of a new hospice: The relief of symptoms in cancer patients in the first year. Palliative Medicine 3: 135–140

Maruta T, Swanson D W, Finlayson R E 1979 Drug abuse and dependency in patients with chronic pain. Mayo Clinic Proceedings 54: 241–244

Misra A L, Pontani R B, Vadlamani N L 1989 Blockade of tolerance to morphine analgesia by cocaine. Pain 38: 77–84

Portenoy R K, Foley K M 1986 Chronic use of opioid analgesics in non-malignant pain: report of 38 cases. Pain 25: 171–186

Porter J, Jick J 1980 Addiction rare in patients treated with narcotics. New England Journal of Medicine 302: 123

Regnard C F B, Badger C 1987 Opioids, sleep and the time of death. Palliative Medicine 1: 107–110

Rigg J R A 1978 Ventilatory effects and plasma concentration of morphine in man. British Journal of Anaesthesia 50: 759–764

Robins L N, Davis D H, Nurco D N 1974 How permanent was Vietnam drug addiction? American Journal of Public Health 64: 38–43

Saunders C 1989 Pain and impending death. In: Wall P D, Melzack R (eds) Textbook of pain, 2nd edn. Churchill Livingstone, Edinburgh, pp 624–631

Scott J F, Viola R A, Buckley G 1992 Pain control during the last week of life in a palliative care unit. Journal of Palliative Care 8 (3): 73

Smith G M, Beecher H K 1962 Subjective effects of heroin and morphine in normal subjects. Journal of Pharmacology and Experimental Therapeutics 136: 47–52

Taub A 1982 Opioid analgesics in the treatment of chronic intractable pain of non-neoplastic origin in Narcotic Analgesics. In: Kitahata L M, Collins J D (eds) Anaesthesiology. Williams and Wilkins, Baltimore, pp 199–208

Tennant F S, Rawson R A 1982 Outpatient treatment of prescription opioid dependence. Archives of Internal Medicine 142: 1845–1847

Tennant F S, Uelman G F 1983 Narcotic maintenance for chronic pain: medical and legal guidelines. Postgraduate Medicine 73: 81–94

Twycross R G 1974 Clinical experience with diamorphine in advanced malignant disease. International Journal of Clinical Pharmacology Therapy and Toxicology 9: 184–198

Twycross R G, Wald S J 1976 Longterm use of diamorphine in advanced cancer. In: Bonica J J, Albe-Fessard D G (eds) Advances in pain research and therapy vol 1. Raven Press, New York, pp 653–661

Twycross R G, Lichter I 1993 The terminal phase. In: Doyle D, Hanks G W, MacDonald N (eds) Oxford Textbook of Palliative Medicine. Oxford University Press, Oxford, pp 649–661

Van der Mass P J, van Delden J J M, Pijnenborg L 1991 Medische beslissingen rond het levenseinde. The Hague, SDU 57–62

Ventafridda V, Ripamonti C, deConno F, Tamburini M, Cassileth B R 1990 Symptom prevalence and control during cancer patients' last days of life. Journal of Palliative Care 6 (3): 7–11

Walsh T D 1984 Opiates and respiratory function in advanced cancer. Recent Results in Cancer Research 89: 115–117

Weissman D E, Dahl J L 1990 Attitudes about cancer pain: a survey of Wisconsin's first year medical students. Journal of Pain and Symptom Management 5: 345–349

Weissman D E, Haddox J D 1989 Opioid pseudoaddiction: an iatrogenic syndrome. Pain 36: 363–366

World Health Organization 1969 Expert committee on drug dependence, 16th report. Technical report series no 407. World Health Organization, Geneva

Writer W D R, Hurtig J B, Evans D 1985 Epidural morphine prophylaxis of postoperative pain: report of a double-blind multicentre study. Canadian Anaesthesiological Society Journal 32: 330–338

Zylicz Z 1993 Opiophobia and cancer pain. Lancet 341: 1473–1474

CHAPTER

18

Alternative routes of administration

CHOICE OF ROUTE

Two surveys found that 11–16% of patients receiving morphine never required injections and 42–50% needed injections for < 24 h (Walsh 1985, Lombard & Oliver 1989). In one of the surveys, the median number of injections was two (Lombard & Oliver 1989).

It may be necessary, of course, to convert from tablets to oral solutions as swallowing becomes more difficult, and the administration of the last few doses may require patience and perseverance. Giving morphine in a concentrated solution into the mouth (sublingual, lingual or cheek) is a time honoured method in this situation, particularly at home.

In comatose patients, reliance on an opioid alone for pain relief is often satisfactory. Some patients, however, experience a return of severe diffuse pain 24–36 h after stopping a nonsteroidal anti-inflammatory drug (NSAID) such as flurbiprofen and naproxen, or 12–24 h after stopping diclofenac or ibuprofen. Thus, if the patient is likely to survive more than 24 h, consideration should be given to the use of NSAID suppositories (Table 18.1) or injections. Because diclofenac and ketorolac are incompatible with other commonly administered SC drugs, it is necessary to use a separate second syringe driver if administering by SC infusion.

Where a syringe driver is available, its use is less disturbing to the patient than repeated injections or the insertion of suppositories. The use of the syringe driver also eliminates the fear associated with administering the injection after which the patient dies. At one palliative care unit, opioids are administered by syringe driver to about two thirds of patients in the terminal phase (Lichter I 1991 Personal Communication).

Before the advent of the portable syringe driver, however, many patients were maintained satisfactorily on rectal medication when the oral route was no longer feasible. At one palliative care unit where the rectal route was the

Table 18.1 Analgesic, anti-emetic and psychotropic suppositories

Drug	Available strengths
UK and USA	
Aspirin	120/130, 195/200, 300, 600/650, 1200 mg (USA)
	300, 600 mg (UK)
Indomethacin	50 mg (USA)
	100 mg (UK)
Morphine	5, 10, 20, 30 mg (USA)
	15, 30 mg (UK)
Domperidone	30 mg
Paracetamol (acetaminophen)	120/125, 325, 650 mg (USA)
	125, 500 mg (UK)
Prochlorperazine	2.5 mg (USA)
	5, 25 mg
UK only	
Flurbiprofen	100 mg
Naproxen	500 mg
Oxycodone pectinate	30 mg[a]
Cyclizine	50 mg
Diazepam	10 mg[b]
USA only	
Opium and belladonna 15 mg	
(B & O supprettes No. 15A, 16A) }	30, 60 mg
Oxymorphone	5 mg
Hydromorphone	3 mg
Thiethylperazine	10 mg
Trimethobenzamide	100, 200 mg
Chlorpromazine	25, 100 mg

[a] Available on a named patient basis, i.e. supplied by manufacturers on receipt of a special order.
[b] Also available as a rectal solution.

routine alternative, 37% of the total *quantity* (not doses) of opioids used were given PR, and only 2% by injection (Henteleff & Fingerote 1983).

TRANSDERMAL

This route is now being used with fentanyl (see p. 286). The major problem is the latent period before the fentanyl starts working. If converting from a very high dose of morphine, the number of patches needed may be a disincentive (Herbst & Strause 1992).

BUCCAL AND SUBLINGUAL

By convention, 'buccal route' refers to the tablet placed on the lining of the gum above the upper teeth and held in position by the upper lip. In moribund patients it may be easier to place tablets or solution in the dependent cheek, rather than under the tongue.

The lining of the mouth is rich in blood vessels and lymphatics. Direct entry into the systemic circulation avoids hepatic first pass metabolism. The best SL preparations are tablets because liquids and pastes may be swallowed inadvertently. Hydrophilic drugs are poorly absorbed whereas lipophilic

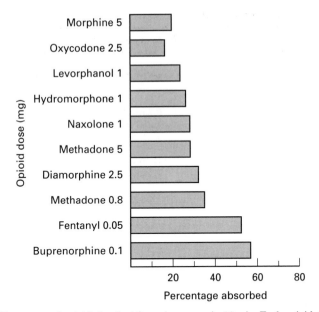

Fig. 18.1   Percentage of opioid absorbed from the tongue in 10 min. Each opioid dissolved in 1 ml.

drugs are relatively well absorbed (Beckett & Triggs 1976). Absorption varies considerably (Fig. 18.1), and is affected by changes in pH. Thus, one third of the content of 1 ml of a methadone solution is absorbed from the tongue in 10 min but, if the pH is raised from neutral to 8.5, the absorption increases to three quarters (Weinberg et al 1988). Changing the pH, however, does not affect the absorption of levorphanol so much and has no affect on hydromorphone.

A study which concluded that the absorption of morphine was nearly 50% greater after SL morphine compared with IM is generally considered erroneous (Bell et al 1985). Another study gave a mean maximum concentration of morphine after SL administration eight times lower than after IM injection, and it occurred several hours later (Fisher et al 1987). A figure of about 20% absorption would seem to be representative (Fig. 18.1). In practice, however, when converting from PO to SL, a 1:1 dose conversion ratio should be used initially, and the dose adjusted according to outcome.

Three quarters of 150 cancer patients obtained 'adequate to good pain relief' by the SL route (Whitman 1984). Morphine tablets containing 10 mg were used and doses were 10–30 mg q3h–q4h. The main adverse effect was the bitter taste of the morphine. This is less troublesome if the buccal route is used instead. Hard candy has been used to mask the taste.

Some centres use buprenorphine when the SL route is indicated, or phenazocine in the UK (Table 18.2). Relative systemic availability for buprenorphine SL compared to IM is 55% (range 16–94%). Although phenazocine is not marketed as a SL preparation, the 5 mg tablets dissolve readily in the mouth and are effective (Blane & Robbie 1972). As the tablets are scored,

Table 18.2 Sublingual (SL) formulations used in palliative care (UK)

Drug	Preparation	Strength	Comment
Analgesics			
Aspirin-glycine[a]	Tablet	500 mg	The glycine enhances the solubility of aspirin. For some patients it is too gritty.
Buprenorphine	Tablet	0.2 mg, 0.4 mg	
Dextromoramide[a]	Tablet	5 mg, 10 mg	Rapid onset of action; relatively short acting and may need to be used q3h.
Diamorphine	Tablet	10 mg	
Morphine	Liquid	20 mg/ml	Supplied with calibrated dropper. SL administration feasible because of small volume; probably absorbed mainly from stomach. Useful for moribund patients at home.
Phenazocine[a]	Tablet	5 mg	Bitter tasting like other opioids.
Anti-emetics and psychotropics			
Hyoscine hydrobromide	Tablet	0.3 mg	An 'over the counter' preparation (Quick Kwells).
Lorazepam[a]	Tablet	1 mg, 2.5 mg	Five times more potent than diazepam. Tablets are scored, permitting use of 0.5 mg.

[a] Oral tablets that can be taken SL.

it is possible to administer a smaller dose. Like other opioids, phenazocine has a bitter taste. In the UK, diamorphine 10 mg tablets are available for SL use.

RECTAL

The surface area of the rectum is small because of the absence of villi. Absorption is mainly by passive diffusion. Venous drainage from the rectum is by:

• superior rectal vein into the portal system
• middle and inferior rectal veins into the systemic circulation.

Extensive anastomoses between the three veins make it impossible to predict how much of the absorbed drug avoids hepatic first pass metabolism.

The absorption of aqueous and alcoholic solutions from the rectum is rapid but absorption from suppositories is slower (De Boer et al 1982). Absorption depends on:

• presence or absence of faeces
• volume inserted into the rectum
• position of suppository in the rectum
• nature of suppository base
• whether surfactants are used.

Studies of morphine absorption from the rectum show that absorption is the same or better than PO (Ripamonti & Bruera 1991). A figure of $53 \pm 18\%$ was obtained in eight patients (Johnson et al 1988). Rectal absorption of morphine is also dependent on pH. Absorption is best if the morphine is administered in a solution of pH 7–8 (Moolenaar et al 1985). M/r morphine tablets can be administered PR (Wilkinson et al 1992). Compared with PO (Fig. 18.2):

- the peak plasma concentration is lower
- the peak plasma concentration is delayed from < 3 h to about 5 h
- after 24 h, 90% has been absorbed.

Some centres administer m/r morphine tablets per vaginum with good results (Maloney et al 1989). Administration per colostomy has also been studied (Hojsted et al 1990). Compared to PR, the mean value was 43% with a range of 0–127%. Because of such a wide variation, administration per colostomy cannot be recommended. Reasons for poor absorption probably include:

- poor vascularity
- insertion into faeces
- hepatic first pass metabolism.

In the UK, morphine 15 mg and 30 mg suppositories are commercially available; in the USA, 5 mg, 10 mg, 20 mg and 30 mg suppositories are available. In practice, a PO:PR potency ratio for morphine of 1 can be used, i.e. the same dose is given by both routes (Hanning et al 1985).

Oxycodone pectinate 30 mg suppositories are available in the UK and Canada. These need be given only q8h. Oxycodone pectinate 30 mg q8h is equivalent to morphine 15 mg q4h. Oxymorphone 5 mg suppositories are available in the USA, and are equivalent to morphine 10 mg.

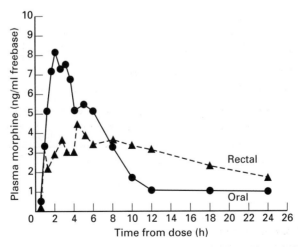

Fig. 18.2 Comparative single dose bio-availability of 30 mg MST tablets administered PO and PR. (Reproduced with permission from Kaiko et al 1989.)

CONTINUOUS SUBCUTANEOUS INFUSION

There are three main reasons for continuous SC infusion:

- persistent nausea and vomiting
- severe dysphagia
- patient too weak for oral drugs shortly before death.

Patients with inoperable intestinal obstruction may need parenteral medication for several weeks. The advantages of an infusion include:

- less nausea and vomiting because medication is retained and effective
- constant drug delivery without peaks or troughs
- no need for injection q4h
- syringe reloaded only once in 24 h.

Syringe driver

Portable battery driven syringe drivers are often used to deliver a continuous SC infusion of morphine or diamorphine together with an anti-emetic and other drugs (Walsh et al 1992). A survey of 97 palliative care units in the UK showed that 28 different drugs are given by SC infusion. Only eight are used by more than one third of the units (Tables 18.3, 18.4).

Several different models of syringe drivers are available. The Graseby Medical Model MS16A and MS26 have a variable speed and a battery with a running life of about 3 months (Fig. 18.3). The syringe drivers are calibrated in mm/h rather than ml/h to allow different types of syringe to be used (Table 18.5). The rate switch and start button are flush with the surface and cannot be accidentally operated; adjustment is made with a screwdriver.

The manufacturers provide instruction booklets. Videotapes providing a visual demonstration of the setting up and use of a portable syringe driver are available from St Christopher's Hospice, London and the Department of Medical Education, Southampton University. A personal workbook about syringe drivers is available from Sobell House.

The use of a syringe driver is not always trouble free (Table 18.6). It is important to check that the plunger is advancing at the set rate. With in-

Tablet 18.3 Drugs given by SC infusion at more than one third of 97 palliative care units (UK)

	Percentage of units using drug	Range of mean maximum dose (mg/24 h)	Median dose (mg/24 h)
Diamorphine	99	300–10 000	2200
Haloperidol	95	5–100	12.5
Methotrimeprazine	93	25–400	150
Cyclizine	85	50–150	150
Midazolam	64	10–160	40
Metoclopramide	64	10–200	30
Dexamethasone	39	4–30	15.5
Hyoscine hydrobromide	39	0.4–4	1.2

Modified from Johnson & Patterson 1992

Table 18.4 Drugs given by SC infusion in less than one sixth of 97 palliative care units (UK)

	Percentage of units using drug
Hyaluronidase	16
Hyoscine butylbromide	8
Chlorpromazine	4
Glycopyrronium bromide	4
Salbutamol	3
Atropine	3
Prochlorperazine	2
Diclofenac	2
Morphine	2
Orphenadrine	2
Codeine phosphate	2
Betamethasone	2
Frusemide	1
Droperidol	1
Pamidronate	1
Ondansetron	1
Pethidine	1
Trifluperazine	1
Diazepam	1
Papaveretum	1

Modified from Johnson & Patterson 1992

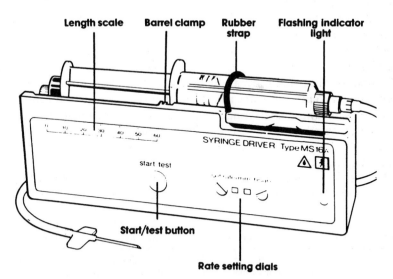

Fig. 18.3 A Graseby Medical syringe driver MS16A is a portable, battery-operated variable speed syringe driver. It allows SC infusion of small volumes over periods ranging from 30 min–50 h. A 10 ml syringe is normally used. MS26 (not shown) takes either a 10 ml or 20 ml syringe and can be set to run for 10 days or more. This pump has a boost button. Each boost delivers 0.23 mm. If held down continuously, the boost button cuts out after 10 boosts.

patients, this can be done on the regular drug rounds; at home, the patient can do this at mealtimes and bedtime. Patients at home should have an emergency telephone number to use if the pump stops working properly.

Table 18.5   Differences between Graseby MS16A and MS26 syringe drivers

	MS16A	MS26
Colour	Blue	Green
Rate settings	1–99 mm/h	1–99 mm/day
Boost button	No	Yes (0.23 mm)
Indicator light frequency	1 second	25 seconds

Table 18.6   Care of syringe driver and injection site

Routine	When things go wrong
Choice of infusion sites	*Infusion stopped or too slow*
Upper chest (intercostal plane)	Inflamed injection site?
Upper arm (outer aspect)	Cannula kinked?
Abdomen	Start button not pressed?
Thighs	Battery failure?
	If none of above true, the machine needs servicing
Each day	*Infusion too fast*
Examine site: change if inflamed	Check rate setting
Check rate	Check rate calculation
Press operation test button where applicable	
Fill new syringe	If both correct, the machine is faulty and needs servicing

Perfusor

The Braun Perfusor is similar to the syringe driver. It is powered by clockwork. There is a choice of three speeds, namely, 6, 12 or 24 h. It can only use a special 10 ml disposable syringe. The Perfusor is fitted with an electronic alarm which sounds after about 1 min if the clockwork mechanism stops.

Pharmacia pump

The Pharmacia 5200 is a battery operated, computer controlled pump. It is widely used in North America and some other countries (Bruera 1990). It works with 50 ml and 100 ml bags. It is a complex device, however, and very expensive. Nurses and patients need careful instruction in its use. Some centres have a specially trained nurse to co-ordinate and supervise the use of the pumps. It is unsuitable for small centres.

Infusors

Several types of portable infusors are also available (Bruera 1990). The Travenol-Baxter models infuse 0.5, 2 or 5 ml/h and have a capacity of 65 ml. Thus, provided the boost facility is not used, the 0.5 ml/h model will deliver medication for 5 days. Alternatively, with 2 ml/h, the patient receives 48 ml/24 h and has a reserve of 17 ml (Fig. 18.4). The infusor weighs only 90 g when full and patients usually pin it to their clothing. A new infusor

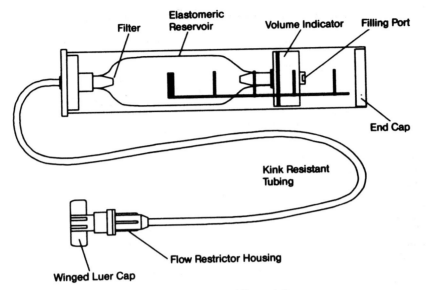

Fig. 18.4   The Travenol-Baxter infusor.

is attached each day, the contents having been prepared by the pharmacy. Empty infusors are discarded.

Each infusor costs £13. In contrast to an infusion pump, there is no initial heavy financial outlay and no possibility of power failure. For patients requiring a boost facility, a boost button (the shape and size of a wrist watch) is available for £7. This is not discarded with the infusor, i.e. it can be used indefinitely.

Mixing medication

Two or more different drugs are commonly given at the same time in one syringe. The following, therefore, need to be considered:

- drug compatibility
- drug stability
- tissue irritability.

Compatibility

Compatibility means miscibility. If compatible, diamorphine or morphine and the chosen anti-emetic will give a clear solution initially and crystals will not form during the period of administration. Most drugs given by SC infusion are miscible. Drugs in oily solution (e.g. diazepam and phenytoin) need to be given separately; also phenobarbitone which is made up in 90% propylene glycol. Some water soluble drugs, however, cause precipitation of certain other water soluble drugs:

- diamorphine and cyclizine are immiscible at high concentrations (Regnard 1986)

- metoclopramide and cyclizine precipitate unless mixed at body temperature and diluted in 16–20 ml (metoclopramide should not normally be given with anticholinergic drugs)
- dexamethasone is precipitated by other drugs unless mixed at body temperature and diluted in 16–20 ml
- midazolam does not mix with betamethasone, dexamethasone or methylprednisolone
- diclofenac and ketorolac must be given alone.

Stability

Stability refers to the chemical integrity of the mixed drugs. Diamorphine is unlikely to cause degradation of the commonly used anti-emetics. High pressure liquid chromatography has confirmed that when diamorphine is mixed with a range of anti-emetics, no loss through hydrolysis occurs in the 24 h (Allwood 1984). After 48 h, hydrolysis is greatest in a solution of diamorphine hydrochloride alone (Table 18.7). Most syringe drivers used in palliative care, however, are refilled every 24 h. Diamorphine hydrolyzes to mono-acetylmorphine in the first instance. This is equipotent with diamorphine (Wright & Barbour 1935).

Irritability

Although some centres recommend changing the butterfly needle every 2 days (Ventafridda et al 1986), this is not always necessary. The frequency with which the needle site needs to be changed depends almost entirely on the drugs infused. In the UK, with diamorphine alone ± metoclopramide or haloperidol, the injection site may need changing only every 1–3 weeks. If cyclizine or a phenothiazine is added, however, it may be necessary to change the site daily.

In patients who experience a painful inflammatory reaction the following steps should be considered:

- change needle site prophylactically (e.g. daily)

Table 18.7 Use of syringe driver: compatability of diamorphine hydrochloride 50 mg/ml with selected anti-emetic drugs[a]

Added drug	Quantity[b] in 20 ml	Diamorphine content (%)	
		24 h	48 h
Cyclizine	50 mg	105	100
Hyoscine	600 μg	106	98
Haloperidol	5 mg	105	98
Prochlorperazine	12.5 mg	105	98
Metoclopramide	50 mg	100	93
Control	–	100	84

[a] Comparable stability figures were obtained with methotrimeprazine in a parallel experiment.
[b] 1 g of diamorphine was dissolved in sterile water, mixed with anti-emetic (already in solution), and made up to 20 ml (as in clinical practice). 2 ml samples were then kept in standard disposable plastic syringes until subsequently assayed.
From Allwood 1984

- use a teflon cannula instead of a butterfly needle (Ventafridda et al 1986)
- reduce the concentration of the irritant drug
- change to an alternative drug (e.g. cyclizine ⟶ hyoscine)
- give the irritant drug by IM injection or PR
- place needle IM rather than SC
- add hyaluronidase 1500 units to the syringe (to facilitate SC diffusion)
- add hydrocortisone 50–100 mg to the syringe.

Although less irritant, teflon cannulae have a tendency to kink. If giving IM, the butterfly needle is inserted through the skin at right angles into an intercostal muscle. The butterfly is then laid flat on the skin and strapped into position in the usual way. In patients with marked inflammation, the local application of 1% hydrocortisone cream t.i.d.–q.i.d. may help.

SUBCUTANEOUS INJECTION

Edmonton injector

The Edmonton injector is a low cost metal device which allows a patient, relative or nurse to administer SC drugs in a fixed volume every 4 h (Fig. 18.5; Bruera 1990). The injector incorporates a series of metal rings around a 3 ml syringe, making it possible to vary the dose from 0.5–3 ml. Medication is dissolved in 100 ml of water in the pharmacy and inserted into the plastic reservoir. By means of a unidirectional valve, each dose is drawn into the syringe and then injected SC through an indwelling needle or cannula. The daily operational cost is over 10 times less than any other SC system.

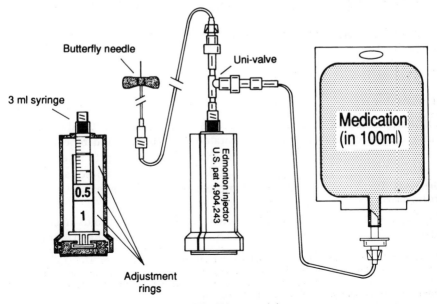

Fig. 18.5 The Edmonton injector.

Other alternatives

An even cheaper approach is a syringe attached to a SC needle or cannula with sufficient medication for 24 h. The patient, family or nurse then injects the correct amount every 4 h. Although this is not as foolproof as the Edmonton injector, it too avoids the need for 'needling' every 4 h. At some centres, for reasons of safety, each dose is made up and injected separately through the injection cap on the cannula.

HYPODERMOCLYSIS

Morphine and other drugs can be infused SC at a rate of 20–80 ml/h if hyaluronidase 600 units/L is added to the infusion fluid (Hayes 1985, Bruera 1990). Hyaluronidase causes rapid diffusion and absorption of injected fluids by temporarily disrupting connective tissue. This method was used extensively 50 years ago but was then replaced by IV infusions (Abbot et al 1952, Butler 1953). It has now been re-introduced in geriatric departments (Shen & Singer 1981, Shen & Arieli 1982). Hypodermoclysis can also be used for hydration, up to 2 L/day.

If dextrose is used, fluid is drawn from the surrounding tissues into the site of injection. This effect may last for several hours and cause pain and a reduction in plasma volume. This can be avoided by using dextrose saline. Hyaluronidase is expensive, and occasional sensitivity reactions occur (Bruera et al 1989). Even without hyaluronidase, 1 L/day can be infused.

INTRAMUSCULAR

The SC route is the preferred parenteral route (Consensus Statement 1983). With morphine or diamorphine, the IM route is used only when these are being given as a bolus dose combined with an irritant second drug, for example chlorpromazine, cyclizine, prochlorperazine. Because it is irritant, however, pethidine is given IM.

INTRAVENOUS

An increasing number of cancer patients have a permanent indwelling silicone central venous catheter to facilitate chemotherapy and repeated blood sampling. Catheters have been kept in place for periods up to 3 years, with a median duration of 40 days (McCredie & Lawson 1984). These catheters can be used for morphine and other symptom relief drugs by either continuous infusion or intermittent bolus (Portenoy et al 1986).

Acute tolerance to the analgesic effect of repeated IV bolus injections of diamorphine and morphine has been reported. On the other hand, continuous IV infusions of morphine have been used for up to 10 weeks without an increase in dose (Holmes 1978).

■ CASE HISTORY

A 30 year-old woman with advanced cancer of the cervix was admitted because of vomiting and abdominal colic caused by subacute intestinal obstruction. She was treated with an IV infusion and nasogastric suction. A bolus of IV diamorphine 10 mg was given for pain. This gave good relief for about 2 h, after which it was repeated. By the end of 24 h, the duration and quality of pain relief was less and the dose of diamorphine was increased to 15 mg. Pain relief was better but again over 24 h each bolus became progressively less effective. The diamorphine was increased to 20 mg and the next day to 30 mg. At this dose the patient slept for 30–60 min after each injection and awoke in severe pain. She was referred to a palliative care unit for advice about pain management.

The IV diamorphine was discontinued and she was given 120 mg morphine q4h PR because she was still vomiting and the rectum was empty. Within 24 h the patient was essentially painfree, alert and beginning to mobilize. She remained on morphine 100–120 mg q4h with good effect and remained mobile until her death two and a half weeks later (Hanks & Thomas 1985).

The conservative dose of rectal morphine should be noted. A total daily dose of diamorphine 360 mg IV (and poor pain relief) was replaced by morphine 720 mg PR (and good pain relief). The authors of the above case history state that, in dealing with acute IV tolerance, they give morphine PO if possible. If this is not feasible because of continued vomiting, morphine is given PR or diamorphine by SC infusion. Relief is generally obtained with a smaller dose of morphine/diamorphine than expected, as in this case. It seems that reducing the fluctuations in plasma opioid concentration by an alternative route of administration increases both the duration and the degree of pain relief.

PATIENT CONTROLLED ANALGESIA

Some centres have machines which permit patient controlled analgesia (PCA). These were developed principally for postoperative use (Kleiman et al 1988). They can be used, of course, in patients with advanced cancer. PCA machines are often cumbersome. A continuous SC infusion using a portable pump with a 'boost' facility has effectively superseded the use of PCA machines in palliative care.

REFERENCES

Abbot W, Levey S, Foreman R et al 1952 The danger of administering parenteral fluids by hypodermoclysis. Surgery 32: 305–315
Allwood M C 1984 Diamorphine mixed with antiemetic drugs in plastic syringes. British Journal of Pharmaceutical Practice 6 (3): 88–90
Beckett A H, Triggs E J 1976 Buccal absorption of basic drugs and its application as an in vivo model of passive drug transfer through lipid membranes. Journal of Pharmacy and Pharmacology 19 (Suppl): S31
Bell M D D, Mishra P, Weldon B D et al 1985 Buccal morphine: a new route for analgesia? Lancet i: 71–73
Blane G F, Robbie D S 1972 Agonist and antagonist actions of narcotic analgesic drugs. In: Kosterlitz H W, Collier A O J, Villareal J E (eds) Proceedings of the Symposium of the British Pharmaceutical Society. Macmillan, London, pp 120–127

Bruera E 1990 Subcutaneous administration of opioids in the management of cancer pain. In: Foley K M, Bonica J J, Ventafridda V (eds) Advances in pain research and therapy, vol 16. Raven Press, New York, 203–217

Bruera E, Legris M A, Kuehn N, Miller M J 1989 Hypodermoclysis for the administration of fluids and narcotic analgesics in patients with advanced cancer. Journal of the National Cancer Institute 81: 1108–1109

Butler J 1953 Peripheral vascular collapse after the subcutaneous use of hypertonic non-electrolyte solution. New England Journal of Medicine 249: 990–999

Consensus Statement 1993 Use of morphine for cancer pain. European Association for Palliative Care

De Boer A G, Moolenaar F, De Leede L G J et al 1982 Rectal drug administration: clinical pharmacokinetic considerations. Clinical Pharmacokinetics 7: 285–311

Fisher A P, Fung C, Hanna M 1987 Serum morphine concentrations after buccal and intramuscular morphine administration. British Journal of Clinical Pharmacology 24: 685–687

Hanks G W, Thomas E A 1985 Intravenous opioids in chronic cancer pain. British Medical Journal 291: 1124–1125

Hanning C D, Smith G, McNeill M, Graham N B 1985 Rectal administration of morphine from a sustained release hydrogel suppository. British Journal of Anaesthesia 57: 236–237

Hayes H 1985 Hypodermoclysis for symptom control in terminal care. Canadian Family Physician 31: 1253–1257

Henteleff P, Fingerote E 1983 Submission to Canadian Advisory Committee on the Management of Pain

Herbst L H, Strause L G 1992 Transdermal fentanyl use in hospice home-care patients with chronic cancer pain. Journal of Pain and Symptom Management 7 (Suppl 3): S54–S57

Hojsted J, Rubeck-Petersen K, Raik H, Bigler D, Broem-Christiansen C 1990 Comparative bioavailability of a morphine suppository given rectally and in a colostomy. European Journal of Clinical Pharmacology 39: 49–50

Holmes A H 1978 Morphine IV infusion for chronic pain. Drug Intelligence and Clinical Pharmacology 12: 556–557

Johnson I, Patterson S 1992 Drugs used in combination in the syringe driver: a survey of hospice practice. Palliative Medicine 6: 125–130

Johnson T, Christensen C B, Jordening H et al 1988 The bioavailability of rectally administered morphine. Pharmacology and Toxicology 62: 203–205

Kaiko R F, Healy N, Pav J, Thomas G B, Goldenheim P D 1989 The comparative bioavailability of MS Contin tablets (controlled release oral morphine) following rectal and oral administration. In: Twycross R G (ed) The Edinburgh Symposium on Pain Control and Medical Education. Royal Society of Medicine Services, London, pp 235–241

Kleiman R L, Lipman A G, Hare B D, MacDonald S D 1988 A comparison of morphine administered by patient-controlled analgesia and regularly scheduled intramuscular injection in severe, postoperative pain. Journal of Pain and Symptom Management 3: 15–22

Lombard D J, Oliver D J 1989 The use of opioid analgesics in the last 24 hours of life of patients with advanced cancer. Palliative Medicine 3: 27–29

McCredie K B, Lawson M 1984 Percutaneous insertion of silicone central venous catheters for long term intravenous access in cancer patients. Internal Medicine 5: 100–105

Maloney C M, Kesner R K, Klein G et al 1989 The rectal administration of MS Contin: clinical implications of use in end-stage cancer. American Journal of Hospice Care 6 (4): 34–35

Moolenaar F, Yska J P, Visser J et al 1985 Drastic improvement in the rectal absorption profile of morphine in man. European Journal of Clinical Pharmacology 29: 119–121

Portenoy R K, Moulin D E, Rogers A, Inturrisi C E, Foley K M 1986 Intravenous infusion of opioids for cancer pain: clinical review and guidelines for use. Cancer Treatment Reports 70: 575–581

Regnard C F B 1986 Antiemetic/diamorphine mixture compatibility in infusion pumps. British Journal of Pharmaceutical Practice 8: 218–220

Ripamonti C, Bruera E 1991 Rectal, buccal, and sublingual narcotics for the management of cancer pain. Journal of Palliative Care 7 (1): 30–35

Shen R, Singer M 1981 Subcutaneous infusions in the elderly. Journal of the American Geriatric Society 29: 583–585

Shen R, Arieli S 1982 Administration of potassium by subcutaneous infusion in elderly patients. British Medical Journal 285: 1167–1168

Ventafridda V, Spoldi E, Caraceni A, Tamburini M, De Conno F 1986 The importance of continuous subcutaneous morphine administration for cancer pain control. The Pain Clinic 1: 47–55

Walsh T D, Smyth E M S, Currie K, Glare P A, Schneider J 1992 A pilot study, review of the literature, and dosing guidelines for patient-controlled analgesia using subcutaneous morphine sulphate for chronic cancer pain. Palliative Medicine 6: 217–226

Weinberg D S, Inturrisi C E, Reidewberg B et al 1988 Sublingual absorption of selected opioid analgesics. Clinical Pharmacology and Therapeutics 44: 335–342

Whitman H H 1984 Sublingual morphine: a novel route of narcotic administration. American Journal of Nursing 84: 939–940

Wilkinson T J, Robinson B A, Begg E J, Duffull S B, Ravenscroft P J, Schneider J J 1992 Pharmacokinetics and efficacy of rectal versus oral sustained-release morphine in cancer patients. Cancer Chemotherapy and Pharmacology 31: 251–254

Wright C I, Barbour F A 1935 The respiratory effects of morphine, codeine and related substances. Journal of Pharmacology and Experimental Therapeutics 54: 25–33

Spinal analgesia

RATIONALE FOR SPINAL ANALGESIA

The presence of opioid receptors in high density in the substantia gelatinosa of the spinal cord provides the logical basis for spinal opioid use (Pert & Snyder 1973, Sabbe & Yaksh 1990). Compared with conventional routes, epidural (ED) and intrathecal (IT) administration have a potentially higher morbidity. The use of the spinal route, therefore, can be justified only if it results in (Hogan et al 1991, Sjoberg et al 1991):

- equal or greater pain relief than conventional routes *and*
- less troublesome or fewer adverse effects.

INDICATIONS FOR SPINAL ANALGESIA

The indications for spinal analgesia and the drugs used vary from centre to centre. Current practice at Sobell House is summarized in Table 19.1.

Table 19.1 Indications for spinal analgesia (Sobell House)

Pain syndrome	Drugs used				Mode	
	Morphine	Bupivacaine	Clonidine	Corticosteroid	Infusion	Bolus
Lumbosacral plexopathy	+	+	±	−	+	+
Visceral neuropathic pain	+	+	±	−	+	+
Fractured femur in patient close to death	±	+	−	−	+	+
Systemic morphine intolerance	+	±	−	−	+	+
Vertebral metastasis (periradiotherapy)	−	−	−	+	−	+

A hierarchy of responsiveness to spinal morphine has been noted (Arner 1991):

- deep somatic continuous
- visceral continuous
- deep somatic intermittent
- visceral intermittent
- neuropathic
- cutaneous.

In one series of 37 cancer patients, mean pain relief was 92% for bone pain but only 42% for neuropathic pain (Kiss et al 1989). The response in neuropathic pain is increased by the addition of bupivacaine (Hogan et al 1991, Sjoberg et al 1991) and clonidine (Eisenach et al 1989, Motsch et al 1990).

PHARMACOKINETIC CONSIDERATIONS

The onset of analgesia after lumbar IT morphine is about 30 min. In contrast, after an injection into a cerebral ventricle, onset may be as fast as 2 min (Lobato et al 1984). Opioids spread rostrally in the circulating cerebrospinal fluid (CSF) and the effects of lumbar IT injection may be partly cerebral (Moulin et al 1986). Lipid solubility is an important determinant of the rate at which opioid enters the spinal cord from the CSF. In CSF, morphine has a longer terminal halflife than diamorphine which is 100 times more lipid soluble (73 and 43 min respectively; Moore et al 1984, Kotob et al 1986). Rostral spread is less with more lipid soluble opioids.

IT doses of less than morphine 0.5 mg have an effect in postoperative pain (Nordberg et al 1984). A dose-response curve has been demonstrated between 0.625 mg and 1.25 mg with a plateau after that (Paterson et al 1984). IT morphine 0.5–1 mg has also been used in chronic pain (Wang 1985), and the dose increased as the disease progressed or tolerance developed (Arner & Arner 1985). Good relief has also been reported in more than 1000 patients with diamorphine 0.5–1 mg (Barron & Strong 1984).

Duration of analgesic effect after spinal opioids is considerably longer than after IM injection. In patients having cardiac surgery, analgesia lasted about 36 h after lumbar IT morphine 2–4 mg (Mathews & Abrams 1980). In patients having total hip replacement, lower doses produced analgesia for 24–48 h (Kalso 1983, Peterson et al 1984). Diamorphine gives an equivalent duration of analgesia to morphine at the same dose.

Bio-availability is less with the ED route. Systemic absorption adds another dimension to both pharmacokinetic and pharmacodynamic considerations. *Only 10–20% of an ED dose of morphine diffuses into the CSF.* This is reflected in the higher doses used by this route. ED morphine 5 mg b.i.d. is equivalent to IT morphine 1 mg once a day (Watson et al 1984).

In a postoperative study of lumbar ED analgesia, morphine 5 mg gave a median duration of relief of 10 h (Watson et al 1984). A second study gave comparable results (Nordberg 1984). Doses used with infusions, however, have been as low as 0.3 mg/h (Cullen et al 1985). This suggests that the dose-response for morphine differs with bolus and infusion.

Vascular changes in pregnancy increase systemic uptake. Results in labour have been correspondingly poor, with a high incidence of adverse effects. Systemic uptake can be reduced and analgesia increased by giving adrenaline concurrently (Jamous et al 1986).

Spinal analgesia in palliative care, in fact, is very different from obstetric use. In palliative care:

- the drug given is usually an opioid and not, as in obstetrics, a local anaesthetic which also blocks motor and sympathetic function
- the pain is chronic rather than acute, and the patient is not opioid naive
- major adverse effects, e.g. severe hypotension with a local anaesthetic and apnoea with an opioid, are much less likely to occur with chronic use
- if the catheter subsequently penetrates the dura mater, the speed of onset of adverse effects is slower when a continuous infusion is being used than with bolus injections (Leykin et al 1985)
- epidurals are used as a last resort, whereas in obstetrics there are several other options still available (e.g. paracervical and pudendal blocks; nitrous oxide and pethidine).

DELIVERY SYSTEMS

Spinal opioids can be administered in several ways (Box 19.A). They can be injected into an external catheter either intermittently or by infusion. Alternatively, a totally implanted system can be used with either an injection port or reservoir (Cherry & Gourlay 1987), and this reduces further the already low infection rate. The additional cost, however, is considerable. An indwelling intracerebroventricular catheter has been used at some centres (Lobato et al 1984).

A small volume can often be used, for example, 6–8 ml/24 h (Tanelian & Cousins 1989). Some portable pumps, however, deliver up to 100 ml (Barkas & Duafala 1988). Choice depends on several factors, particularly prognosis

---

BOX 19.A
SPINAL DRUG DELIVERY SYSTEMS (Waldman 1990a)

Percutaneous ED or IT catheter
Direct percutaneous
Lateral SC tunnelling

Totally implanted ED or IT catheter
SC injection port
Implanted manually activated pump
Implanted infusion pump
Implanted programmable infusion pump

and cost. SC ports are very durable; they are made to take many thousands of injections before leaking.

Guidelines for intermittent self-administration of epidural opioids from prefilled syringes are available (Gove et al 1985). Epidural opioids have been used for periods over 6 months, and sometimes for more than a year (Crawford et al 1983, Cousins & Mather 1984, Gove et al 1985, Van Lee 1986, Ventafridda et al 1987, Arner et al 1988).

TECHNICAL CONSIDERATIONS

Practice differs between centres (Box 19.B). The advantage of the ED route is the potentially lower morbidity, i.e. headache secondary to CSF leak and infection (meningitis). On the other hand, the catheter tip may occlude (it is not bathed in CSF) or migrate intrathecally.

Other problems include kinking, accidental removal and infection (Zenz et al 1981, Crawford et al 1983). Tunnelling the catheter laterally under the skin reduces the infection rate (Coombs 1986) and the technical complications (Table 19.2). Generally, the catheter is left in position indefinitely, and replaced only if it blocks (Box 19.C). The site of insertion is relatively stereotyped:

- thoracic for upper body and upper limb pain
- lumbar for lower body and lower limb pain.

Insertion of catheter

The catheter is inserted using an aseptic technique. The spine is normally fully flexed to ensure easy access between the vertebrae, and the level of entry is determined by the site of the pain.

A Tuohy needle is inserted by the anaesthetist into the ED space. With

---

BOX 19.B
CONTROVERSIES IN SPINAL ANALGESIA

Route, regimen and choice of drugs
Intrathecal (IT) v. epidural (ED)
Infusion v. bolus
Preservative in morphine v. no preservative
Morphine v. morphine and local anaesthetic
Dose of morphine when combining with local anaesthetic
Stopping v. tapering previous PO/SC morphine therapy

Technical considerations
Tunnelling catheter under skin away from midline
Suturing catheter to skin
Bacterial filter
Sterile dressing over skin puncture site (under adhesive plaster)
Changing adhesive plaster (Hypafix) weekly

Table 19.2   Technical complications of chronic ED morphine (n = 110)

	Catheter	
	Tunnelled (n = 15)	Nontunnelled (n = 95)
Obstruction of the catheter	4	43
Dislocation of the catheter	–	23
Pain during injection	–[a]	34
Subcutaneous leak of injected fluids	2	17
Local skin infection	1	4
Total	7	121[b]

[a] These 15 patients had a low infusion rate.
[b] No technical complications occurred in 24 patients; one complication in 44; more than one complication in 27.
From Crul & Delhaas 1991

BOX 19.C
PROBLEMS ASSOCIATED WITH A PERCUTANEOUS CATHETER

Catheter leaks (care of percutaneous site becomes difficult because of wetness and/or infusion loses effect)

Catheter kinks (occasionally deep to skin entry site)

Catheter blocks

Catheter falls out

Catheter breaks (externally)

Infection (erythema ± bead of pus at percutaneous site should not cause concern, though more diffuse painful erythema indicating cellulitis calls for action)

Migration to IT space (this is rare; the effect of the infusion becomes much greater)

---

a syringe of air or saline attached to the needle, resistance can be felt as the needle passes through the interspinous ligament. The resistance drops once the needle is in the ED space, and the air or saline can be easily injected.

A catheter is threaded through the needle to 3–4 cm beyond the tip. Once the catheter is in position, the needle is removed and the catheter aspirated to ensure there is no blood or CSF. If blood is withdrawn, the catheter may be in an ED vessel, and should be moved slightly or withdrawn. If the placement seems satisfactory, a test bolus dose of local anaesthetic is injected. The patient's blood pressure is taken every 5 min for 20 min to detect significant hypotension. If no adverse reactions are noted, further injections may then be given or an infusion started (Wildsmith & Armitage 1987).

Maintenance of catheter

The external portion of the catheter is looped to reduce the risk of dislodging the catheter tip. The loop must be large enough to prevent kinking. The external portion of the catheter is then secured to the skin with adhesive plaster (e.g. Hypafix).

Some centres use a bacterial filter on the assumption that this will decrease the likelihood of infection. There is no evidence that this is so. However, if a bacterial filter is used:

- place a gauze pad beneath it
- cover with a gauze dressing
- secure with adhesive plaster
- check that there is no leakage onto the gauze because of a loose or faulty connection.

The filter and extension line is changed every week, maintaining asepsis. The new extension line and filter are primed with the analgesic solution from the infusion system. The old filter is then removed and the new one attached to the catheter.

Some centres change the adhesive plaster once a week but this is unnecessary. The plaster should be removed only if there is:

- pain at the percutaneous site
- a saturated dressing as a result of catheter leakaqe
- loss of analgesic effect and catheter displacement is a possible cause.

A saturated dressing also raises the question of outward migration of the catheter. The marks on the catheter should be checked in relation to point of entry through the skin and compared with the position recorded at the time of insertion.

When a catheter is to be removed:

- place the patient in a comfortable position
- remove plaster
- withdraw the catheter without using excessive force
- clean the puncture site with an antiseptic and cover with a sterile plaster
- check that the full length of catheter has been removed.

SPINAL ANALGESIA PROTOCOLS

Many centres have standing orders covering the use of spinal opioids (Box 19.D). St Oswald's Hospice, Newcastle, has a comprehensive 10 page 'Spinals policy' document which includes a chart for recording observations. In practice, however, the risk of severe adverse effects is small because patients will have been receiving PO/SC opioids for some time and are no longer 'opioid naive'.

DRUGS AND DOSES

Many drugs can be given by the spinal route (Box 19.E). In this section those commonly used in Sobell House are discussed.

BOX 19.D
SPINAL OPIOIDS: EXAMPLE OF STANDING ORDERS (Waldman 1990b)

Measure vital signs every 15 min for 1 h → every 30 min for 1 h → every hour for 4 h → every 4 h for 24 h.

Check and record respiratory rate every hour for 24 h.

Patient to remain supine with head of bed up 30° for 30 min after the initial injection.

For respirations < 6/min administer IV/IM naloxone:

- dilute 400 μg (one ampoule) with 8 ml of saline
- give 2 ml every 5 min until respirations > 10/min
- notify doctor if this is necessary.

For severe itching administer antihistamine IM q4h–q6h as needed, e.g. chlorpheniramine 10 mg, diphenhydramine 50 mg, promethazine 25–50 mg.

For nausea (in the absence of an existing anti-emetic standing order) administer haloperidol 1–1.5 mg PO or 2.5 mg SC q4h as needed.

If the patient develops hypotension (a drop of diastolic blood pressure > 20 mm Hg), administer ephedrine 10 mg IV every 3 min up to a total of 50 mg. Notify doctor if this is necessary.

If drowsy, patient may get up with assistance 30 min after the initial injection of spinal opioids.

Urinary retention: may catheterize if necessary. Notify doctor if this is done.

Document pain on pain chart when measuring vital signs.

If any problems or questions arise, contact . . . . .
[Signed by doctor with date]

BOX 19.E
DRUGS USED FOR SPINAL ANALGESIA

Opioid
Buprenorphine
Butorphanol (Hurley & Johnson 1990)
Diamorphine (Barron & Strong 1984)
Fentanyl (Sabbe & Yaksh 1990)
Hydromorphone (Coombs et al 1986)
Methadone (Shir et al 1991)
Morphine (Crul & Delhaas 1991, Erdine & Aldemir 1991)
Tramadol (Baraka et al 1993)

Nonopioid
Baclofen (Jones et al 1988, Penn et al 1989)
Clonidine (Motsch et al 1990)
Corticosteroids (Bezon 1986)
Local anaesthetics (Akerman et al 1988, Du Pen et al 1992)
Midazolam (Rigoli 1983, Serrao et al 1992)
Octreotide (Chrubasik 1985, Penn et al 1992)

Corticosteroids

Depot methylprednisolone 80 mg in 2 ml or triamcinolone hexacetonide 40–80 mg in 2–4 ml are the preparations normally used. Either a single ED injection is given or daily for three days via an indwelling catheter. Further injections can be given at monthly or longer intervals. Depot corticosteroids cannot be injected through a bacterial filter.

The effect of ED corticosteroids is unpredictable and may not peak until a week after injection. Some patients, however, obtain benefit for weeks from one injection. Benefit probably relates to the ability of corticosteroids to reduce spontaneous activity in injured nerves (see p. 444).

Morphine

A standard ampoule of morphine sulphate 10 mg/ml (with preservative) is used. The dose depends on previous opioid medication. This will be higher than the dose used in opioid naive postoperative patients (De Leon-Casasola et al 1993). The following conversion factors are used at many centres:

PO → ED, *divide 24 h dose by 10*
SC → ED, *divide 24 h dose by 5*
ED → IT, *divide 24 h dose by 10*

Some centres use a smaller starting dose of IT morphine, i.e. 1% and not 2% of the previous SC dose (Coombs 1986). Preservative-free morphine is used at some centres.

Although some patients with neuropathic pain obtain complete relief with ED morphine, total success with morphine alone is unlikely if there are well established central generating mechanisms.

A few patients convert back to oral morphine after several weeks of successful treatment with spinal morphine. One centre recommends multiplying the dose of epidural morphine by 5 rather than 10 in this circumstance (Hanks G W 1992 Personal Communication). The reason for the symmetry is because, on occasion, a 10–fold increase has proved to be excessive. Accordingly, a smaller conversion factor is used and the dose adjusted upwards if necessary.

Bupivacaine

At some centres morphine and morphine plus bupivacaine are given sequentially (Table 19.3; Van Dongen et al 1993). In Sobell House, however, morphine is no longer given alone. Spinal morphine and spinal local anaesthetics have a synergistic analgesic effect (Penning & Yaksh 1992, Krames 1993).

The starting dose of bupivacaine varies according to centre and circumstances (Table 19.4). Higher concentrations of bupivacaine cause numbness and weakness or paralysis. Although such concentrations are sometimes necessary to provide adequate relief, this is not normally the case.

Local anaesthetics have a weak antimicrobial effect. This partly explains

Table 19.3 ED morphine and bupivacaine

Type of pain[a]	Success with	
	Morphine alone	Morphine & bupivacaine
Nociceptive	5	2 + 1[b]
Neuropathic	–	3 + 2[c]
Mixed	1	1 + 1[b]
	6	6 + 4

[a] Seven of nociceptive and mixed pains were intermittent.
[b] Relief obtained but heavy legs (weakness) not acceptable to patient.
[c] In two patients continuous infusion not pursued after success with bolus injection, because pump not available (1) and no reason given (1).
From Hogan et al 1991

Table 19.4 Starting doses for continuous spinal infusion

Drug	Epidural	Intrathecal
Morphine *or* diamorphine alone	24 h oral morphine dose ÷ 10 = 24 h ED dose in *mg*	24 h oral morphine dose ÷ 100 = 24 h IT dose in *mg*
Fentanyl	24 h oral morphine dose × 10 = 24 h ED dose in *µg*	24 h oral morphine dose ÷ 2 = 24 h IT dose in *µg*
Bupivacaine alone (0.25% = 2.5 mg/ml)	Bupivacaine dose: lumbar = 20 ml/24 h thoracic = 10 ml/24 h *Do not exceed 5 ml/h*	Bupivacaine dose: lumbar = 10 ml/24 h thoracic = 5 ml/24 h *Do not exceed 2 ml/h*
Bupivacaine (0.25% = 2.5 mg/ml) with morphine or diamorphine	Bupivacaine dose: lumbar = 5 ml/24 h thoracic = 2.5 ml/24 h *Do not exceed 5 ml/h*	Bupivacaine dose: lumbar = 2 ml/24 h thoracic = 1 ml/24 h *Do not exceed 2 ml/h*

Based on St. Oswald's Hospice 1993

why it is relatively safe to leave an ED indwelling catheter in place for days or weeks.

Clonidine

ED clonidine has been used to relieve nonmalignant pain, usually with morphine or a local anaesthetic (Coombs et al 1984, Tamsen & Gordh 1984, Mendez et al 1990, Motsch et al 1990). It has also been used in cancer patients (Eisenach et al 1989).

Clonidine is a mixed $alpha_1$ and $alpha_2$ adrenergic agonist (mainly $alpha_2$). It reduces the responsiveness of peripheral blood vessels to vasoconstrictor and vasodilator substances, and to sympathetic nerve stimulation. These actions led to its use in prophylaxis against migraine and in the treatment of hypertension (Anonymous 1990). Clonidine may cause a reduction in venous return and mild bradycardia, resulting in a reduced cardiac output. Clonidine has also been used to attenuate the opioid withdrawal syndrome, thereby demonstrating an interaction with the opioid system at some level.

Hypotension is the most likely adverse effect after bolus injection. Sedation and dry mouth may also occur initially. Dizziness, headache, euphoria, nocturnal unrest, nausea, constipation, rash and impotence have all been reported. Long term use has occasionally precipitated depression. Agitation may occur after stopping long term treatment.

Typically, for ED use, clonidine 150 µg is diluted to 5 ml in normal saline and injected slowly as a bolus. If relief is obtained, an infusion is set up containing clonidine 150–300 µg/24 h. Clonidine is discussed further in Chapter 23.

Midazolam

Spinal midazolam is sometimes used. Animal studies indicate that midazolam enhances the affinity of spinal opioid receptors for opioid agonists and decreases the affinity for naloxone (Tejwani et al 1990).

CLINICAL EXPERIENCE

The following three case histories relate to the early experience at Sobell House of the use of ED analgesia (Ottesen et al 1990).

■ CASE HISTORY

A 74 year-old man was admitted with a history of disseminated cancer of the bladder. A pulmonary metastasis in the apex of the left lung resulted in Pancoast syndrome. He had severe pain in the left shoulder and arm, together with dysfunction of the lower brachial plexus. The pain was sharp and worse on movement, and he did not obtain adequate relief from a NSAID, co-proxamol, buprenorphine, morphine, dexamethasone or amitriptyline. Morphine made him confused, while radiotherapy was started but not completed because of his poor general condition.

An ED catheter was inserted at T4–5. After injection of 5 mg of morphine sulphate in normal saline, he was painfree without adverse effects. The catheter was attached to a portable syringe driver and morphine 10 mg/24 h was infused. This was subsequently reduced to 8 mg. He died painfree 2 weeks later.

■ CASE HISTORY

A 36 year-old woman with cancer of the bronchus was admitted with incapacitating pains in the left side of her neck and down her right leg. An isotope bone scan showed metastases in the cervical spine, sacrum and pelvis. The pain in the neck responded well to radiotherapy and a combination of a NSAID, morphine and amitriptyline, but the leg pain persisted. The distribution of the leg pain, with associated numbness of the back of the thigh and absent ankle jerk, suggested infiltration of S1–2 nerve roots. The pain was completely relieved by a bolus dose of ED morphine 10 mg injected at L2–3. Radiotherapy to the sacrum was started.

Given the option of having morphine by infusion or injecting the catheter herself t.i.d., the patient chose the latter because she was reluctant to carry a portable syringe driver. She remained painfree at home on morphine 8 mg t.i.d. The pain recurred after 11 days when the ED infusion was temporarily stopped. Ten days later, however, it proved possible to stop the morphine completely, presumably as a result of the previous radiotherapy.

■ CASE HISTORY

A 55 year-old woman with metastatic cancer of her left breast was admitted because of incapacitating pain in her right hip and leg. An isotope bone scan showed progressive metastases in the lumbar spine, pelvis and femora. The hip pain responded to radiotherapy but she still complained of pain in the L5–S1 distribution. A combination of morphine, dexamethasone and amitriptyline yielded little benefit.

An ED catheter was inserted at L2–3. Injection of 10 mg of morphine sulphate in normal saline gave good relief. Depot methylprednisolone 80 mg was injected daily for 3 days because of a previous good response in this patient with ED corticosteroids (Bezon 1986). She remained painfree on an infusion of morphine 20 mg/24 h from a portable syringe driver.

Two weeks later a new pain in the right lateral pelvis suddenly developed. She did not improve significantly when the morphine was increased to 30 mg/ 24 h. A radiograph revealed pathological fractures of the right pubis and right ischium. Morphine 30 mg and bupivacaine 215 mg were mixed to make a 60 ml solution and infused over 24 h from a nonportable syringe driver. This combination relieved the pain completely without causing orthostatic hypotension, and without adverse effects on motor and bladder function. The morphine was reduced to 20 mg/24 h because of drowsiness but later was gradually increased to 40 mg.

ADVERSE EFFECTS

Adverse effects are related to:

- drugs used
- doses given
- route administered (IT or ED)
- whether or not the patient is opioid naive.

Local anaesthetic

Local anaesthetics block sympathetic nerve fibres and, therefore, can cause *hypotension*. This will develop within 10 min of a bolus injection or commencing an infusion. It is unlikely, however, with the doses recommended. As already noted, in higher concentrations, local anaesthetics cause numbness, paralysis and urinary retention. If injected into an ED vein, several serious adverse effects may occur:

- CNS excitement: tremor of lips, twitching of corner of mouth
- CNS depression (rare)

- hypotension: faintness, lightheadedness
- cardiac arrhythmia: pallor, sweating.

If the local anaesthetic is injected into the CSF, it is likely to cause a 'total spinal' (i.e. a total spinal anaesthetic):

- total paralysis from the neck down
- numbness
- hypotension
- apnoea.

Opioid

Adverse effects are generally less with chronic use compared with acute (Tables 19.5, 19.6). Naloxone 400 mg IM reverses most adverse effects associated with ED morphine without reducing analgesia (Korbon et al 1985, Ueyama et al 1992). Nalbuphine 5 mg IM/IV may be a better option. In postcaesarean patients who had received morphine 5 mg ED, it decreased nausea, vomiting and pruritus significantly whereas naloxone had no effect

Table 19.5 Adverse effects in opioid naive postoperative patients after ED morphine 5 mg (n = 128)

Effect	Incidence (%)
Nausea	48
Vomiting	30
Pruritus	41
Urinary retention	34
Hypotension	4
Respiratory depression	4

From Writer et al 1985

Table 19.6 Complications and adverse effects of chronic ED morphine (n = 225)

	n	%
Catheter related	40	18
Displacement	16	7
Infection	9	4
Occlusion	8	4
Leakage	5	2
Epidural haematoma	2	1
Drug related	70	31
Burning pain	22	10
Constipation	16	7
Urinary retention	8	4
Nausea and vomiting	10	4
Pruritus	8	4
Tolerance	4	2
Hypotension	2	1

From Erdine & Aldemir 1991

(Cohen et al 1992). Sedation increased after nalbuphine but pain scores were unchanged; the reverse was true for naloxone.

Rectovaginal muscle spasms have been reported in one patient with IT morphine which necessitated the continuing concurrent use of midazolam by patient controlled analgesia (PCA) (Littrell et al 1992).

Although very high concentrations of opioid are seen in the CSF 30 min after IT injection (Moore et al 1984), toxicity has not been a problem in monkeys after 14–16 months of continuous infusion with ED morphine (Yaksh 1981), and in man after 6 months (Meier et al 1982). Dural thickening after chronic IT administration (Coombs et al 1985) and pain on ED injection (Zenz 1984) may be attributable to disease rather than the spinal opioids.

Respiratory depression

Life threatening respiratory depression up to 12 h after ED use has been reported (Etches et al 1989). With opioid naive patients, summation of the systemic effects of an ED dose with an earlier dose administered by a conventional route (oral or injection) should be avoided as far as possible, particularly in the elderly (Gustafsson et al 1982).

Respiratory depression was not seen in a series of over 1000 patients given IT diamorphine (Barron & Strong 1984) or in 2500 patients given one of several ED opioids (Rawal & Sjostrand 1986). Even so, the risk cannot be ignored, particularly when repeated injections are required. In acute care, 12 h should elapse after spinal injection before a patient is moved from an intensive care area. In chronic use, respiratory depression is not a problem with either spinal route (Wang 1985, Coombs 1986).

Urinary retention

Postoperatively, urinary retention occurs in 15–30% of patients (Moulin et al 1986). Animal studies suggest that inhibition of bladder function by spinal opioids is mediated by spinal mechanisms involving mu and delta receptors (Dray & Metsche 1984). Oral phenoxybenzamine (an alpha adrenergic antagonist) given before and after elective caesarean section reduced the incidence of urinary retention from about 50% to 10% (Evron et al 1984). If the patients are catheterized, however, this is of limited importance. Spinal opioids also inhibit ejaculation, a function controlled by the autonomic nervous system (Pybus et al 1984).

Pruritus

Pruritus has been reported with all the opioids administered by the spinal route (McQuay et al 1980), and also enkephalin analogues (Moulin et al 1984). The pruritus is not relieved by antihistamines or phenothiazines. After lumbar injection, the pruritus may be experienced in the lower half of the body or may be more generalized. Occasionally, it is limited to the face. The severity of the pruritus can be such that the patient refuses further spinal opioids, despite previous good analgesia.

In a randomized controlled trial in postoperative patients, hydromorphone caused significantly less pruritus than morphine; 44% had severe pruritus with morphine compared with 11% on hydromorphone. Nausea and sedation were equal in the two groups.

TOLERANCE

Tolerance to spinal opioids may occur with chronic use. It is a predictable consequence of the very high local CSF concentrations. Tolerance develops more rapidly with infusions than with on demand bolus injections (Erickson et al 1984). It is not an insuperable problem because increasing the dose corrects the reduced response. Abstention for about a week leads to a reversal of tolerance.

NURSES AND SPINAL ANALGESIA

In the past, trained nurses in the UK could not give bolus spinal injections or, without specific training, fill and change the syringe of a spinal infusion. The same nurses, however, could give 'as needed' SC injections, and fill and change the syringe of a SC infusion. This was because the spinal administration of drugs represented an 'extended role' for the nurse (Derrick 1989). It led to the absurd situation whereby patient and families were changing the syringe (and sometimes filling it) because the community nurse (trained and experienced in other respects) was not allowed to be involved.

The situation has become more flexible since the UK Central Council for Nursing Midwifery (UKCC) issued a new code of professional practice (UKCC 1992). The code explicitly warns nurses to 'honestly acknowledge' any limitations of knowledge and skill and take steps to remedy them. It is also their responsibility to ensure any extension of their roles does not adversely affect patient care or push them outside the UKCC's Code of Professional Conduct. The Code also reminds nurses of their personal accountability in every area of their work and warns them to avoid any 'inappropriate delegation' of duties to other staff. It is, therefore, no longer necessary for nurses to obtain extended role certificates to carry out extra duties. Instead, it places responsibility for competence in the hands of the individual nurse (Hand 1992).

In some countries nurses have handled ED injections for years. In a Danish multicentre study of over 100 outpatients, district nurses shared responsibility in about one fifth and were solely responsible in two fifths of the cases (Crawford et al 1983). District nurses are responsible for the administration of injections or the reloading of the syringe driver in several other countries (Howard et al 1981, Arner et al 1988, Tanelian & Cousins 1989). At some centres, patients and relatives are taught the management of ED drugs at home (Gove et al 1985, Malone et al 1985, Van Lee 1986, Ahlgren & Ahlgren 1987, Cherry & Gourlay 1987, Fisher et al 1987, Tanelian & Cousins 1989).

SUMMARY

Spinal analgesia has a definite place in the relief of pain after major surgery and after injuries such as multiple rib fractures (Ullman et al 1989). In these situations the use is self-limiting and is unlikely to exceed 14 days. With chronic pain, the spinal route is used only after systemically administered opioids and other drugs have been shown to be ineffective or associated with intolerable adverse effects (Sjostrand & Rawal 1986).

Before instituting long term treatment, it is essential to determine whether the pain is opioid responsive. Ideally, a test injection of an appropriate dose of ED morphine should be given and compared with the effect of normal saline (Erickson et al 1984). This is rarely done in cancer patients.

The concurrent use of morphine and bupivacaine has greatly enhanced the value of epidural analgesia. Bupivacaine relieves the opioid resistant component of the pain, typically seen in many cases of lumbosacral plexopathy.

REFERENCES

Ahlgren F I H, Ahlgren M B E 1987 Epidural administration of opiates by a new device. Pain 31: 353–357

Akerman B, Arwestrom E, Post C 1988 Local anesthetics potentiate spinal morphine antinociception. Anesthesia and Analgesia 67: 943–948

Anonymous 1990 Clonidine in migraine prophylaxis: Now obsolete. Drug and Therapeutics Bulletin 28: 79–80

Arner S 1991 Differentiation of pain and treatment efficacy. Disertation Karolinska Institute. Stockholm, p 31

Arner S, Arner B 1985 Differential effects epidural morphine in the treatment of cancer-related pain. Acta Anaesthesiologica Scandinavica 29: 32–36

Arner S, Rawal N, Gustafsson L L 1988 Clinical experience of long-term treatment with epidural and intrathecal opioids: a nationwide survey. Acta Anaesthesiologica Scandinavica 32: 253–259

Baraka A, Jabbour S, Ghabash M, Nader A, Khoury G, Sibai A 1993 A comparison of epidural tramadol and epidural morphine for postoperative analgesia. Canadian Journal of Anaesthesia 40: 308–313

Barkas G, Duafala M E 1988 Advances in cancer pain management: a review of patient-controlled analgesia. Journal of Pain and Symptom Management 3: 150–160

Barron D W, Strong J E 1984 The safety and efficacy of intrathecal diamorphine. Pain 18: 279–285

Bezon H T 1986 Epidural steroid injections for low back pain and lumbosacral radiculopathy. Pain 27: 277–295

Cherry D A, Gourlay G K 1987 The spinal administration of opioids in the treatment of acute and chronic pain: bolus doses, continuous infusion, intraventricular administration and implanted drug delivery systems. Palliative Medicine 1: 89–106

Chrubasik J 1985 Spinal infusion of opiates and somatostatin. Hygieneplan, Germany

Cohen S E, Ratner E F, Kreitzman T R, Archer J H, Mignano L R 1992 Nalbuphine is better than naloxone for treatment of side effects after epidural morphine. Anesthesia and Analgesia 75: 747–752

Coombs D 1986 Management of chronic pain by epidural and intrathecal opioids: newer drugs and delivery systems. In: Sjostrand U H, Rawal N (eds) International Anesthesiology Clinics 24 (2): regional opioids in anesthesiology and pain management. Little Brown, Boston, pp 59–74

Coombs D W, Saunders R, Gaylor M et al 1984 Clinical trial of intrathecal clonidine for cancer pain. Journal of Regional Anesthesia 9: 34–35

Coombs D W, Fratkin J D, Meier F et al 1985 Neuropathologic lesions and CSF morphine concentrations during chronic continuous intraspinal morphine infusion: a clinical and post mortem study. Pain 22: 337–351

Coombs D W, Saunders R L, Fratkin J D, Jensen L E, Murphy C A 1986 Continuous intrathecal hydromorphone and clonidine for intractable cancer pain. Journal of Neurosurgery 64: 890–894

Cousins M J, Mather L E 1984 Intrathecal and epidural administration of opioids. Anesthesiology 61: 276–310

Crawford M E, Anderson H B, Augustenberg G et al 1983 Pain treatment on outpatient basis using extradural opiates: a Danish multicentre study comprising 105 patients. Pain 16: 41–47

Crul B J P, Delhaas E M 1991 Technical complications during long term subarachnoid or epidural administration of morphine in terminally ill cancer patients: A review of 140 cases. Regional Anesthesia 16: 209–213

Cullen M L, Staren E D, El-Ganzouri A, Logas W G, Ivkanovich A D, Economou S G 1985 Continuous epidural infusion for analgesia after major abdominal operations: a randomised prospective double-blind study. Surgery 98: 718–726

De Leon-Casasola O A, Myers D P, Donaparthi S et al 1993 A comparison of postoperative epidural analgesia between patients with chronic cancer taking high doses of oral opioids versus opioid-naive patients. Anesthesia and Analgesia 76: 302–307

Derrick S 1989 What are the legal implications of extended nursing roles? The Professional Nurse April: 350–352

Dray A, Metsch R 1984 Inhibition of urinary bladder contractions by a spinal action of morphine and other opioids. Journal of Pharmacology and Experimental Therapeutics 231: 254–260

Du Pen S L, Kharasch E D, Williams A et al 1992 Chronic epidural bupivacaine-opioid infusion in intractable cancer pain. Pain 49: 293–300

Eisenach J C, Rauck R L, Buzzanell C, Lysak S Z 1989 Epidural clonidine analgesia for intractable cancer pain: phase I. Anesthesiology 71: 647–652

Erdine S, Aldemir T 1991 Long term results of peridural morphine in 225 patients. Pain 45: 155–159

Erickson D L, Lo J, Michaelson M 1984 Intrathecal morphine for treatment of pain due to malignancy. Pain (suppl) 2: S19

Etches R C, Sandler A N, Daley M D 1989 Respiratory depression and spinal opioids. Canadian Journal of Anaesthesiology 36: 165–185

Evron S, Magora F, Sadovsky E 1984 Prevention of urinary retention with phenoxybenzamine during epidural morphine. British Medical Journal 288: 190

Fisher A P, Simpson D, Hanna M 1987 A role for epidural opioid in opioid-insensitive pain? The Pain Clinic 1: 233–236

Gove L F, Gordon N H, Miller J, Scott W 1985 Pre-filled syringes for self-administration of epidural opiates. Pharmaceutical Journal 234: 378–379

Gustafsson L L, Friberg-Nielson S, Garle M et al 1982 Extradural and parenteral morphine: kinetics and effects in postoperative pain. A controlled clinical study. British Journal of Anesthesia 54: 1167–1174

Hand D 1992 Taking a giant leap towards freedom. Nursing Standard 6 (42): 23

Hogan Q, Haddox J D, Abram S, Weissman D, Taylor M L, Janjan N 1991 Epidural opiates and local anesthetics for the management of cancer pain. Pain 46: 271–279

Howard R P, Milne L A, Williams N E 1981 Epidural morphine in terminal care. Anaesthesia 36: 51–53

Hurley R J, Johnson M D 1990 Spinal opioids in the management of obstetric pain. Journal of Pain and Symptom Management 5: 146–153

Jamous M A, Hand C W, Moore R A, Teddy P J, McQuay H J 1986 Epinephrine reduces systemic absorption of extradural diacetylmorphine. Anesthesia and Analgesia 65: 1290–1294

Jones R F, Anthony M, Torda T A, Poulos C 1988 Epidural baclofen for intractable spasticity. Lancet i: 527

Kalso E 1983 Effects of intrathecal morphine injected with bupivacaine on pain after orthopaedic surgery. British Journal of Anaesthesia 55: 415–422

Kiss I E, Simini B, May J W 1989 Effect of epidural morphine on various kinds of cancer pain. Palliative Medicine 3: 217–221

Korbon G A, James D J, Verlander J M et al 1985 Intramuscular naloxone reverses the side effects of epidural morphine while preserving analgesia. Regional Anesthesia 10: 16–20

Kotob H I M, Hand C W, Moore R A et al 1986 Intrathecal morphine and heroin in man: 6 hour drug analysis in spinal fluid and plasma. Anaesthesia and Analgesia 65: 718–722

Krames E S 1993 The chronic intraspinal use of opioid and local anaesthetic mixtures for the relief of intractable pain: when all else fails! Pain 55: 1–4

Leykin Y, Rudik V, Niv D, Geller E 1985 Delayed respiratory depression following extradural injection of morphine. Israeli Journal of Medical Science 21: 855–857

Littrell R A, Kennedy L D, Birmingham W E, Leak W D 1992 Muscle spasms associated with intrathecal morphine therapy: treatment with midazolam. Clinical Pharmacy 11: 57–59

Lobato R D, Madrid J L, Fatela L V, Rivas J J, Gozalo J, Barcena A 1984 Analgesia elicited by low-dose intraventricular morphine in terminal cancer patients. Pain (suppl) 2: S342

McQuay H J, Bullingham R E S, Evans P J D, Lloyd J W, Moore R A 1980 Demand analgesia to assess pain relief from epidural opiates. Lancet i: 768–769

Malone B T, Beye R, Walker J 1985 Management of pain in the terminally ill by administration of epidural narcotics. Cancer 55: 438–440

Mathews E T, Abrams L D 1980 Intrathecal morphine in open heart surgery. Lancet i: 543

Meier F A, Coombs D W, Saunders R L, Pageau M G 1982 Pathologic anatomy of constant morphine infusion by intraspinal silastic catheter. Anesthesiology 57: A206

Mendez R, Eisenach J C, Kashtan K 1990 Epidural clonidine analgesia after caesarean section. Anesthesiology 73: 848–852

Moore R A, Bullingham R E S, McQuay H J, Allen M C, Cole A 1984 Spinal fluid kinetics of morphine and heroin. Clinical Pharmacology and Therapeutics 35: 40–45

Motsch J, Graber E, Ludwig K 1990 Addition of clonidine enhances postoperative analgesia from epidural morphine: a double-blind study. Anesthesiology 73: 1067–1073

Moulin D E, Max M, Kaiko R, Inturrisi C, Maggard J, Foley K 1984 The analgesic efficacy of intrathecal D-Ala2-D-Leu5 enkephalin (DADL) in cancer patients with chronic pain. Pain (suppl) 2: S343

Moulin D E, Inturrisi C E, Foley K M 1986 Epidural and intrathecal opioids: cerebrospinal fluid and plasma pharmacokinetics in cancer pain patients. In: Foley K M, Inturrisi C E (eds) Advances in pain research and therapy, vol 8. Raven Press, New York, pp 369–383

Nordberg G 1984 Pharmacokinetic aspects of spinal morphine analgesia. Acta Anaesthesiologica Scandinavica (suppl 79) 28: 7–38

Nordberg G, Hedner T, Mellstrand T, Dahlstrom B 1984 Pharmacokinetic aspects of intrathecal morphine analgesia. Anesthesiology 60: 448–454

Ottesen S, Minton M, Twycross R G 1990 The use of epidural morphine at a palliative care centre. Palliative Medicine 4: 117–122

Paterson G M C, McQuay H J, Bullingham R E S, Moore R A 1984 Intradural morphine and diamorphine dose-response studies. Anaesthesia 39: 113–117

Penn R D, Paice J A, Kroin J S 1992 Octreotide: A potent new non-opiate analgesic for intrathecal infusion. Pain 49: 13–19

Penn R D, Savoy S M, Corcos D et al 1989 Intrathecal baclofen for severe spinal spasticity. New England Journal of Medicine 329: 1517–1521

Penning J P, Yaksh T L 1992 Interaction of intrathecal morphine with bupivacaine and lidocaine in the rat. Anesthesiology 77: 1186–1200

Pert C B, Snyder S H 1973 Opiate receptor: demonstration in nervous tissue. Science 179: 1011–1014

Pybus A, Torda T, McQuay H J, Moore R A 1984 Opiates and sexual function. Nature 310: 636

Rawal N, Sjostrand U H 1986 Clinical application of epidural and intrathecal opioids for pain management. In: Sjostrand U H, Rawal N (eds) Regional opioids in anesthesiology and pain management. International anaesthesiology clinics 24. Little Brown, Boston, pp 43–57

Rigoli M 1983 Epidural analgesia with benzodiazepines. In: Tiengo M, Cousins M J (eds) Pharmacological basis of anesthesiology: clinical pharmacology of new analgesics and anesthetics. Raven Press, New York, pp 69–76

Sabbe M B, Yaksh T L 1990 Pharmacology of spinal opioids. Journal of Pain and Symptom Management 5: 191–203

St Oswald's Hospice 1993 Spinals policy. St Oswald's Hospice, Newcastle-upon-Tyne

Serrao J M, Marks R L, Morley S J, Goodchild C S 1992 Intrathecal midazolam for the treatment of chronic mechanical low back pain: a controlled comparison with epidural steroid in a pilot study. Pain 48: 5–12

Shir Y, Shapira S S, Shenkman Z, Kaufman B, Magora F 1991 Continuous epidural methadone treatment for cancer pain. The Clinical Journal of Pain 7: 339–341

Sjoberg M, Appelgren L, Einarsson S et al 1991 Long-term intrathecal morphine and bupivacaine in 'refractory' cancer pain. Results from the first series of 52 patients. Acta Anaesthesiologica Scandinavica 35: 30–43

Sjostrand U H, Rawal N 1986 Regional opioids in anaesthesiology and pain management. International anesthesiology clinics 24 (2). Little Brown, Boston, pp 135

Tamsen A, Gordh T 1984 Epidural clonidine produces analgesia. Lancet ii: 231–232

Tanelian D L, Cousins M J 1989 Combined neurogenic and nociceptive pain in a patient with Pancoast tumour managed by epidural hydromorphone and oral carbamazepine. Pain 36: 85–88

Tejwani G A, Rattan A K, McDonald J S 1990 Anesthesiology 73: A1270

Ueyama H, Nishimura M, Tashiro C 1992 Naloxone reversal of nystagmus associated with intrathecal morphine administration (letter). Anesthesiology 76: 153

Ullman D A, Fortune J B, Greenhouse B B, Wimpy R E, Kennedy T M 1989 The treatment of patients with multiple rib fractures using continuous thoracic epidural narcotic infusion. Regional Anesthesia 14: 43–47

Van Dongen R T M, Crul B J P, De Bock M 1993 Long term intrathecal infusion of morphine and morphine-bupinacaine mixture in the treatment of cancer pain: a retrospective analysis of 51 cases. Pain 55: 119–123

Van Lee A 1986 Epidural morphine in the terminally ill: How long and how high? The Pain Clinic 1: 69–70

Ventafridda V, Spoldi E, Caraceni A, de Conno F 1987 Intraspinal morphine for cancer pain. Acta Anaesthesiol Scand 31 (suppl 85): 47–53

Waldman S D 1990a Implantable drug delivery systems: practical considerations. Journal of Pain and Symptom Management 5; 169–174

Waldman S D 1990b The role of spinal opioids in the management of cancer pain. Journal of Pain and Symptom Management 5: 163–168

Wang J K 1985 Intrathecal morphine for intractable pain secondary to cancer of pelvic organs. Pain 21: 99–102

Watson P J Q, Moore R A, McQuay H J et al 1984 Plasma morphine concentrations and analgesic effects of lumbar extradural morphine and heroin. Anesthesia and Analgesia 63: 629–634

Wildsmith J A W, Armitage E N 1987 Principles and practice of regional anaesthesia. Churchill Livingstone, Edinburgh

Writer W D R, Hurtig J B, Evans D 1985 Epidural morphine prophylaxis of postoperative pain: report of a double-blind multicentre study. Canadian Medical Association Journal 32: 330–338

Yaksh T L 1981 Spinal opiate analgesia: characteristics and principles of action. Pain 11: 293–346

Zenz M 1984 Epidural opiates for the treatment of cancer pain. In: Zimmermann M, Drings P, Wagner G (eds) Pain in the cancer patient: pathogenesis, diagnosis and therapy. Springer-Verlag, Berlin, pp 107–115

Zenz M, Schappler-Scheele B, Neuhans R, Piepenbrock S, Hilfrich J 1981 Long term peridural morphine analgesia in cancer pain. Lancet i: 91

Morphine and dyspnoea

Comprehensive accounts of the treatment of dyspnoea in advanced cancer are available elsewhere (Cockcroft & Guz 1987, Stark 1988, Wasserman & Casaburi 1988, Cowcher & Hanks 1990, Cohen et al 1992, Ahmedzai 1993).

THE EXTENT OF THE PROBLEM

In the National Hospice Study (USA), dyspnoea occurred in 70% of patients at some time during the last 6 weeks of life (Reuben & Mor 1986). The prevalence increased as patients approached death. In the week immediately before death, dyspnoea was the main symptom in 21% of 86 patients associated with a district palliative care team in the UK (Higginson & McCarthy 1989). Staff-rated scores for dyspnoea increased in the final week of the patient's life (Fig. 20.1). Dyspnoea was also noted in the last 48 h in 22% of 200 patients associated with a palliative care unit in New Zealand (Lichter & Hunt 1990). The dyspnoea was relieved adequately in all but 2%. In stark contrast, 28% of 120 patients associated with an Italian palliative care unit had 'unendurable dyspnoea' at the end of life which necessitated heavy sedation (Ventafridda et al 1990).

The more encouraging New Zealand data, however, are similar to those reported by a palliative care unit in the UK, where only one patient in a consecutive series of 100 died with uncontrolled dyspnoea (Saunders 1989). The patient in question had been an inpatient for only one day and steps were still actively being taken to ease his distress at the time of death.

These figures are perhaps the best. Severe or very severe dyspnoea was reported by the key carer in more than 50% of 80 patients in the UK during the last week of life (Addington-Hall et al 1991). These patients died mainly at home or in hospital; only eight died in a palliative care unit. Of those with dyspnoea, less than half received treatment which helped. In other words, 29% of patients had severe or very severe dyspnoea for which no effective

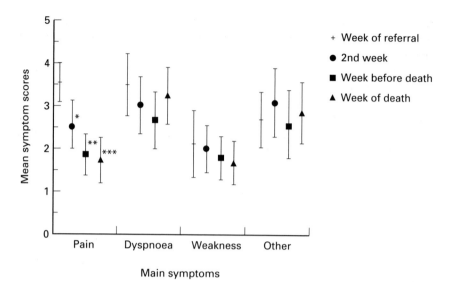

Fig. 20.1 Mean scores (and 95% confidence intervals) for main symptoms while receiving palliative care from a district support team. Asterisks indicate a significant difference from the initial score. (Reproduced with permission from Higginson & McCarthy 1989.)

treatment was offered. This percentage is virtually identical with that reported from Milan.

GENERAL CONSIDERATIONS

Dyspnoea in advanced cancer is usually multifactorial. Whereas reversible causes such as bronchospasm, cardiac failure, pleural effusion or massive ascites are usually treated specifically, dyspnoea associated with irreversible causes requires symptomatic measures. The aim of such treatment is to relieve the perception of breathlessness. Dyspnoea is usually associated with tachypnoea and, if severe, accompanied by anxiety. Companionship, a comforting hand and a soothing voice all help to contain the anxiety provoked by an exacerbation. Relaxation techniques and breathing exercises help to prevent respiratory panic attacks.

A cool draft of air on the face is beneficial, and can be achieved by opening a window or by the use of a fan. A fan often provides as much relief as nasal oxygen and, at the end of life, does not impede bedside companionship. On the other hand, oxygen has a place in management, particularly if the patient is hypoxic (Bruera et al 1992). It is important, however, not to encourage oxygen dependence unnecessarily.

In practice, few dyspnoeic patients in palliative care units in the UK receive oxygen. Reliance is placed instead on psychological approaches and the use of drugs, particularly morphine.

RELEVANT PHYSIOLOGY

The sensation of breathlessness is not fully understood. The basic fault is an imbalance between a demand for ventilation and the ability of the respiratory system to respond. Endogenous opioids are said to be involved in the regulation of respiratory function (Shook et al 1990). Evidence for this comes from the observation that the increase in respiratory effort seen with increased airways resistance is blunted in patients with chronic obstructive airways disease (COAD) and is restored by naloxone (Santiago et al 1981). Increased airways resistance in COAD can be likened to a noxious stimulus which triggers the production of endogenous opioids. These findings, however, have been disputed (Kirsch et al 1988).

Morphine reduces the ventilatory response to:

- carbon dioxide (Eckenhoff & Oech 1960)
- hypoxia (Santiago et al 1977)
- exercise (Santiago et al 1979).

Morphine also reduces oxygen consumption at rest and on exercise in normal subjects (Santiago et al 1979) and may alter the central perception of breathlessness (Johnson et al 1983).

CLINICAL TRIALS IN DYSPNOEA

Opioids

Healthy volunteers

In six healthy volunteers, codeine 60 mg PO had an effect on exercise induced dyspnoea but no greater than that obtained with placebo (Stark et al 1983). The codeine, however, did permit higher levels of carbon dioxide to be tolerated during breath holding.

Chronic obstructive airways disease (COAD)

The results of several trials of opioids in 'pink puffers' are summarized in Table 20.1. In addition to subjective ratings of dyspnoea (McGavin et al 1978), measurements included:

- spirometry
- exercise tests
- psychological tests for anxiety and depression.

Several patients in the long term study of dihydrocodeine stopped treatment because of adverse effects (Woodcock et al 1982). Because of this, a further study was undertaken with a lower dose of dihydrocodeine, i.e. 15 mg t.i.d. (Johnson et al 1983). This provided benefit without adverse effects (Table 20.1).

Studies with diamorphine demonstrated no benefit, even though in terms of analgesia the dose of diamorphine used was comparable to or greater than those of dihydrocodeine (Eiser et al 1991). This suggests that analgesic and antidyspnoea potency may not be the same.

Hydromorphone rectal suppositories (3 mg b.i.d.–q.i.d.) were used to

Table 20.1 Randomized controlled trials of opioids and dyspnoea in patients with chronic obstructive airways disease

Number of patients	Opioid	Oral dose	Schedule	Main results — Subjective	Main results — Objective	Comments	Authors
11	Codeine	30 mg q.i.d.	4 weeks	No change	Exercise tolerance unchanged	2/11 withdrawn because of respiratory deterioration; one case of acute urinary retention	Rice et al 1987
12	Dihydrocodeine	1 mg/kg	Single dose	Dyspnoea reduced 20%	Exercise tolerance increased by 18%	Oxygen gave comparable benefit; dyspnoea reduced 32% when both given	Woodcock et al 1981b
16	Dihydrocodeine	30 mg t.i.d. 60 mg t.i.d. } 2 weeks each		Improvement *at lower dose* (oxygen cost diagram)	p_aCO_2 rose (≤ 40 mm Hg)	5 withdrew because of nausea and vomiting; 2 constipated and drowsy	Woodcock et al 1982
18	Dihydrocodeine	15 mg t.i.d.	1 week	Dyspnoea reduced 18%	Pedometer increased 17%; treadmill walking increased 12%	No adverse effects reported	Johnson et al 1983
13	Morphine	0.8 mg/kg	Single dose	Dyspnoea no greater despite increased workload	Maximum workload increased by 18% and oxygen uptake by 19%	One patient became markedly hypotensive after exercise test ($140 \rightarrow 60$ mm Hg) and was given naloxone	Light et al 1989
14	Diamorphine	2.5 or 5 mg q.i.d.	2 weeks	No change	Exercise tolerance unchanged	4/18 withdrew because of chest infection, pruritus, constipation, headache	Eiser et al 1991
8	Diamorphine	7.5 mg	Single dose	No change	Exercise tolerance unchanged		Eiser et al 1991

control dyspnoea in a single patient double-blind trial (Robin & Burke 1986). The patient was a 63 year-old woman with COAD with a $p_a CO_2$ of about 40 mm Hg. Hydromorphone or placebo were alternated every 3 days after an initial unblinded period during which the appropriate hydromorphone dose was determined. The patient had a dramatic improvement in dyspnoea rating during hydromorphone treatment and returned to her baseline status when taking placebo.

Terminal cancer

Twenty cancer patients with dyspnoea were given SC morphine. The dose in five patients not previously receiving opioids was 5 mg. In the rest it was the equivalent of two and a half times their regular analgesic dose (Bruera et al 1990). The causes of dyspnoea included:

- progressive lung tumour
- lung metastases
- pleural effusion
- carcinomatous lymphangitis
- pneumonia
- pulmonary fibrosis.

None of the patients had COAD, and all patients were receiving continuous oxygen.

No significant differences before and 45 min after morphine were recorded in:

- respiratory rate
- respiratory effort
- oxygen saturation
- end-tidal $p_a CO_2$.

Subjective ratings of dyspnoea, however, improved significantly ($p < 0.001$). Mild nausea and sedation occurred only in patients who had not received opioids before. The duration of action of the morphine on dyspnoea was shorter than its analgesic effect (Fig. 20.2). The results indicate that, in dyspnoeic patients without COAD, SC morphine improves dyspnoea at doses which do not compromise respiratory function.

At another centre, eight patients with terminal lung cancer and severe dyspnoea despite oxygen, nonopioid drugs and intermittent opioid injections were studied (Cohen et al 1991). Morphine 1–2 mg IV was administered every 5–10 min until the patient reported relief. A continuous IV morphine infusion was then started, with the hourly dose equal to 50% of the initial cumulative bolus dose. Six patients experienced good relief, one moderate and one poor. Serial blood gas estimations showed a variable $p_a CO_2$ but a steadily rising $p_a CO_2$ to greater than 50 mm Hg after 24 h in 5/7 patients. Pulse and blood pressure changed little and only one patient had a respiratory rate of < 10/min. The major adverse effect was sedation. This was

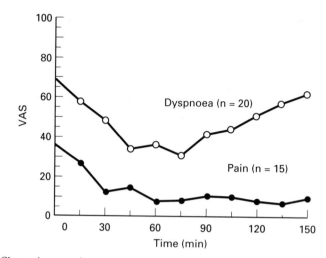

Fig. 20.2   Change in mean dyspnoea and mean pain after SC morphine. Results expressed as mean ± SE. (Reproduced with permission from Bruera et al 1990.)

treated by discontinuing the infusion until the patient's mental state improved. It was then restarted at half the rate. Seven of the patients died during the study period of 3–4 days. The shortest survival was 16 h.

Benzodiazepines

An early report of the use of diazepam in 'pink puffers' suggested that patients obtained a 'striking' reduction in dyspnoea and an improvement in exercise tolerance (Mitchell-Heggs et al 1980). Subsequent reports have emphasized, however, that such drugs are ineffective unless the patient is anxious (Woodcock et al 1981a, Eimer et al 1985, Man et al 1986, Greene et al 1989). Further, in debilitated patients, there is a risk of toxic cumulation with benzodiazepines such as diazepam. Thus, in one study over 2 weeks, diazepam 5 mg t.i.d. and 10 mg nocte was associated with the following adverse events (Woodcock et al 1981a):

- falling downstairs
- falling off motorcycle
- repeated oversleeping
- repeated late arrival at work
- unable to continue job in machine instruction.

In an open study in three 'pink puffers', diazepam ≤ 25 mg/day doubled the exercise tolerance from about 20 m to 40 m in two. In the third, exercise tolerance decreased from nearly 100 m to 25 m (Sen et al 1983). The first patient, however, subsequently became drowsy and ataxic, and his exercise tolerance returned almost to its original level. The above doses, however, are much higher than most doctors would recommend.

A trial of alprazolam 0.5 mg b.i.d. for 1 week in 24 patients with COAD showed no benefit (Man et al 1986). Drowsiness was a common adverse effect.

Sedative antihistamines

Promethazine was compared with placebo and with diazepam in a trial in 15 'pink puffers' (Woodcock et al 1981a). Each treatment period was 2 weeks and patients received promethazine 25 mg t.i.d. and 50 mg nocte. Other sedative drugs were withdrawn 2 weeks before the study. Compared with placebo, patients on promethazine had:

- significant improvement in dyspnoea grade ($p < 0.05$)
- significantly greater walking distance in 12 min
- beneficial trend with daily dyspnoea rating
- no significant changes in spirometry results.

Many patients complained of drowsiness, although this was not statistically significant for the whole group. Only one dose reduction of promethazine was made.

In a subsequent study, promethazine 25 mg q.i.d. for 1 month was compared with codeine 30 mg q.i.d. in 11 patients with COAD (Rice et al 1987). Seven patients completed both arms of the study. No significant changes from the baseline were observed, although there was a trend toward improvement in exercise tolerance and dyspnoea. The study was stopped because of concerns about its safety. Three patients complained of drowsiness and one patient receiving promethazine was admitted to hospital because of deterioration in respiratory function.

Neuroleptics

In 12 young healthy volunteers who received chlorpromazine 25 mg PO, dyspnoea was reduced by almost one third during an exercise test compared with placebo (O'Neill et al 1985a). Although sedation was not a problem in the volunteers, the impact of regular chlorpromazine in elderly debilitated patients has not been evaluated.

Cannabinoids

The effects of cannabinoids on respiratory function have been studied (Ahmedzai et al 1984). In normal subjects, nabilone 2 mg b.i.d. results in:

- bronchodilatation
- increased ventilatory response to carbon dioxide
- relaxation
- sedation.

No controlled data are available in either COAD or advanced cancer. Even so, nabilone has been used in very anxious cancer patients with severe dyspnoea who were considered to be in danger of developing hypercapnic respiratory failure if given other respiratory sedatives, for example in carcino-matous lymphangitis and severe COAD (Ahmedzai 1993).

The initial dose of nabilone was 100 µg b.i.d., increasing if necessary up to 250 µg q.i.d. Above this dose, most patients complained of unacceptable sedation, and some of dysphoria. The use of nabilone is also limited by hypotension and tachycardia.

Nonsteroidal anti-inflammatory drugs (NSAIDs)

As with other tissues, prostaglandins (PGs) are produced in the lungs and act as a local hormone mediating various effects (Said 1982). Indomethacin has been shown to reduce the perception of dyspnoea during submaximal exercise in healthy volunteers (O'Neill et al 1985b). A study with a single dose of indomethacin 50 mg in patients with COAD, however, failed to detect a significant difference (Schiffman et al 1988). NSAIDs were also unhelpful in patients with chronic interstitial lung disease (O'Neill et al 1986).

CLINICAL USE OF MORPHINE FOR DYSPNOEA

Morphine and other opioids affect respiration in several ways (Table 20.2). The studies in patients with COAD, as well as those in cancer patients, provide a scientific basis for the use of opioids in dyspnoeic cancer patients. Many doctors, however, are reluctant to use morphine for dyspnoea. This probably relates to the following factors (Johanson 1990):

- unfamiliarity with published data about opioids and dyspnoea
- general lack of experience in treating dyspnoea
- working in a setting where there is a reflex avoidance of any drug with a potential for respiratory depression
- a perception that dyspnoea is a relatively low treatment priority
- doctor's fear that the use of morphine in terminally ill patients hastens death and is tantamount to euthanasia.

The trials of *low dose* dihydrocodeine (15 mg t.i.d.), morphine PO and hydro-morphone PR in patients with COAD, however, should be re-assuring to doctors coming from a respiratory medicine background. Information is not enough, however, and many doctors will need both encouragement and

Table 20.2   Effects of opioids on respiratory sensation

Effect	Unique to opioids
Cerebral sedation	No
Reduced anxiety	No
Reduced sensitivity to hypercapnia	No
Improved cardiac function	Yes
Inhaled route — act on opioid receptors in airways	Yes
Analgesia	Yes

From Ahmedzai 1993

support to begin to feel comfortable with the use of morphine for dyspnoea. The data at the beginning of this chapter demonstrate the need for better management. Early intervention and continuing supervision will prevent 'unendurable dyspnoea' at the end of life.

The question as to whether morphine hastens death in dyspnoeic patients is important. Rather like morphine in pain relief, however, it is a matter of timing. Early use might, in fact, *prolong* survival by reducing physical and psychological distress and exhaustion. In this situation, the ethical considerations discussed in Chapter 27 will help enable the doctor to distinguish between risk taking in the relief of extreme suffering and deliberate death acceleration (i.e. euthanasia).

Morphine or an alternative opioid should be considered for dyspnoea in advanced cancer in the following situations:

- increasing dyspnoea in an ambulant patient
- increasing dyspnoea in patients already receiving morphine for pain relief
- increasing dyspnoea in the bedfast/nonambulant patient
- acute respiratory emergencies at the very end of life.

Anxiety is an invariable concomitant of increasing or acute dyspnoea. This does not mean, however, that an anxiolytic should automatically be prescribed for dyspnoeic patients. The results of the use of diazepam in patients with COAD indicate the need for caution (see p. 388). Anxiety provoked by dyspnoea can be reduced in various ways:

- explanation
- breathing exercises
- advice about changing the pattern of one's life
- relaxation techniques.

A benzodiazepine should be considered only as an adjunct to psychological intervention. The latter may obviate the need for an anxiolytic — whereas continued use of a benzodiazepine may result in drowsiness, delirium and ataxia. On the other hand, a benzodiazepine should be used at the very end of life or with marked anxiety associated with rapidly increasing dyspnoea.

Morphine for dyspnoea in the ambulant patient

The following is a typical situation:

■ CLINICAL CHALLENGE
A 70 year-old man with advanced lung cancer and a history of moderate COAD complains of increasing shortness of breath on exertion. His haemoglobin concentration is 11.5 g/dl. He is not in congestive cardiac failure, nor does he have an infection or pleural effusion. Psychological and other nondrug measures have already been initiated and have helped considerably for several months. Over the last 2 weeks the dyspnoea has worsened significantly.

Generally, the dose of morphine to reduce dyspnoea is smaller than those used to relieve pain:

- begin with a test dose of 3–5 mg PO and review response
- if no adverse effect, continue with 3–5 mg q4h PO and 6–10 mg nocte
- if there is no benefit at all, and no adverse effects: increase the dose next day by about 50%
- if there is benefit but the resting respiratory rate is still 24/min or more: increase the dose after 2 or 3 days and review
- consider further adjustment to morphine after 2 or 3 more days.

At each stage, benefit must be weighed against adverse effects. The primary aim is a less dyspnoeic patient who, ideally, is neither sedated nor cyanosed. At a centre using IV morphine, the mean morphine dose for dyspnoea relief was 6 mg/h compared with 20 mg/h for pain relief (Cohen et al 1992).

Sometimes a patient may already be on oral morphine for pain relief. In this circumstance, a further upward adjustment of 33–50% in the dose of morphine may be considered.

Morphine for dyspnoea in the nonambulant patient

■ CLINICAL CHALLENGE
An emergency home visit is requested for a 39 year-old woman with disseminated cancer of the ovaries. She is sitting propped up in bed and looks terrified. Her respiration rate is 50/min and she has a tachycardia of 110/min. She has not slept for 3 nights and is exhausted.

Dyspnoea at rest is rare and always frightening. Thus, in terms of drug management, the right first step in the above case would be to give a benzodiazepine. The dose depends on several factors including current use of anxiolytic-sedative drugs. For example, in an old person who had not been taking regular diazepam, midazolam 5 mg SC would be appropriate. Alternatively, 2 mg IV could be given, followed by 1 mg/min until the patient is more settled. In practice, however, a SC injection can be given more quickly and easily, and it begins to act within minutes, during which time an opioid injection can be prepared for possible IV use.

The choice of route for administering morphine (or diamorphine) in this situation is partly determined by personal choice and partly by the clinical situation. It may be possible to use oral morphine if the patient is much improved with the benzodiazepine, or to increase an existing morphine regimen (for pain relief) by 50%. If a cannula has been inserted the IV route will be used for the opioid. The initial regimen referred to earlier is conservative (see p. 387); other centres would give an initial bolus dose of 2 mg, followed by 1 mg every 2 or 3 min until relief was obtained. A typical cumulative bolus dose of morphine would be 7–8 mg.

Again, the next step depends on personal choice and circumstances. An IV infusion of morphine can be used (Cohen et al 1991). In the UK, a SC infusion would normally be used if parenteral medication was indicated. In many patients, oral morphine will be acceptable and effective. In this situation, ordinary morphine preparations should be used, and not m/r forms, until a stable pattern of prescribing is achieved.

Nebulized morphine

There are several reports of the use of nebulized morphine (Masters et al 1985, Masters et al 1988). Systemic bio-availability by this route is low. Compared with IM morphine, a mean figure of 17% has been reported, ranging from 9–35% (Chrubasik et al 1988). In volunteers comparing nebulized morphine with IV morphine, bio-availability was found to be approximately 5% (Davis et al 1992). In a further study with 10 mg, 20 mg and 30 mg doses of nebulized morphine, comparable figures were obtained with all three doses (Davis et al 1994). In patients with severe COAD, nebulized morphine 5 mg increased exercise tolerance time by a mean of 65 seconds, compared with 9 seconds for placebo (Young et al 1989). Others have not demonstrated clear benefit in COAD, however, with such small doses (Beauford et al 1993).

Taken together, these data suggest that:

- nebulized morphine should not be used for pain relief because of low systemic bio-availability
- the effect on dyspnoea is probably a local one.

Nebulized morphine is now the route of choice for dyspnoea at many centres (Box 20.A). A dose-response curve has not been established. Patients should be allowed to determine their own optimal frequency. A few use the nebulizer only once or twice a day. The benefit experienced by a patient is occasionally dramatic. More often the effect is less marked. Most patients who have had a test dose, however, want to continue using it. It is not known which patients derive greatest benefit. Those with carcinomatous lymphangitis, small pleural

---

BOX 20.A
GUIDELINES FOR THE USE OF NEBULIZED MORPHINE

Most patients prefer a mouthpiece rather than a mask.

Start with morphine sulphate 20 mg diluted to 4–5 ml in normal saline.

Nebulize with air or oxygen at 8 L/min for 10 min or until most of the solution has disappeared.

Repeat q4h.

Consider increasing dose to 40 mg, then 80 mg.

Consider increasing frequency to q3h (40 mg) or even q2h (80 mg) if benefit obtained but shortlasting.

As the putative receptors are in the larger airways, particle size is immaterial.

effusions, large intrapulmonary masses or pneumonia *may* derive more benefit than patients with large pleural effusions, mesothelioma or anaemia. Nebulized morphine may also be of benefit in patients already taking even large doses of oral morphine for pain. Opinions differ about the value of nebulized morphine for dry cough. Some centres regard this as an indication for nebulized lignocaine, if unresponsive to systemic morphine.

MORPHINE INDUCED RESPIRATORY DEPRESSION

Occasionally a patient does develop obvious symptoms and/or signs of opioid excess, manifesting as drowsiness, confusion and a slow respiratory rate (< 10/min). Provided the patient is not agitated or cyanosed the best course of action is to omit the next one or two scheduled doses of morphine and then restart on half the previous dose if the adverse effects have largely or completely resolved. One reason for unintentional overdosing is cumulation of morphine-6-glucuronide (M6G) in renal failure. Another is an error in drug dispensing. The latter, although alarming, usually does not require the use of naloxone.

■ CASE HISTORY

An 82 year-old man with cancer of the prostate and COAD was admitted for pain relief. He was treated with diamorphine 120 mg and cyclizine 200 mg/24 h by SC infusion. Following admission, a nurse unfamiliar with the syringe driver, reset the rate from 2 mm/h to 48 mm/h. When the error was discovered 45 min later, the patient had received diamorphine 90 mg/h instead of 5 mg/h (O'Neill 1989).

■ CASE HISTORY

A 69 year-old woman with lung cancer was admitted for respite care. She complained of breathlessness and a nonproductive cough, for which she took diamorphine solution 'as needed'. Her total daily dose varied between 7.5 mg and 20 mg. On her second day in hospital, the patient was inadvertently given diamorphine 50 mg; i.e. 5 ml of 10 mg/ml instead of 5 ml of 1 mg/ml (O'Neill 1989).

Both patients had normal renal and hepatic function. They complained of nausea and vomited once 2–4 h after the overdose. Both patients were drowsy but were easily roused during the subsequent 24 h. Their observations were otherwise normal. Neither patient showed any clinical evidence of respiratory depression. Naloxone was available but was not used. Their normal regimen was restarted after 24 h (O'Neill 1989).

The need for caution if using naloxone has already been emphasized (see p. 299). A standard dose of 400 µg is usually too much and results in an agitated patient in severe pain and/or dyspnoea, necessitating further immediate treatment with morphine (Cohen et al 1992).

On the other hand, one elderly patient without pain or dyspnoea and no previous exposure to either weak or strong opioids, became bradypnoeic, cyanosed and comatose after m/r morphine 30 mg. After admission to a palliative care unit, he required three doses of naloxone 400 μg IV over several hours (Lovel T 1993 Personal Communication).

A similar situation has been reported with an 83 year-old woman with renal failure and chronic pancreatitis (Bigler et al 1984). She became bradypnoeic, cyanosed and comatose after three doses of m/r morphine 30 mg q8h. The woman required naloxone 200 μg/h by IV infusion *for nearly 4 days* to maintain respiration and level of consciousness.

MORPHINE INDUCED DYSPNOEA?

A 75 year-old man taking m/r morphine 30 mg nocte for bone pain complained of orthopnoea at night (Kerr 1988). Because of an attack in the dentist's chair, he went to the local hospital for a check up. He had a resting respiratory rate of 22/min, and blood gases and pH demonstrated respiratory alkalosis secondary to hyperventilation (Goldenheim 1988). He discontinued the morphine and the episodes of orthopnoea stopped.

An explanation for the discrepancy between symptoms and findings might relate to the dissociation between the time of the orthopnoea and the time of the investigations. The symptoms were generally at night; the tests were during the day by which time morphine and M6G would have been largely eliminated from the body. The patient, however, may represent an example of a syndrome seen occasionally in which a patient wakes up almost apnoeic as a result of a bedtime dose of morphine. The occasional deep respiration is rightly perceived as abnormal and the long silent gaps can be very frightening. It is not too difficult to see how this could be reported as 'orthopnoea'. The subsequent episode of 'acute breathlessness' in the dentist's chair could have been psychogenically induced.

There are anecdotal reports of another form of morphine related dyspnoea, namely, bronchospasm secondary to opioid induced bronchial histamine release. The fact that the increasing use of nebulized morphine has not led to a plethora of cases suggests that this syndrome must be very rare.

OPIOID INDUCED PULMONARY OEDEMA

It is over 100 years since William Osler published the first report of opioid induced pulmonary oedema (Osler 1880). It is now an accepted syndrome which has been described in association with various opioids (Bogartz & Miller 1971, Frand et al 1972a, Gottlieb & Boylen 1974, Presant et al 1975, Shanies 1977). Most reports involve diamorphine (Steinberg & Karliner 1968, Frand et al 1972b). Pulmonary oedema is a consistent autopsy finding in individuals who die of diamorphine overdose (Helpern & Rho 1966). Pulmonary oedema has also been reported with salicylates (Hrnicek et al 1976, Bowers et al 1977), chlordiazepoxide (Richman & Harris 1972) and barbiturates (Schoenfeld 1964).

Symptoms of pulmonary oedema occur within 2 h of injection (Frand et al 1972a). In some fatal cases, the needle has still been in the victim's vein at the time of death (Helpern & Rho 1966). Clinical manifestations vary; patients may be awake, somnolent or comatose. Respiratory patterns range from profound dyspnoea to apnoea. There may be frothy sputum, cyanosis and hypotension. Crepitations may or may not be present (Steinberg & Karliner 1968, Frand et al 1972b).

Arterial blood gas determinations usually reveal marked hypoxaemia and slight hypercapnia, with acidosis of mixed respiratory and metabolic origin. Central venous pressure is nearly always low (Frand et al 1972b). Chest radiographs generally display bilateral poorly defined fluffy opacities. Occasionally, only a single lung or portion of a lung is involved (Jaffe & Koschmann 1970). The heart is usually of normal size.

The pathogenesis of opioid induced pulmonary oedema is unclear. As in other forms of pulmonary oedema, increased capillary permeability results in fluid being exuded into the alveoli. The instigating factor, however, is unknown. Hypoxia, a hypersensitivity reaction, toxic effects of drug contaminants, and neurogenic stimuli have all been postulated to play a role but no proof has been forthcoming (Frand et al 1972b).

Treatment of opioid induced pulmonary oedema consists of oxygen and naloxone. Mechanical ventilation may be necessary. Response to treatment is usually rapid; physical findings of pulmonary oedema clear within 24 h. Radiographic improvement lags behind clinical improvement, and takes 3–4 days to resolve (Frand et al 1972b).

As is the case in other forms of noncardiogenic pulmonary oedema, treatment aimed at reducing intravascular volume, diminishing venous return, and stimulating inotropic cardiac function has no place in the treatment of this syndrome. Diuretics, rotating tourniquets, morphine, and digitalis (all used in cardiogenic pulmonary oedema) are not indicated and may be harmful.

REFERENCES

Addington-Hall J M, MacDonald L D, Anderson H R, Freeling P 1991 Dying from cancer: the views of bereaved family and friends about the experience of terminally ill patients. Palliative Medicine 5: 207–214

Ahmedzai S 1993 Palliation of respiratory symptoms. In: Doyle D, Hanks G W C, MacDonald N (eds) Oxford textbook of palliative medicine. Oxford University Press, Oxford, pp 349–378

Ahmedzai S, Carter R, Mills R J, Moran F 1984 Effects of nabilone on pulmonary function. Marihuana 1984: Proceedings of the Oxford Symposium on Cannabis. IRL Press, Oxford, pp 371–378

Beauford W, Saylor T T, Stansbury D W, Avalos K, Light R W 1993 Effects of nebulized morphine sulphate on the excercise tolerance of the ventilatory limited COPD patient. Chest 104: 175–178

Bigler D, Eriksen J, Christensen C B 1984 Prolonged respiratory depression caused by slow release morphine. Lancet i: 1477

Bogartz L J, Miller W C 1971 Pulmonary oedema associated with propoxyphene intoxication. Journal of the American Medical Association 215: 259–262

Bowers R E, Brigham K L, Owen P J 1977 Salicylate pulmonary oedema: the mechanism in sheep and review of the clinical literature. American Reviews of Respiratory Diseases 115: 261–268

Bruera E, Macmillan K, Pither J, MacDonald N 1990 Effects of morphine on the dyspnoea of terminal cancer patients. Journal of Pain and Symptom Management 5: 341–344

Bruera E, Schoeller T, Tun N, Maceachern T, Suarez-Almazor M 1992 Symptomatic benefit of supplemental oxygen in hypoxemic patients with advanced cancer. Journal of Palliative Care 8 (3): 68

Chrubasik J, Wust H, Friedrich G, Geller E 1988 Absorption and bioavailability of nebulized morphine. British Journal of Anaesthesia 61: 228–230

Cockcroft A, Guz A 1987 Breathlessness. Postgraduate Medical Journal 63: 637–641

Cohen M H, Johnston-Anderson A, Krasnow S H et al 1991 Continuous intravenous infusion of morphine for severe dyspnea. Southern Medical Journal 84: 229–234

Cohen M H, Johnston-Anderson A, Krasnow S H, Wadleigh R G 1992 Treatment of intractable dyspnea: clinical and ethical issues. Cancer Investigation 10: 317–321

Cowcher K, Hanks G W 1990 Long-term management of respiratory symptoms in advanced cancer. Journal of Pain and Symptom Management 5: 320–330

Davis C L, Lam W, Butcher M, Joel S P, Slevin M L 1992 Low systemic bioavailability of neublised morphine: potential therapeutic role for the relief of dyspnoea. British Journal of Cancer 65 (Suppl 16): 12

Davis C L, Lam W, Roberts M, Daniels J, Joel S P, Slevin M L 1994 The pharmacokinetics of nebulised morphine. [in press]

Eckenhoff J E, Oech S R 1960 The effects of narcotics and antagonists upon respiration and circulation in man. Clinical Pharmacology and Therapeutics 1: 701–708

Eimer M, Cable T, Gal P, Rothenberger L A, McCue J D 1985 Effects of clorazepate on breathlessness and exercise tolerance in patients with chronic airflow obstruction. Journal of Family Practice 21: 359–362

Eiser N, Denman W T, West C, Luce P 1991 Oral diamorphine: lack of effect on dyspnoea and exercise tolerance in the 'pink puffer' syndrome. European Respiratory Journal 4: 926–931

Frand U I, Shim C S, Williams M H Jr 1972a Methadone-induced pulmonary oedema. Annals of Internal Medicine 76: 975–979

Frand U I, Shim C S, Williams M H Jr 1972b Heroin-induced pulmonary oedema. Annals of Internal Medicine 77: 29–35

Goldenheim P D 1988 Comment: dyspnoea with controlled-release morphine sulfate tablets. Drug Intelligence and Clinical Pharmacy 22: 1005

Gottlieb L S, Boylen T C 1974 Pulmonary complications of drug abuse. Western Journal of Medicine 120: 8–16

Greene J G, Pucino F, Carlson J D, Storsved M, Strommen G L 1989 Effects of alprazolam on respiratory drive, anxiety, and dyspnoea in chronic airflow obstruction: a case study. Pharmacotherapy 9: 34–38

Helpern M, Rho Y M 1966 Deaths from narcotism in New York City. New York State Journal of Medicine 66: 2391–2408

Higginson I, McCarthy M 1989 Measuring symptoms in terminal cancer: are pain and dyspnoea controlled? Journal of the Royal Society of Medicine 82: 264–267

Hrnicek G, Skelton J, Miller W C 1976 Pulmonary edema and salicylate intoxication. Journal of the American Medical Association 230: 866–867

Jaffe R B, Koschmann E G 1970 Intravenous drug abuse: pulmonary, cardiac and vascular complications. American Journal of Roentgenology 109: 107–120

Johanson G A 1990 Should opioids or sedatives be used for dyspnoea in end-stage disease? American Journal of Hospice and Palliative Care 7 (4): 12–13

Johnson M A, Woodstock A A, Geddes D M 1983 Dihydrocodeine for breathlessness in 'pink puffers'. British Medical Journal 286: 675–677

Kerr H D 1988 Dyspnoea possibly associated with controlled-release morphine sulfate tablets. Drug Intelligence and Clinical Pharmacy 22: 397–399

Kirsch J L, Muro J R, Mahutte C K, Stansbury D W, Fischer C A, Light R W 1988 Effect of naloxone on maximal exercise performance and control of ventilation in chronic obstructive pulmonary disease. American Review of Respiratory Diseases 137: 439s

Lichter I, Hunt E 1990 The last 48 hours of life. Journal of Palliative Care 6 (4): 7–15

Light R W, Muro J R, Sato R J, Stansbury D W, Fischer C E, Brown S E 1989 Effects of oral morphine on breathlessness and exercise tolerance in patients with chronic obstructive pulmonary disease. American Review of Respiratory Diseases 139: 126–133

McGavin C R, Artvinli M, Nade H et al 1978 Dyspnoea, disability and distance walked: comparison of estimates of exercise performance in respiratory disease. British Medical Journal ii: 241–243

Man G C W, Hsu K, Sproule B J 1986 Effect of alprazolam on exercise and dyspnea in patients with chronic obstructive pulmonary disease. Chest 90 (6): 833–836

Masters N J, Bennett M R, Wedley J R 1985 Nebulised morphine: a new delivery method for pain relief. Practitioner 229: 649–650, 653

Masters N J, Heap G, Wedley J, Moore A 1988 Inhaled nebulised morphine and diamorphine: useful in general practice? Practitioner 232: 910–914

Mitchell-Heggs P, Murphy K, Minty K et al 1980 Diazepam in the treatment of dyspnoea in the 'pink puffer' syndrome. Quarterly Journal of Medicine, 49: 9–20

O'Neill W M 1989 Safety of diamorphine in overdosage. Palliative Medicine 3: 307–309

O'Neill P A, Morton P B, Stark R D 1985a Chlorpromazine: a specific effect on breathlessness? British Journal of Clinical Pharmacology 19: 793–797

O'Neill P A, Stark R D, Morton P B 1985b Do prostaglandins have a role in breathlessness? American Review of Respiratory Diseases 132: 22–24

O'Neill P A, Stretton T B, Stark R D, Eillis S H 1986 The effect of indomethacin on breathlessness in patients with diffuse parenchymal disease of the lung. British Journal of Diseases of the Chest 80: 72–79

Osler W 1880 Oedema of the left lung: morphia poisoning. In: Montreal General Hospital reports clinical and pathological, vol 1. Dawson Bros, Montreal, pp 291–292

Presant S, Knight L, Klassen G 1975 Methadone-induced pulmonary oedema. Canadian Medical Association Journal 113: 966–967

Reuben D B, Mor V 1986 Dyspnea in terminally ill cancer patients. Chest 89: 234–236

Rice K L, Kronenberg R S, Hedemark L L, Niewoehner D E 1987 Effects of chronic administration of codeine and promethazine on breathlessness and exercise tolerance in patients with chronic airflow obstruction. British Journal of Diseases of the Chest 81: 287–292

Richman S, Harris R D 1972 Acute pulmonary oedema associated with Librium abuse. Radiology 103: 57–58

Robin E D, Burke C M 1986 Single patient randomized clinical trial: opiates for intractable dyspnea. Chest 90: 888–891

Said S I 1982 Metabolic functions of the pulmonary circulation. Circulation Research 50: 325–333

Santiago T V, Pugliesi A C, Edelman N H 1977 Control of breathing during methadone addiction. American Journal of Medicine 62: 347–354

Santiago T V, Johnson J, Riley D J, Edelman N H 1979 Effects of morphine on ventilatory response to exercise. Journal of Applied Physiology 47: 112–118

Santiago T V, Remolina C, Scoles V, Edelman N H 1981 Endorphins and the control of breathing: ability of naloxone to restore flow resistive load compensation in chronic obstructive pulmonary disease. New England Journal of Medicine 304: 1190–1195

Saunders C 1989 Pain and impending death. In: Wall P D, Melzack R (eds) Textbook of pain, 2nd edn. Churchill Livingstone, Edinburgh, pp 624–631

Schiffman G L, Stansbury D W, Fischer C E, Sato R I, Light R W, Brown S E 1988 indomethacin and perception of dyspnea in chronic airflow obstruction. American Review of Respiratory Diseases 137: 1094–1098

Schoenfeld M R 1964 Acute pulmonary oedema caused by barbiturate poisoning. Angiology 15: 445–453

Sen D, Jones G, Leggat P O 1983 The response of the breathless patient treated with diazepam. British Journal of Clinical Practice June: 232–233

Shanies H M 1977 Noncardiogenic pulmonary oedema. Medical Clinics of North America 61: 1319–1337

Shook J E, Watkins W D, Camporesi E M 1990 Differential roles of opioid receptors in respiration, respiratory disease, and opiate-induced respiratory depression. American Review of Respiratory Diseases 142: 895–909

Stark R D 1988 Dyspnoea: assessment and pharmacological manipulation. European Respiratory Journal 1: 280–287

Stark R D, Morton P B, Sharman P, Percival P G, Lewis J A 1983 Effects of codeine on the respiratory responses to exercise in healthy subjects. British Journal of Clinical Pharmacology 15: 355–359

Steinberg A D, Karliner J S 1968 The clinical spectrum of heroin pulmonary oedema. Archives of Internal Medicine 122: 122–127

Ventafridda V, Ripamonti C, de Conno F, Tamburini M, Cassileth B R 1990 Symptom prevalence and control during cancer patients' last days of life. Journal of Palliative Care 6 (3): 7–11

Wasserman K, Casaburi R 1988 Dyspnea: physiological and pathophysiological mechanisms. Annuals of Review Medicine 39: 503–515

Woodcock A A, Gross E R, Geddes D M 1981a Drug treatment of breathlessness: contrasting effects of diazepam and promethazine in pink puffers. British Medical Journal 283: 343–345

Woodcock A A, Gross E R, Gellert A, Shah S, Johnson M, Geddes D M 1981b Effects of dihydrocodeine, alcohol, and caffeine on breathlessness and exercise tolerance in patients with chronic obstructive lung disease and normal blood gases. New England Journal of Medicine 305: 1611–1616

Woodcock A A, Johnson M A, Geddes D M 1982 Breathlessness, alcohol and opiates. New England Journal of Medicine 306: 1363–1364

Young I H, Daviskas E, Keena V A 1989 Effect of low dose nebulised morphine on exercise endurance in patients with chronic lung disease. Thorax 44: 387–390

Psychotropic drugs

In this chapter, the WHO classification of psychotropic drugs will be used (Box 21.A). 'Neuroleptic' (i.e. antipsychotic) is used rather than the older term 'major tranquillizer'. With the advent of more powerful benzodiazepines, the division of tranquillizers into major and minor is anachronistic. The word tranquillizer on its own, however, is still a useful umbrella term for both neuroleptics and anxiolytic sedatives.

PSYCHOTROPIC DRUGS AND PAIN RELIEF

The use of psychotropic drugs in the management of pain raises several questions (Breitbart 1992, Cameron 1992):

- do these drugs have specific analgesic activity?
- do they work by depressing the general level of arousal or by modifying sensory perception?
- is the apparent analgesic effect of tranquillizers and antidepressants secondary to a reduction of anxiety or an improvement in depression.

The first two questions will be discussed subsequently in relation to each of the five classes of psychotropic drugs. The following comments provide a short answer to the third.

Given that pain is an *unpleasant sensory and emotional experience* (IASP Subcommittee on Taxonomy 1980), there will be occasions when a highly anxious or deeply depressed patient in pain will benefit from an anxiolytic or an antidepressant. Indeed, there are times when pain remains resistant to analgesics until the concurrent psychological morbidity is dealt with.

Diazepam is also used to relieve recurrent or persistent cramp. Many patients troubled by cramp are also anxious. Diazepam, therefore, is of double benefit; it relaxes both muscles and mind.

BOX 21. A
WHO CLASSIFICATION OF PSYCHOTROPIC DRUGS

Neuroleptics

- butyrophenones
- phenothiazines

Anxiolytic sedatives

- barbiturates
- benzodiazepines
- buspirone
- hydroxyzine
- meprobamate

Antidepressants

- tricyclics
- mianserin
- selective serotonin re-uptake inhibitor (SSRI)
- mono-amine oxidase inhibitors (MAOIs)
- reversible inhibitors of mono-amine oxidase A (RIMA)

Psychostimulants

- caffeine
- cocaine
- dexamphetamine
- methylphenidate

Psychodysleptics (hallucinogens)

- cannabis (marihuana, hashish)
- lysergide (lysergic acid diethylamide, LSD)

The mind is sometimes the sole cause of the pain. Such pain is termed psychogenic and may well require a combination of psychotherapy and psychotropic medication to achieve relief. The classic example is atypical facial pain as a manifestation of depression. Psychogenic pain, however, is not restricted to clearly defined syndromes (Feinmann et al 1984). This may lead to difficulties in diagnosis and treatment (Kuhn & Bradman 1979).

NEUROLEPTICS

These drugs are marketed primarily as antipsychotics and include the phenothiazines and the butyrophenones. Except in the anxious, psychotic or delirious patient, there is little place for neuroleptic drugs in pain management. Anecdotal reports suggest, however, that neuroleptic drugs may have a specific place in the relief of phantom viscus pain.

Phenothiazines

In a volunteer study, most phenothiazines were found to be either mildly or markedly *algesic* (Moore & Dundee 1961). Nine phenothiazines were given IM in doses commonly employed in anaesthesia with atropine 600 µg as a premedication in women undergoing uterine curettage. Pain thresholds were measured 60–90 min later by applying increasing pressure to the anterior surfaces of the tibia. The results indicated that the phenothiazines could be classified into three groups, listed here in rank order of effect:

- some analgesic activity:
  — trimeprazine
  — chlorpromazine
  — promazine
- mildly algesic:
  — prochlorperazine
  — perphenazine
  — trifluoperazine
  — triflupromazine
- markedly algesic:
  — promethazine
  — pecazine

There was no clear relationship between analgesic action and chemical structure. Thus, while those with analgesic properties all have a dimethylamino-propyl side chain, so does promethazine which is markedly algesic. There is no evidence, however, that promethazine is algesic in cancer patients with pathological pain when taken as a night sedative. Likewise, prochlorperazine is often used concurrently with morphine as an anti-emetic without apparent loss of analgesic effect. Surprisingly, despite it heading the list, little interest has been shown in the use of trimeprazine as a co-analgesic.

In chronic pain, the combination of a neuroleptic with an antidepressant appears to be no more effective than treatment with an antidepressant alone (Getto et al 1987). Further, in a comparison of morphine and chlorpromazine in postoperative cancer patients, chlorpromazine was no better than placebo, and morphine and chlorpromazine together were no better than morphine alone (Fig. 21.1). The incidence of sedation was several times greater for the combination of morphine and chlorpromazine than for morphine alone. Despite these results, phenothiazines are still considered by some doctors to have an opioid sparing effect. But, as one observer commented:

> 'If a criterion of analgesia is that a patient is not bothering the staff by pushing the button and requesting more analgesic, a phenothiazine could be said to 'spare' analgesics. But if the patient is asked how bad the pain is, the reply will indicate that the phenothiazine seems not to be improving the situation, at least when administered on a single dose basis' (Beaver 1980).

Methotrimeprazine

Methotrimeprazine is the one exception: by injection, 20 mg is as potent as 10 mg of morphine, although it acts for only about 3 h (Beaver et al

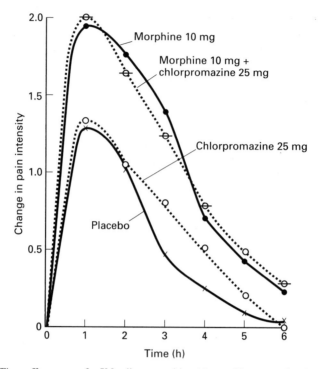

Fig. 21.1 Time-effect curves for IM saline, morphine 10 mg, chlorpromazine 25 mg and a combination of morphine 10 mg and chlorpromazine 25 mg. Randomized order of treatments on a complete crossover basis to 34 patients with cancer pain. (Reproduced with permission from Houde 1966.)

1966, Bonica & Halpern 1972). The oral to parenteral potency ratio for methotrimeprazine has not been determined. When allowance is made for differences in the first pass effect of the liver and in plasma halflife, methotrimeprazine by mouth is perhaps about 2/3 as potent as morphine on a weight for weight basis.

In many patients, methotrimeprazine causes unacceptable drowsiness. It is used at some centres solely in moribund patients. In this circumstance, however, it is being used primarily for sedation.

Methotrimeprazine also causes orthostatic (postural) hypotension, and some consider its use should be limited to nonambulant patients. A rigid limitation is unnecessary, however, provided one is aware of this effect.

Butyrophenones

Haloperidol is a butyrophenone neuroleptic. Compared with chlorpromazine, it is a more potent anti-emetic but causes less sedation and less anticholinergic and cardiovascular effects (Ayd 1976). On the other hand, it has a greater propensity for causing extrapyramidal reactions.

It has been claimed that haloperidol is able to relieve chronic cancer pain, either alone or in combination with opioids (Cavenar & Maltebie 1976,

Maltebie & Cavenar 1977). The six patients on which this claim is based all suffered from prolonged pain complicated by insomnia and physical and mental exhaustion. In other words, they were suffering from overwhelming pain (see p. 20). Patients received 10–30 mg of haloperidol nocte, usually starting with 10 mg and increasing rapidly if sleep remained disturbed. Benzhexol 5 mg b.i.d. was given prophylactically to prevent extrapyramidal effects. Other medication (including analgesics) was also modified.

These cases merely show that haloperidol is a useful alternative to diazepam or a phenothiazine in overwhelming pain. They do not support the contention that haloperidol has specific analgesic properties (Hanks et al 1983, Glazier 1990). As noted in Chapter 2, the most important step in the treatment of overwhelming pain is to ensure that the patient has a good night's sleep. The interaction between haloperidol and indomethacin, causing profound drowsiness, has already been noted (see p. 205).

ANXIOLYTIC SEDATIVES

Barbiturates

Barbiturates are contra-indicated in pain management. Subanaesthetic doses of thiopentone antagonize the analgesic effects of both the opioids and nitrous oxide (Clutton-Brock 1961). Although anticonvulsants, barbiturates are not of benefit in neuropathic pain (Tasker 1987). The algesic effect of barbiturates is probably mediated via the reticular formation in the brain stem (Brazier 1954). Sedative doses are needed to achieve an impact on the cerebral cortex. IV amylobarbitone and thiopentone are helpful in patients with overwhelming pain at the end of life (see p. 563).

Benzodiazepines

Benzodiazepines exert their effects on the CNS primarily by facilitating GABA (gamma-aminobutyric acid) binding to GABA receptors (Richter et al 1985). Benzodiazepines have anxiolytic, sedative, muscle relaxant, anticonvulsant and amnesic properties. Benzodiazepines also have an anti-emetic effect in patients receiving chemotherapy (Bishop et al 1984) and in volunteers receiving morphine by IV infusion (Coda et al 1992). Although it was originally thought that the effect was secondary to the amnesic effect, it is probable that benzodiazepines have a primary anti-emetic effect in certain circumstances (Coda et al 1992).

Although there is considerable overlap in the properties of individual benzodiazepines, the pharmacological profiles are not all identical (Ansseau et al 1984); hence the marketing of some benzodiazepines as anxiolytics and others as anticonvulsants. There is also considerable variation in pharmacokinetic properties:

- some are soluble in water, e.g. midazolam, flunitrazepam; others are not, e.g. diazepam
- some are prodrugs, e.g. flurazepam

Table 21.1   Classification of benzodiazepines

Short acting (halflife < 5 h)	Intermediate acting (halflife 5–25 h)	Long acting (halflife > 25 h)
Midazolam	Temazepam	Chlordiazepoxide[a]
Triazolam	Oxazepam	Clonazepam
	Lorazepam	Chlorazepate
	Flunitrazepam	Diazepam
		Flurazepam[b]
		Nitrazepam

[a] Halflife of active metabolite nordiazepam = 30–200 h.
[b] Halflife of active metabolite desalkylflurazepam = 40–250 h.

- some have one or more active metabolites
- including active metabolites, plasma halflives vary from 1–250 h (Table 21.1).

It is generally considered that benzodiazepines do not have a direct analgesic effect in nociceptive pain (Coda et al 1992). In one study, however, benefit was seen with alprazolam combined with an opioid in neuropathic pain (Fernandez et al 1987). Alprazolam, inhibits serotonin re-uptake (Zarcone et al 1989). It may, therefore, differ from other benzodiazepines.

Clonazepam is used at many centres as a second line anticonvulsant in neuropathic pain. The usual starting dose is 500 µg nocte for 1 week, with weekly increments of 500 µg up to a daily dose of 3 mg. Above 2 mg, it is probably better to give additional tablets at breakfast and/or lunch. The main limiting effect is sedation. A clear dose-response relationship is found in the treatment of trigeminal neuralgia (McQuay 1988). The situation is less clear with other causes of neuropathic pain. A threshold dose, or even a therapeutic window, may exist rather than a true dose-response curve (McQuay 1988).

Administration of midazolam by IV 'patient controlled anxiolysis' did not decrease postoperative morphine requirements, nor did it affect patients' pain scores (Egan et al 1992). On the other hand, intrathecal (IT) midazolam in animals potentiates morphine analgesia, probably by enhancing the affinity of spinal opioid receptors for opioids (Liao & Takemori 1990, Tejwani et al 1990).

Other animal studies have also shown an interaction between benzodiazepines and opioids (Britton et al 1983, Cooper 1983). In rats, benzodiazepines inhibit morphine glucuronidation (Pacifici et al 1986). Clonazepam and diazepam were the most potent inhibitors, and oxazepam and nitrazepam the least. Temazepam and midazolam were not examined. Whether this has any clinical significance is not known.

The following three case histories illustrate the benefit of an anxiolytic in the right circumstances (Richtsmeier et al 1992).

■ CASE HISTORY

A 17 year-old adolescent with a bone tumour required repeated debridement for a skin flap. He had severe pain (10/10) whenever his leg was manipulated.

Patient controlled analgesia (PCA) with morphine failed to relieve the pain. IV diazepam was then tried. After this he became relaxed enough to discuss his anxiety and the details of his care. He subsequently refused opioids and had only minimal pain during further debridement.

■ CASE HISTORY

An 11 year-old girl with chondroblastoma of the tibia was treated with curettage of the lesion and iliac bone graft. IV morphine was administered by patient controlled analgesia (PCA). The pain remained 8/10 and she was also troubled by nausea and insomnia. Medication was changed to oral hydrocodone and paracetamol, which resulted in less nausea and improved comfort. The next day, however, the patient complained of severe abdominal pain, leg spasms, and nausea. She was distressed and refused to participate in physical therapy. She was given lorazepam 0.5 mg IV and oral paracetamol. Within 30 min her pain, anxiety and nausea abated, and she was able to participate in physical therapy without difficulty. She received one more dose of lorazepam but subsequently required only paracetamol for mild pain.

■ CASE HISTORY

An 18 year-old adolescent with sickle cell disease presented with severe pain (8/10). He had already received two doses of pethidine 75 mg IM and hydroxyzine 25 mg IM, as well as morphine 8 mg IV. He had had minimal pain relief. The patient was then given levorphanol 2 mg IV without benefit. Subsequently, alprazolam 0.25 mg PO was given. Within 1 h the patient stated, 'Now my muscles feel relaxed'. Pain relief improved dramatically and he slept moderately well. He was discharged on oral analgesics within 16 h of receiving alprazolam.

Diazepam is probably the benzodiazepine most commonly used for pain relief. It is used as a combined anxiolytic and night sedative in patients who are very anxious or fearful and in those who have cramp or myofascial pain.

The prescription of diazepam is sometimes discouraged because of its potential for causing depression if used for prolonged periods. In my experience, it is not notably depressing, possibly because the relief of anxiety and pain has a counteracting effect and because of the relatively short periods it is generally used for in palliative care (i.e. weeks rather than months). As with phenothiazines, however, it is important to be aware that depression may develop and that an antidepressant may need to be substituted.

Sedative and respiratory depressant effects are increased by the concurrent use of opioids. Respiratory depression, however, is a serious risk only when a potent benzodiazepine such as midazolam is given IV.

Concern is often expressed about benzodiazepine dependence (Adams 1989). Indeed, in New York State for example, prescriptions for benzodiazepines must be written on the same triplicate forms as strong opioids (King & Strain 1990). There is less need for concern in patients with advanced cancer because of their short prognosis. Even so, benzodiazepines should not be used as the panacea for anxiety. All psychotropic drugs, when used for psychological reasons, must form only one component of a multimodal strategy.

Hydroxyzine

Hydroxyzine is an anxiolytic-sedative with antihistaminic, antispasmodic and anti-emetic properties. In postoperative patients, hydroxyzine 100 mg IM has been shown to have analgesic activity approaching that of morphine 8 mg IM. Given together, hydroxyzine and morphine have additive effects (Fig. 21.2). The sedative effect of the combination was only slightly greater than that of morphine alone. In a second postoperative study, morphine 5 mg IM and hydroxyzine 100 mg IM gave comparable relief to morphine 10 mg alone (Hupert et al 1980).

Some centres in the USA routinely prescribe hydroxyzine 25 mg PO q4h during the day and 50–100 mg PO nocte with oral morphine (Rumore & Schlichting 1986). These doses, however, are much less than 100 mg IM. Even so, hydroxyzine offers several theoretical advantages:

- if opioid sparing, it could reduce adverse opioid effects

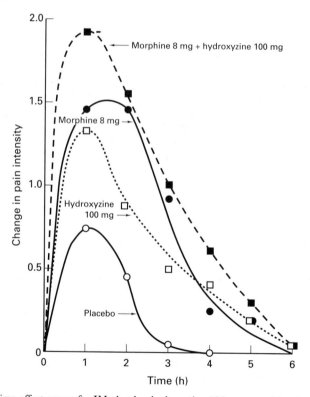

Fig. 21.2   Time-effect curves for IM placebo, hydroxyzine 100 mg, morphine 8 mg and a combination of hydroxyzine 100 mg and morphine 8 mg as single treatments to patients with postoperative pain. (Reproduced with permission from Beaver & Feise 1976.)

- separate anti-emetic, anxiolytic and night sedative drugs might not be needed.

These potential benefits have not been evaluated.

ANTIDEPRESSANTS

The place of the antidepressants in pain management is well established (Max 1990, Onghena and Van Houdenhove 1992). Most studies have been in patients with postherpetic neuralgia or diabetic neuropathy, predominantly with tricyclic antidepressants (Box 21.B). Antidepressants appear to act in two main ways:

- potentiating opioid analgesia (an 'opioid sparing' effect), probably through both noradrenergic and serotonergic mechanisms (Botney and Fields 1983, Levine et al 1986, Ventafridda et al 1990)
- a direct analgesic effect, which is most apparent in tension headaches and neuropathic pain (Spiegel et al 1983, Zitman et al 1990, Onghena and Van Houdenhove 1992).

An 'opioid sparing' effect has been demonstrated in cancer patients receiving morphine and imipramine 50–75 mg nocte (Walsh 1986). Patients receiving imipramine needed, on average, 20% less morphine. Perhaps the most dramatic example of an interaction, however, is the synergistic effect between morphine and desipramine in the tail flick test in the rat (Driessen et al 1990).

BOX 21.B
ANTIDEPRESSANTS AND CHRONIC NONMALIGNANT PAIN (Getto et al 1987, Onghena & Van Houdenhove 1992)

Although the analgesic effect is distinct from the antidepressant effect, patients with depression and chronic nonmalignant pain are more likely to benefit from the use of an antidepressant drug.

Most effective in chronic headache and neuropathic pain.

Least effective in patients with chronic musculoskeletal pain or chronic pain syndrome (see Chapter 2).

Although amitriptyline is the antidepressant most often studied, benefit is seen with most antidepressants.

Mixed serotonin and noradrenaline re-uptake inhibitors provide greatest relief (e.g. amitriptyline, imipramine).

The dose required for pain relief is usually lower than that required for major depression.

In nondepressed patients, it is advisable to start with lower doses to reduce the likelihood of distressing anticholinergic effects.

In patients with pain related insomnia, a sedative antidepressant should be given in a single dose in the evening or at bedtime.

The combination of a neuroleptic with an antidepressant is no more effective than an antidepressant alone.

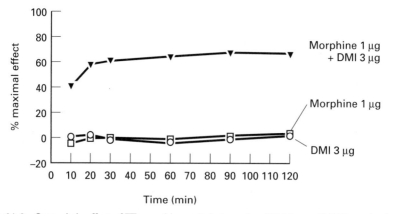

Fig. 21.3 Synergistic effect of IT morphine and desipramine (DMI) on tail flick test in the rat, represented as % of maximum achievable effect. (Reproduced with permission from Driessen et al 1990.)

In the given doses, both substances alone were ineffective but together produced a definite antinociceptive effect (Fig. 21.3).

The direct analgesic effect is independent of any antidepressant effect (Watson et al 1982, Max et al 1987) and becomes apparent several days before the antidepressant effect (Hameroff et al 1982). The mixed serotonin-noradrenaline re-uptake blockers are the most effective (Table 21.2; Kishore-Kumar et al 1989, Onghena and Van Houdenhove 1992). In neuropathic pain, maprotiline, a selective noradrenaline re-uptake blocker, is less effective than amitriptyline, a mixed re-uptake blocker (Watson et al 1992. A selective serotonin re-uptake blocker, paroxetine 40 mg/day, is less effective than another mixed re-uptake blocker, namely, imipramine in individualized doses (Sindrup et al 1990).

In the maprotiline study, there was a suggestion that there may be sub-groups of patients which respond better to a particular drug (Watson et al 1992). This could be because of genetic differences in the balance and type of neurotransmitters. It has therefore been suggested that, if amitriptyline fails to relieve, maprotiline (or desipramine) should be tried. Antidepressants, are still widely regarded as the drugs of choice for neuropathic pain. They are, however, not the whole story (Box 21.C).

A synopsis of possible underlying mechanism for this direct analgesic effect is given in Box 21.D. It is sometimes suggested that antidepressants are better for superficial burning pain and anticonvulsants better for stabbing pain. Amitriptyline, however, relieves burning and stabbing pains equally well (Max et al 1987, Watson et al 1992).

Most antidepressants except mono-amine oxidase inhibitors (MAOIs) act by inhibiting the presynaptic re-uptake of serotonin or noradrenaline or both (Fig. 21.4). A meta-analysis of 39 controlled trials indicated that mixed serotonin and noradrenaline re-uptake inhibitors were the most effective for pain relief (Onghena & Van Houdenhove 1992). Indeed, specific serotonin re-uptake inhibitors (SSRI) such as fluoxetine and zimelidine failed to pro-

Table 21.2 Pharmacological properties of some antidepressant drugs

Antidepressant drugs	Type	Plasma halflife (h)	Noradrenaline uptake inhibition	Serotonin uptake inhibition	Anticholinergic effects	Sedative effects
Tricyclic compounds						
Imipramine[a]	Tertiary amine	4–18	++	+++	++	++
Amitriptyline[b]	Tertiary amine	10–25	+	+++	+++	++
Clomipramine	Tertiary amine	16–20	+	+++	++	++
Nortriptyline	Secondary amine	13–93	+++	+	++	0
Desipramine	Secondary amine	12–61	+++	0	+	0
Protriptyline	Secondary amine	54–198	+++	++	++	0
Doxepin[c]	Tertiary amine	8–25	+	+	+++	++
Dothiepin	Tertiary amine	14–40	++	+	+	++
Related compounds						
Viloxazine (bicyclic)	Secondary amine	2–5	+++	0	0	0
Maprotiline (bridged tricyclic)	Secondary amine	27–58	+++	+	+	+
Mianserin[d]	Tertiary amine	8–19	0	0	0	++
Unrelated compounds						
Trazodone[d]		4	0	+	0	++

[a] Metabolized to desipramine.
[b] Metabolized to nortriptyline.
[c] Metabolized to desmethylodoxepin (beta halflife 33–81 h).
[d] Inhibits presynaptic alpha$_2$ receptors.
Pharmacological activity: 0 = none; + = slight; ++ = moderate; +++ = marked.
From Ashton 1987

BOX 21.C
APPROACH TO NEUROPATHIC PAIN

Nerve compression pain is generally more responsive to opioids than neural injury pain.

A combination of morphine and a corticosteroid may well relieve nerve compression pain resistant to morphine alone.

Most pure neural injury pains (e.g. chronic postoperative scar pains, postherpetic neuralgia) are best treated with secondary analgesics in the first instance:

- antidepressant (see Chapter 21) $\left.\right\}$ generally regarded as drugs of choice
- anticonvulsant (see Chapter 23)
- alprazolam (see Chapter 21)
- mexiletine (see Chapter 23)
- flecainide (see Chapter 23)

Spinal analgesia (see Chapter 19) will be needed for some patients, particularly those with cancer related plexopathy:

- morphine
- morphine and bupivacaine
- clonidine
- morphine and clonidine
- morphine, bupivacaine and clonidine

SC ketamine with PO/SC morphine is an alternative to spinal analgesia (see Chapter 23).

Nondrug treatments include:

- TENS (see Chapter 26)
- dorsal column stimulation (see Chapter 25)
- hypnosis (see Chapter 26)

BOX 21.D
POSSIBLE MECHANISMS FOR THE DIRECT ANALGESIC EFFECT OF ANTIDEPRESSANTS (Breitbart 1992)

Serotonin re-uptake blockade
Noradrenaline re-uptake blockade
Desensitization of alpha$_2$- and beta-adrenergic receptors
Potentiation of alpha,-adrenergic and serotonin receptor agonists
Decreasing sensitivity of adrenergic receptors on injured nerve sprouts
Inhibiting paroxysmal neuronal discharges
Adenosinergic effects
Antihistamine effects

vide relief in patients with diabetic neuropathy and postherpetic neuralgia responsive to amitriptyline (Watson & Evans 1985, Lynch et al 1990). On the other hand, paroxetine (another SSRI) was shown to be effective in a trial in diabetic neuropathy (Sindrup et al 1990). In patients with a paroxetine plasma concentration above 150 nM, pain relief was similar to that obtained with imipramine and with fewer adverse effects.

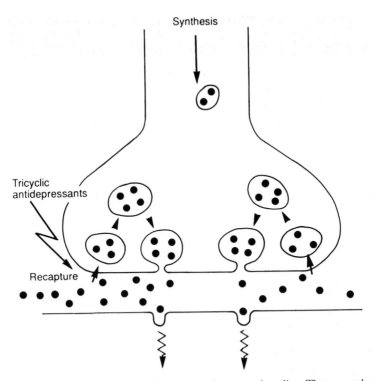

Fig. 21.4 Dots represent molecules of either serotonin or noradrenaline. These are released from the presynaptic nerve fibres and act as neurotransmitters, i.e. activate postsynaptic transmission via a specific receptor. Unused molecules are recycled. Re-uptake is blocked by tricyclic antidepressants, thereby maintaining a higher level of postsynaptic activity.

One explanation for this disparity is that high degrees of serotonin re-uptake inhibition may be needed for analgesia, and that the doses of fluoxetine and zimelidine were insufficient. The poor results with patients with low paroxetine concentrations would be consistent with this view. An alternative explanation is that paroxetine has a second unidentified action in addition to serotonin re-uptake inhibition.

If further studies confirm that paroxetine is generally effective in neuropathic pain, it will herald less toxic treatment for serotonin responsive neuropathic pain. That said, it should be pointed out that desipramine is as effective as amitriptyline and causes less severe adverse effects (Lynch et al 1990). For reasons of fashion, however, amitriptyline continues to be used at many centres.

The following questions need to be asked about antidepressant analgesia:

- what is the correct dose of an antidepressant when used to relieve neuropathic pain?
- is there a dose-response curve for the analgesic effect of antidepressants?

The time course for antidepressant analgesia permits weekly upward adjustments in the dose. Rapid oral loading with imipramine 50–350 mg/day in diabetic patients produced near maximal analgesia after 6 days (Sindrup et al

1990). In a study of dothiepin in chronic pain, outpatients were started on 75 mg nocte and only a few found it intolerable (McQuay H J 1990 Personal Communication). Because tricyclics have plasma halflives of about 24 h, the drug will cumulate for at least a week after each dose increment. Poor metabolizers are at risk of severe toxicity.

Although there are anecdotal reports of responses to doses as low as 25–40 mg, most doctors move arbitrarily up to 50–75 mg as soon as possible. Using a less toxic drug than amitriptyline facilitates dose escalation.

Amitriptyline

At many centres, amitriptyline is still regarded as the antidepressant of choice for neuropathic pain. A clear dose-response effect has been shown for its analgesic effect (Max et al 1987, McQuay et al 1993; Fig. 21.5). At some centres the dose of amitriptyline is raised on a weekly basis until either the pain is relieved or adverse effects prevent a further increase.

Treatment with amitriptyline is limited by its adverse effects:

- sedation
- orthostatic hypotension
- anticholinergic effects (Box 21.E)
- aggravation of pre-existing heart block.

The use of amitriptyline is associated with a doubling of the incidence of femoral fractures (Ray et al 1987).

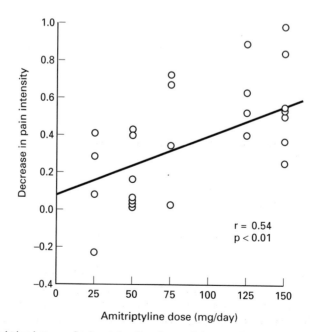

Fig. 21.5 Relation between final amitriptyline dose and decrease in pain intensity over the 6 week treatment period. (Reproduced with permission from Max et al 1987.)

BOX 21.E
ANTICHOLINERGIC EFFECTS

Caused by
Belladonna alkaloids

- atropine
- hyoscine

Neuroleptics

- haloperidol
- phenothiazines

Antidepressants

- mianserin
- tricyclics

Antihistamines

- chlorpheniramine
- cyclizine
- hydroxyzine
- promethazine

Antispasmodics

- mebeverine
- oxybutynin
- propantheline

Effects
'dry as a bone,
blind as a bat,
red as a beet,
hot as a hare,
mad as a hatter'

Visual

- mydriasis   } blurred
- loss of accommodation } vision

Cardiovascular

- palpitations   } also related to noradrenaline
- extrasystoles   } potentiation and a
- arrhythmias   } quinidine-like action

Gastro-intestinal

- dry mouth
- heartburn (reduced tone in lower oesophageal sphincter)
- constipation

Urinary

- hesitancy of micturition
- retention of urine

There appears to be a 'therapeutic window' for amitriptyline in some patients (Watson 1984). Seven patients with postherpetic neuralgia or painful diabetic neuropathy had good relief with amitriptyline 20–100 mg (median 50 mg). With this dose the pain was reduced from severe to mild. When the dose was increased, the pain became severe again; when decreased the pain became mild again. Most patients do not manifest this effect.

Nortriptyline is the major active metabolite of amitriptyline and a 'therapeutic window' was noted for its antidepressant effect in one trial (Kragh-Sorensen et al 1976). Thus, if a patient given a loading dose of a tricyclic drug reports increased pain, lowering the dose to 25–50 mg nocte might bring relief.

The maximum total dose should be maintained for 3 weeks before concluding that the drug is ineffective. Because sudden discontinuation may cause insomnia, amitriptyline should be tapered over 2 weeks when stopping treatment.

Desipramine

Desipramine is not sedative and has only mild anticholinergic properties. It can, however, cause marked orthostatic hypotension and exacerbate heart block (Blackwell 1987). Because desipramine is a selective noradrenaline re-uptake blocker it is likely to be less effective than amitriptyline. In one trial in diabetics given a mean dose of over 200 mg/day, no patient reported complete relief and 7/20 had none. There was no relationship between relief and drug dose or plasma concentration. These results were not as good as those seen with amitriptyline in another trial. On the other hand, in postherpetic neuralgia, desipramine produced better analgesia than had been previously obtained with amitriptyline (Kishore-Kumar et al 1990). Thus, until a crossover trial is completed, it will not be possible to be certain about the relative efficacy of amitriptyline and desipramine. Even so, desipramine is a useful alternative in patients unable to tolerate amitriptyline.

Several studies have examined the interaction of desipramine and morphine in humans. In one, although it had no analgesic effect alone, desipramine 50 mg nocte for 7 days before operation resulted in significantly better relief with morphine postoperatively (Levine et al 1986). In another, desipramine 50 mg nocte for 3 nights beginning one week before operation had a similar effect to the 7 day course (Gordon et al 1993). If given for the final 3 nights before the operation, however, desipramine made no difference (Fig. 21.6). These results reflect the known latency in humans in relation to the antidepressant effect of tricyclic drugs.

PSYCHOSTIMULANTS

Psychostimulants have been shown to enhance analgesia (Forrest et al 1977, Bruera et al 1989, Bruera et al 1992b). Clinical experience suggests, however, that such drugs should be used very selectively. Many cancer patients are anxious because of physical deterioration and uncertainty, and a psychostimulant may well exacerbate anxiety and make matters worse.

Dexamphetamine

Dexamphetamine potentiated the action of opioid analgesics in 450 young patients after abdominal and orthopaedic operations (Forrest et al 1977). Pain

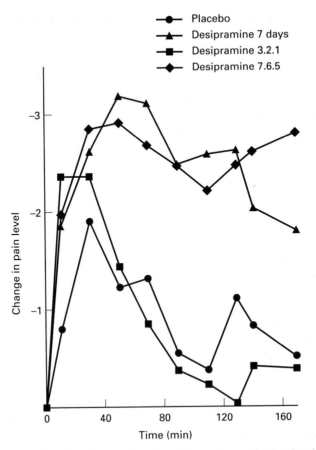

Fig. 21.6 Change in intensity after morphine 6 mg IV in postoperative dental patients who had previously received desipramine. ▲ = patients who received desipramine 50 mg PO for 7 days pre-operatively; ■ = patients who received desipramine 50 mg PO for the immediate 3 pre-operative days; ◆ = patients who received desipramine 50 mg PO for 3 days starting 7 days pre-operatively; ● = patients who received placebo. (Reproduced with permission from Gordon et al 1993.)

relief scores definitely improved when amphetamine was added. The effect on wakefulness was less marked. Many patients complained of sweating, however, and there was a tendency towards more dizziness and nausea. Other adverse effects included visual disturbance, body tremors and flushing. This study raises several questions:

- how would the combination work in the elderly, in whom the adverse psychological effects of drugs are more easily evoked, and in whom myocardial stimulation may more readily cause an arrhythmia?
- could the combined smooth muscle depressant properties of the two drugs result in a higher rate of urinary retention and ileus?

The place of dexamphetamine in advanced cancer is limited because most patients appear to do better on a mildly sedative regimen. In patients with continued troublesome drowsiness or lack of concentration, the addition of dexamphetamine 2.5–5 mg in the morning and at midday may well be of benefit. Tolerance may occur. Thus, the dose should be increased if, after several weeks, the patient complains that 'it is no longer working'. Dexamphetamine antagonizes drug induced sedation and is itself antagonized by sedative drugs. The concurrent use of a sedative and a psychostimulant is, therefore, pharmacological nonsense.

Methylphenidate

Methylphenidate is an amphetamine with a short halflife. It is well tolerated by elderly ill patients (Kaplitz 1975, Katon & Raskind 1980). In a controlled trial, 10 mg each morning improved cognitive function in 20 cancer patients receiving morphine $\geq$ 150 mg/24 h by SC infusion (Bruera et al 1992a). No changes were observed, however, in pain, nausea and activity scores.

In a subsequent open study in 14 cancer patients with severe incident pain, methylphenidate 10 mg was given at 0800 h and 5 mg at 1200 h (Bruera et al 1992b). This enabled the daily dose of morphine to increase to a higher level before sedation was complained of (Table 21.3). The causes of the incident pain were bone metastasis in 13 and inguinal lymphadenopathy in one. In 12, weight bearing and walking provoked the pain and in the other two, sitting did. Patients with a history of drug or alcohol dependence, psychiatric conditions, agitated delirium or paranoia were not prescribed methylphenidate. In consequence only two thirds of patients with severe incident pain received it. One patient, not included in the results, developed acute dysphoria and agitation after the first test dose. This settled after haloperidol 2 mg SC and the patient did not receive further methylphenidate. Previous experience with methylphenidate suggests that if toxicity occurs it will usually do so within 2 days of starting treatment (Bruera et al 1987).

The 14 patients received methylphenidate for a mean of 37 ± 14 days. The dose of methylphenidate was subsequently increased if sedation occurred with no recent dose increase of morphine. As a result, the final mean daily dose was 42 ± 15 mg. This suggests that tolerance occurs.

Cocaine

As noted in Chapter 14, the effect of cocaine 10 mg was evaluated in two controlled trials of the Brompton cocktail in cancer patients (Melzack et al 1979, Twycross 1979). Neither showed any lasting benefit from the addition

Table 21.3 Effect of methylphenidate on morphine tolerance and pain in 14 cancer patients with severe incident pain

	Mean daily dose of morphine (mg)	Mean pain score (VAS)	Mean sedation (VAS)
Before methylphenidate	248	55	65
After methylphenidate	405	38	42

From Bruera et al 1992b

of cocaine. Some patients, notably older ones, develop an agitated delirium with hallucinations when given morphine and cocaine, particularly if the dose of cocaine is > 10 mg q4h. Symptoms abate when cocaine is withdrawn.

There is no longer any justification for using the Brompton cocktail. Indeed, the *routine* use of any psychostimulant is to be deplored. When starting oral morphine, elderly patients should be told that they may feel drowsy for several days but that the drowsiness will clear during the first week. If troublesome drowsiness persists, other reasons should be looked for before ascribing it solely to morphine (see p. 322). In *rare* instances, it may be appropriate to prescribe a psychostimulant for persistent drowsiness, either dexamphetamine 2.5–5 mg or methylphenidate 10 mg once or twice in the first half of the day.

PSYCHODYSLEPTICS

Cannabis

Cannabis is a weak psychodysleptic. Tetrahydrocannabinol (THC), the active principle in cannabis (marihuana), possesses euphoriant, analgesic, appetite stimulant and anti-emetic effects. Controlled trials have shown that in patients with previous cannabis exposure, THC can provide comparable relief to codeine (Noyes et al 1975). In patients without previous exposure, THC carries with it a risk of unacceptable adverse effects, including (Noyes et al 1975, Noyes et al 1976):

- sedation
- thought impairment
- depersonalization.

Nabilone is a THC homologue with anxiolytic properties (Lemberger & Rowe 1975).

The main thrust behind moves in the USA in the 1980s to legalize cannabis for medicinal use lay in its potential role as an anti-emetic for patients receiving chemotherapy. The anti-emetic effect is closely related to the euphoriant effect, suggesting that the mechanism of action is mediated via the psychological component of nausea and vomiting. Patients say, however, that THC capsules are not as effective as cannabis cigarettes, even though the capsule contains three times as much THC.

With the use of dexamethasone and high dose IV metoclopramide, and latterly $5HT_3$ receptor antagonists, there is little justification for encouraging the use of THC or nabilone.

Lysergide

Lysergide (lysergic acid diethylamide/LSD) is a potent psychodysleptic. It is a Schedule 1 Controlled Drug. This means that it is *not* available for use medicinally. It has been used successfully in a small number of cancer patients, however, more as an aid to psychotherapy than as an analgesic.

In one study, the following criteria were used in patient selection (Richards et al 1972). The patient must:

- be suffering from physical pain, depression, anxiety or psychological isolation associated with his malignancy
- have a life expectancy of at least 3 months
- have no evidence of brain metastases or organic brain disease
- have no gross psychopathology nor be prepsychotic.

The treatment procedure consisted of three phases:

- a series of interviews totalling 6–12 h over a period of 2–3 weeks in which rapport was established and the patient was prepared for the drug session
- the lysergide session
- several subsequent drug free interviews for the integration of the lysergide session experiences.

Pain relief following lysergide assisted psychotherapy often lasted weeks or months. There was no clear dose-response relationship and the effect of lysergide was not predictable. The relief almost certainly resulted from a change in the patient's psychological outlook.

REFERENCES

Adams J E 1989 News from the council on research: task force on benzodiazepine dependency. Psychiatric Research Reports 4: 3

Ansseau M, Doumont A, Diricq St 1984 Methodology required to show clinical differences between benzodiazepines. Current Medical Research and Opinion 8 (Suppl 4): 108–113

Ashton C H 1987 Brain systems, disorders and psychotropic drugs. Oxford Medical Publications, Oxford

Ayd F J 1976 Haloperidol update: 1975. Proceedings of the Royal Society of Medicine 69: 14–18

Beaver W T 1980 Combination analgesics. In: The Use of Analgesics. Postgraduate Medicine Publications, Riker Laboratories, Northridge, California, pp 27–37

Beaver W T, Feise G 1976 Comparison of the analgesic effects of morphine, hydroxyzine and their combination in patients with postoperative pain. In: Bonica J J, Albe-Fessard D G (eds). Advances in pain research and therapy, vol 1. Raven Press, New York, pp 553–557

Beaver W T, Wallenstein S L, Houde R W, Rogers A 1966 A comparison of the analgesic effects of methotrimeprazine and morphine in patients with cancer. Clinical Pharmacology and Therapeutics 5: 436–446

Bishop J F, Oliver I N, Wolf M M et al 1984 Lorazepam: a randomized, double-blind, crossover study of a new antiemetic in patients receiving cytotoxic chemotherapy and prochlorperazine. Journal of Clinical Oncology 2: 691–695

Blackwell B 1987 Side effects of antidepressant drugs. In: Hales R E, Frances A J (eds) Psychiatry update: The American Psychiatry Association Annual, vol 6. American Psychiatry Association, Washington, pp 724–745

Bonica J J, Halpern L M 1972 Analgesics. In: Modell W (ed) Drugs of Choice 1972–1973. Mosby, St Louis, pp 185–217

Botney M, Fields H L 1983 Amitriptyline potentiates morphine analgesia by a direct action on the central nervous system. Annals of Neurology 13: 160–164

Brazier M A B 1954 Brain mechanisms and consciousness. Oxford University Press, Oxford, p 163

Breitbart W 1992 Psychotropic adjuvant analgesics for cancer pain. Psycho-Oncology 1: 133–145

Britton K T, Stewart R D, Risch S C 1983 Benzodiazepines attenuate stimulated B-endorphin release. Psychopharmacology Bulletin 19: 759–760

Bruera E, Brenneis C, Chadwick S, Hanson J, MacDonald R N 1987 Methylphenidate associated with narcotics for the treatment of cancer pain. Cancer Treatment Reports 71: 67–70

Bruera E, Brenneis C, Paterson A H, MacDonald R N 1989 Use of methylphenidate as an adjuvant to narcotic analgesics in patients with advanced cancer. Journal of Pain and Symptom Management 4: 3–6

Bruera E, Miller M J, Macmillan K, Kuehn N 1992a Neuropsychological effects of methylphenidate in patients receiving a continuous infusion of narcotics for cancer pain. Pain 48: 163–166

Bruera E, Fainsinger R, MacEachern T, Hanson J 1992b The use of methylphenidate in patients with incident cancer pain receiving regular opiates: a preliminary report. Pain 50: 75–77

Cameron L B 1992 Neuropsychotropic drugs as adjuncts in the treatment of cancer pain. Oncology 6: 65–80

Cavenar J O, Maltebie A A 1976 Another indication for haloperidol. Psychosomatics 17(3): 128–130

Clutton-Brock J 1961 Pain and the barbiturates. Anaesthesia 16: 80–88

Coda B A, Mackie A, Hill H F 1992 Influence of alprazolam on opioid analgesia and side effects during steady-state morphine infusions. Pain 50: 309–316

Cooper S J 1983 GABA and endorphin mechanisms in relation to the effects of benzodiazepines on feeding and drinking. Progress in Neuropsychopharmacology and Biological Psychiatry 7: 495–503

Driessen B, Schlutz H, Reimann W 1990 Evidence for a non-opioid component in the analgesic action of tramadol. Naunyn Schmiedeberg's Archives of Pharmacology 341: R104

Egan K J, Ready L B, Nessly M, Greer B E 1992 Self-administration of midazolam for postoperative anxiety: a double-blinded study. Pain 49: 3–8

Feinmann C, Harris M, Cawley R 1984 Psychogenic pain: presentation and treatment. British Medical Journal 288: 436–438

Fernandez F, Adams F, Holmes V F 1987 Analgesic effect of alprazolam in patients with chronic organic pain of malignant origin. Journal of Clinical Psychopharmacology 7: 167–169

Forrest W H, Brown B W, Brown C R et al 1977 Dextroamphetamine with morphine for the treatment of post-operative pain. New England Journal of Medicine 296: 712–715

Getto C J, Sorkness C A, Howell T 1987 Antidepressants and chronic nonmalignant pain: a review. Journal of Pain and Symptom Management 2: 9–18

Glazier H S 1990 Potentiation of pain relief with hydroxyzine: a therapeutic myth? DICP, The Annals of Pharmacotherapy 24: 484–488

Gordon N C, Heller P H, Gear R W, Levine J D 1993 Temporal factors in the enhancement of morphine analgesia by desipramine. Pain 53: 273–276

Hameroff S R, Cork R C, Scherer K et al 1982 Doxepin effects on chronic pain, depression and plasma opioids. Journal of Clinical Psychiatry 43: 22–27

Hanks G W, Thomas P J, Trueman T, Weeks E 1983 The myth of haloperidol potentiation. Lancet ii: 523–524

Houde R W 1966 On assaying analgesics in man. In: Knighton R S, Dumke P R (eds), Pain. Little Brown, Boston, pp 183–196

Hupert C, Yacoub M, Turgeon L R 1980 Effect of hydroxyzine on morphine analgesia for the treatment of postoperative pain. Anaesthesia and Analgesia 59: 690–696

IASP Subcommittee on Taxonomy 1980 Pain terms: a list with definitions and notes on usage. Pain 8: 249–252

Kaplitz S E 1975 Withdrawn apathetic geriatric patients responsive to methylphenidate. Journal of the American Geriatric Society 23: 271–276

Katon W, Raskind M 1980 Treatment of depression in the medically ill elderly with methylphenidate. American Journal of Psychology 137: 963–965

King S A, Strain J J 1990 Benzodiazepines and chronic pain. Pain 41: 3–4

Kishore-Kumar R, Schafer S C, Lawlor B A, Murphy D L, Max M B 1989 Single doses of the serotonin agonists buspirone and m-chlorophenylpiperazine do not relieve neuropathic pain. Pain 37: 223–227

Kishore-Kumar R, Max M B, Schafer S C et al 1990 Desipramine relieves postherpetic neuralgia. Clinical Pharmacology & Therapeutics 47: 305–312

Kragh-Sorensen P, Hansen C E, Baastrup P C, Hvidberg E F 1976 Self-inhibiting action of nortriptylin's antidepressive effect at high plasma levels: a randomized double-blind study controlled by plasma concentrations in patients with endogenous depression. Psychopharmacologia 45: 305–312

Kuhn C C, Bradman W A 1979 Pain as a substitute for the fear of death. Psychosomatics 20: 494–495

Lemberger L, Rowe H 1975 Clinical pharmacology of nabilone, a cannabinol derivative. Clinical Pharmacology and Therapeutics 18: 720–726

Levine J D, Gordon N C, Smith R, McBryde R 1986 Desipramine enhances opiate postoperative analgesia. Pain 27: 45–49

Liao J-C, Takemori A E 1990 Quantitative assessment of antinociceptive effects of midazolam, amitriptyline and carbamazepine alone and in combination with morphine in mice. Anesthesiology 73: A753

Lynch S, Max M B, Muir J, Smoller B, Dubner R 1990 Efficacy of antidepressants in relieving diabetic neuropathy pain: amitriptyline vs. desipramine and fluoxetine vs. placebo. Neurology 40 (suppl 1): 437

McQuay H J 1988 Pharmacological management of neuropathic pain. In: Hanks G W (ed) Pain and cancer. Cancer Survey Series, vol 7. Oxford University Press, Oxford, pp 141–159

McQuay H J, Carroll D, Glynn C J 1993 Dose-response for analgesic effect of amitriptyline in chronic pain. Anaesthesia 48: 281–285

Maltebie A A, Cavenar J O 1977 Haloperidol and analgesia: case reports. Military Medicine 142: 946–948

Max M B 1990 Towards physiologically based treatment of patients with neuropathic pain. Pain 42: 131–133

Max M B, Culnane M, Schafer S C et al 1987 Amitriptyline relieves diabetic neuropathy pain in patients with normal or depressed mood. Neurology (NY) 37: 589–596

Melzack R, Mount B M, Gordan J M 1979 The Brompton mixture versus morphine solution given orally: effects on pain. Canadian Medical Association Journal 120: 435–439

Moore J, Dundee J W 1961 Alterations in response to somatic pain associated with anaesthesia. VII: the effects of nine phenothiazine derivatives. British Journal of Anaesthesia 33: 422–431

Noyes R, Brunk S, Avery D 1975 The analgesic effects of oral delta-9-tetrahydrocannabinol and codeine. Clinical Pharmacology and Therapeutics 18: 84–89

Noyes R, Brunk S, Avery D 1976 The analgesic effects of oral delta-9-tetrahydrocannabinol in far advanced cancer patients. Comparative Psychiatry 17: 641–646

Onghena P, Van Houdenhove B 1992 Antidepressant-induced analgesia in chronic non-malignant pain: a meta-analysis of 39 placebo-controlled studies. Pain 49: 205–219

Pacifici G-M, Gustafsson L L, Sawe J, Rane A 1986 Metabolic interaction between morphine and various benzodiazepines. Acta Pharmacologica et Toxicologica 58: 249–252

Ray W A, Griffin M R, Schaffner W, Baugh D K, Melton L J 1987 Psychotropic drug use and the risk of hip fracture. New England Journal of Medicine 316: 363–369

Richards W, Grof S, Goodman L, Kurland A 1972 LSD-assisted psychotherapy and the human encounter with death. Clinical Pharmacology and Therapeutics 18: 84–89

Richter O, Klatte A, Abel J, Freye E, Haag W, Hartung E 1985 Pharmacokinetic data analysis of alfentanil after multiple injections and etomidate-infusion in patients undergoing orthopaedic surgery. International Journal of Clinical Pharmacology, Therapeutics and Toxicology 23: 11–15

Richtsmeier A J, Barkin R L, Alexander M 1992 Benzodiazepines for acute pain in children. Journal of Pain and Symptom Management 7: 492–495

Rumore M M, Schlichting D A 1986 Clinical efficacy of antihistamines as analgesics. Pain 25: 7–22

Sindrup S H, Gram L F, Brosen K, Eshoj O, Mogensen E F 1990 The selective serotonin re-uptake inhibitor paroxetine is effective in the treatment of diabetic neuropathy symptoms. Pain 42: 135–144

Spiegel K, Kalb R, Pasternak G W 1983 Analgesic activity of tricyclic antidepressants. Annals of Neurology 13: 462–465

Tasker R 1987 The problem of deafferentation pain in the management of the patient with cancer. Journal of Palliative Care 2 (2): 8–12

Tejwani G A, Rattan A K, McDonald J S 1990 Involvement of spinal opioid receptors in midazolam induced antinociception. Anesthesiology 73: A1270

Twycross R G 1979 The effect of cocaine in the Brompton Cocktail. In: Bonica J J, Liebeskind J C, Albe-Fessard D G (eds), Pain Research and Therapy, vol 3. Raven Press, New York, pp 927–932

Ventafridda V, Bianchi M, Ripamonti C et al 1990 Studies on the effects of antidepressant drugs on the antinociceptive action of morphine and on plasma morphine in rat and man. Pain 43: 155–162

Walsh T D 1986 Controlled study of imipramine and morphine in advanced cancer. Proceedings of the American Society of Clinical Oncology 5 (929): 237

Watson C P N 1984 Therapeutic window for amitriptyline analgesia. Canadian Medical Association Journal 130: 105–106

Watson C P N, Evans R J 1985 A comparative trial of amitriptyline and zimelidine in postherpetic neuralgia. Pain 23: 387–394

Watson C P N, Evans R J, Reed K, Merskey H, Goldsmith L, Warsh J 1982 Amitriptyline versus placebo in postherpetic neuralgia. Neurology (NY) 32: 671–673

Watson C P N, Chipman M, Reed K, Evans R J, Birkett N 1992 Amitriptyline versus maprotiline in postherpetic neuralgia: a randomized double-blind crossover trial. Pain 48: 29–36

Zarcone V P, Benson K L, Csernansky J G, Faull K F 1989 Alprazolam: treatment response. CSF metabolites, and sleep variables. Biological Psychiatry 25: A54

Zitman F G, Linssen A C G, Edelbroek P M, Stijnen T 1990 Low dose amitriptyline in chronic pain: the gain is modest. Pain 42: 35–42

CHAPTER 22 | Corticosteroids

INDICATIONS FOR USE

In this chapter, the use of corticosteroids in advanced cancer will be discussed generally as well as dealing more specifically with their role in pain relief. In one survey, nearly 60% of some 400 palliative care unit inpatients were prescribed a corticosteroid (Hanks et al 1983).

In the section on corticosteroids in the British National Formulary over 20 indications are given for their use, none specific to advanced cancer. In a separate section entitled 'Prescribing in terminal care', however, six indications are given (BNF 1993):

- bone pain
- nerve compression pain
- raised intracranial pressure
- dyspnoea with bronchospasm or partial obstruction
- anorexia
- dysphagia caused by a tumour mass.

There are, in fact, many more reasons for prescribing corticosteroids to patients with advanced cancer (Box 22.A; Walsh & Avashia 1992). These can be grouped into four categories:

- specific
- pain relief
- hormone therapy
- general.

The first two categories, with few exceptions, relate to the anti-inflammatory effect of corticosteroids. Hence their use, for example, in raised intracranial pressure, spinal cord compression, and obstruction of the superior vena cava or other hollow organ (Galicich et al 1961, Gilbert et al 1978, Carter et al 1982, Flombaum et al 1986).

BOX 22.A
INDICATIONS FOR USE OF CORTICOSTEROIDS IN ADVANCED CANCER

Specific
Hypercalcaemia
Incipient paraplegia
Carcinomatous neuropathy
Dyspnoea:

- pneumonitis (after radiotherapy)
- carcinomatous lymphangitis
- tracheal compression/stridor

Superior vena caval obstruction
Pericardial effusion
Haemoptysis
Obstruction of hollow viscus:

- bronchus
- ureter
- [intestine]

Rectal discharge (give PR)
Sweating/diaphoresis
To reduce radiation induced
Inflammation
Leuco-erythroblastic anaemia

Pain relief
Raised intracranial pressure
Nerve compression
Spinal cord compression
Metastatic arthralgia
[Bone pain]

Hormone therapy
Replacement
Anticancer

General
To improve appetite
To enhance sense of wellbeing
To improve strength

When used as hormone therapy, corticosteroids result in regression or cessation of progression in one third of elderly patients with breast cancer for as long as 1 year (Minton et al 1981). Patients with prostate cancer may obtain similar benefit (Tannock et al 1989). Finally, the general use of corticosteroids stems from their known beneficial effect on appetite, mood and strength.

COMPARISON OF CORTICOSTEROIDS

Different centres and different doctors favour different preparations. It is important, therefore, to be aware of the relative anti-inflammatory potency of the commonly used corticosteroids (Table 22.1). The use of prednisone is obsolete; it is a prodrug which is metabolized to prednisolone in the liver. Similarly cortisone is a prodrug of hydrocortisone. Dexamethasone is seven times more potent than prednisolone; thus 2 mg is approximately equivalent to 15 mg of prednisolone.

Corticosteroids differ not only in potency but also in duration of effect (Table 22.1). Because this is much longer than the plasma halflife, the term 'biological halflife' has been coined. This is conventionally defined as the duration of suppression of the hypothalamopituitary-adrenal axis after a single dose. This in turn mirrors the duration of the anti-inflammatory effect. Given such durations of action, only hydrocortisone (and cortisone) need be given more than once a day. The time honoured 'three times a day' for prednisolone is clearly unnecessary. The only reason for dividing the daily dose of dexamethasone, for example, is to reduce the number of tablets to be swallowed at any one time.

REPLACEMENT THERAPY

Normal replacement therapy in deficiency states (i.e. Addison's disease or postadrenalectomy) is hydrocortisone (cortisol) 20–30 mg PO/day, given in two doses — the larger in the morning and the smaller in the evening to mimic the normal diurnal rhythm. Fludrocortisone, a potent mineralocorticosteroid, is also given in a dose of 50–300 µg daily.

In normal circumstances, major physical stress leads to the endogenous secretion of up to 300 mg of hydrocortisone per 24 h. Thus, when providing additional exogenous hydrocortisone in patients with possible adrenal suppression, hydrocortisone 100 mg should be given IM or IV q6h–q8h. After the period of acute stress is over, the dose of hydrocortisone can be halved every day until normal maintenance doses are once again achieved.

DISADVANTAGES OF CORTICOSTEROIDS

The BNF devotes a whole section under corticosteroids to their disadvantages (Section 6.3.3). Box 22.B is based on this section. Mineralocorticosteroid effects are, however, negligible with high potency glucocorticosteroids such as dexamethasone and bethamethasone.

In a retrospective review of 59 patients with brain tumours or epidural spinal cord compression, one half developed one or more adverse effects and one fifth required hospital admission for diagnosis and/or management of corticosteroid related complications (Weissman et al 1987). The reasons for hospital admission are not stated, but almost certainly included hyperglycaemia. One patient developed diabetic keto-acidosis. The highest incidence of toxicity was seen in patients with a plasma albumen concentration of less than 25 g/L.

Patients receiving dexamethasone for more than 3 weeks had a toxicity incidence of 76%, compared with 5% for those treated for shorter periods.

Table 22.1 Adrenal corticosteroids

Drug	Anti-inflammatory potency	Equivalent dose (mg)	Sodium retaining potency	Daily dose (mg) above which HPA axis suppression possible[a]		Plasma halflife (min)	Biological halflife (h)
				Males	Females		
Hydrocortisone	1	20	++	20–30	15–25	90	8–12
Cortisone	0.8	25	++	25–35	20–30	90	8–12
Prednisone	3.5	5	+	7.5–10	7.5	⩾ 200	18–36
Prednisolone	4	5	+	7.5–10	7.5	⩾ 200	18–36
Methylprednisolone	5	4	–	7.5–10	7.5	⩾ 200	18–36
Triamcinolone	5	4	–	7.5–10	7.5	⩾ 200	18–36
Paramethasone	10	2	–	2.5–5	2.5–5	⩾ 300	36–54
Betamethasone	25–30[b]	0.7–0.8	–	1–1.5	1–1.5	⩾ 300	36–54
Dexamethasone	25–30[b]	0.7–0.8	–	1–1.5	1–1.5	⩾ 300	36–54

[a] A general guide only; the dose varies according to total body surface area,
[b] Different sources give different values (Gilman et al 1985, Grahame-Smith & Aronson 1992, BNF 1993).
Based on Swartz & Dluhy 1978

BOX 22.B
DISADVANTAGES OF CORTICOSTEROIDS

Glucocorticosteroid effects
Diabetes
Osteoporosis
Avascular bone necrosis
Mental disturbances:

- paranoid psychosis
- depression
- euphoria

Muscle wasting
Peptic ulceration (if given with NSAIDs)
Infection:

- septicaemia (may delay recognition)
- tuberculosis

Suppression of growth in child

Mineralocorticosteroid effects
Hypertension
Sodium and water retention
Potassium loss

Cushing's syndrome
Moon-face
Striae
Acne

Steroid cataract
If prednisolone 15 mg (or equivalent) taken daily for several
years = 75% risk

Similarly, patients receiving a total of dexamethasone 400 mg had a toxicity incidence of 75%, compared with 13% for those treated with smaller total doses.

The risk of peptic ulceration is described as 'weakly linked' to corticosteroid use in the BNF. This statement is supported by published data which indicate that any risk is almost entirely related to the concurrent use of nonsteroidal anti-inflammatory drugs (NSAIDs) rather than to corticosteroids themselves (Piper et al 1991, Guslando & Titobello 1992). Postmortem studies in cancer patients have demonstrated that death may be precipitated by complicated peptic ulceration (i.e. haemorrhage, perforation) in 5% of patients receiving corticosteroids compared with 1% in others (Schell 1966). Data about concurrent NSAID consumption, however, was not provided. Even so, while a risk of this order is acceptable in patients with a specific ongoing need for a corticosteroid, it cannot be ignored in other circumstances.

Recent data from dermatological patients receiving corticosteroids indicate a very low risk of serious upper gastro-intestinal haemorrhage (Carson et al 1991). In another study in which corticosteroids were associated with increased mortality, the association was with infection and not peptic ulceration (Henry et al 1987).

Oropharyngeal candidiasis is a common adverse effect. In a prospective survey of several hundred patients with advanced cancer who received corticosteroids, nearly one third developed oral candidiasis, accounting for 80% of all such cases in the unit in question. 20% developed ankle oedema and 18% a moon-face — an effect dreaded by many women. In addition, some 10% experienced hypomania, agitation, hyperkinesia or insomnia, and in 5% the corticosteroid was withdrawn because of unacceptable effects (Hanks et al 1983).

Corticosteroid hypersensitivity

Hypersensitivity to hydrocortisone is well documented (Chan & O'Brien 1993). Reports include urticaria, angio-oedema, bronchospasm and ana-phylaxis (Fulcher & Katelaris 1991). A case of urticaria and bronchospasm with dexamethasone has also been reported.

■ CASE HISTORY

A 39 year-old woman presented with inflammatory breast cancer, which was treated with combination chemotherapy followed by surgery and radio-therapy. Local recurrence and bone metastases a year later were treated with tamoxifen. Further local recurrence was subsequently treated with amino-glutethimide and hydrocortisone. Six months later the patient developed pleural and liver metastases. Ibuprofen 400 mg q.i.d. failed to relieve pain, and dexamethasone 2 mg t.i.d. and cimetidine 800 mg once daily were started. Four days later the patient developed a generalized urticarial rash with bronchospasm, which was treated with IV hydrocortisone and chlorphenir-amine. Ibuprofen and cimetidine were stopped and dexamethasone continued. She had two further attacks in the next 2 days. One week after starting dexamethasone, she received chemotherapy with anti-emetic cover of IV dexamethasone 8 mg and metoclopramide 10 mg followed by dexamethasone 4 mg PO q.i.d. and had a further urticarial attack associated with broncho-spasm. At this point dexamethasone hypersensitivity was suspected and the drug discontinued. There were no further attacks. Intradermal injections of hydrocortisone and dexamethasone both gave negative results, suggesting that the urticaria and bronchospasm were a pseudo-allergic drug reaction (Chan & O'Brien 1993).

It has been suggested that the release of vaso-active mediators from plasma proteins may be the underlying mechanism (Williams 1993). NSAIDs, ionic cholegraphic contrast media, IV hydrocortisone, benzylpenicillin, and sulphonamides release prostaglandin F_{2a} from plasma proteins. IV prepara-tions of basic drugs (e.g. neuromuscular blocking agents, metoclopramide, procainamide, and desferrioxamine) displace histamine.

These in vitro observations suggest that pseudo-allergic drug reactions may be regulated not by pharmacological specificity but by relatively non-specific protein binding properties. The displacement properties of acidic or basic protein binding drugs and the effects of released vaso-active mediators are probably additive. The adverse reactions experienced by the patient above may, therefore, be attributable to the drug regimen as a whole and not solely to dexamethasone.

Corticosteroid myopathy

Muscle weakness develops in 50–80% of patients with Cushing's syndrome (Golding et al 1961, Eidelberg 1991). It is also a feature of corticosteroid therapy. The minimal dose which induces myopathy is not known. For any given dose, however, women are more susceptible than men (Bunch et al 1980). In a group of asthmatic patients who received prednisolone ≥ 40 mg per day, two thirds had detectable hip flexor weakness when formally tested (Bowyer et al 1985). In contrast, weakness was detectable in only 3% receiving 30 mg a day or less. Some cases have occurred only after a cumulative dose of prednisolone 5000–15 000 mg. Others have developed much sooner, for example, after only 10 days and a total dose of 400 mg (Askari et al 1976).

Over the years many cases of corticosteroid myopathy have been seen at Sobell House, notably in elderly men with prostatic cancer who have been taking dexamethasone 4 mg daily for 4 weeks or more. The incidence in a retrospective review of patients with primary brain tumours was 11% (Dropcho & Soong 1991). The peak period of onset was in the third month of treatment. In 2/23 affected patients, the respiratory muscles were involved.

The pathogenesis of corticosteroid induced myopathy is still a matter of speculation. Selective immobilization of certain muscles in rats, however, results in more marked myopathy in the immobilized muscles (Goldberg & Goodman 1969). This observation led to the suggestion that corticosteroids exacerbate disuse atrophy in some way. Animal studies also suggest that fluorinated corticosteroids, for example dexamethasone, cause more atrophy and weakness than nonfluorinated corticosteroids, for example hydrocortisone and prednisolone (Dropcho & Soong 1991). Converting to an equivalent dose of a nonfluorinated corticosteroid might, therefore, result in stabilization or improvement in strength.

Electromyographic studies give confusing results. They have been interpreted as showing (Askari et al 1976):

- myopathy
- neuropathy
- neuromyopathy
- normal muscle.

Features of corticosteroid myopathy are shown in Box 22.C. An appropriate level of suspicion is perhaps the main prerequisite for diagnosis. For example, a patient may walk into the consultation room with no difficulty but subsequently have difficulty getting up from the sitting position. If the chrono-

BOX 22.C
CORTICOSTEROID MYOPATHY

Symptoms
Generally insidious onset
Diffuse myalgia may occur (Askari et al 1976)
Difficulty with:

- climbing stairs
- standing up   } early
- arm elevation
- holding head up   } late
- distal extremities

Signs
Weakness   } usually
Wasting   } symmetrical
Hypercortisolism:

- moon-face
- abdominal striae
- ankle oedema

Normal
Reflexes
Sensation
Enzymes (AST, CPK, aldolase)

Differential diagnosis
Hpokalaemia
Hypophosphataemia
Nonmetastatic carcinomatous neuropathy/myopathy
Lumbosacral plexopathy
Spinal cord compression

logical sequence fits with corticosteroid myopathy, a presumptive diagnosis should be made and the following steps taken:

- explanation to patient and family
- discuss need to compromise between maximizing therapeutic benefit and minimizing adverse effects
- halve corticosteroid dose (normally possible as a single step)
- arrange for physiotherapy
- emphasize that weakness will not worsen and should improve somewhat after 3–4 weeks
- review after 2–3 weeks to ensure that there is no further deterioration and to give encouragement
- consider changing from dexamethasone to prednisolone.

Acute hydrocortisone myopathy

Reference to this rare syndrome is included for general interest. Given its association with high dose parenteral hydrocortisone, it is unlikely to be seen in palliative care. On the other hand, unless specific to hydrocortisone, it could occur with short term high dose dexamethasone. The following case history illustrates the features of this devastating syndrome:

■ CASE HISTORY

A 37 year-old housewife with a history of asthma since childhood was admitted to hospital cyanosed with intense bronchospasm. She was treated with IV bronchodilators and commenced on IV hydrocortisone 1 g q6h. Despite these measures she required mechanical ventilation, which was continued for 6 days. She continued to receive bronchodilators and a reducing dose of hydrocortisone, later changed to oral prednisolone.

Myopathy became evident when the patient was slow to resume spontaneous respiration despite resolution of her bronchospasm. She was unable to raise her limbs from the bed because of profound weakness of both proximal and distal muscles. There were no sensory or reflex changes and the cranial nerves were intact. When first measured, plasma creatine phosphokinase (CPK) concentration was 888 U/L (normal female range 0–65) and aspartate transaminase 168 U/L (normal range 5–30). Electromyography showed no specific abnormalities. A biopsy specimen of the left deltoid muscle showed vacuolar changes in all fibre types and regenerating basophil fibres throughout the specimen. There was no evidence of denervation.

Plasma CPK returned to normal over the next 2–3 weeks, and muscle power began to improve. Recovery was almost complete after 6 months despite continuing to take prednisolone 5–10 mg daily to control her asthma (Van Marle & Woods 1980).

A few other cases have been published (Sury et al 1988). Resolution takes several months and distal limb muscles are as severely affected as proximal ones. It is recommended that, even in severe status asthmaticus, the dose of hydrocortisone should not exceed 1 g in 24 h by continuous infusion (Van Marle & Woods 1980, Sury et al 1988); in the above case the patient received 4 g.

Avascular bone necrosis

Avascular bone necrosis is a well documented adverse effect of corticosteroid treatment (Box 22.D). Most cases are bilateral. The femoral head is the area most commonly affected. Here, and in the humeral head, bone collapse is likely. In one series of nearly 200 postrenal transplant patients, the incidence was over 20% (Ibels et al 1978). Symptoms began 1 month to 10.5 years (mean = 1.5 years) after transplant surgery during which time most patients had taken prednisolone 15 mg/day together with azathioprine. All had had much larger doses, however, in the immediate postoperative weeks.

Avascular bone necrosis has also been reported after relatively short courses of dexamethasone (18–37 days) with a total cumulative dose of about 200 mg following neurosurgery (McCluskey & Gutteridge 1982).

BOX 22.D
CAUSES OF AVASCULAR BONE NECROSIS (Ibels et al 1978)

Traumatic disruption of blood supply:

- subcapital fracture of neck of femur
- slipped femoral capital epiphysis
- traumatic dislocation

Arterial obstruction:

- Gaucher's disease
- sickle cell anaemia
- nitrogen bubbles (compressed air workers)
- atheroma
- emboli
- postradiation fibrosis
- neoplastic infiltration
- osteomyelitis (inflammation)

Corticosteroid therapy

Alcoholism

Gout

■ CASE HISTORY

A 36 year-old man underwent transfrontal removal of a craniopharyngioma. Because there were signs of corticosteroid deficiency postoperatively, he received IV hydrocortisone for several days as well as prophylactic dexamethasone to prevent oedema of the CNS. When the hydrocortisone was stopped dexamethasone was continued. For 32 days after the operation he received the equivalent of almost 200 mg dexamethasone, before he was finally stabilised on 7–9 mg of prednisolone daily for replacement. Hip pain developed 7 months after the operation and shoulder pain a few months later. Radiological examination showed avascular necrosis of the heads of both femurs and humeri. Within 2 years of operation he underwent bilateral total hip replacement.

Avascular bone necrosis has also been reported in patients receiving corticosteroids as part of a chemotherapeutic regimen, notably in lymphoma (Editorial 1982). It is, however, a rare complication — only 12 cases were identified in 3500 lymphoma patients, i.e. 0.34% (Thorne et al 1981).

Radiological changes are not immediately apparent. Intra-osseous pressure is, however, consistently raised up to four times above normal in stage 1 (Box 22.E). Corticosteroid avascular bone necrosis should be regarded, therefore, as a compartment syndrome affecting the intra-osseous compartment, and depriving the bone of its blood supply. Many theories have been advanced to explain why treatment with corticosteroids should predispose to avascular necrosis (e.g. fat embolism, hypercoagulability, fat cell swelling), but the question remains unanswered.

BOX 22.E
RADIOGRAPHIC CHANGES IN AVASCULAR BONE NECROSIS (Nixon 1984)

Plain radiographs (positive in about 40% of cases)
Stage 1

- no changes on plain radiographs *or*
- nonspecific osteoporosis

Stage 2

- abnormal or irregular bone density
- lucent subchondral crescent
  (often best seen on lateral film)

Stage 3

- irregular bone density (mottling)
- obvious collapse of femoral head (flattening)

Stage 4

- severe deformity of femoral head
- extensive destruction of joint

Bone scan (positive in > 90% of cases)
Changes most likely in stages 1 and 2

- 'cold spot' surrounded by 'hot halo' (if area of necrosis large)
- 'hot spot' alone (represents reactive bone around small area of necrosis)

Magnetic resonance imaging (Zizic 1990)
Will demonstrate early changes, i.e. incipient damage with oedema

Several conservative orthopaedic approaches have been used to arrest the development of the syndrome (Nixon 1984), but the likelihood is that the diagnosis will be too late for such interventions in patients with advanced cancer. The majority of patients with femoral head collapse will require hip joint replacement within 3 years — perhaps not relevant in palliative care.

Skin changes

Systemic corticosteroids and potent topical corticosteroids may cause a range of skin changes (Box 22.F). The use of small systemic doses or low potency topical preparations generally avoids adverse skin effects (Table 22.2).

Flushing

Facial and upper trunk flushing has been reported with intra-articular injection of triamcinolone acetonide 40 mg (equivalent to methylprednisolone 40 mg). In one survey, it occurred in about one third of patients and was more common in women than men (Pattrick & Doherty 1987). In half of those affected it was considered unpleasant. It occurred between 2 and 30 h after the injection and lasted for between 6 and 96 h (mean 36 h). It is not

> **BOX 22.F**
> **SKIN CHANGES ASSOCIATED WITH HIGH POTENCY TOPICAL**
> **CORTICOSTEROIDS AND HIGH DOSE SYSTEMIC CORTICOSTEROIDS (BNF 1993).**
>
> Spread and worsening of untreated infection
>
> Thinning of the skin (which may be restored over a period of time after stopping treatment although the original structure may never return)
>
> Irreversible atrophic striae
>
> Increased hair growth
>
> Peri-oral dermatitis (an inflammatory papular disorder on the face of young women)
>
> Acne at the site of application in some patients
>
> Mild depigmentation and vellus hair

Table 22.2 Potency classification of topical corticosteroids

Class	Potency	Examples
I	Very potent	Clobetasol proprionate 0.05% (Dermovate)
II	Potent	Betamethasone 0.1% (Betnovate); Hydrocortisone butyrate (Locoid)
III	Moderately potent	Clobetasone butyrate 0.05% (Eumovate)
IV	Mild	Hydrocortisone 1%

known whether the corticosteroid itself, its side chain or the vehicle is responsible for the flushing. Although it has not been reported with methylprednisolone, it is clearly something to be aware of.

WITHDRAWAL PHENOMENA

The dangers of sudden cessation of corticosteroids are universally known, namely, acute adrenal insufficiency, hypotension and death. Less well known are a group of minor withdrawal phenomena (BNF 1993):

- rhinitis
- conjunctivitis
- loss of weight
- arthralgia
- painful pruritic skin nodules.

STEROID PSEUDORHEUMATISM

As noted in Chapter 5, patients receiving corticosteroids for rheumatoid arthritis occasionally develop diffuse pains, malaise and pyrexia (Box 22.G). This syndrome, called steroid pseudorheumatism, is also sometimes seen in cancer patients receiving large doses of corticosteroids, or when a very high

---

BOX 22.G
STEROID WITHDRAWAL PAIN OR PSEUDORHEUMATISM (Rotstein & Good 1957)

Myalgia and cramps	Malaise
Arthralgia	Pyrexia
Tendon pains	Tachycardia
Bone pains	Restlessness
Weakness	Emotional lability
Fatigue	Memory deficit

---

dose is reduced rapidly to a lower maintenance level. Thus, cancer patients most likely to be affected are those:

- receiving 100 mg of prednisolone daily for several days in association with chemotherapy
- with spinal cord compression given dexamethasone 100 mg for several days (Greenberg et al 1979)
- on high doses of dexamethasone to reduce raised intracranial pressure associated with brain metastases
- reducing from a high dose to a low dose
- reducing an ordinary maintenance dose after a prolonged course.

DRUG INTERACTIONS

Corticosteroids antagonize the effects of:

- antidiabetic therapy (both oral hypoglycaemics and insulin)
- antihypertensives (because of their mineralocorticosteroid effect)
- diuretics (because of their mineralocorticosteroid effect).

There is an increased risk of hypokalaemia if high doses of corticosteroids are prescribed with:

- beta$_2$ sympathomimetics (e.g. salbutamol, terbutaline)
- carbenoxolone.

It is also important to be aware that the metabolism of corticosteroids is accelerated by a number of drugs:
- aminoglutethimide (dexamethasone only)
- anticonvulsants
  — carbamazepine
  — phenobarbitone
  — phenytoin
  — primidone
- ripamficin.

The interaction with anticonvulsants is the most important one in advanced cancer (Table 22.3). It must be taken into account when deciding an appropriate dose of, for example, dexamethasone in patients with a symptomatic

Table 22.3 Interaction between corticosteroids and anticonvulsants

Drug combination	Plasma halflife (% decrease)	Clearance (% increase)
Hydrocortisone + phenytoin	14	27
Prednisolone + phenytoin	45	77
Prednisolone + phenobarbitone	23	?
Methylprednisolone + phenytoin	56	130
Methylprednisolone + phenobarbitone	53	90
Dexamethasone + phenytoin	51	140
Dexamethasone + phenobarbitone	44	88

From Gambertoglio 1983

cerebral tumour. The increase in clearance is proportional to the initial halflife; thus the rate of metabolism of the longer acting corticosteroids (e.g. dexamethasone) is affected more than prednisolone or hydrocortisone (Avery 1987). As a working rule, it is best to assume that phenytoin and phenobarbitone halve the pharmacological effect of dexamethasone. This means that the anticipated dose should be doubled.

GENERAL USES OF CORTICOSTEROIDS IN ADVANCED CANCER

Thirty years ago, an enthusiast commented that the use of corticosteroids may allow 'the breast cancer patient to walk to the necropsy room' (Stoll 1963). However, as already noted, some patients develop crippling adverse effects, notably myopathy and avascular bone necrosis, and many others develop distressing oropharyngeal candidiasis. Fortunately, studies published more recently provide a more objective evaluation of the potential benefits of corticosteroids in patients with advanced cancer.

In a controlled trial in 40 terminal cancer patients of methylprednisolone 32 mg/day for 2 weeks, appetite increased in 77%, mood in 71% and activity in 68% (Table 22.4). All patients continued on methylprednisolone for a further 20 days. Most measures had deteriorated by the end of this time, although there was still significant benefit compared with baseline. The deterioration could reflect either loss of corticosteroid effect or disease progression or both.

Table 22.4 Randomized controlled trials of methylprednisolone 32 mg daily for 2 weeks

Feature (n = 31)	% better with methylprednisolone	% better with placebo	No difference
Pain intensity (28)	68	14	18
Analgesic consumption (28)	57	14	32
Appetite	77	10	13
Activity	61	16	23
Depression	71	13	16
Anxiety	19	23	58
Patient's selection	74	10	16
Investigator's selection	71	18	16

From Bruera et al 1985

A loss of effect with time was also seen in another controlled trial. In this, dexamethasone 3 mg and 6 mg daily were comparable with placebo — the higher dose being comparable with methylprednisolone 32 mg. Subjective improvement in appetite and strength was noted after 2 weeks but had disappeared by 4 weeks (Moertel et al 1974).

The figures for benefit seen in time limited trials are much better than those reported in a recent survey (Needham et al 1992). These authors surveyed 100 terminal cancer patients about corticosteroid use when admitted to a palliative care unit, using a standardized questionnaire. At the time of admission, 33 patients were taking corticosteroids and seven had in the past. Of the 28 who were well enough to complete the questionnaire:

- about one third said they had benefited
- one third were undecided
- one third said they had not.

Half of the latter had started treatment more than 1 month before; in one case 4 months. Among the doubtful was a woman who had been taking prednisolone 30 mg daily for 2 years. Of the corticosteroid receiving patients, 95% suffered from anorexia ± weight loss ± weakness, compared with 88% of patients who had never received corticosteroids!

Some doctors have used IV methylprednisolone as the corticosteroid of choice for general purposes (Pierquin et al 1978). A dose of 125 mg IV is given daily for 30 days, followed by oral maintenance therapy with prednisolone 15 mg daily. There is no evidence that the IV regimen is superior to the use of oral dexamethasone or prednisolone in terms of pain relief or general benefit. It is therefore not recommended.

CORTICOSTEROIDS AND PAIN RELIEF

Corticosteroids are used as 'co-analgesics' more often by some doctors than others. This may relate more to fashion than to science. Certainly in the early 1970s corticosteroids were used more often in metastatic bone pain than today. As the role of PGs in osteolysis became more fully appreciated, there was a major shift to using a NSAID as the analgesic or co-analgesic of choice in this situation (see Chapters 11 & 12).

A number of studies have shown, however, that corticosteroids reduce pain in various situations — and not just that associated with bone metastasis. Selected studies are summarized in Box 22.H. The regimen for spinal cord compression comes from the USA (Greenberg et al 1979). The author is unaware of any objective evidence for the benefits of such a high dose. At Sobell House, dexamethasone 12 mg PO is given at diagnosis, followed by 16–32 mg daily during the initial phase of palliative radiotherapy. The dose is reduced in the light of response to treatment and adverse effects. The aim is to achieve a dose in single figures within 2 weeks.

Because corticosteroids have a major impact on the inflammatory process, it is possible that the main analgesic effect is anti-inflammatory. Corticosteroids reduce the production of PGs by inhibiting phospholipase

BOX 22.H
CORTICOSTEROIDS AND PAIN RELIEF: SELECTED STUDIES

Animal studies (Brown & Garrett 1972)
Radiant heat tail flick in 150 rats:

- aim to determine the dose of morphine [or methadone] that increased reaction time 4 seconds in 50% of rats (mean time in control group = 6 seconds)
- morphine given daily in escalating doses for 2 weeks
- in the rats receiving dexamethasone, the amount of morphine needed was 36% (day 0) and 45% (day 14) of the control figures

Postoperative analgesia (Korman & McKay 1985)
Fallopian tube surgery via Pfannenstiel incision:

- 15 women received dexamethasone 15–20 mg IV q4h for 2 days peri-operatively; 48 women acted as controls
- controls needed a mean of 617 mg of pethidine equivalents (given as pethidine or papaveretum); corticosteroid group needed 344 mg (56%)

Cancer patients (Bruera et al 1985)
Randomized controlled crossover trial:

- compared methylprednisolone 32 mg/day with placebo in 31 patients
- analgesic consumption (capsules of propoxyphene + dipyrone) decreased in 16/28 (57%) with methylprednisolone
- pain intensity decreased in 19/28 (68%)

Metastatic prostate cancer (Tannock et al 1989)
Progressive disease despite oestrogens ± orchidectomy:

- 37 men received prednisolone 7.5–10 mg daily
- 14 patients (38%) had less pain 1 month later; 7 patients (19%) maintained improvement for median of 4 months (range 3–30)
- symptomatic response was associated with decrease in plasma androgen concentration

Epidural spinal cord compression (Greenberg et al 1979)
High dose dexamethasone:

- 100 mg IV bolus before commencing radiotherapy, then 96 mg PO for 3 days and 48 mg for 2 days, tapering to zero after 2 weeks
- 'dexamethasone substantially ameliorated pain in the majority of patients, with relief often coming within hours'

activity, and thereby prevent the formation of arachidonic acid from cell membrane phospholipids. Arachidonic acid is the stem precursor substance of PGs. Studies in rats with experimentally induced injuries of molar teeth suggest other modes of actions, such as a reduction in injury induced nerve sprouting and a reduction in the calcitonin gene-related peptide and substance P content of sensory fibres (Hong et al 1993).

Other animal studies point to a possible central analgesic effect for cortico-steroids (Pieretti et al 1992). Seemingly contradictory results, however, suggest that there may be differences between species. A central effect mediated via improved mood is also possible. Paradoxically, however, corticosteroids inhibit the release of beta-endorphin.

There is clearly a theoretical case for using both a corticosteroid and a NSAID in the management of certain pains, for example bone metastasis. However, more tablets may lead to reduced compliance or more adverse gastro-intestinal effects. Maximal relief may sometimes be obtained only by using an opioid, a NSAID, and a corticosteroid concurrently, for example intrapelvic malignancy invading muscle and bone, and compressing nerves.

Thus, although a corticosteroid is likely to improve pain relief in most patients, such drugs should not be used indiscriminately because of their propensity for causing serious adverse effects. It is recommended, therefore, that a corticosteroid should be considered as a co-analgesic only when there is a large tumour mass within a relatively confined space. There is often an area of inflammation around a tumour and pressure on neighbouring veins and lymphatics may lead to further local or regional swelling, i.e. total mass = neoplasm + surrounding inflammation. Corticosteroids reduce the inflammation and thereby reduce the total mass and associated pain (Fig. 22.1).

The classical situation is that of headache caused by raised intracranial pressure secondary to a cerebral neoplasm. There may be other central nervous symptoms or signs, and patients often show improvement lasting for

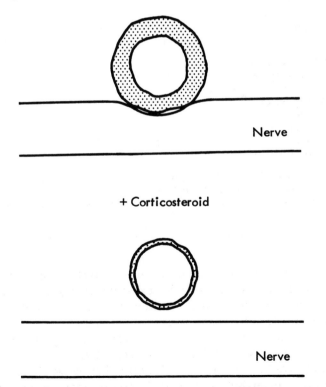

Fig. 22.1 Possible mechanism of action of corticosteroids in pain relief. For explanation see text.

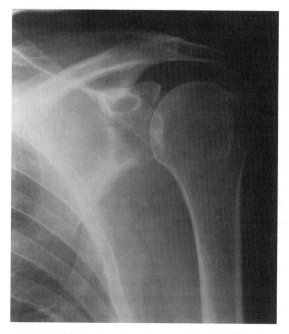

Fig. 22.2   Radiograph of the left shoulder of a 68 year-old man with cancer of the penis. He had excruciating pain if his arm was abducted more than a few mm. The glenoid fossa is totally replaced by a metastasis.

several weeks or months after starting treatment. Analgesics and elevating the head of the bed may help the pain when headache is the main symptom. Corticosteroids are also of benefit in relieving nerve compression pain. Some nerve compression pains respond to opioids alone. Most respond to a combination of an opioid and a corticosteroid. Those which do not will need one of the following:

- an antidepressant (Chapter 21)
- another alternative drug for opioid resistant neuropathic pain (Chapter 23) *or*
- epidural morphine and bupivacaine (Chapter 20).

Metastatic arthralgia refers to pain caused by metastatic involvement of the acetabulum (relatively common) or glenoid fossa (uncommon)). It occurs mostly in patients with cancer of the breast, bronchus or prostate (Fig. 22.2). In addition to radiation therapy, sometimes maximum relief is obtained only by the combined use of opioid, NSAID and corticosteroid. Alternatively, injection into the joint space of a long acting preparation of either methylprednisolone (Depo-Medrone) or triamcinolone hexacetonide (Lederspan) may be considered.

INTRALESIONAL INJECTION OF CORTICOSTEROIDS

Solitary rib metastasis

Pain from a rib metastasis is often eased by a local injection of bupivacaine

Table 22.5 Pain relief with intralesional methylprednisolone

Response	Number of patients
Complete abolition of pain	11
Pain much improved but not abolished	3
Small improvement only	3
No improvement	3
Not evaluated	2
	22

From Rowell 1988

0.5% and depot methylprednisolone. Having located the tender spot, the skin and subcutaneous tissues are infiltrated with local anaesthetic as the needle is advanced onto the rib. Then, 2 ml (80 mg) of depot methyl-prednisolone is injected with the tip of the needle pressing against the tender spot in the rib — or in some instances into a pathological fracture. Then the needle is repositioned under the rib and 5 ml of bupivacaine 0.5% is injected to anaesthetize the intercostal nerve.

This technique has resulted in relief for several months in some patients, particularly those with breast cancer and myeloma. Sometimes no benefit is obtained or only a transient one related to the effect of the intercostal local anaesthetic block. In these cases, the existing drug regimen may need to be modified. Radiation therapy or the use of thoracic intrathecal chlorocresol should also be considered (see p. 513).

The benefit of intralesional methylprednisolone for rib metastases has been quantified in 22 patients (Table 22.5). Half the patients had breast cancer and four multiple myeloma. All had well localized persistent rib pain and tenderness. One patient had three painful ribs and six had two. Thirty one ribs were injected on 23 occasions. Of the 20 patients who could be evaluated, 14 obtained complete or good relief after 2–10 days, a success rate of 70%.

In two patients the pain recurred after 10 days and 3 months respectively. Length of follow up was 3 weeks to 14 months. There were no significant complications. On three occasions an intercostal vein was entered. In this circumstance, an intercostal block was not proceeded with.

Sacro-iliac pain

The use of local anaesthetic and a corticosteroid in sacro-iliac pain is discussed later (see p. 511).

PERINEURAL INJECTION OF CORTICOSTEROIDS

Corticosteroids are also injected epidurally to relieve chronic low back pain. This technique has also been used in advanced cancer (see p. 372). The question arises as to how corticosteroids relieve pain when injected in this way. The traditional explanation has been that the corticosteroid reduces inflammation and thereby reduces the local concentrations of algesic substances which stimulate or sensitize nerve endings. It has been shown in patients with osteo-arthritis however that, whereas intrasynovial injection of corticosteroids is generally unsatisfactory, injecting corticosteroid into tender spots along nerves supplying painful joints often results in impressive joint pain relief (Pybus 1984). This suggests that corticosteroids may have a direct inhibitory effect on abnormally excitable damaged nerve fibres.

Supporting evidence for this hypothesis comes from animal experiments (Devor et al 1985). Rats had one of three commercially available parenteral corticosteroid preparations injected around the stump of a sciatic nerve shortly after the nerve had been ligated and cut. Single doses of all three preparations (two depot, one ordinary) markedly reduced the incidence of spontaneous discharge from the cut ends of the nerve, and continued to do so for the 14 day period of observation. Corticosteroids injected intraperitoneally or applied to the contralateral nerve had no effect.

This study strongly supports a local action of corticosteroids on damaged nerve endings. Further, in view of the minimal inflammation associated with the technique of experimental neuroma formation, it is unlikely that reduction in spontaneous neuronal discharge is mediated via an anti-inflammatory effect. It seems likely, therefore, that corticosteroids affect the impulse generating mechanism in the neuroma fibres. It has been shown, for example, that corticosteroids can hyperpolarize nerve cells by activating the electrogenic sodium ion pump (Devor et al 1985).

These data encourage the use of depot corticosteroid injections at sites of ectopic impulse generation (e.g. tender spots) in the treatment of pains and paraesthesias associated with nerve injury.

SPECIFIC USES OF CORTICOSTEROIDS IN ADVANCED CANCER

This section will be limited to three indications, namely symptomatic brain tumours, hypercalcaemia, and anti-emesis. Spinal cord compression has already been referred to under pain relief. The use of corticosteroids in developing superior vena caval obstruction, pending radiotherapy, should also be emphasized.

Symptomatic brain tumours

The use of corticosteroids to relieve symptoms and signs caused by brain tumours stretches back over 40 years (Kirkham 1988). The original dexamethasone regimen of 10 mg IV followed by 4 mg IM q.i.d. was undoubtedly arbitrary (Galicich et al 1961). It has, however, given rise to the fashion of prescribing 16 mg PO daily for most patients.

Benefit derives in part from reducing the reactive oedema around the tumour (Box 22.I). Benefit also results from a reduction in cerebral blood flow (Beaney et al 1987). Corticosteroids sometimes have a cytostatic or cytotoxic effect (Freshney et al 1980, Pilkington 1989). This possibly explains why some patients with a fairly high grade glioma live several years after

---

BOX 22.I
EFFECT OF CORTICOSTEROIDS ON BRAIN METASTASES

Clinical improvement (Ehrenkranz & Posner 1981):

- focal signs
- mental status

Decrease in intracranial pressure (Richardson et al 1970):

- plateau waves
- baseline pressure

Electro-encephalographic improvement

Improvement in radionucleotide brain scans and CT scans:

- less oedema
- less isotope or contrast cumulation

Decrease in cerebral blood flow (Beaney et al 1987)

Decrease in peritumour inflammation:

- 'tightening' of blood-brain barrier
- reduced tumour capillary permeability to water, ions and low molecular weight substances

Reduction in tumour cell proliferation (Mealey et al 1971, Pilkington 1989)

---

diagnosis, palliative radiotherapy and continued low dose dexamethasone (Posner et al 1977).

The maximum beneficial dose is not known, although one author suggested 96 mg/day (Renaudin et al 1973). This figure was arrived at by doubling the dose if symptoms and signs failed to resolve on a lower dose. It was not appreciated, however, that almost all those who reached the top dose were also receiving an anticonvulsant. This would suggest that the dose ceiling in normal circumstances is likely to be in the region of 48 mg.

The British Brain Tumour Therapy Group undertook a trial of dexamethasone 'up to 16 mg a day' and methylprednisolone *500 mg* on alternate days, equivalent to 100 mg of dexamethasone (Capildeo 1989, Jamous 1989). The endpoint was relapse, death or completion of a year of treatment. Of those receiving methylprednisolone:

- > 50% complained of dyspepsia
- > 50% developed a moon-face
- 30% developed infections (commonly a chest infection)
- 8% became hirsute.

The investigators concluded:

> 'Adverse effects were remarkably few and not different from those usually encountered in patients on long term corticosteroid therapy using conventional doses.'

That said, the likelihood of unacceptable adverse effects with higher doses is sufficiently great to suggest that doubling and redoubling the dose is unlikely to be in the patient's best interests. A maintenance dose of dexamethasone in single figures, unless the patient is also taking an anticonvulsant, would seem to be a sensible working rule.

Corticosteroids are also prescribed to reduce the adverse effects of cranial irradiation for brain metastases. One centre recommends 16 mg daily for 4 days, then 8 mg daily for a further 4 days, followed by 4 mg daily until the end of the course of radiotherapy. In a series of 14 patients, only one required re-institution of corticosteroid therapy for corticosteroid reversible symptoms within 30 days of completing radiotherapy (Weissman et al 1991).

Hypercalcaemia

Because of poor results, corticosteroids are not the treatment of choice for hypercalcaemia associated with malignant disease (Thalassinos & Joplin 1970, Percival et al 1984). The bisphosphonates are now used increasingly instead (see p. 496). It is important, however, not to lose sight of the fact that corticosteroids are still of value in hypercalcaemia in breast cancer (Box 22.J).

Anti-emesis

Dexamethasone has been shown to have a powerful anti-emetic effect in patients receiving highly emetogenic chemotherapeutic regimens (Gralla 1989, Grunberg 1989, Editorial 1991, Sridhar et al 1992). It is usually given with metoclopramide ± diphenhydramine or lorazepam (Table 22.6). Now it

---

BOX 22.J
CORTICOSTEROIDS AND HYPERCALCAEMIA

Study 1 (Thalassinos & Joplin 1970)

- 13 cancer patients (8 with breast cancer)
- all had failed to respond to rehydration alone
- given cortisone acetate 150 mg or prednisolone 30 mg/day PO
- only one patient responded (breast)

Study 2 (Percival et al 1984)

- 28 cancer patients (17 with breast cancer)
- rehydration ± prednisolone 20–60 mg/day PO
- the addition of prednisolone did not confer additional benefit

Study 3 (Mannheimer 1965)

- 59 hypercalcaemic episodes treated
- 40 breast cancer patients and osteolytic metastases
- all had failed rehydration alone
- prednisolone 60–80 mg daily PO or methylprednisolone up to 80 mg daily IV
- benefit in 46/59 episodes; 32/40 patients
- mean plasma calcium concentration = 3.9 ⟶ 2.8 mmol/L
- mean urinary calcium concentration = 11 ⟶ 5 mmol/24 h

Table 22.6 Combination anti-emetic regimens for chemotherapy

Chemotherapy	Anti-emetics	Timing
Cisplatin (40, 40–70, $\geq$ 100 mg/m²)	Dexamethasone 20 mg IV	40 min before
	Lorazepam 1.5 mg/m² IV	35 min before
	(*or* diphenhydramine 50 mg IV)	
	Metoclopramide 1–2–3 mg/kg IV[a]	30 min before + 2 h later
Cyclophosphamide + doxorubicin	Dexamethasone 20 mg IV	40 min before
	Metoclopramide 3 mg/kg	30 min before + 2 h later
	or	then 40 mg PO q3h p.r.n.
	Metoclopramide 2 mg/kg	30 min before + 2 & 4 h later
	Diphenhydramine 50 mg IV/PO	with first and alternate doses of metoclopramide
Dacarbazine	As for cisplatin 40–70 mg/m²	

[a] Higher doses used with higher cisplatin doses.
From Gralla 1989

is increasingly used in conjunction with a 5HT$_3$ receptor antagonist, for example ondansetron, granivetron (Hursti et al 1993).

The recommended dose is dexamethasone 20 mg IV 30–40 min before chemotherapy (Gralla 1989, Parry & Martin 1991). No significant differences have been noted between this and multiple doses totalling 50–60 mg or even 60 mg/m². Lower doses, such as 10 mg, have not been examined. In the USA, where the trials were carried out, a 20 mg dose is convenient; it comprises one ampoule and costs less than $1. The largest ampoule size in the UK is, however, only 8 mg and costs nearly £2. It is not clear why the dexamethasone is given IV; it is possible that an oral dose would be equally effective. The datasheet for dexamethasone recommends doubling or trebling the dose for oral administration.

One study indicates that tetracosactrin (synthetic adrenocorticotrophic hormone/ACTH) 0.5 mg IM is as effective as methylprednisolone 40 mg IV as a chemotherapeutic anti-emetic (Bonneterre et al 1991).

Suppression of PG synthesis may underlie the effectiveness of corticosteroids as anti-emetics (Aapro & Alberts 1981, Cairnie & Leach 1982) but there is no evidence available to support this. There is, therefore, currently no good hypothesis to explain the anti-emetic effects of corticosteroids (Leslie et al 1990).

GENERAL CONSIDERATIONS

Which corticosteroid?

The choice of corticosteroid is arbitrary. Dexamethasone has less mineralocorticosteroid effect than prednisolone which, in turn, has less than hydrocortisone. This could be an important consideration. It is more likely, however, that the choice between dexamethasone and prednisolone will be determined by fashion, cost and availability (Table 22.7).

Table 22.7   Selected preparations of prednisolone and dexamethasone (UK)

Prednisolone	Dexamethasone
Tablets[a]	
1 mg, 5 mg	0.5 mg, 2 mg
5 mg soluble	
2.5 mg, 5 mg enteric coated	
25 mg	
Suppositories	
5 mg	
Retention enemas[b]	
20 mg/100 ml	
Injections	
	5 mg/ml, 10 mg/2 ml as sodium phosphate (= dexamethasone 8 mg)
	8 mg/2 ml as sodium phosphate (= dexamethasone 6.66 mg)

[a] Nonenteric coated tablets are all available *scored* to facilitate breaking into halves.
[b] For use in local inflammatory conditions of the rectum and lower colon, including acute radiation proctitis. Of no benefit, however, in chronic (ischaemic) radiation proctitis.

Table 22.8   Cost of betamethasone and dexamethasone injections (UK)[a]

Preparation	Cost (pence/mg)
Betamethasone	
4 mg/1 ml	16
Dexamethasone	
5 mg/1 ml (= dexamethasone 4 mg)	21
8 mg/2 ml (= dexamethasone 6.66 mg)	26
10 mg/2 ml (= dexamethasone 8 mg)	16
100 mg/5 ml	15

[a] Based on BNF No. 25 (1993)

For example, dexamethasone is commonly used but betamethasone is not, despite the fact that, in the UK, the equipotent betamethasone 0.5 mg tablet is significantly cheaper. Whether betamethasone is cheaper by injection depends on the preparation purchased (Table 22.8). On the other hand, the dexamethasone 2 mg tablet is the preparation most commonly used, and a corresponding betamethasone tablet is not presently manufactured.

Dexamethasone tablets dissolve readily in water. A large number can be given, therefore, in a small volume of fluid. Some patients prefer this.

Dose of corticosteroid

The choice of starting dose remains arbitrary in many cases. In controlled trials to treat anorexia, the daily dose used varied between the equivalent of 15 and 40 mg of prednisolone (Moertel et al 1974, Willox et al 1984, Bruera et al 1985, Twycross & Guppy 1985). As noted in relation to hypercalcaemia and breast cancer, it is perhaps better to start with a relatively high dose in order not to miss a treatment effect and to reduce to a lower maintenance dose if treatment continues beyond 7 days.

In relation to anorexia, it should not be forgotten that there are well documented alternative treatments. For example, many patients benefit from megestrol acetate and the effect is still detectable after 2 months (Tchekmedyian et al 1986, Loprinzi et al 1990, Feliu et al 1992). Megestrol is, however, considerably more expensive. Given the 50% response to placebo (Wilcox et al 1984), the best initial step may well be dietary advice + multivitamin tablets.

SC infusion

At Sobell House, if a patient becomes moribund and can no longer swallow tablets, corticosteroids are discontinued. There may be occasions, however, when it is appropriate to give a corticosteroid by SC infusion, for example, in a patient with intestinal obstruction, troublesome vomiting and another specific reason for receiving a corticosteroid. In this circumstance, it will not be the only drug used. There is, however, danger of precipitation with dexamethasone:

> 'Our nurses have mastered the skill of including dexamethasone in syringe driver solutions. They make up the rest of the cocktail to the calculated volume (50 mm of syringe barrel length minus the volume of prescribed corticosteroid) and then very slowly draw in the dexamethasone. Doing it any other way seems to produce precipitation or clouding of the solution' (Dover S 1987 Personal Communication).

This technique may indeed minimize the risk of precipitation but clearly the dexamethasone is not being fully mixed with the other drugs. Most of the dexamethasone, therefore, will be administered as an initial bolus each 24 h. Given the prolonged duration of action of the drug, this is acceptable. On the other hand, a separate SC or IM injection might be better.

Precipitation can be avoided, however, simply by mixing the dexamethasone and other drugs at body temperature (37°C) rather than room temperature (18–22°C). The correct temperature is easily obtained by holding and warming the syringe in the palm of one's hand (Moyle J 1993 Personal Communication).

MONITORING CORTICOSTEROID USE

It is disturbing to note that a survey of patients newly admitted for palliative care found that more than 50% of patients receiving a corticosteroid did not know the reason for prescription nor how long it was intended they should continue (Needham et al 1992). More than two thirds did not have a Steroid Card and a comparable proportion did not know that long term corticosteroid treatment should not be stopped suddenly. If this sample is representative, it appears that, in advanced cancer, corticosteroids are stopped only infrequently and that their effects are not adequately monitored. The authors of the survey concluded that many doctors appear not to exercise the same care with corticosteroids in patients with advanced cancer as they do in other situations.

It would seem an essential safeguard, therefore, for doctors to state clearly in their notes why a corticosteroid is being prescribed and to communicate this to the patient. Except where tumour control is the objective, the corticosteroid should be prescribed initially on a trial basis for 1 week because the chances of obtaining a better response after this time are poor (Bruera et al 1985). Treatment will be continued only if benefit is perceived subjectively or objectively. Corticosteroids for general purposes should be avoided as far as possible in anxious patients and in diabetics because of the likelihood of a worsening of the associated condition.

If the equivalent of prednisolone 40 mg a day or less is used (methylprednisolone 32 mg, dexamethasone 6 mg), it is safe to stop the corticosteroid abruptly at the end of the week (Byyny 1976). Short courses of larger doses, and longer courses of lower doses, however, will lead to prolonged suppression of the hypothalamopituitary-adrenal axis, and doses must be tapered over several days or weeks according to circumstances.

Advanced cancer and polypharmacy tend to go hand in hand. Thus to discontinue drugs which are not yielding benefit will help ease the patient's tablet burden and possibly enhance compliance with other medication. Further, as already noted, unless the number of tablets preclude single administration, corticosteroids other than hydrocortisone should be given once a day at breakfast.

REFERENCES

Aapro M S, Alberts D S 1981 Dexamethasone as an anti-emetic in patients treated with cisplatin. New England Journal of Medicine 305: 520

Askari A, Vignos P J, Moskowitz R W 1976 Steroid myopathy in connective tissue disease. The American Journal of Medicine 61: 485–491

Avery 1987 Characteristics of some adrenocorticosteroid preparations in Avery's drug treatment, principles and practice of clinical pharmacology and therapeutics. 3rd edn. pp 564

Beaney R P, Leenders K L, Brooks D J 1987 Effects of dexamethasone in brain tumour patients. Lancet i: 571–572

Bonneterre J, Kerbrat P, Fargeot P et al 1991 Tetracosactrin vs methylprednisolone in the prevention of emesis in patients receiving FEC regimen for breast cancer. European Journal of Cancer 27: 849–852

Bowyer S L, LaMothe M P, Hollister J R 1985 Steroid myopathy: incidence and detection in a population with asthma. Journal of Allergy and Clinical Immunology 76: 234–242

British National Formulary 1993 A Joint Publication of the British Medical Association and the Royal Pharmaceutical Society of Great Britain, London, No 26 (September 1993) pp 12–13

Brown J H, Garrett R L 1972 Relative degree of tolerance to morphine sulfate and methadone hydrochloride in the rat and the interaction of dexamethasone. Archives of Internal Pharmacodynamics 196: 176–183

Bruera E, Roca E, Cedaro L, Carraro S, Chacon R 1985 Action of oral methylprednisolone in terminal cancer patients: a prospective randomized double-blind study. Cancer Treatment Reports 69: 751–754

Bunch T W, Worthington J W, Combs J J, Iestrup D M , Engel A G 1980 Azathioprine with prednisone for polymyositis: a controlled clinical trial. Annals of Internal Medicine 92: 365–369

Byyny R L 1976 Withdrawal from glucocorticoid therapy. New England Journal of Medicine 295: 30–32

Cairnie A B, Leach K E 1982 Dexamethasone: a potent blocker for radiation-induced taste aversion in rats. Pharmacology, Biochemistry and Behaviour 17: 305–311

Capildeo R 1989 High-dose methylprednisolone for the treatment of malignant brain tumours. In: Capildeo R (ed) Steroids in diseases of the central nervous system. John Wiley, Chichester, pp 103–112

Carson J L, Strom B L, Schinnar R, Duff A, Sim E 1991 The low risk of upper gastrointestinal bleeding in patients dispensed corticosteroids. American Journal of Medicine 91: 223–228

Carter R L, Pittam M R, Tanner N S B 1982 Pain and dysphagia in patients with squamous carcinomas of the head and neck: the role of perineural spread. Journal of the Royal Society of Medicine 75: 598–606

Chan A T C, O'Brien M E R 1993 Hypersensitivity to dexamethasone. British Medical Journal 306: 109

Devor M, Govrin-Lippmann R, Raber P 1985 Corticosteroids reduce neuroma hyperexcitability. In: Fields H L, Dubner R, Cervero F (eds) Advances in pain research and therapy, vol 9. Raven Press, New York, pp 451–455

Dropcho E J, Soong S-J 1991 Steroid induced weakness in patients with primary brain tumors. Neurology 41: 1235–1239

Editorial 1982 Osteonecrosis caused by combination chemotherapy. Lancet i: 433–444

Editorial 1991 Ondansetron versus dexamethasone for chemotherapy-induced emesis. Lancet 338: 478

Eidelberg D 1991 Steroid myopathy. In: Rottenberg D A (ed) Neurological complications of cancer treatment. Butterworth-Heinemann, Boston, pp 185–191

Ehrenkranz J R L, Posner J B 1981 Adrenocorticosteroid hormones. In: Weiss L, Gilbert H A, Posner J B (eds). Brain metastasis, Martinus Nijhoff Publishers, Hague, pp 340–363

Feliu J, Gonzales-Baron M, Berrocal A et al 1992 Usefulness of megestrol acetate in cancer cachexia and anorexia: a placebo controlled study. American Journal of Clinical Oncology 15: 436–440

Flombaum C D, Schroy P, Watson R, Vanamee P 1986 Treatment of acute obstructive renal failure with high-dose methylprednisolone. Archives of Internal Medicine 146: 58–61

Freshney R I, Sherry A, Hassanzadah M, Freshney M, Crilly P, Morgan D 1980 Control of cell proliferation in human glioma by glucocorticoids. British Journal of Cancer 41: 857–866

Fulcher D A, Katelaris C H 1991 Anaphylactoid reaction to intravenous hydrocortisone sodium succinate: a case report and literature review. The Medical Journal of Australia 154: 210–214

Galicich J H, French L A, Melby J C 1961 Use of dexamethasone in the treatment of cerebral edema resulting from tumours and brain surgery. Journal Lancet 81: 46–53

Gambertoglio J G 1983 Corticosteroids and anticonvulsants. Drug Interactions Newsletter 12: 55–58

Gilbert R W, Kim J H, Posner J B 1978 Epidural spinal cord compression from metastatic tumours: diagnosis and treatment. Annals of Neurology 3: 40–51

Gilman A G, Goodman L S, Rall T W, Murad F (eds) 1985 Goodman and Gilman's The pharmacological basis of therapeutics, 8th edn. Pharmaceutical Press, London p 1447

Goldberg A L, Goodman H M 1969 Relationship between cortisone and muscle work in determining muscle size. Journal of Physiology 200: 667–675

Golding D N, Murray S M, Pearce G W et al 1961 Corticosteroid myopathy. Annals of Physiology and Medicine 5: 171

Grahame-Smith D G, Aronson J K 1992 The Oxford textbook of clinical pharmacology and drug therapy, 2nd edn. Oxford University Press, Oxford, pp 585–586

Gralla R J 1989 An outline of anti-emetic treatment. European Journal of Cancer and Clinical Oncology 25: S7–S11

Greenberg H S, Kim J-H, Posner J B 1979 Epidural spinal cord compression from metastatic tumour: results with a new treatment protocol. Annals of Neurology 8: 361–366

Grunberg S M 1989 Advances in the management of nausea and vomiting induced by non-cisplatin containing chemotherapeutic regimens. Blood Reviews 3: 216–221

Guslando M, Titobello A 1992 Steroid ulcers: a myth revisited. British Medical Journal 304: 655–656

Hanks G W, Trueman T, Twycross R G 1983 Corticosteroids in terminal cancer: a prospective analysis of current practice. Postgraduate Medical Journal 59: 702–706

Henry D A, Johnston A, Dobson A, Duggan J 1987 Fatal peptic ulcer complications and the use of nonsteroidal anti-inflammatory drugs, aspirin, and corticosteroids. British Medical Journal 295: 1227–1229

Hong D, Byers M R, Oswald R J 1993 Dexamethasone treatment reduces sensory neuropeptides and nerve sprouting reactions in injured teeth. Pain 55: 171–181

Hursti T J, Fredrikson M, Steineck G, Borjeson S, Furst C J, Peterson C 1993 Endogenous cortisol exerts antiemetic effect similar to that of exogenous corticosteroids. British Journal of Cancer 68: 112–114

Ibels L S, Alfrey A C, Huffer W E, Weil R 1978 Aseptic necrosis of bone following renal transplantation: experience in 194 transplant recipients and review of the literature. Medicine (Baltimore) 57: 25–45

Jamous M A 1989 High-dose methylprednisolone for malignant gliomas: safety and side-effects. In: Capildeo R (ed) Steroids in diseases of the central nervous system. John Wiley, Chichester, pp 113–122

Kirkham S R 1988 The palliation of cerebral tumours with high-dose dexamethasone: a review. Palliative Medicine 2: 27–33

Korman B, McKay R J 1985 Steroids and postoperative analgesia. Anaesthesia and Intensive Care 13: 395–398

Leslie R A, Shah Y, Thejomayen M, Murphy K M, Robertson H A 1990 The neuropharmacology of emesis: the role of receptors in neuromodulation of nausea and vomiting. Canadian Journal of Physiology and Pharmacology 68: 279–288

Loprinzi C L, Ellison N M, Schaid D J et al 1990 Controlled trial of megestrol acetate for the treatment of cancer anorexia and cachexia. Journal of the National Cancer Institute 82: 1127–1132

McCluskey J, Gutteridge D H 1982 Avascular necrosis of bone after high doses of dexamethasone during neurosurgery. British Medical Journal 284: 333–334

Mannheimer I H 1965 Hypercalcaemia of breast cancer: management with corticosteroids. Cancer 18: 679–691

Mealey J, Chen T T, Schanz G P 1971 Effects of dexamethasone and methylprednisolone on cell cultures of human glioblastomas. Journal of Neurosurgery 34: 324–334

Minton M J, Knight R K, Rubens R D, Hayward J L 1981 Corticosteroids for elderly patients with breast cancer. Cancer 48: 883–887

Moertel C G, Schutt A J, Reitemeier R J, Hahn R G 1974 Corticosteroid therapy of preterminal gastrointestinal cancer. Cancer 33: 1607–1609

Needham P R, Daley A G, Lennard R F 1992 Steroids in advanced cancer: a survey of current practice. British Medical Journal 305: 999–1000

Nixon J E 1984 Early diagnosis and treatment of steroid induced avascular necrosis of bone. British Medical Journal 288: 741–744

Parry H, Martin K 1991 Single-dose IV dexamethasone: an effective anti-emetic in cancer chemotherapy. Cancer Chemotherapy and Pharmacology 28: 231–232

Pattrick M, Doherty M 1987 Facial flushing after intra-articular injection of steroid. British Medical Journal 295: 1380

Percival R C, Yates A J P, Gray R E S, Neal F E, Forrest A R W, Kanis J A 1984 Role of glucocorticoids in management of malignant hypercalcaemia. British Medical Journal 289: 287

Pieretti S, Di Giannuario A, Loizzo A et al 1992 Dexamethasone prevents epileptiform activity induced by morphine in in vivo and in vitro experiments. Journal of Pharmacology and Experimental Therapeutics 263: 830–839

Pierquin B, Baillet F, Maylin C 1978 Corticotherapie en Cancerologie. Malaine, Paris

Pilkington G J 1989 Steroids and gliomas: experimental and in vitro studies. In: Capildeo R (ed) Steroids in diseases of the central nervous system. John Wiley, Chichester, pp 83–97

Piper J M, Ray W A, Daugherty J R, Griffin M R 1991 Corticosteroid use and peptic ulcer disease: role of nonsteroidal anti-inflammatory drugs. Annals of Internal Medicine 114: 735–740

Posner J B, Howieson J, Cvitkovic E 1977 Disappearing spinal cord compression: oncolytic effect of glucocorticoids (and other chemotherapeutic agents) on epidural metastases. Annals of Neurology 2: 409–413

Pybus P K 1984 Osteoarthritis: a new neurological method of pain control. Medical Hypothesis 14: 413–422

Renaudin J, Fewer D, Wilson C B, Boldrey E B, Calogero J, Enot K J 1973 Dose dependency of Decadron in patients with partially excised brain tumours. Journal of Neurosurgery 39: 302–305

Richardson A, Hide T A H, Eversden I D 1970 Longterm continuous intracranial-pressure monitoring by means of a modified subdural pressure transducer. Lancet ii: 687–689

Rotstein J, Good R A 1957 Steroid pseudorheumatism. AMA Archives of International Medicine 99: 545–555

Rowell N P 1988 Intralesional methylprednisolone for rib metastases: an alternative to radiotherapy? Palliative Medicine 2: 153–155

Schell H W 1966 This risk of adrenal corticosteroid therapy in far-advanced cancer. American Journal of the Medical Sciences 252: 641–649

Sridhar K S, Hussein A M, Hilsenbeck S, Cairns V 1992 Five-drug antiemetic combination for cisplatin chemotherapy. Cancer Investigation 10: 191–199

Stoll B A 1963 Corticosteroids in therapy of advanced mammary cancer. British Medical Journal 2: 210–214

Sury M R J, Russell G N, Heaf D P 1988 Hydrocortisone myopathy. Lancet ii: 515

Swartz S L, Dluhy R G 1978 Corticosteroids: clinical pharmacology and therapeutic use. Current Therapeutics Sept: 145–170

Tannock J, Gospodarowicz M, Meakin W, Panzarella T, Stewart L, Rider W 1989 Treatment of metastatic prostatic cancer with low-dose prednisolone: evaluation of pain and quality of life as pragmatic indices of response. Journal of Clinical Oncology 17: 590–597

Tchekmedyian N S, Tait N, Moody M, Greco F A, Aisner J 1986 Appetite stimulation with megestrol acetate in cachectic cancer patients. Seminars in Oncology 13: 37s–43s

Thalassinos N C, Joplin F G 1970 Failure of corticosteroid therapy to correct the hypercalcaemia of malignant disease. Lancet ii: 537–539

Thorne J C, Evans W K, Alison R E, Fournasier V 1981 Avascular necrosis of bone complicating treatment of malignant lymphoma. American Journal of Medicine 71: 751–758

Twycross R G 1992 Corticosteroids in advanced cancer. British Medical Journal 305: 969–970

Twycross R G, Guppy D 1985 Prednisolone in terminal breast and bronchogenic cancer. Practitioner 229: 57–59

Van Marle W, Woods K L 1980 Acute hydrocortisone myopathy. British Medical Journal 281: 271–272

Walsh D, Avashia J 1992 Glucocorticoids in clinical oncology. Cleveland Clinic Journal of Medicine 59: 505–515

Weissman D E, Dufer D, Vogel V, Abeloff M D 1987 Corticosteroid toxicity in neuro-oncology patients. Journal of Neuro-Oncology 5: 125–128

Weissman D E, Janjan N A, Erickson B et al 1991 Twice-daily tapering dexamethasone treatment during cranial radiation for newly diagnosed brain metastases. Journal of Neuro-Oncology 11: 235–239

Willox J, Corr J, Shaw J et al 1984 Prednisolone as an appetite stimulant in patients with cancer. British Medical Journal 288: 27

Williams W R 1993 Hypersensitivity to dexamethasone. British Medical Journal 306: 585–586

Zizic T M 1990 Avascular necrosis of bone. Current Opinion in Rheumatology 2: 26–37

Miscellaneous drugs

In this chapter, various other drugs which relieve pain in specific circumstances are discussed. It is not possible to arrange the drugs in order of importance because their usefulness is limited to one or a few pain syndromes. Consequently, the order chosen follows the systematic classification of the British National Formulary. This begins with drugs acting on the gastro-intestinal system and ends with drugs used in anaesthesia.

DRUGS ACTING ON THE GASTRO-INTESTINAL SYSTEM

Drugs for stomatitis and mucositis

Stomatitis (painful mouth) is common in advanced cancer (Box 23.A). Many cases relate to infection with *Candida albicans* and respond to treatment with an antifungal antibiotic. Ketoconazole 200 mg daily for 7 days is used at many centres on the grounds of efficacy, cost and ease of administration. Courses of more than 10 days have been associated with hepatotoxicity. Other centres use fluconazole. Unlike ketoconazole, this has negligible effect on the P450-mediated enzymes involved in the synthesis of adrenal steroids. In recommended doses, however, it is more expensive.

In one trial, 95% of patients responded to ketoconazole 200 mg daily for 5 days compared with 87% with a single dose of fluconazole 150 mg (Regnard 1993). White patches on the buccal mucosa cleared in a median of 2 days with both treatments. More patients on ketoconazole relapsed so that the number remaining clinically free of candidiasis was identical in both groups, i.e. two thirds. These data make single dose fluconazole a convenient option.

Patients with painful aphthous ulcers should be treated with a combination of an antibiotic or an antiseptic and a corticosteroid (Box 23.B). Symptomatic measures for nonspecific stomatitis are listed in Box 23.C.

Radiotherapy and chemotherapy induced mucositis are the most severe

BOX 23.A
CAUSES OF STOMATITIS IN ADVANCED CANCER

Malnutrition:

- hypovitaminosis
- anaemia
- protein deficiency

Altered immunity
Drugs:

- chemotherapy
- corticosteroids
- antibiotics

Infection:

- candidiasis
- aphthous ulcers

Dry mouth

BOX 23.B
DRUG TREATMENT OF APHTHOUS ULCERS

Antibiotics and antiseptics:

- tetracycline suspension
- chlorhexidine gluconate gel (Corsodyl dental gel)

Inflammatory and immune suppression:

- hydrocortisone
- triamcinolone acetonide
- betamethasone-17-benzoate

BOX 23.C
SYMPTOMATIC MEASURES FOR NONSPECIFIC STOMATITIS

Mouthwashes
Topical analgesics:

- choline salicylate (Bonjela gel)
- benzydamine (Difflam)
- diphenhydramine local application

Mucosal coating agents:

- sucralfate 1 g tablet (crush and spread around mouth with tongue)

Local anaesthetics:

- lignocaine viscous 2%
- benzocaine
- dyclonine

forms of oropharyngeal mucositis seen in cancer patients. Fortunately, such hazards are usually in the past by the time a patient is referred for palliative care. Energetic treatment is called for because the pain can be extremely severe when eating or drinking. In addition to local treatment, morphine is usually necessary. This can often be taken orally but some centres recommend IV patient controlled analgesia (PCA). Opioids alone usually achieve no more than 50–60% relief. The role of antibiotics in the relief of mucositis is under investigation.

Diphenhydramine

Diphenhydramine hydrochloride, an antihistamine, is a mild topical mucosal analgesic (Douglas 1985). It is used in many cancer centres in local applications to soothe a painful buccal mucosa. If significant amounts of diphenhydramine are swallowed, they may cause drowsiness. Diphenhydramine is no longer available in the UK as a single preparation. It is present in several cough medicines and, therefore, can presumably be bought in powder form from the manufacturers.

Diphenhydramine in kaopectate comprises equal parts of diphenhydramine solution (12.5 mg/5 ml) and kaopectate. The pectin in the kaopectate is thought to help the diphenhydramine adhere to the mucosal surface. It is spread around the mouth with the tongue and then swallowed. Up to 30 ml q2h is used.

Stomatitis cocktail (National Cancer Institute, USA) comprises lignocaine viscous 2%, diphenhydramine solution (12.5 mg/5 ml) and Maalox (a proprietary antacid) in equal parts. It is spread around the mouth with the tongue, held for 2 min and then spat out. Up to 30 ml q2h is used.

NSAIDs

Benzydamine hydrochloride is a nonsteroidal anti-inflammatory drug (NSAID) which is absorbed through skin and mucosae (see p. 207). It also has a mild local anaesthetic action. Benzydamine oral rinse used as a gargle (15 ml) is of proven value in radiation induced oral mucositis (Kim et al 1985, Epstein et al 1989). It may sting initially. A spray is also available. The recommended dose is four to eight puffs onto painful areas every 1.5–3 h.

Choline salicylate gel can also be used.

Corticosteroids

Topical corticosteroids are of benefit in severe radiation induced mucositis. One approach is to dissolve a 2 mg tablet of betamethasone sodium phosphate in 15 ml water. This is then spread around the mouth with the tongue for 2 min before being spat out. In patients receiving radical radiotherapy for parotid tumours, it has been administered q.i.d. the day before and throughout the course of treatment (Abdelaal et al 1989):

'The ipsilateral oral mucosa that received the full dose of irradiation (60 Gy in 30 treatments over 6 weeks) showed progressive whitening as radiation treatment progressed, in contrast to the erythema that usually occurs. The mucosa remained virtually ulcer free. The most impressive result was the absence of any discomfort or bleeding of the oral mucosa, even at the end of treatment . . . Histological examination of a specimen of the oral mucosa of one of the patients taken at completion of irradiation showed absence of the inflammatory component of irradiation induced mucositis and some thickening and keratinisation of the buccal epithelium' (Abdelaal et al 1989).

Mucosa adhesive film

Another approach is to cover the mucosa with an adhesive protective film. One report speaks of dissolving grade M hydroxypropylcellulose 600 mg in 3% ethanol and adding tetracaine 10 mg, thiamphenicol 5 mg and triacetin 24 mg. The ethanolic solution was cast in teflon 6 × 10 cm and dried overnight in a glovebox, forming a pliant translucent film about 0.1 mm thick. When applied to a wet mucosal surface, the film adhered firmly. In a preliminary evaluation in two patients, pain relief lasted 4–6 h (Yotsuyanagi et al 1985). This is longer than the relief obtained from lignocaine gel. New films can be substituted as necessary. The two patients each used five or six films over several days.

Compound antacids

Activated dimethicone (simethicone) and oxethazaine are both available as compound antacids. Dimethicone is an antifoaming agent of value in gassy dyspepsia. Oxethazaine is a local anaesthetic of value in the management of painful oesophagitis.

Activated dimethicone (simethicone)

Squashed stomach syndrome (see p. 100) is common in patients with hepato-megaly and/or marked ascites. Small stomach syndrome is common after partial gastrectomy or associated with linitis plastica of the stomach. Post-prandial epigastric discomfort and/or pain is a feature of these syndromes. They are helped by:

- explanation
- dietary advice (meals 'small and often')
- an antacid containing an antifoaming agent
- a prokinetic agent such as metoclopramide.

In the UK, Asilone suspension (containing activated dimethicone 135 mg/5 ml, together with aluminium and magnesium salts) is a good choice of compound antacid. In the USA, Maalox Plus can be used.

Squashed/small stomach syndrome causes epigastric fullness more often than pain and the patient may complain of 'wind' and hiccup. In the following case history, retrosternal pain caused by acid regurgitation through an endo-oesophageal tube was the main symptom.

■ CASE HISTORY

A 54 year-old woman with cancer of the gastro-oesophageal junction had an endo-oesophageal tube inserted. A few days later she began to experience lower retrosternal and epigastric pain for which dihydrocodeine was prescribed. This helped a little. Ten days later she was re-admitted as an emergency with severe lower abdominal colic caused by severe constipation and rectal impaction. She was treated with enemas and oral laxatives. The reason for the original pain was explained to her, and she was treated with metoclopramide 10 mg before meals and Asilone 10 ml after meals with good effect. She learned to distinguish between gastric distension pain, for which she took additional Asilone, and an intermittent epigastric pain probably caused by the cancer itself, for which she took paracetamol 1 g about once every other day.

Endoscopy and oesophageal biopsy have shown that an antacid containing activated dimethicone is superior to a plain antacid in the management of reflux oesophagitis (Ogilvie & Atkinson 1986). Further, in reflux oesophagitis, an antacid containing dimethicone is at least as effective as one containing alginic acid (Smart & Atkinson 1990). These findings suggest that antacids containing dimethicone can be regarded as 'broad-spectrum' antacids for all patients troubled by acid dyspepsia, whether gastric or oesophageal.

Antacids containing alginic acid are still often prescribed for patients with acid reflux. Such preparations, however, are:

- weak antacids
- often high in sodium content
- more expensive.

Much of the antacid content adheres to the alginate matrix which floats on the surface of the gastric contents. Thus, neutralization of gastric acid is localized to the proximal stomach contents which is, of course, the portion refluxed. All things considered, an antacid containing dimethicone would seem to be preferable.

Oxethazaine

Oxethazaine is a surface anaesthetic. It has a prolonged action after a relatively slow onset. It is poorly absorbed from mucous membranes. It is administered by mouth in the treatment of painful oesophagitis caused, for example, by acid reflux ± candidiasis or radiotherapy. It is available in the UK with aluminium and magnesium hydroxides as Mucaine. It does not diminish oesophageal reflux. Mucaine should be used in patients with distressing retrosternal discomfort when drinking or eating as a *temporary* topical analgesic until other measures have taken effect.

Table 23.1   Drugs and the lower oesophageal sphincter

Decrease tone	Increase tone
Alcohol	Prokinetic agents:
Nicotine	metoclopramide
Carminatives:	cisapride
mint	domperidone
anise	Antacids
dill	Bethanechol
Anticholinergics	
Pethidine	
Diazepam	
Oestrogens	
Theophylline	
Nitrates and nitrites	
Calcium channel blockers:	
verapamil	
nifedipine	
diltiazem	
Hydralazine	
Isoproterenol	

In the normal oesophagus, little of the oxethazaine adheres to the oeso-phageal mucosa because of rapid transit from pharynx to stomach. In pathological states, however, peristalsis is often significantly impaired. This, together with an injured (more adhesive) mucosa, allows time for absorption and consequential local anaesthesia. Mucaine should be taken in a dose of 10–15 ml about 15 min before meals, and at bedtime if necessary, without any additional fluid. Concomitant measures to reduce acid reflux and oesophageal mucosal injury should be considered. This includes reviewing drug therapy (Table 23.1).

H$_2$-receptor antagonists

The story of cimetidine and acute herpes zoster is included as a cautionary tale. Several cases of 'dramatic improvement in pain and pruritus' were re-ported in the 1980s when patients with acute herpes zoster were prescribed cimetidine (Mavlight & Talpaz 1984). In an uncontrolled study 18/21 patients benefited (Van der Spuy et al 1980). The rationale for the benefit was as follows:

- herpes zoster is associated with depressed cellular immune function
- because thymus dependent T-lymphocytes possess H$_2$-receptors, antagonists may modify cell mediated responses (Rockin 1976)
- H$_2$-receptor antagonists may also have a direct antitumour effect (Van der Spuy 1980).

However, when a randomized controlled trial was undertaken in 63 patients (cimetidine 200 mg t.i.d. and 400 mg nocte v. placebo for 28 days), no be-nefit was seen. The rate of healing was identical, as was the incidence of postherpetic neuralgia 3 and 6 months later (Levy et al 1985).

Prokinetic agents

This group of drugs is useful in dyspeptic conditions associated with gastric distension or opioid induced delayed gastric emptying. The prokinetic effect of metoclopramide and cisapride is mediated by a $5HT_4$ agonist effect which, in turn, triggers a cholinergic mechanism. The prokinetic effect is therefore antagonized by anticholinergic drugs, as well as by opioids. The prokinetic mechanism of action of domperidone is different. It is possibly acting as a dopamine antagonist but details are obscure.

Metoclopramide

Metoclopramide 20 mg IV and a compound preparation of papaverine 20 mg, morphine 6.6 mg, noscapine 3 mg, codeine 0.4 mg and methylscopolamine 0.15 mg are equally effective in relieving ureteric colic (Table 23.2). Papaverine and methylscopolamine are both antispasmodics. An equal number of patients in each group needed supplementary opioid analgesia. A subsequent trial of metoclopramide 20 mg SC and morphine 20 mg with atropine 0.5 mg also showed equal relief with metoclopramide (Muller et al 1990).

In a trial in prostaglandin (PG) induced labour for second trimester termination of pregnancy, metoclopramide 10 mg IV was compared with placebo as an adjunct to IV patient controlled analgesia (PCA) in 15 patients (Rosenblatt et al 1991). The metoclopramide group:

- used half as much PCA morphine (24 mg v. 52 mg)
- registered lower pain scores
- were delivered of the foetus more rapidly ($p < 0.05$).

It is possible, therefore, that metoclopramide relieves cramp by restoring normal peristalsis in the fallopian tubes and uterus, and in consequence improves the expulsive force (Rosenblatt et al 1991).

Whether $5HT_4$ receptors are involved at these sites is unclear. Metoclopramide is also a dopamine antagonist, and dopamine receptors have been identified along the length of the human fallopian tube (Helm et al 1982).

In summary, metoclopramide enhances normal peristaltic contractions in both the upper gastro-intestinal and the genito-urinary tracts, and alleviates painful muscular dysfunction in both organs.

Table 23.2 IV metoclopramide and ureteric colic

Time after injection (min)	Mean VAS pain scores	
	Metoclopramide	Opioid-antispasmodic
0	78	73
10	71	62
20	64	54
30	55	51

From Hedenbro & Olsson 1988

Antispasmodics

Antispasmodics are used for the treatment of intestinal colic, notably in irritable bowel syndrome (IBS). Most antispasmodic drugs used in IBS have a direct action on smooth muscle, e.g. enteric coated peppermint oil and mebeverine.

Peppermint oil

Peppermint oil is a naturally occurring agent which has been used for many years in the upper gastro-intestinal tract, both as an antispasmodic and to reduce flatulence. This latter effect is related to reduction in the tone of the lower oesophageal sphincter.

Studies in man have demonstrated that peppermint oil significantly reduces colonic motility for periods of 10–20 min (Duthie 1981). In vitro studies suggest that menthol, (the active constituent in peppermint oil) acts as a calcium channel blocker (Taylor et al 1985). Abdominal symptoms improved in two placebo controlled trials with peppermint oil capsules (Rees et al 1979, Dew et al 1984). Another study, however, failed to demonstrate superiority to a placebo (Nash et al 1986). Because menthol is absorbed in the small bowel, the site of release of the peppermint oil is critical if it is to affect colonic motility; commercial preparations are entericcoated in order to delay release.

Mebeverine

Mebeverine in doses ranging from 135–270 mg t.i.d. has been shown to be effective in reducing pain in IBS over 3–8 weeks (Anonymous 1986). *Alverine* may be as effective as mebeverine, but evidence is limited.

Anticholinergic antispasmodics

Anticholinergic antispasmodics, e.g. hyoscine butylbromide and mepenzolate, have not been shown to benefit patients with IBS and have an unacceptable incidence of adverse effects. *Dicyclomine* has both direct smooth muscle and anticholinergic effects. Dicyclomine 10 mg t.i.d. is probably less effective, however, than mebeverine 135 mg t.i.d. (Grillage et al 1990).

Antispasmodics and cancer pain

Antispasmodics are of value in advanced cancer in patients with moderate colic associated with low grade intestinal obstruction. Many patients, however, have intermittent colic with a background of continuous abdominal cancer pain. These patients do better on regular morphine. Some patients, however, need a combination of morphine and hyoscine butylbromide. This quaternary salt of hyoscine is not well absorbed from the gastro-intestinal tract and should be given parenterally by SC injection or infusion (Wick 1951, Herxheimer & Haefeli 1966).

CARDIOVASCULAR SYSTEM DRUGS

Drugs from this category which are useful in morphine resistant pain include:

- drugs for arrhythmias (lignocaine, flecainide, mexiletine)
- clonidine
- calcium channel blockers (e.g. nifedipine).

Drugs for arrhythmias

Class I anti-arrhythmics are membrane stabilizing drugs and include ligno-caine, flecainide and mexiletine. Local anaesthetics have been shown to have an analgesic effect which is independent of their local anaesthetic action (De Jong & Nace 1968). Thus, IV lignocaine and procaine:

- block the nociceptive response to laryngoscopy (Gefke et al 1983)
- decrease the cough reflex (Steinhaus & Gaskin 1963)
- reduce postoperative pain (Keats et al 1951, DeClive-Lowe et al 1958, Bartlett & Hutaserani 1961).

IV infusions of local anaesthetic have been successful in treating chronic pain (Schnapp et al 1981, Boas et al 1982, Edwards et al 1985, Kastrup et al 1986). The duration of pain relief is generally longer than the corresponding local anaesthetic effect. Other studies have shown that IV local anaesthetics decrease spontaneous discharges from a neuroma (Chabal et al 1989) and from acutely injured corneal A-delta and C nerve fibres (Tanelian & MacIver 1991).

Orally administered lignocaine analogues are a more practical option. For example, tocainide is as effective as carbamazepine in treating trigeminal neuralgia (Lindblom & Lindstrom 1984, Lindstrom & Lindblom 1987). Unfortunately, tocainide can cause severe blood dyscrasias (Gertz et al 1986, Soff & Kadin 1987) and interstitial pneumonitis (Perlow et al 1981). Mexil-etine is free of these adverse effects and, in a dose of 10 mg/kg per day, is an effective analgesic in painful diabetic neuropathy (Dejgaard et al 1988). Mexiletine is also effective in nerve injury pain (Chabal et al 1992). Subjects received mexiletine:

- 150 mg b.i.d. for 3 days
- 150 mg t.i.d. for 2 weeks
- if still in pain, 150 mg q.i.d. for 1 week
- if still in pain, a further increase to 750 mg/day.

Only two patients complained of mild nausea. The minimal adverse effects were possibly related to the gradual increase in dose and to the moderate maximum dose. For most subjects, the maximum dose is ≤ 10 mg/kg, whereas in the treatment of arrhythmias, the dose is normally 10–15 mg/kg.

Benefit has also been reported in an open study in 8/9 patients with poststroke pain (Awerbuch & Sandyk 1990).

Use of anti-arrhythmics in cancer pain

An increasing number of palliative care centres are using flecainide or mexiletine for neuropathic pain, usually when an antidepressant and/or an anticonvulsant has failed (Dunlop et al 1988). In one report, 9/21 patients with neuropathic pain obtained a good sustained response with flecainide over 1–14 weeks (Sinnott et al 1991). With a maximum daily dose of 100 mg b.i.d. only 5/15 had good relief, compared with 4/6 with 200 mg b.i.d. Only one patient experienced adverse effects (confusion and nocturnal hallucinations) which cleared when flecainide was discontinued.

In most cases flecainide was second line treatment when anticonvulsant therapy had failed (eight cases) or caused unacceptable drowsiness (six cases). All patients were also receiving opioids. Only two patients had been treated previously with a tricyclic antidepressant.

Flecainide, however, has acquired a bad reputation because of results from the Cardiac Arrhythmia Suppression Trial (CAST investigators 1989). This study showed an increased incidence of sudden death in patients with symptom free ventricular arrhythmias treated with flecainide after myocardial infarction. To date, however, no such complication has been observed in cancer patients treated with flecainide for neuropathic pain.

It is, however, a general rule that, under certain circumstances, anti-arrhythmic drugs may become pro-arrhythmic. Tricyclic antidepressants also have arrhythmic potential. Thus, it would seem a sensible precaution to discontinue treatment with a tricyclic antidepressant before commencing flecainide or mexiletine. Theoretically, a washout period of at least 3 days would be sensible. Some centres, however, do not do this; they change drugs without an interval.

Because of the CAST report, it is likely that more centres will opt for mexiletine. It was originally developed as an anticonvulsant and an anorexiant, and the most frequent adverse effects are nausea and tremor. Peak plasma concentrations can be reduced by taking smaller doses at greater frequency or by delaying absorption by taking it after food.

Clonidine

Clonidine is a mixed alpha$_1$- and alpha$_2$-adrenergic agonist (mainly alpha$_2$). It reduces the responsiveness of peripheral blood vessels to vasoconstrictor and vasodilator substances, and to sympathetic nerve stimulation (Hieble & Ruffolo 1991). These actions led to its use in prophylaxis against migraine and in the treatment of hypertension (Anonymous 1990). Clonidine may cause a reduction in venous return and mild bradycardia, resulting in a reduced cardiac output.

Hypotension is the most likely adverse effect after bolus injection. Sedation and dry mouth may also occur initially. Dizziness, headache, euphoria,

BOX 23.D
POSSIBLE MECHANISMS OF ACTION OF CLONIDINE ANALGESIA

Agonist effect at alpha$_2$-adrenergic receptor or imidazoline receptors resulting in:

- peripheral and/or central suppression of sympathetic transmitter release (Langer et al 1980, Davis et al 1991)
- presynaptic inhibition of nociceptive afferents (Calvillo & Ghignone 1986)
- postsynaptic inhibition of spinal cord neurones (Yaksh 1985, Michel & Insel 1989)
- facilitation of brain stem pain modulating systems (Sagen & Proudfit 1985).

nocturnal restlessness, nausea, constipation, rash and impotence have all been reported. Long term use has occasionally precipitated depression. Agitation may occur after stopping long term treatment, or even a hypertensive crisis.

Clonidine and related alpha$_2$-adrenergic agonists modify nociception in animal models (Yaksh 1985, Nakamura & Ferreira 1988). Early anecdotal reports in humans of benefit from clonidine (Tamsen & Gordh 1984) have since been substantiated in controlled studies (Coombs et al 1984, Glynn et al 1986, Glynn et al 1988, Max et al 1988, Zeigler et al 1992). Possible mechanisms of action are listed in Box 23.D.

In a randomized double-blind crossover study, 40 patients with post-herpetic neuralgia of 3 months to 7 years duration were given single oral doses of clonidine 200 µg, codeine 120 mg, ibuprofen 800 mg or placebo (Max et al 1988). Patients reported significantly more pain relief after clonidine than after the other three treatments. Codeine and ibuprofen were ineffective (Fig. 23.1). Sedation, dizziness, and other adverse effects were more frequent after clonidine (74%) and codeine (69%) than after placebo (36%) and ibuprofen (28%). Pain relief tends to be greater in trials in which drugs cause adverse effects. Thus, clonidine's superiority over codeine (which had a similar incidence of adverse effects) can be taken as further evidence of a specific analgesic effect.

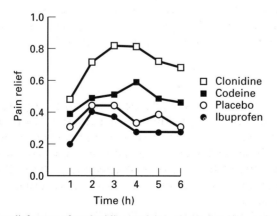

Fig. 23.1   Hourly relief scores after clonidine, codeine, placebo, and ibuprofen (category scale). (Reproduced with permission from Max et al 1988.)

Table 23.3 Results of epidural clonidine and morphine in 15 spinally injured patients with neuropathic pain

Drug giving relief	Number of patients
Morphine	5
Clonidine	10
Both	3
Neither	3

From Glynn et al 1986

In a single-blind crossover epidural (ED) study, 15 patients with spinal injuries and neuropathic pain of 1–26 years duration were given clonidine 150 mg and morphine 5 mg (Table 23.3). The interval between injections was 24 h or longer. The first patient investigated obtained pain relief from ED clonidine which lasted 6 *weeks*. When the pain returned a repeat injection of clonidine was given rather than morphine. The second dose was equally effective. The patient subsequently took intermittent courses of oral clonidine. Previously, ED local anaesthetic had failed to provide relief.

Subsequently, 9/10 patients who obtained relief with ED clonidine were given clonidine orally in doses of up to 100 µg t.i.d. Five patients were still taking clonidine with good effect 9 months later. Two others continued taking clonidine because if they stopped it the pain got worse, even though with clonidine the pain was no better than before the trial. The other two stopped taking clonidine because of, respectively, no benefit and severe depression. Two patients who obtained relief from ED morphine and one who had relief from both drugs were maintained satisfactorily on oral morphine.

Of the three double drug failures, two obtained relief from ED buprenorphine 0.3 mg. This suggests that failure with morphine related to the dose being too low. One of the two continued to take and benefit from sublingual (SL) buprenorphine; the other could not because of nausea and vomiting. Perhaps of relevance is the fact that the patient who did not respond even to buprenorphine was the eldest (74 years), had had pain the longest (26 years), and had a cervical lesion (C5–C6).

Transdermal clonidine (Langley & Heel 1988) has been evaluated in 24 patients with painful diabetic neuropathy (Zeigler et al 1992). In a randomized double-blind crossover study, patients received clonidine 300 µg/day or placebo patches, each for 6 weeks separated by a 2 week washout period. On a group basis, clonidine could not be distinguished from placebo at conventional levels of statistical significance. Nine patients, however, felt that they obtained sufficient benefit to undergo further cycles of testing with clonidine alone. Seven of the nine consistently reported return of pain when clonidine was stopped. One patient was equivocal and one had no benefit with retreatment. The seven consistent responders appeared similar to the other 17 patients in terms of pain quality and neurological signs. At the time of the report, benefit had been maintained for between 3 and 17 months.

The observation of reproducible pain relief in a minority of patients is consistent with the view that clonidine counteracts one or more, but not all, of the diverse mechanisms involved in neuropathic pain.

Calcium channel blockers

Calcium channel blockers interfere with the inward displacement of calcium ions through the slow channels of active cell membranes. Currently available calcium channel blockers are classified according to their cardiovascular properties (Table 23.4).

Table 23.4   Cardiovascular properties of calcium channel blockers

Class	Example	Anti-arrhythmic	Anti-anginal	Antihypertensive
I	Verapamil	++	++	++
II	Nifedipine	–	++	++
III	Diltiazem	(+)	++	++

Verapamil

Verapamil has moderate effects on smooth muscle contraction but a marked effect on cardiac calcium channels. It prolongs gastro-intestinal transit time and commonly causes constipation.

Nifedipine

Nifedipine has a marked relaxant effect on smooth muscle, particularly in the arterioles. It tends to cause a reflex tachycardia. Principal adverse effects are ankle oedema, flushing and postural hypotension. The oedema reflects increased peripheral vasodilatation, not cardiac failure. It may also cause facial flushing and sweating.

Diltiazem

Diltiazem, from the third class of calcium channel blockers, has properties intermediate between verapamil and nifedipine. It does not cause a reflex tachycardia.

In cardiology, calcium channel blockers are generally second line drugs or 'add on' ones. Nifedipine has been used to relieve troublesome hiccup (Anonymous 1990). It has also been used to relieve oesophageal spasm.

DRUGS ACTING ON THE CENTRAL NERVOUS SYSTEM

This group of drugs includes analgesics and psychotropic drugs which are discussed elsewhere. The focus in this section is on anticonvulsants.

Table 23.5   Drugs used in the treatment of epilepsy

Drug	Membrane effects	Neurotransmitter effects
Phenytoin	+	+ (serotonin)
Phenobarbitone	–	+ (GABA)
Valproate	–	+ (?GABA)
Carbamazepine	+	?
Benzodiazepines	–	+ (GABA)
Ethosuximide	?	–
Paraldehyde	+	– ?
Vigabatrin	–	+ (GABA)

From Grahame-Smith & Aronson 1992

Anticonvulsants

Anticonvulsants prevent the spread of the neuronal excitation in epilepsy by poorly understood mechanisms (Table 23.5). These mechanisms involve:

- a stabilizing effect on excitable cell membranes
- blocking the spread of seizure activity by enhancing GABA inhibition of synaptic transmission.

The N-methyl D-aspartate (NMDA) receptor-ion complex has also been implicated (Richens 1991). The benzodiazepines and the barbiturates enhance GABA function by interacting with GABA receptors at the $GABA_A$/benzodiazepine receptor complex. Valproate enhances GABA function by an unknown mechanism, but it may enhance GABA synthesis and/or release. Vigabatrin (gamma-vinyl-GABA) increases GABA function by competitive inhibition of GABA transaminase, which is responsible for the breakdown of GABA. Four anticonvulsants have been studied in relation to neuropathic pain (Swerdlow 1984, McQuay 1988):

- phenytoin (not now used)
- carbamazepine
- sodium valproate
- clonazepam (Chapter 21).

The anticonvulsant properties are not necessarily the determining factor in pain relief because, at anticonvulsant drug concentrations, barbiturates are not analgesic (Bonduelle et al 1964). Clinical observations suggest that different patients with stabbing pain may respond to different anticonvulsants (Swerdlow & Cundill 1981). Clonazepam appeared to be the most frequently effective drug.

Carbamazepine

Carbamazepine was first shown to be effective in trigeminal neuralgia. In an open study, 36/40 patients became painfree within 24 h of starting therapy (Blom 1963). The remaining four became painfree when phenytoin was added. Phenytoin, however, has generally been superseded by carbamazepine in trigeminal neuralgia because carbamazepine is more effective long term provided the dose is individually optimized (McQuay 1988).

Carbamazepine has also been shown to be effective in diabetic neuropathy. At a daily dose of 600 mg in a double-blind crossover trial, carbamazepine produced relief in 28/30 patients (Rull et al 1969).

Carbamazepine commonly causes a number of adverse effects, including nausea, ataxia and nystagmus. These can be minimized by initially prescribing only 100 mg b.i.d. and increasing the daily dose by no more than 200 mg a week. Of patients who initially respond, however, 20% subsequently become refractory to carbamazepine.

Oxcarbazepine is a derivative of carbamazepine which causes fewer adverse effects and should be used in patients intolerant of carbamazepine. Oxcarbazepine and carbamazepine are equally efficacious (Reinikainen et al 1987).

Oxcarbazepine is rapidly absorbed after oral ingestion (Theisohn & Heimann 1982, Schutz et al 1986). The primary metabolite is 10-hydroxycarbazepine; this too has anticonvulsant properties (Baltzer & Schmutz 1977). Oxcarbazepine is also of value in affective disorders (Emrich et al 1985) and spasticity (Bittencourt & Silvado 1985).

Sodium valproate

Sodium valproate is increasingly widely used but the evidence for its efficacy is mainly anecdotal (Peiris et al 1980). Although often prescribed b.i.d. or t.i.d., it has a long halflife and can conveniently be given in a single dose at bedtime. It may take 2 weeks to achieve a stable plasma concentration. Many patients obtain benefit with 500–600 mg/day. Others need higher doses, possibly 1 g or more. Sedation may be a problem with higher doses. In the frail elderly, a starting dose of 200 mg at bedtime is advisable. Sodium valproate may cause dyspepsia and/or nausea as a result of gastric irritation. It may also cause weight gain.

Anticonvulsants and cancer pain

Opinions differ as to whether these are first or second line drugs for neuropathic pain. At some centres they are first line (Sinnott et al 1991) but, at most, tricyclic antidepressants are. It is often said that a tricyclic should be used if the pain is mainly superficial and burning, but an anticonvulsant if the pain is solely or mainly stabbing in character. Results in patients with diabetic neuropathic pain, however, indicate that it is incorrect to limit anticonvulsants in this way. They have an effect on all forms of neuropathic pain.

My present practice is to use a tricyclic antidepressant (e.g. amitriptyline) initially and to *add* sodium valproate after some 2 weeks if there is residual stabbing pain despite a dose of 75 mg nocte for at least a week.

Table 23.6 Pain exacerbated by infection

Patient	Fever	Site of ulceration	Anbibiotic	Daily dose of morphine	
				Before antibiotics	After antibiotics
1	No	Under chin	Cephalexin PO	440 mg PO	240 mg PO
2	No	Mouth	Penicillin IV	360 mg IV	120 mg PO
3	No	Neck	Cephalexin PO	80 mg IV	90 mg PO
4	Yes	Neck	Cephalothin IV	144 mg IV	120 mg PR
5	No	Mouth	Penicillin IV + gentamicin IV	48 mg IV	150 mg PO[a]
6	No	Neck	Cephalexin PO	77 mg IV	180 mg PO[a]
7	No	Mouth	Metronidazole IV[b]	72 mg IV	20 mg PO

[a] See author's comment in text.
[b] Patient was allergic to penicillin.
From Bruera & MacDonald 1986

ANTIBIOTICS

Secondary infection is sometimes the cause of worsening pain in ulcerated tumours. One report gives details of seven patients with locally recurrent cancers of the tongue or the floor of the mouth (Bruera & MacDonald 1986). All had had good pain relief with oral opioids for extended periods. Then severe pain recurred without definite new signs. All had large tumour masses with ulceration and necrosis, induration, swelling and surrounding erythema. Pain relief improved markedly in all patients within 3 days of starting an antibiotic (Table 23.6). Given an IV:PO potency ratio for morphine of 3:1, patients 5 and 6 continued to need much the same dose of morphine. In the other five patients, however, dramatic reductions in morphine requirements were witnessed.

Because of necrosis, ulceration and the location of the tumour, cultures are not very helpful. Fever, leucocytosis and signs of local infection may be absent. A trial of antibiotics, therefore, should be started if circumstances suggest that infection may be a factor.

At Sobell House, we have had similar experiences in patients with infection in the sacral and perineal regions. Here, it is best to assume that there is a mixed infection of aerobic and anaerobic bacteria. Treatment in these circumstances should be with both flucloxacillin and metronidazole PO.

CALCITONIN

Calcitonin is a polypeptide hormone which inhibits osteoclast activity by binding to osteoclast receptors. Calcitonin is used in Paget's disease of the bone (Martin 1979) and also in the prevention of postmenopausal osteoporosis (MacIntyre et al 1988, Meunier et al 1990). It is given by injection or nasally.

Animal studies suggest that calcitonin injected into the lateral ventricle of the brain may have a specific analgesic effect. This is independent of any effect on plasma calcium. This analgesic effect is reversible by doses of naloxone 10–100 times greater than that required to reverse the effects of morphine (Bates et al 1981).

Calcitonin relieves acute postoperative phantom limb pain. When an IV infusion of 200 IU was administered over 20 min, the median pain score fell from seven to four, whereas after a placebo infusion the pain was unchanged (Jaeger & Maier 1992). One week after the calcitonin infusion, 76% were painfree and another 14% had more than 50% relief. After 1 year 71% were still painfree. In contrast, in a longitudinal study of patients with phantom limb pain, 72% had pain 1 week postoperatively, 65% at 6 months and 59% at 2 years (Jensen et al 1983).

■ CASE HISTORY

A 38 year-old woman had an above knee amputation for sarcoma. She was treated effectively with carbamazepine 800 mg/day for phantom limb pain and methotrimeprazine 20 mg/day for intolerable itching in the phantom foot from the second postoperative day. A year later, she underwent disarticulation of the hip because of a scar recurrence. Phantom limb pain recurred postoperatively and carbamazepine did not relieve it. In addition, she had neuropathic pain associated with lumbosacral plexopathy. Two infusions of calcitonin eased the phantom limb pain and the burning neuralgia. She continued to take m/r morphine tablets 120 mg/day for pains associated with the operation and the cancer itself. She died a year later.

Calcitonin and cancer pain

Several open studies indicate that calcitonin can relieve metastatic bone pain in some patients (Simone & Racanelli 1980, Di Silverio et al 1981, Serrou et al 1981, Leyland & Hindley 1982, Allan 1983). This effect has been confirmed in a double-blind placebo controlled trial (Gennari et al 1985).

■ CASE HISTORY

A patient who had had a mastectomy for breast cancer developed bone metastases. She was treated with stilboestrol. Two years later, she complained of severe pain in the right side of her pelvis. She received palliative radiotherapy and her pain completely abated for another 2 years. She then began to experience pain again which remained severe despite taking morphine 30 mg q4h.

She was given injections of calcitonin 200 IU b.i.d. for 4 days, with definite relief. The pain subsequently eased completely. Eight months later she was still completely painfree, and needed no analgesics, even though there was radiographic evidence of disease progression. She died 2 months later still painfree (Allan 1983).

It is unlikely that the relief was a placebo response. On the other hand, the patient was not receiving a NSAID. It is possible, therefore, that the need for calcitonin and the response to it might have been different if peripheral neural sensitization had been blocked by a cyclo-oxygenase inhibitor.

The mechanism by which calcitonin modulates pain perception, however, is still hypothesis. Interactions with opioid receptors have been reported

(Laurian et al 1986) but not confirmed (Wiesenfeld-Hallin & Persson 1984, Morton et al 1986). The analgesic effect can be reversed by serotonin antagonists such as methysergide (Guidobono et al 1986). Binding sites for calcitonin have been identified near brain areas rich in serotonin, i.e. the hypothalamus and limbic system (Olgiati et al 1983). In animal experiments, calcium injections reverse the analgesic effects of intraventricular calcitonin, but there is no relationship between its analgesic potency and plasma calcium concentrations in man (Gennari et al 1985).

Although calcitonin is a peptide of high molecular weight, it may be transported across the blood-brain barrier by special carrier proteins, as described for somatostatin (Pardridge 1988). The fast onset of pain relief after calcitonin administration could be explained in this way. IV administration may be necessary to obtain relief in phantom limb pain (Jaeger et al 1988). A nasal spray has been used with good effect in metastatic bone pain (Szanto et al 1992).

DRUGS FOR URINARY TRACT DISORDERS

Bladder spasms

Treatment of bladder spasms depends on the cause (Table 23.7). Anticholinergic drugs are, however, the mainstay of drug treatment. These act

Table 23.7 Treatment of bladder spasms

Cause	Treatment
Infection (cystitis)	Bladder washouts (if catheterized)
	Change indwelling catheter
	Intermittent catheterization q4–6h
	Encourage oral fluids
	Urinary antiseptics[a]:
	hexamine (methenamine) hippurate
	Antibiotics:
	systemic
	by instillation
Catheter irritation	Change catheter
	Reduce volume of balloon
Catheter sludging	Bladder washouts:
	tap water
	chlorhexidine and benzocaine (Hibitane)
	Noxyflex ⎫ if cheaper alternative ineffective
	Renacidin ⎭
	Continuous bladder irrigation
Cancerous irritation or infiltration of bladder or trigone	Anticancer treatment:
	chemotherapy
	hormone therapy
	Anticholinergic drugs:
	oxybutynin
	amitriptyline
Radiation fibrosis	Anticholinergic drugs

[a] Hexamine effective only in acid urine.

by reducing detrusor (bladder muscle) tone and by enhancing bladder sphincter tone (Bissada et al 1979). Although detrusor muscle sensitivity is increased by PGs and decreased by cyclo-oxygenase inhibitors (Abdel-Rahman et al 1981), the use of NSAIDs in this condition is usually not noticeably beneficial. In the past, phenazopyridine was used with good effect in some patients (see below). Coeliac axis plexus block and lumbar sympathetic block have also been used to relieve intractable bladder spasms.

Anticholinergic drugs

All these drugs cause unwanted as well as wanted anticholinergic effects, e.g. dry mouth, blurred vision. These tend to limit the clinical usefulness of anticholinergic drugs.

Amitriptyline 25–50 mg nocte is probably the simplest and most effective regimen.

Oxybutynin is marketed specifically for detrusor overactivity. In a dose of 5 mg PO t.i.d., over half of those treated will obtain a good response (Gajewski & Awad 1986). This dose, however, is too toxic for many patients. Particularly in the elderly, a dose of 2.5 mg b.i.d. may be sufficient. The maximum recommended dose is 5 mg q.i.d.

Propantheline The response to propantheline is variable (Gajewski & Awad 1986).

Belladonna alkaloids are sometimes used 'as needed'. Useful preparations include:

- hyoscine hydrobromide 0.3 mg SL
- belladonna and opium suppositories (USA only; see p. 268).

Several preparations containing hyoscyamine (laevo-atropine) are available in the USA (Twycross & Lack 1990). Hyoscyamine can be regarded as double strength atropine.

Flavoxate

Flavoxate has a selective action on smooth muscle fibres and a weak anticholinergic effect (Ruffman 1988). It is as effective as oxybutynin in the treatment of urge incontinence (Milani et al 1993). Adverse effects are seen in about one quarter of patients taking 400 mg t.i.d, compared with 90% of patients taking oxybutynin 5 mg t.i.d.

Phenazopyridine

Phenazopyridine, no longer available in the UK, exerts an analgesic effect on the mucosa of the urinary tract. It is used to provide symptomatic relief of dysuria in conditions such as cystitis, prostatitis, and urethritis. The usual dose is 200 mg PO t.i.d., preferably after food.

Phenazopyridine discolours urine either orange or red, and underclothes are apt to be stained. Phenazopyridine stains may be removed from fabric by soaking in a solution of sodium dithionite 0.25%. Phenazopyridine hydrochloride is contra-indicated in patients with impaired renal function (Martindale 1989).

OCTREOTIDE

Octreotide is a long acting analogue of somatostatin, a hypothalamic hormone (Editorial 1992). Its prime use is in the relief of symptoms associated with gastro-enteropancreatic endocrine tumours and for the short term treatment of acromegaly before surgical intervention. Because it reduces intestinal and pancreatic secretions, octreotide is also useful in the treatment of intractable vomiting associated with inoperable intestinal obstruction (Khoo et al 1992, Mercadante et al 1993), and in the management of pancreatic fistulae (Tulassay et al 1992).

Octreotide may also be of value in chronic nonmalignant pancreatic pain (Donnelly et al 1991). Chronic pancreatic pain is caused by hypertension in the scarred pancreatic ducts (Okazaki et al 1988). Suppressing exocrine function by administering pancreatic supplements reduces pain in 50–75% of patients with chronic pancreatitis (Mossner et al 1989). The benefit reported with octreotide is likely, therefore, to relate to its ability to suppress exocrine secretion (Lembcke et al 1987).

Octreotide has also been administered intrathecally (Chrubasik 1985).

DISTIGMINE

Distigmine, an anticholinesterase, has been used as adjuvant pain medication (Hampf et al 1989). In a 'ragbag' of chronic pain patients, pain was reduced on average by about:

- 15% by amitriptyline 25–75 mg
- 30% by amitriptyline and sodium valproate 200–600 mg
- 45% by amitriptyline and sodium valproate with distigmine 5 mg daily–b.i.d.

Curiously, unless the distigmine was started simultaneously with the other medication, no benefit was seen. The mechanism of action is unknown. Distigmine counteracts the anticholinergic properties of amitriptyline.

SKELETAL MUSCLE RELAXANTS

These are used for the relief of chronic muscle spasm or spasticity; they are not indicated for spasm associated with minor injuries. They act principally on the CNS with the exception of dantrolene which has a peripheral site of action. They differ in action from the muscle relaxants used in anaesthesia which block transmission at the neuromuscular junction.

The underlying cause of spasticity should be treated and any aggravating factors (e.g. pressure sores, infection) remedied. The major disadvantage of treatment with these drugs is that reduction in muscle tone can cause a loss of the splinting action of the spastic leg and trunk muscles and may, therefore, result in decreased mobility.

Dantrolene

Dantrolene acts directly on skeletal muscle and produces fewer central adverse effects. This makes it a good choice, particularly if drowsiness is a problem. The dose should be increased slowly (BNF 1993).

Baclofen

Baclofen inhibits transmission at spinal level and also depresses the CNS (Faigle et al 1980). Its plasma halflife is about 3.5 h increasing to 4.5 h in the elderly (Kochak et al 1985). The dose should be increased slowly to avoid sedation and hypotonia. Other adverse events are uncommon.

Diazepam

Diazepam is used in palliative care particularly if there is concomitant anxiety. Sedation and, occasionally, hypotonia are disadvantages. Other benzodiazepines also have muscle relaxant properties. Muscle relaxant doses of benzodiazepines are similar to anxiolytic doses. Benzodiazepines are also used in myoclonus.

Quinine

Quinine is an antimalarial drug given in a dose of 200–300 mg nocte to relieve nocturnal leg cramps (Warburton et al 1987). It is toxic in overdose and accidental fatalities have occurred in children.

In one study, compared with placebo, quinine reduced the frequency of cramps and sleep disturbance but did not affect cramp severity (Connolly et al 1992). A 50% reduction in the number of cramps was also noted in 13/27 patients while receiving placebo; this response was usually seen within 3 days. A mild increase in adverse effects was also noted when patients received placebo.

Thrombocytopenia has been reported in men taking quinine sulphate 200 mg at supper and 300 mg nocte. It is rare but can be fatal. Cinchonism, a syndrome comprising nausea and vomiting, tinnitus and deafness, occurs at toxic quinine levels. Other adverse effects include headache, visual disturbance, diarrhoea, pruritus, dermatitis, easy bruising, fatigue, and weakness. Smoking may block the effect of quinine (Connolly et al 1992).

CAPSAICIN

Capsaicin is a naturally occurring alkaloid found in the fruits of various species of the nightshade family (Solanaceae) and in chilli peppers. Capsaicin 0.075% cream is available for topical use. Capsaicin affects the synthesis, storage, transport and release of substance P (SP) in nociceptive fibres. In animals, capsaicin has also been shown to be neurotoxic, principally affecting nociceptive C fibres (Chung et al 1993).

Application of capsaicin causes an initial release of SP from C-fibres with subsequent depletion on continued use. Axonal transport of SP to synaptic terminals is reduced and synthesis inhibited (Gamse et al 1982). Capsaicin may also elevate the thresholds for the release of SP and other neurotransmitters. Reduced availability of SP diminishes pain transmission. Following cessation of capsaicin application, SP stores revert to pretreatment levels and neuronal sensitivity returns to normal (Gamse et al 1981, Fitzgerald 1983, LaMotte et al 1988).

Topical capsaicin has been available for some years in the USA, Canada and Australia. Clinical trials involving treatment for up to 2 years have shown capsaicin cream to be well tolerated without systemic adverse effects (Watson et al 1988, Bernstein et al 1989, Watson et al 1993).

The most frequently reported adverse effect of capsaicin cream is tingling, stinging or burning at the site of application. This effect is thought to be related to the initial release of SP from C fibres. The stinging and burning usually decreases with continued applications, often clearing in a few days. In others, dysaesthesiae may persist for 4 weeks or more. Temperature, humidity and occlusion influence the dysaesthesiae. Patients should avoid excessive sweating, and not take a hot bath immediately before or after application. Occlusion and tight bandaging should be avoided.

Application less frequently than t.i.d. is associated with a greater incidence or prolongation of the burning sensation. If the burning is severe, topical lignocaine can be applied before capsaicin in the first few weeks of treatment. Capsaicin cream should not be put on broken skin. It should also be kept away from eyes or mucous membranes. Patients should wash their hands after applying capsaicin cream.

In an open study of topical capsaicin 0.025% in postaxillary dissection pain, 14/18 women continued treatment (Watson et al 1989). Twelve had benefit after 4 weeks, eight of whom had good or excellent responses. After 6 months most of these patients still had good relief. A randomized placebo controlled trial of capsaicin cream 0.075% for 6 weeks gave comparable results (Watson & Evans 1992). Thus, 8/13 patients had 50% or more improvement; five of these were categorized as having a good or excellent result. Benefit was seen mainly in relation to stabbing pains.

KETAMINE

Ketamine is used principally as a dissociative anaesthetic (Boulton 1985). It activates the limbic system and depresses the cerebral cortex. Ketamine has a plasma halflife of about 3 h (Clements et al 1982). It is given IV or IM and provides anaesthesia for short surgical procedures. More commonly, it is used as an anaesthetic induction agent. In addition, subanaesthetic doses have been used as an analgesic in injured, postoperative and cancer patients by SC, IM, IV, ED and IT routes (Sadove et al 1971, Owen et al 1987, Kanamura et al 1990, Oshima et al 1990). It has also been given PO (Grant et al 1981).

Oral bio-availability is < 20%. Norketamine is the main metabolite and is about 1/3 as potent as ketamine. The maximum blood concentration of norketamine is greater after oral administration than after IV or IM (Clements et al 1982).

The analgesic effect is mediated at spinal level where ketamine acts as a NMDA receptor antagonist. There may also be an effect on the medial thalamic nuclei. NMDA receptors in the dorsal horn are activated by ongoing activity in nociceptive afferents (see p. 43). Activation is relatively rapid. Ketamine is of value, therefore, in acute pain. Its use may obviate the need for opioids (Ito & Ichiyanagi 1974). Combined use with morphine is generally preferable (Bristow & Orlikowski 1989). When ketamine 5–20 mg/h was combined with an IV infusion of morphine 1 mg/h after laparotomy, however, no additional benefit was reported when compared with a control group (Edwards et al 1993). Ketamine has, however, been used successfully in amputees with phantom limb pain (Stannard & Porter 1993).

Several reports of SC ketamine infusions in cancer patients have been published. In one 'analgesics such as morphine and pentazocine had become ineffective' (Oshima et al 1990). Initially, ketamine 10 mg SC was given as a bolus followed by an infusion of 10 mg/h using a portable syringe driver. Two increments of 2.5 mg/h were made after 24 h and 48 h respectively if pain was still reported. The maximum dose of 15 mg/h was based on pharmacokinetic considerations (Idvall et al 1979, Nimmo & Clements 1981).

Pain relief was obtained in 13/18 patients with infusion rates of 2.5–15 mg/h (60–360 mg/24 h) (Oshima et al 1990). Ketamine was not effective in three patients and dubious in two. In four patients ketamine was the sole analgesic for 10–48 days and two patients received ketamine for 5–7 months. Adverse effects comprised:

- injection site inflammation (6 patients)
- salivation (2)
- insomnia (2).

In a second group of 26 patients, ketamine was administered as either IV or SC bolus, or by SC infusion with morphine (Luczak et al 1992). Pain relief was achieved in each case. Indications for ketamine and doses used are given in Table 23.8. Bedbound patients requiring ketamine to prevent movement induced pain also received IV diazepam 2–10 mg or IV haloperidol 1–3 mg 2–3 min before ketamine in order to prevent the hallucinosis or bad dreams commonly seen as 'emergent' phenomena after ketamine anaesthesia. One patient continued to experience bad dreams despite IV midazolam 7.5 mg or IV haloperidol 2.5 mg. She refused further IV ketamine but subsequently tolerated SC ketamine 120 mg/24 h for 30 days.

Table 23.8   Ketamine analgesia in 26 cancer patients

Indication for use	Number of patients[a]	Route	Dose
To relieve pain on movement (turning and washing bedbound patients)	17	IV bolus	40–120 mg initially 20–40 mg subsequently
	1	PO bolus	0.5 mg/kg[b]
For immediate relief of neuropathic pain	8	IV bolus	20–40 mg (once only)
SC morphine infusion inadequate	9	SC infusion	60–180 mg/24 h
	1	IT infusion[c]	? mg/24 h

[a] Some patients received ketamine by more than one route.
[b] Woman aged 44 with breast cancer, bone metastases and spinal cord compression. Analgesia obtained 30 min after ingestion of ketamine.
[c] SC ketamine and morphine inadequate; 'dramatic relief' when given IT.
From Luczak et al 1992

At Sobell House, we have not used repeat IV bolus ketamine to relieve movement induced pain. We have, however, used several SC infusions. The first was in a woman with lumbosacral plexopathy who declined ED analgesia:

■ CASE HISTORY
A 75 year-old woman developed right sided sciatic pain. CT confirmed recurrent cancer of the sigmoid colon adherent to the posterior pelvic muscles and involving the right sciatic nerve. Multifraction palliative radiotherapy was commenced. Oral morphine up to 100 mg q4h gave little relief, nor did the addition of dexamethasone 8 mg/day. She then began to experience left sciatic pain and, 2 weeks later, severe right groin pain when getting out of bed if her legs were not held closely together. This movement induced pain was considered to be L1 nerve pain caused by nerve entrapment as it passed over the brim of the pelvis.

It was concluded that the pain was mainly neuropathic and an antidepressant was prescribed (dothiepin 75 mg nocte) but did not help. ED morphine and bupivacaine was suggested, but the patient declined this option. After another week with no improvement, she was treated with ketamine 60 mg and diamorphine 200 mg in 24 h by continuous SC infusion. The dose of ketamine was increased over 6 days to 300 mg/24 h; and the diamorphine halved. At the end of this time there was:

● no right sciatic pain
● minimal left sciatic pain (a tugging pain in the posterior lower thigh when walking)
● intermittent severe right L1 nerve pain when she got out of bed unless she held her legs together.

The left sciatic pain remitted completely over the next 2–3 weeks, and the L1 pain became both minimal and inconstant.

The diamorphine was changed to m/r morphine 200 mg b.i.d. but the ketamine remained unchanged. She also received flurbiprofen 100 mg b.i.d.

and dexamethasone 4 mg daily, together with longstanding atenolol 100 mg daily for hypertension. She required an enema three times a week.

The patient returned home with suitable support (including an electrically powered invalid chair). After about 2 months the dose of ketamine was reduced slowly to 50 mg/24 h without a return of the pain. She died from renal failure 6 months after starting ketamine.

It is possible that the dose of ketamine could have been reduced sooner and more rapidly if good pain management resulted in desensitization of the dorsal horn. On the other hand, the pain was neuropathic and spontaneous neuronal activity would probably persist.

Ketamine, is not just of value for movement induced and neuropathic pain. In the following case history, ketamine was used to treat intractable pain associated with *en cuirass* metastatic breast cancer.

■ CASE HISTORY

A 49 year-old woman was admitted with constant severe burning pain, affecting the upper half of her torso and her left arm to the elbow. Its site corresponded to cutaneous recurrence of breast cancer. On admission she was in severe pain despite > 10 000 mg of oral morphine daily, together with a tricyclic antidepressant and a corticosteroid. Within 24 h of starting a SC infusion of ketamine at a rate of 0.5 mg/kg/h she said she was comfortable. *The morphine was reduced to 100 mg daily.*

She remained on ketamine infusion for 48 days, had improved mobility and slept well. The infusion was maintained between 0.25–0.5 mg/kg/h with boosts of SC ketamine before the dressing was changed. She died peacefully 7 weeks after starting ketamine (Laird & Lovel 1993).

Assuming that the woman weighed between 50 and 60 kg, the daily dose of ketamine (excluding boluses) varied from 300–360 mg to 600–720 mg. She did not, however, experience any psychotomimetic effects, nor was her liver function affected.

It is probably best to start treatment with ketamine with a relatively low dose, for example 100 mg/day, and increase by 100 mg/day up to 500–600 mg. Some centres, however, start with a relatively high rate of infusion (500 µg/kg/h, i.e. 500–600 mg/day or more) and then reduce rapidly to 50% of the starting dose. If this approach is used, the dose of morphine should be halved when the ketamine is commenced. Further reductions may be necessary to correct sedation.

Because ketamine is irritant, a more dilute solution of ketamine may be preferable (i.e. 10 mg/ml rather than 50 mg/ml). This can be diluted if necessary with an equal volume of physiological saline.

NITROUS OXIDE

Given in subanaesthetic doses, certain inhalational anaesthetics produce complete relief of moderate pain and partial relief of severe pain without causing loss of consciousness or affecting cardiovascular or respiratory function. The most common agents used in this way are:

- nitrous oxide in oxygen
- 0.35–0.5% trichlorethylene in air
- 0.35–0.5% methoxyflurane in air.

They are administered by means of simple demand-flow inhalers. The Entonox apparatus available in the UK contains premixed 50% nitrous oxide and 50% oxygen. It has been used for the relief of severe pain (Baskett & Withnell 1970):

- at the site of accidents and disasters
- during ambulance transport
- in the emergency room.

A major theoretic limitation of the use of a nitrous oxide-oxygen mixture is in patients with acute respiratory problems or COAD, in whom the retention of nitrous oxide would be undesirable. Because of this, pulmonary disorders are considered by some people to be a contra-indication for this therapy (Marvin et al 1984).

Severe neurological symptoms have been reported in 15 patients (all but one of whom were dentists) following prolonged heavy exposure to nitrous oxide associated with professional use and/or self-administration (Layzer 1978). Initial symptoms were usually numbness or tingling in the hands or legs. Later symptoms included:

- L'hermitte sign (12)
- impairment of equilibrium or gait (12)
- trunk numbness (10)
- inability to walk unaided (7)
- mental changes (7)
- impotence (7)
- sphincter impairment (4)
- dysarthria (2)
- impairment of smell or taste (1).

Ten patients had to stop work. Symptoms resembled those of subacute combined degeneration of the spinal cord, and it was considered possible that nitrous oxide interfered with the action of vitamin B_{12} on the nervous system. All improved on stopping exposure to nitrous oxide and regained the ability to walk unaided but six followed a relapsing course associated with re-exposure to nitrous oxide. Administration of corticosteroids to six and vitamin B_{12} to four did not appear to influence the extent of recovery (Layzer 1978). Neurological effects have not been observed in nurses intermittently assisting patients with the use of nitrous oxide.

REFERENCES

Abdelaal A S, Barker D S, Fergusson M M 1989 Treatment for irradiation-induced mucositis. Lancet i: 97

Abdel-Rahman M, Coulombe A, Elhilali M M 1981 Detrusor dynamics II. Effect of prostaglandins and their synthesis inhibitor on stress relaxation time course. Inventative Urology 18: 281–284

Allan E 1983 Calcitonin in the treatment of intractable pain from advanced malignancy. Pharmatherapeutica 3: 482–486

Anonymous 1986 Some antispasmodic drugs for the irritable bowel syndrome. Drug and Therapeutics Bulletin 24: 93–95

Anonymous 1990 Clonidine in migraine prophylaxis: now obsolete. Drug and Therapeutics Bulletin 28: 79–80

Anonymous 1990 Intractable hiccup: baclofen and nifedipine are worth trying. Drug and Therapeutics Bulletin 28: 36

Awerbuch G I, Sandyk R 1990 Mexiletine for thalamic pain syndrome. International Journal of Neuroscience 55: 129–133

Baltzer V, Schmutz M 1977 Anticonvulsive properties of GP 47680 and GP 47779, its main human metabolite; compounds related to carbamazepine. In: Meinardi H, Rowan A J (eds) Advances in epileptology. Swetz & Zeitlinger, Amsterdam, pp 295–299

Bartlett E E, Hutaserani O 1961 Xylocaine for the relief of postoperative pain. Anesthesia and Analgesia 40: 296–304

Baskett P J F, Withnell A 1970 Use of Entonox in the ambulance services. British Medical Journal ii: 41

Bates R L F, Buckley G A, Eglen R M, Strettle R J 1981 The interaction of naloxone and calcitonin in the production of analgesia in the mouse. British Journal of Pharmacology 74: 280p

Bernstein J E, Korman N J, Bickers D R, Dahl M V, Millikan L E 1989 Topical capsaicin treatment of chronic postherpetic neuralgia. Journal of the American Academy of Dermatology 21: 265–270

Bissada N K, Finkbeiner A E, Welch L T 1979 Uropharmacology: X. Central nervous system stimulants and depressants. Urology 13: 464–473

Bittencourt P R, Silvado C E 1985 Oxcarbazepine, GP 47779 and spasticity. Lancet i: 676

Blom S 1963 Tic douloureu treated with new anticonvulsant. Experience with G32883. Archives of Neurology 9: 285

Boas R A, Covino B G, Sahnarian A 1982 Analgesic response to IV lignocaine. British Journal of Anaesthesia 54: 501–505

Bonduelle M, Houdart R, Sigwald J, Bouygues P, Lormeau G 1964 Traitement medical efficace de la nevralgie faciale par un derive de l'iminostilbene. Nouvelle Presse Medicale 72: 1905–1908

Boulton T B 1985 Anaesthesia beyond the major medical centre: current techniques with ketamine. Blackwell Scientific Publications, Oxford

Bristow A, Orlikowski C 1989 Subcutaneous ketamine analgesia: postoperative analgesia using subcutaneous infusions of ketamine and morphine. Annals of the Royal College of Surgeons of England 71: 64–66

British National Formulary 1993 Dantrolene Sodium. BNF No 25. British Medical Association and Royal Pharmaceutical Society of Great Britain, London, p 382

Bruera E & MacDonald N 1986 Intractable pain in patients with advanced head and neck tumours: a possible role of local infection. Cancer Treatment Reports 70: 691–692

Calvillo O, Ghignone M 1986 Presynaptic effect of clonidine on unmyelinated afferent fibers in the spinal cord of the cat. Neuroscience Letters 64: 335–339

Cardiac arrhythmia suppression trial (CAST) investigators 1989 Preliminary report: effect of encainide and flecainide on mortality in a randomized trial of arrhythmia suppression after myocardial infarction. New England Journal of Medicine 321: 406–412

Chabal C, Russell L C, Burchiel K J 1989 The effect of intravenous lidocaine, tocainide, and mexiletine on spontaneously active fibres originating in rat sciatic neuromas. Pain 38: 333–338

Chabal C, Jacobson L, Mariano A, Chaney E, Britell C W 1992 The use of oral mexiletine for the treatment of pain after peripheral nerve injury. Anesthesiology 76: 513–517

Chrubasik J 1985 Spinal infusion of opiates and somatostatin. Hygieneplan, Germany

Chung J M, Paik K S, Kim J S et al 1993 Chronic effects of topical application of capsaicin to the sciatic nerve on responses of primate spinothalamic neurons. Pain 53: 311–321

Clements J A, Nimmo W S, Grant I S 1982 Bio-availability, pharmacokinetics and analgesic activity of ketamine in humans. Journal of Pharmaceutical Sciences 71: 539–542

Connolly P S, Shirley E A, Wasson J H, Nierenberg D W 1992 The treatment of nocturnal leg cramps: a crossover trial of quinine vs. vitamin E. Archives of Internal Medicine 152: 1877–1880

Coombs D W, Saunders R, Gaylor M et al 1984 Clinical trial of intrathecal clonidine for cancer pain. Journal of Regional Anesthesia 9: 34–35

Davis K D, Treede R B, Raja S N, Meyer R A, Campbell J N 1991 Topical application of clonidine relieves hyperalgesia in patients with sympathetically maintained pain. Pain 47: 309–318

DeClive-Lowe S G, Desmond J, North J 1958 Intravenous lignocaine anesthesia. Anesthesiology 13: 138–146

Dejgaard A, Petersen P, Kastrup J 1988 Mexiletine for treatment of chronic painful diabetic neuropathy. Lancet i: 9–11

De Jong R H, Nace R A 1968 Nerve impulse conduction during intravenous lidocaine injection. Anesthesiology 29: 22–28

Dew M J, Evans B K, Rhodes J 1984 Peppermint oil for the irritable bowel syndrome: a multicentre trial. British Journal of Clinical Practice 38: 394–398

Di Silverio F, Galfano G, Zezza A, Cruciani E, Giabobini S, Tanaglia R 1981 The use of calcitonin in the treatment of metastasizing prostatic carcinoma. In: Pecile A (ed) International Symposium on Calcitonin, Milan 1980. Excerpta Medica, Amsterdam, pp 295–301

Donnelly P K, Parry A, Hanning C 1991 Somatostatin for chronic pancreatic pain. Journal of Pain and Symptom Management 6: 349–350

Douglas W W 1985 Histamine and 5-hydroxytryptamine (serotonin) and their antagonists. In: Gilman A G, Goodman L S, Rall T W, Murad F (eds). Goodman and Gilman's the pharmacological basis of therapeutics, 7th edn. Macmillan, New York pp 605–638

Dunlop R, Davies R J, Hockley J, Turner P 1988 Analgesic effects of oral flecainide. Lancet i: 420–421

Duthie H L 1981 The effect of peppermint oil on colonic motility in man. British Journal of Surgery 68: 820

Editorial 1992 Octreotide steaming ahead. Lancet 339: 837–839

Edwards W T, Habib F, Burney R G, Begin G 1985 Intravenous lidocaine in the management of various chronic pain states. Regional Anesthesia 10: 1–6

Edwards N D, Fletcher A, Cole J R, Peacock J E 1993 Combined infusions of morphine and ketamine for postoperative pain in elderly patients. Anaesthesia 48: 124–127

Emrich H M, Dose M, von Zerssen D 1985 The use of sodium valproate, carbamazepine and oxcarbazepine in patients with affective disorders. Journal of Affective Disorders 8: 243–250

Epstein J B, Stevenson-Moore P, Jackson S et al 1989 International Journal of Radiation, Oncology, Biology and Physics 16: 1571–1575

Faigle J W, Keberle H, Degen P H 1980 Chemistry and pharmacokinetics of baclofen. In: Feldman R G, Young R R, Koella W P (eds) Spasticity: disordered motor control. Symposia Specialists, Miami, pp 461–475

Fitzgerald M 1983 Capsaicin and sensory neurones: a review. Pain 15: 109–130

Gajewski J B, Awad S A 1986 Oxybutynin versus propantheline in patients with multiple sclerosis and detrusor hyperreflexia. Journal of Urology 135: 966–968

Gamse R, Leeman S E, Holzer P, Lembeck F 1981 Differential effects of capsaicin on the content of somatostatin, substance P, and neurotensin in the nervous system of the rat. Naunyn Schmiedebergs Archives of Pharmacology 317: 140–148

Gamse R, Petsche U, Lembeck F, Jancso G 1982 Capsaicin applied to peripheral nerve inhibits axoplasmic transport of substance P and somatostatin. Brain Research 239: 447–462

Gefke K, Andersen L W, Friesel F 1983 Lidocaine given intravenously as a suppressant of cough and laryngospasm in connection with extubation after tonsillectomy. Acta Anaesthesiologica Scandinavica 27: 111–112

Gennari C, Chierichetti S M, Piolini M et al 1985 Analgesic activity of salmon and human calcitonin against cancer pain: a double-blind, placebo-controlled clinical study. Current Therapeutic Research 38: 298–303

Gertz M A, Garton J P, Jennings W H 1986 Aplastic anemia due to tocainide. New England Journal of Medicine 314: 583–584

Glynn C J, Jamous M A, Teddy P J, Moore R A, Lloyd J W 1986 Role of spinal noradrenergic system in transmission of pain in patients with spinal cord injury. Lancet ii: 1249–1250

Glynn C, Dawson D, Sanders R 1988 A double-blind comparison between epidural morphine and epidural clonidine in patients with chronic noncancer pain. Pain 34: 123–128

Grahame-Smith D G, Aronson J K 1992 Oxford textbook of clinical pharmacology and drug therapy, 2nd edn. Oxford University Press, Oxford

Grant I S, Nimmo W S, Clements J A 1981 Pharmacokinetics and analgesic effects of IM and oral ketamine. British Journal of Anaesthesia 53: 805–810

Grillage M G, Nankani J N, Atkinson S N, Prescott P 1990 A randomised double-blind study of mebeverine versus dicyclomine in the treatment of functional abdominal pain in young adults. British Journal of Clinical Practice 44: 176–179

Guidobono F, Netti C, Pagani F et al 1986 Relationship of analgesia induced by centrally injected calcitonin to the CNS serotonergic system. Neuropeptides 8: 259–271

Hampf G, Bowsher D, Nurmikko T 1989 Distigmine and amitriptyline in the treatment of chronic pain. Anesthesia Progress 36: 58–62

Hedenbro J L, Olsson A M 1988 Metoclopramide and ureteric colic. Acta Chirurgica Scandinavica 154: 439–440

Helm G, Owman C, Rosengren E, Sjoberg N O 1982 Regional and cyclic variations in catecholamine concentration of the human fallopian tube. Biology of Reproduction 26: 553–558

Herxheimer A, Haefeli L 1966 Human pharmacology of hyoscine butylbromide. Lancet ii: 418–421

Hieble J P, Ruffolo R R 1991 Therapeutic applications of agents interacting with alpha-adrenoceptors. In: Ruffolo R R (ed) Alpha-adrenoceptors: molecular biology, biochemistry and pharmacology, vol 8. Karger, Basel, pp 180–220

Idvall J, Ahlgren I, Aronsen K F, Stenberg P 1979 Ketamine infusions: pharmacokinetics and clinical effects. British Journal of Anaesthesia 51: 1167–1173

Ito Y, Ichiyanagi K 1974 Post-operative pain relief with ketamine infusion. Anaesthesia 29: 222–229

Jaeger H, Maier C 1992 Calcitonin in phantom limb pain: a double-blind study. Pain 48: 21–27

Jaeger H, Maier C, Wawersik K 1988 Postoperative behandlung von phantomschmerzen und kausalgien mit calcitonin. Anasthesist 37: 71–76

Jensen T S, Krebs B, Nielsen J, Rasmussen P 1983 Phantom limb, phantom pain and stump pain in amputees during the first six months following limb amputation. Pain 17: 243–256

Kanamaru T, Saeki S, Katsumata N, Mizuno K, Ogawa S, Suzuki H 1990 Ketamine infusion for control of pain in patients with advanced cancer. Masui 39: 1368–1371

Kastrup J, Petersen P, Dejgard A, Hilsted J, Angelo H R 1986 Treatment of painful diabetic neuropathy with intravenous lidocaine infusion. British Medical Journal 292: 173

Keats A A, D'Alessandro G L, Beecher H K 1951 A controlled study of pain relief by intravenous procaine. Journal of the American Medical Association 147: 1761–1763

Khoo D, Riley J, Waxman J 1992 Control of emesis in bowel obstruction in terminally ill patients. Lancet 339: 375–376

Kim J H, Chu F, Lakshmi V, Houde R 1985 A clinical study of benzydamine for the treatment of radiotherapy induced mucositis of the oropharynx. International Journal of Tissue Reaction 7: 215–218

Kochak G M, Rakhit A, Wagner W E, Honc F, Waldes L, Kershaw R A 1985 The pharmacokinetics of baclofen derived from intestinal infusion. Clinical Pharmacology and Therapeutics 38: 251–257

Laird D, Lovel T 1993 Paradoxical pain. Lancet 341: 241

LaMotte R H, Simone D A, Baumann T K, Shain C N, Alreja M 1988 Hypothesis for novel classes of chemoreceptors mediating chemogenic pain and itch. In: Dubner R, Gebhart G F, Bond M R (eds) Proceedings of the Vth World Congress on Pain. Elsevier, New York, pp 529–535

Langer S Z, Cavero I, Massingham R 1980 Recent developments in noradrenergic neurotransmission and its relevance to the mechanism of action of certain antihypertensive agents. Hypertension 2: 372–382

Langley M S, Heel R C 1988 Transdermal clonidine: a preliminary review of its pharmacodynamic properties and therapeutic efficacy. Drugs 35: 123–142

Laurian L, Oberman Z, Graf E, Gilad S, Hoerer E, Simantow R 1986 Calcitonin induced increase in ACTH, beta-endorphin and cortisol secretion. Hormone and Metabolic Research 18: 268–271

Layzer R B 1978 Myeloneuropathy after prolonged exposure to nitrous oxide. Lancet ii: 1227

Lembcke B, Creutzfeldt W, Schlescer S et al 1987 Effect of the Somatostatin Analogue Sandostatin on gastrointestinal, pancreatic and biliary function and hormone release in man. Digestion 36: 108–124

Leyland M J, Hindley A 1982 Calcitonin in the management of malignant bone pain. Clinical Science 62: 43

Levy D W, Banerjee A K, Glenny H P 1985 Cimetidine in the treatment of herpes zoster. Journal of the Royal College of Physicians of London 19: 96–98

Lindblom U, Lindstrom P 1984 Analgesic effect of tocainide in neuralgia. Acta Neurologica Scandinavica 98: 216–217

Lindstrom P, Lindblom U 1987 The analgesic effect of tocainide in trigeminal neuralgia. Pain 28: 45–50

Luczak J, Okupny M, Sopata M 1992 The use of ketamine in palliative care. Paper presented at the Advanced Palliative Care Course, Lad, Poland,

MacIntyre I, Stevenson J C, Whitehead M I, Wimalawansa S J, Banks L M, Healy M J R 1988 Calcitonin for prevention of postmenopausal bone loss. Lancet i: 900–902

McQuay H J 1988 Pharmacological management of neuropathic pain. In: Hanks G W (ed) Pain and cancer. Cancer Survey Series, vol 7. Oxford University Press, Oxford, pp 141–159

Martin T J 1979 Treatment of Paget's disease with the calcitonins. Australian and New Zealand Journal of Medicine 9: 36–43

Martindale 1989 The Extra Pharmacopoeia, 29th edn. Pharmaceutical Press, London

Marvin J A, Engrave L H, Heimbach D M 1984 Self-administered nitrous oxide analgesia for debridement: a five year experience. Presented at the 16th Annual Meeting of the American Burn Association, San Francisco

Mavlight G M, Talpaz M 1984 Cimetidine for herpes zoster. New England Journal of Medicine 310: 318–319

Max M B, Schafer S C, Culnane M, Dubner R, Gracely R H 1988 Association of pain relief with drug side effects in postherpetic neuralgia: a single-dose study of clonidine, codeine, ibuprofen, and placebo. Clinical Pharmacology and Therapeutics 43: 363–371

Mercadante S, Spoldi E, Caraceni A, Maddaloni S, Simonetti M T 1993 Octreotide in relieving gastro-intestinal symptoms due to bowel obstruction. Palliative Medicine 7: 295–299

Meunier P J, Delmas P D, Chaumet-Riffaud P D et al 1990 Intranasal salmon calcitonin for prevention of postmenopausal bone loss: a placebo controlled study in 109 women. In: Christiansen C, Overgaard K (eds) Osteoporosis 1990. Osteopress, Copenhagen, pp 1861–1867

Michel M C, Insel P A 1989 Are there multiple imidazoline binding sites? TIPS 10: 342–344

Milani R, Scalambrino S, Milia R et al 1993 Double-blind crossover comparison of flavoxate and oxybutynin in women affected by urinary urge syndrome. International Urogynaecology Journal 4: 3–8

Morton C R, Maisch B, Zimmermann M 1986 Calcitonin: brain stem microinjection but not systemic administration inhibits spinal nociceptive transmission in the cat. Brain Research 372: 149–154

Mossner J, Wresky H P, Kestel M, Zeeh J, Regner U, Fishbach W 1989 Influence of treatment with pancreatic extracts on pancreatic enzyme secretion. Gut 3: 1143–1149

Muller T F, Naesh O, Svare E, Jensen A, Glyngdal P 1990 Metoclopramide (Primperan) in the treatment of ureterolithiasis. Urology International 45: 112–113

Nakamura M, Ferreira S H 1988 Peripheral analgesic action of clonidine: mediation by release of endogenous enkephalin-like substances. European Journal of Pharmacology 146: 223–228

Nash P, Gould S R, Barnardo D E 1986 Peppermint oil does not relieve the pain of irritable bowel syndrome. British Journal of Clinical Practice 40: 292–293

Nimmo W S, Clements J A 1981 Ketamine on demand for postoperative analgesia. Anaesthesia 36: 826

Ogilvie A L, Atkinson M 1986 Does dimethicone increase the efficacy of antacids in the treatment of reflux oesophagitis? Journal of the Royal Society of Medicine 79: 584–587

Okazaki K, Yamamoto Y, Kagiyama S et al 1988 Pressure of papillary zone and pancreatic main duct in patients with chronic pancreatitis in the early state. Scandinavian Journal of Gastroenterology 23: 501–506

Olgiati V R, Guidobono F, Netti C, Pecile A 1983 Localization of calcitonin binding sites in rat central nervous system: evidence of its neuroactivity. Brain Research 265: 209–215

Oshima E, Tei K, Kayazawa H, Urabe N 1990 Continuous subcutaneous injection of ketamine for cancer pain. Canadian Journal of Anaesthesia 37: 385–392

Owen H, Reekie R M, Clements J A, Watson R, Nimmo W S 1987 Analgesia from morphine and ketamine. Anaesthesia 42: 1051–1056

Pardridge W M 1988 Recent advances in blood brain barrier transport. Annual Review of Pharmacology and Toxicology 28: 25–39

Peiris J B, Perera G L S, Devendra S V, Lionel N D W 1980 Sodium valproate in trigeminal neuralgia. Medical Journal of Australia 2: 278

Perlow G M, Jain B P, Pauker S G, Zarren H S, Wistran D C, Epstein R L 1981 Tocainide-associated interstitial pneumonitis. Annals of Internal Medicine 94: 489–490

Rees W D W, Evans B K, Rhodes J 1979 Treating irritable bowel with peppermint oil. British Medical Journal 2: 835–836

Regnard C F B 1993 Single dose fluconazole versus five day ketoconazole in oral candidiasis. Presented at Palliative Care Research Forum, London

Reinikainen K J, Keranen T, Halonen T, Komulainen H, Riekkinen P J 1987 Comparison of oxcarbazepine and carbamazepine: a double blind study. Epilepsy Research 1: 284–289

Richens A 1991 The basis of the treatment of epilepsy: neuropharmacology. In: Dam M (ed) A practical approach to epilepsy. Pergamon Press, Oxford, pp 75–85

Rockin R E 1976 Modulation of cellular-immune responses in vivo and in vitro by histamine receptor bearing lymphocytes. Journal of Clinical Investigation 57: 1051–1058

Rosenblatt W H, Cioffi A M, Sinatra R, Saberski L R, Silverman D G 1991 Metoclopramide: an analgesic adjunct to patient-controlled analgesia. Anesthesia and Analgesia 73: 553–555

Ruffmann R 1988 A review of flavoxate hydrochloride in the treatment of urge incontinence. Journal of International Medical Research 16: 317–330

Rull J A, Quibrera R, Gonzalez-Millan H, Castaneda O L 1969 Symptomatic treatment of peripheral diabetic neuropathy with carbamazepine. Diabetologia 5: 215–218

Sadove M S, Shulman M, Hatano S, Fevold N 1971 Analgesic effects of ketamine administered in subsissociative doses Anesthesia and Analgesia 50: 452–457

Sagen J, Proudfit H 1985 Evidence for pain modulation by pre- and postsynaptic noradrenergic receptors in the medulla oblongata. Brain Research 331: 285–293

Schnapp M, Mays K S, North W C 1981 Intravenous 2-chloroprocaine in treatment of chronic pain. Anesthesia and Analgesia 60: 844–845

Schutz H, Feldman K F, Faigle J W, Kriemler H P, Winkler T 1986 The metabolism of ^{14}C-oxcarbazepine in man. Xenobiotica 16: 769–778

Serrou B, Cupissol D, Favier F, Caulin F 1981 Efficacy of calcitonin in the treatment of bone metastases pain. Lyon Medit Med — Med Sud-Est Suppl 17 (7): 40–46

Simone C, Racanelli A 1980 Synthetic salmon calcitonin and osteolytic breast cancer metastases. Folia Oncologica 3: 533–543

Sinnott C, Edmonds P, Cropley I, Hanks G 1991 Flecainide in cancer nerve pain. Lancet 337: 1347

Smart H L, Atkinson M 1990 Comparison of a dimethicone/antacid (Asilone gel) with an alginate/antacid (Gaviscon liquid) in the management of reflux oesophagitis. Journal of the Royal Society of Medicine 83: 554–556

Soff G A, Kadin M E 1987 Tocainide-induced reversible agranulocytosis and anemia. Archives of Internal Medicine 147: 598–599

Stannard C F, Porter G E 1993 Ketamine hydrochloride in the treatment of phantom limb pain. Pain 54: 227–230

Steinhaus J E, Gaskin L P 1963 A study of intravenous lidocaine as a suppressant of cough reflex. Anesthesiology 24: 285–296

Swerdlow M 1984 Anticonvulsant drugs and chronic pain. Clinical Neuropharmacology 7: 51–82

Swerdlow M, Cundill J G 1981 Anticonvulsant drugs used in the treatment of lancinating pain: a comparison. Anaesthesia 36: 1129–1132

Szanto J, Ady N, Jozsef S 1992 Pain killing with calcitonin nasal spray in patients with malignant tumors. Oncology 49: 180–182

Tamsen A, Gordh T 1984 Epidural clonidine produces analgesia. Lancet i: 231–232

Tanelian D L, MacIver M B 1991 Analgesic concentrations of lidocaine suppress tonic A-delta and C fiber discharges produced by acute injury. Anesthesiology 74: 934–936

Taylor B A, Duthie H L, Luscombe D K 1985 Mechanism by which peppermint oil exerts its relaxant effect on gastrointestinal smooth muscle. Journal of Pharmacy and Pharmacology 37 (suppl): 104

Theisohn M, Heimann G 1982 Disposition of the antiepileptic oxcarbazepine and its metabolites in healthy volunteers. European Journal of Pharmacology 22: 545–551

Tulassay Z, Flautner L, Fehervari I 1992 Octreotide. Lancet 339: 1428

Twycross R G, Lack S A 1990 Therapeutics in terminal cancer, 2nd edn. Churchill Livingstone, Edinburgh

Van der Spuy S, Levy D W, Levin W 1980 Cimetidine in the treatment of herpes virus infections. South African Medical Journal 58: 112–116

Warburton A, Royston J P, O'Neill C J et al 1987 A quinine a day keeps the leg cramps away? British Journal of Clinical Pharmacology 23: 459–465

Watson C P N, Evans R J 1992 Post-mastectomy pain syndrome and topical capsaicin: a randomized trial. Pain 51: 375–379

Watson C P N, Evans R J, Watt V R 1988 Postherpetic neuralgia and topical capsaicin. Pain 33: 333–340

Watson C P N, Evans R J, Watt C R 1989 The postmastectomy pain syndrome and the effect of topical capsaicin. Pain 38: 177–186

Watson C P N, Tyler K L, Bickers D R, Millikan L E, Smith S, Coleman E 1993 A randomized vehicle-controlled trial of topical capsaicin in the treatment of postherpetic neuralgia. Clinical Therapeutics 15: 510–526

Wick H 1951 The pharmacology of buscopan. Archives of Experimental Pathology and Pharmacology 213: 485–500

Wiesenfeld-Hallin Z, Persson A 1984 Subarachnoid injection of salmon calcitonin does not induce analgesia in rats. European Journal of Pharmacology 104: 375–377

Yaksh T L 1985 Pharmacology of spinal adrenergic systems which modulate spinal nociceptive processing. Pharmacology, Biochemistry and Behaviour 22: 845–858

Yotsuyanagi T, Yamamura K, Akao Y 1985 Mucosa-adhesive film containing local analgesic. Lancet ii: 613

Zeigler D, Lynch S A, Muir J, Benjamin J, Max M B 1992 Transdermal clonidine versus placebo in painful diabetic neuropathy. Pain 48: 403–408

Disease modification and immobilization

INTRODUCTION

In the next three chapters a wide range of approaches to pain relief are discussed (Table 24.1). In this chapter attention is focused on:

- palliative anticancer treatment
- modifying the effects of the disease
- orthopaedic surgery and immobilization.

When palliative anticancer treatment is considered in far advanced cancer, it is important to ensure that the treatment is not worse than the disease. Further, because hormone treatment or chemotherapy has been started, this does not mean that analgesics should be withheld. The analgesic effect of anticancer treatment may be delayed for several weeks and possibly longer. A combined approach is necessary.

Hypercalcaemia and lymphoedema both cause significant morbidity and pain. Treatments to correct or contain these conditions may well form part of the approach to pain relief in affected individuals. Orthopaedic surgical treatment of pathological fractures of the femur and humerus is another important aspect of pain management.

RADIOTHERAPY

Several general points about radiotherapy are listed in Box 24.A. Pain relief is the most common indication for palliative radiotherapy (Box 24.B). Many patients experience adverse effects with radiotherapy, about which they should be warned (Box 24.C). Some patients, however, notice nothing but transient fatigue.

Table 24.1   Disease modifying and nondrug methods of pain relief

Category	Chapter	Examples
Palliative anticancer treatment	24	Radiotherapy Hormone therapy Chemotherapy
Modifying the effects of the disease	24	Correction of hypercalcaemia Treatment of lymphoedema Orthopaedic surgery
Immobilization	24	Rest Slings Splints Cervical collar Surgical corset Walking aids Wheelchair
Nerve blocks	25	Local anaesthetic Neurolytic
Neurosurgery	25	Pituitary ablation Spinothalamic tractotomy Dorsal column stimulation DREZ lesion[a]
Counterirritation	26	Massage Chemical Heat Cold TENS[b] Vibration Acupuncture
Psychological	26	Distraction Creative activity Art therapy Imagery Relaxation Hypnosis Cognitive-behavioural therapy Psychodynamic therapies

[a] DREZ = dorsal root entry zone.
[b] TENS = transcutaneous electrical nerve stimulation.

Certain tumours metastasize more readily to bone:

- myeloma
- melanoma
- breast
- bronchus
- prostate
- kidney
- thyroid.

All tumours can, however, and sometimes do. The sites most frequently affected are the axial skeleton (vertebral bodies, pelvis, ribs, sternum), the proximal ends of the femur and humerus, and the base of the skull (Fig. 24.1).

BOX 24.A
GENERAL POINTS ABOUT RADIOTHERAPY (Ashby 1991)

Radiotherapy is the delivery of ionizing radiation into a defined volume of the body in order to eradicate or substantially depopulate the tumour cells within that volume, without exceeding the tolerance of normal tissues.

The biological effect of radiation on tissues is complex. It is dependent on:

- the volume (how much of the body is treated)
- the dose delivered per fraction (treatment session)
- the overall treatment time
- the type of radiation.

Generally speaking, the larger the volume, the lower the dose tolerated.

The effects of irradiation can be divided into:

- early injury (manifests during and immediately after treatment)
- late injury (becomes apparent months or years later).

The dose per fraction has an important influence on late injury to normal tissue.

For radical (curative) treatments, a large number of small fractions will be delivered to a small or medium sized volume. A standard treatment regimen might be 60 Gy in 30 fractions over 6 weeks.

For palliative treatment, a small number of larger fractions can often be given, e.g., 20 Gy in 5 fractions over 5 days, or a single dose of 6–8 Gy.

Palliative radiotherapy should:

- have a clearly stated palliative endpoint
- have minimal adverse effects
- be convenient for the patient
- minimize the number of hospital visits
- minimize the overall duration of treatment
- minimize the time spent by the patient away from home.

When deciding on an appropriate schedule for any given patient, it is necessary to consider (Gilbert et al 1977):

- the site of the tumour
- the area to be irradiated
- life expectancy
- degree of debility.

Ionizing radiation can be delivered in various ways for the treatment of bone pain. External beam therapy is the form most commonly used.

Open studies

The combined results from 16 surveys, mostly retrospective, of nearly 2500 treatments for bone pain give a mean complete response rate of 52% and a mean overall response rate of 86% (Hoskin 1988). Only four of the surveys include data on duration of response. One year after treatment 65–90% of

---

BOX 24.B
INDICATIONS FOR PALLIATIVE RADIOTHERAPY

Pain

- bone metastases
- plexopathy
  — brachial
  — lumbosacral
- compression
  — spinal cord
  — cauda equina

Compression syndromes

- spinal cord compression
- superior vena caval obstruction
- cerebral tumours

Bleeding

- haemoptysis
- haematuria
- vaginal bleeding
- rectal bleeding

Fungation and ulceration

Blockage of hollow viscus

- bronchus
- ureter

---

patients were still painfree (Table 24.2; Gilbert et al 1977, Garmatis & Chu 1978). Many of the surveys suffer from the usual problems of retrospective data collection, for example incomplete treatment details and lack of formal evaluation of pain (Hoskin 1988).

Randomized studies

The results of three studies evaluating different treatment schedules are shown in Table 24.3. In one, two fifths of the patients with partial response and over one half of the patients with complete response had recurrence of pain at the irradiated site, mostly in the weeks immediately preceding death. Median duration of relief was 12–15 weeks in complete responders and 20–28 weeks in partial responders (Tong et al 1982). In patients surviving more than one year, nearly 60% had continuing relief (Price et al 1986). In one study, breast and prostate cancers had a higher rate of complete response compared with other primary sites (Tong et al 1982); the other two studies failed to detect a difference.

Single treatment versus fractionated treatment

In a randomized study, a single exposure of 8 Gy was compared with a

BOX 24.C
ACUTE ADVERSE EFFECTS OF RADIOTHERAPY (Ashby 1991)

Systemic (not confined to volume irradiated)
Malaise
Nausea and/or vomiting   } partly site specific: not expected with
Anorexia   } therapy to limbs or chest
Fatigue

Specific (confined to volume irradiated)
Skin

- erythema
- pruritus
- moist desquamation

Abdomen and pelvis

- nausea
- vomiting
- diarrhoea
- cystitis (frequency, dysuria, haematuria)

Head and neck

- dry mouth
- altered taste
- oropharyngeal mucositis

Chest

- oesophageal mucositis

Head

- alopecia

Bone marrow

- suppression

course of 30 Gy in 10 daily fractions (Price et al 1986). No difference was found in the speed of onset or duration of pain relief, which was independent of the site of the primary tumour. There was a 25% retreatment need in the 8 Gy group. A higher incidence of gastro-intestinal adverse effects has been reported in patients receiving a single treatment (Cole 1989).

Fractionation is most common when there is:

- a high risk of nausea and vomiting despite prophylactic anti-emetics
  — when irradiating in the region of the stomach (e.g. upper lumbar spine)
  — when treating a large field size (e.g. half or more of the pelvis)
- a risk of spinal cord damage (i.e. when irradiating cervical or thoracic spine)
- a good prognosis with a likelihood of retreatment at a later date (e.g. in breast cancer)
- retreatment.

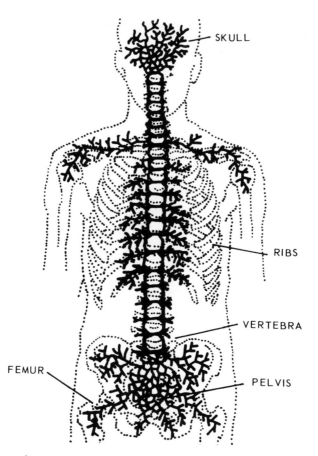

Fig. 24.1   Batson's paravertebral venous plexus. Pathway of spread for many bone metastases.

Table 24.2   Radiation and relief of bone pain in 152 treatment fields[a]

	n	%
Early relief (≤ 2 weeks)	106	70
Early partial relief (≤ 2 weeks)		
Delayed complete relief (2–12 weeks)	33	22
No relief	13	8
Recurrence of pain	20	14
Permanent relief	119	78

[a] Patients received a range of doses: relief identical in all treatment groups.
From Allen et al 1976

Treatment with a single exposure requires more time on the day of treatment, and this has to be allowed for. The patient has to be seen and planned, as well as treated. There is, however, an overall saving of time both for the patient and staff. Objections to single treatments are shown in Table 24.4.

At one centre, departmental audit doubled the number of single treatments for bone pain from 32% to 67% (Dodwell et al 1993). Some radio-

Table 24.3 Prospective studies of localized radiotherapy for bone pain

Number of treatments	Dose fractionation	Overall response rate (%)	Reference
1016	15–40.5 Gy in 1–3 weeks	90	Tong et al 1982
57	24 Gy in 6 fractions in 3 weeks 20 Gy in 2 fractions in 1 week	48	Madsen 1983
288	30 Gy in 10 fractions in 2 weeks 8 Gy in 1 fraction	85	Price et al 1986

Table 24.4 Objections to single dose palliative radiotherapy

Objections (Baughan 1991)	Comments (Kelly et al 1991)
Tumour oedema greater; dangerous if spinal cord or nerve root compression	Neurological deterioration uncommon in patients given 12.5–15 Gy in single dose with corticosteroid cover
More nausea, vomiting and diarrhoea if gastro-intestinal tract included in field	Single treatment causes more nausea but is of shorter duration; diary records over one month show no overall difference (Cole 1989)
Radiographers have less opportunity to counsel and re-assure	
Tumour killing effect in single treatment is considerably less; greater chance of regrowth and renewed pain	Tumour shrinkage is not the major determinant of pain relief. Benefit seen: — < 24 h in some patients after hemibody irradiation (Wilkins & Keen 1987) — after single dose of 4 Gy (Price et al 1988) — with both radiosensitive & radioresistant tumours (Hoskin et al 1989) Single treatment needs more time allocated but overall is less exhausting for the patients

therapists, however, still do not prescribe single treatments (Crellin et al 1989, Dodwell et al 1993).

Wide field irradiation

Because the majority of bone metastases are the result of vascular spread, isolated deposits are unusual. If the patient has pain from multiple sites, hemibody irradiation is an option (Table 24.5). Single fraction hemibody irradiation provides relief in about 75% of patients. An even higher response rate can probably be achieved by increasing the dose (Nag & Shah 1986). Relief occurs within 2 days in many patients with both upper and lower hemibody irradiation. In one study, the mean survival was 30 weeks (Salazar et al 1986).

Almost all patients experience gastro-intestinal toxicity; nausea and vomiting within a few hours and diarrhoea up to one week later. These are severe in about one quarter of the patients. Pretreatment hydration, corticosteroids

Table 24.5 Wide field radiotherapy in bone pain

Dose (single exposure unless stated)	Number of patients	Response rate (%)	Reference
8 Gy (upper and lower)	15	75	Epstein et al 1979
3–6 Gy (upper) 10 Gy (lower)	570	55–72	Fitzpatrick 1981
7.5 Gy (upper) 10 Gy (lower)	96	80	Rowland et al 1981
7–8 Gy (upper and lower) or 3–4 Gy to myeloma	129	76	Qasim 1981
6 Gy (upper) 8 Gy (lower)	168	73	Salazar et al 1986
16 Gy in 2 fractions (upper and lower)	19	100	Nag & Shah 1986
6–7 Gy (upper) 6–8 Gy (lower)	39	82	Hoskin 1988
8 Gy (lower)	141	82	Wilkins & Keen 1987

and anti-emetics are generally recommended. Upper hemibody treatment results in a variable degree of temporary alopecia. Significant bone marrow depression is seen in less than 10% after hemibody irradiation, but occurs in the majority who receive two sequential hemibody treatments.

The lungs are the limiting factor in upper hemibody irradiation. Figures for acute pneumonitis vary from 10–50% for upper hemibody irradiation with 10–11 Gy (Fitzpatrick 1981, Qasim 1981). With doses of 6–8 Gy, the figures are much less, namely, 2–14%. Patients occasionally die from acute pneumonitis and a few develop chronic fibrosis (Hoskin 1988). In consequence, many centres would limit the uncorrected lung dose to 6 Gy (corrected dose = 7–7.5 Gy).

Radio-isotopes

A number of different radio-isotopes have been used to irradiate painful bone metastases. These can either be tumour specific (e.g. ^{131}I for differentiated thyroid cancer) or specific for bone (e.g. ^{32}P and ^{89}Sr). Two studies, for example, have demonstrated the benefit of ^{89}Sr in bone metastases in prostate cancer (Laing et al 1991, Lewington et al 1991).

Marrow suppression, manifesting as a fall in the platelet count, occurs and is maximal 3–5 weeks after treatment. This usually causes no problems provided the platelet concentration was initially above 100×10^5/dl (Laing et al 1991). Repeat treatments should not be given within 3 months. Guidelines for the use of ^{89}Sr are available (Robinson et al 1992).

HORMONE THERAPY

All breast and prostate cancer patients should be reviewed to see if a further hormonal manipulation might be appropriate. Overall, response rates vary from 20–50% in breast cancer (Smith & Macaulay 1985) and from 60–90% in prostate cancer (Lyss 1987), with a median duration of response of 12–20 months. Particularly in breast cancer, a patient who has had a good response to one hormone is more likely to respond well to a second hormone. Considerable pain relief is often reported shortly after starting treatment (Whitehouse 1985). Options in hormone therapy have increased over the last decade. Liaison with local oncological services is necessary, therefore, to determine the state of the art.

Corticosteroids may be of benefit. In one third of elderly patients with breast cancer, corticosteroids result in regression or cessation of progression of their cancer for up to one year (Minton et al 1981). Patients with prostatic cancer obtain similar benefit (Tannock et al 1989).

Medroxyprogesterone acetate (MPA) 750 mg IM was given b.i.d. for 30 days to patients with advanced breast cancer, most of whom had severe bone pain (Pannuti et al 1979). Complete or partial relief of pain was noted in over 90% of patients. Improvement was seen within 1 or 2 weeks in almost all those who responded and was generally maximal in less than a month.

Benefit was more noticeable in patients with multiple bone metastases 'who were forced to keep completely still' in bed before treatment because of intense movement precipitated pain. Between 15% and 20% of patients treated with MPA developed abscesses at the site of injection. Other adverse effects were also noted (Table 24.6). Adverse effects all resolved within 3 weeks of completing the course of treatment.

The mean duration of objective remission was 7 months (compared with 1–2 years for most other hormone therapies). The duration of pain relief after completion of treatment was not stated. The analgesic effect of MPA is thought to be independent of an anticancer effect because:

- the incidence of pain relief is considerably greater than the incidence of objective remission of the tumour (90% compared with about 45%)
- some patients obtain significant relief despite obvious clinical progression of the disease.

Table 24.6 Adverse effects of treatment with IM medroxyprogesterone acetate (MPA) in doses of 500–2000 g/day for 30 days (166 patients)

Side effect		Percentage
Induration	at site of	7
Abscess	injections	18
Moon-face		16
Tremor		16
Sweating		15
Vaginal bleeding		10
Cramps		9
Thrombophlebitis		1

Modified from Pannuti et al 1979

It is possible that MPA acts by producing a selective 'medical hypophysectomy'. The fact that many patients were bedfast because of pain suggests, however, that the use of analgesics and radiotherapy may have been more restricted than is the case in the UK.

CHEMOTHERAPY

Chemotherapy may be helpful in patients with recurrent squamous cell cancers of the head and neck which have already been treated with surgery and/or radiation. About 35% respond to methotrexate or cisplatin, and considerable pain relief is obtained in 1–2 weeks. Methotrexate 25–50 mg/m^2 IV weekly is usually well tolerated, even in elderly debilitated patients. As always, benefits must be weighed carefully against adverse effects (Boop & Fischer 1981).

BISPHOSPHONATES

Necropsy studies show that 85% of those dying of breast and lung cancer, and 60% of those with prostate cancer, have bone metastases (Stoll 1983). The morbidity from skeletal involvement is considerable. Bone metastases are the commonest cause of pain in advanced cancer (Twycross & Fairfield 1982). Bone metastases also cause:

- hypercalcaemia
- nerve root compression
- compression of the spinal cord
- pathological fractures
- immobility
- bone marrow failure (leuco-erythroblastic anaemia).

Bisphosphonates are 'osteoclast blocking agents' (Boonekamp et al 1986, Lowik et al 1988, Bijvoet 1990). Bisphosphonates are used to treat Paget's disease of the bone (Harinck et al 1987). They are also generally very effective in correcting hypercalcaemia, and reduce the incidence of other complications of bone metastases (Fig. 24.2; Coleman et al 1988, Morton et al 1988a).

Mechanism of bone resorption

Bone turnover is a tightly regulated process. Normal resorption and formation of bone (via osteoclasts and osteoblasts respectively) are closely linked. Bone destruction associated with osteolytic metastases is initially mediated by osteoclasts. Subsequently, tumour cells themselves release chemicals which cause bone resorption (Garrett et al 1987).

Mechanism of action of bisphosphonates

The realization that bisphosphonates inhibit osteoclasts led to studies in

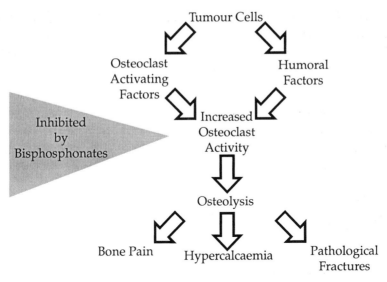

Fig. 24.2   Effects of bisphosphonates in metastatic bone disease.

normocalcaemic patients with osteolytic bone metastases to see if bone destruction could be reduced (Coleman et al 1988, Morton et al 1988a). Pamidronate 30 mg was given every 2 weeks by IV infusion. Radiological healing of metastases occurred in about a quarter of patients with stabilization in another quarter. Pain eased and calcium excretion fell. Studies with clodronate have yielded comparable results (Siris et al 1983, Adami et al 1985). Biochemical improvement and pain relief has also been reported in patients with hormone resistant prostate cancer (Clarke et al 1991). On the other hand, etidronate, which inhibits bone mineralization as well as resorption, does not have a comparable analgesic effect (Fleisch & Felix 1979, Smith 1989).

CORRECTION OF HYPERCALCAEMIA

Hypercalcaemia occurs in 10–20% of all patients with advanced malignant disease. The figure is higher in breast and lung cancer (Watson 1966). In addition to causing nausea, vomiting, constipation, weakness and depression, hypercalcaemia may precipitate or exacerbate pain.

Several reports have been published of patients who have experienced a reduction in bone pain, or complete relief, when hypercalcaemia has been corrected. Relief was noted in 6/7 (Parsons et al 1974), 10/15 (Davies et al 1979) and 5/15 patients (Coombes et al 1979).

A lack of response may relate to differences in the mechanisms responsible for the bone pain. For example, in some patients the pain may relate to rapid bone resorption (considered to be a cause of pain in Paget's disease), whereas in others microscopic buckling or compression of bone when standing could be responsible. In the former, benefit from correction of hypercalcaemia could be anticipated but not in the latter. Despite the unpredictability, if a patient with hypercalcaemia has pain which is not relieved by analgesics, steps should be taken to correct it.

Management

In patients with advanced cancer, correction of hypercalcaemia should not be an automatic response to an elevated plasma calcium concentration. The patient's total situation must be considered. Sometimes, in very debilitated patients, hypercalcaemia may best be seen as a 'terminal event' and left uncorrected (Box 24.D).

A bisphosphonate is now standard treatment for the correction of hypercalcaemia in the UK. Either pamidronate 30–90 mg or clodronate 1500 mg is given by IV infusion in 0.9% saline, usually over 4 h (Ralston et al 1989, O'Rourke 1993). The maximum effect is seen after 3–5 days with clodronate and 5–7 days with pamidronate. Normocalcaemia is maintained for an average of 3 weeks with pamidronate (Morton et al 1988b), but less than 1 week with clodronate (O'Rourke et al 1993).

The main limitation with bisphosphonates is that orally less than 1% is absorbed (Fleisch & Felix 1979, Daley-Yates et al 1991). Even so, clodronate is marketed for oral use as maintenance treatment (Elomaa et al 1985).

In countries where bisphosphonates are not available or too expensive, mithramycin can be used. Mithramycin is a cytotoxic antibiotic and a potent inhibitor of osteoclast activity. It is usually given in a dose of 25 µg/kg, i.e. about 1.5 mg. It is commonly given by IV infusion in normal saline together with a loop diuretic. It can, however, be given by slow IV injection in 20–30 ml over several minutes. In patients with impaired renal function a smaller dose should be used, for example 1 mg. It is effective within 12–36 h in over 80% of patients.

Mithramycin can be repeated every 2 days, up to 150 µg/kg (< 10 mg) during the first week. If renal function is impaired the initial dose should be reduced to 15 µg/kg (1 mg) and the total dose during the first week should be < 7 mg. Mithramycin should not be used if there is bone marrow suppression or an unexplained bleeding tendency.

IM calcitonin is also effective but expensive. Because its effects are transient, it needs to be given q6h until anticancer or other measures have had time to act. If none of the above drugs is available, a corticosteroid or phosphate tablets should be used (Box 24.E).

BOX 24.D
CRITERIA FOR CORRECTING HYPERCALCAEMIA IN A TERMINALLY ILL PATIENT

Severe symptoms attributable to hypercalcaemia
First episode or long interval since previous one
Previous good quality of life (in the patient's opinion)
Patient willing to have IV infusion and blood tests
Medical judgement that correction will achieve a durable effect (based partly on the results of previous treatment)

BOX 24.E
CORRECTION OF HYPERCALCAEMIA WITH CORTICOSTEROIDS OR PHOSPHATE

Encourage ⩾ 3 L daily fluid intake ± diuresis with loop diuretic.

If primary is breast, renal, myeloma, lymphoma, prescribe dexamethasone 8 mg or prednisolone 60 mg daily.

If above ineffective and with other primary sites:

- prescribe phosphate tablets 500 mg b.i.d.
- increase by 500 mg daily every 3–7 days to total of 3 g/day
- nausea and diarrhoea are the main adverse effects
- may accumulate in renal failure; do not use if plasma phosphate > 5 mg/dl.

Aspirin or other NSAID can be added if PG production a possible contributory factor (breast, renal).

TREATMENT OF LYMPHOEDEMA

The most effective way to relieve pain in lymphoedema is to treat the lymphoedema itself. Thus, over a 3 month period, on a scale of 0–3, mean pain scores reduced from 1.8 to 1 (Carroll & Rose 1992). Of 22 patients initially evaluated, 12 became completely painfree, and none had severe pain (compared with three at the initial evaluation).

The conservative (physical) treatment of lymphoedema is beyond the scope of this book. Suffice it to say that it generally comprises skin care, massage, compression garment (sleeve or stocking) and exercise. Some patients require intensive compression bandaging initially to enable a compression garment to be fitted (Rose et al 1993). The rationale for the treatment is:

- skin care to prevent infection with an acute exacerbation of the swelling, and subsequent fibrosis
- light massage to stimulate the superficial lymphatics to contract, thereby bypassing the deep lymphatic obstruction
- compression to prevent overstretching and disruption of elastic tissue in the swollen tissues
- exercise when wearing the compression garment to provide continuing light surface massage, and continued enhanced superficial lymphatic flow.

An increasing number of lymphoedema clinics are being set up in the UK. These are usually run by a clinical nurse specialist or a physiotherapist. Information about these may be obtained from the British Lymphology Interest Group (c/o Sir Michael Sobell House, Churchill Hospital, Oxford, OX3 7LJ).

ORTHOPAEDIC SURGERY

Pathological fracture of a long bone occurs in under 1% of patients with advanced cancer but, when it does, it inflicts a considerable burden on a patient. Only about 1% of such fractures occur distal to the knee or elbow (Galasko 1974). Internal fixation or the insertion of a prosthesis should always be considered, particularly in the case of a femur, because these measures obviate the need for prolonged bedrest. In addition, the pain is either relieved completely or much reduced.

The decision whether to treat surgically depends to a large extent on the patient's general condition. In lung cancer and melanoma, pathological fracture often presages death. This is generally not so in breast cancer, particularly if the tumour is hormone sensitive. The results of several published series indicate that the median survival after the first or only pathological fracture associated with breast cancer is about 6 months, ranging from 2 months to 4 years (Twycross 1977). Internal fixation should generally be followed by irradiation to facilitate healing of the fracture. Radiotherapy is often delayed until the wound has healed and the stitches removed, but this is not essential.

Subcapital fractures of the femur do not unite even when treated in this way because of the irreversible loss of blood supply to the femoral head (Galasko 1974). With these, the treatment of choice is arthroplasty (Fig. 24.3). This relieves the pain and the patient can be mobile again within days.

Consideration should sometimes be given to prophylactic nailing. It is easier than the internal fixation of an established, displaced fracture and is less disturbing for the patient. Further, when over half of the cortex has

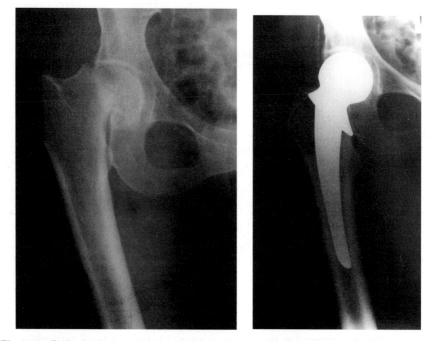

Fig. 24.3 Radiographs showing subcapital fracture of the right femur in a 58 year-old woman with breast cancer, and after treatment with a Thompson's hemi-arthroplasty.

been destroyed, deformity takes place on weight bearing and this causes pain. Prophylactic nailing also facilitates nursing and, should a fracture subsequently occur, it is often symptomless.

Fracture is unlikely when less than 25% of the cortex of a long bone has been eroded, but when erosion is more than 75%, the bone is so weak that it often fractures spontaneously (Fidler 1973). The indications for prophylactic internal fixation of a long bone are, therefore:

- increasing pain
- destruction of over half of the cortex radiologically.

Local irradiation of a long bone metastasis has been considered a further indication because of an increased risk of fracture (Editorial 1981). Irradiation may, however, result in significant recalcification. In other words, irradiation may modify the above criteria, and render surgical intervention unnecessary.

A more extensive procedure may be necessary when bone destruction is widespread or when the fracture is close to the end of the bone and adequate fixation by a nail is not possible (Yablon & Paul 1976). Lesions are first treated by excision and curettage, and then by appropriate internal fixation with the simultaneous insertion of an acrylic cement into the bone defect. In patients with advanced disease, the risk of local or general spread of the tumour as a result of curettage is outweighed by the benefits of the procedure. Of 73 patients submitted to this procedure, only four failed to regain function in the affected limb (Yablon & Paul 1976).

Stabilization of the spine is another area where orthopaedic surgery is of value (Galasko 1988).

IMMOBILIZATION

Some patients continue to experience pain on movement despite the optimal use of analgesics, other drugs and radiotherapy. In these, the situation may be improved by suggesting modifications to daily activity. For example, a man may continue to struggle to stand when shaving unless it is suggested that sitting would be a good idea. Such a suggestion is accepted more readily if accompanied by a simple explanation of why weight bearing precipitates or exacerbates the pain. An individually designed plastic support for patients with multiple collapsed vertebrae or a Thomas splint for femoral fracture pain are occasionally necessary to overcome intolerable pain on movement in bedfast patients. A lumbar plexus block, however, is a better option for femoral fractures (see p. 512). The humerus can be immobilized in the bedfast patient by an arm sling fastened to a torso jacket by means of interlocking Velcro.

■ CASE HISTORY

A 57 year-old woman with breast cancer sustained a pathological fracture of the right femoral neck. Because of the extent of the metastatic bone disease, surgical management was not possible. Relief at night and when sitting in a chair was achieved with oral morphine and a NSAID. She repeatedly said how wonderful it was to be out of pain, yet careless movement of the right thigh was transiently very painful. Before the presence of a fracture was confirmed, she herself had limited weight bearing to a minimum. When transferring from bed to wheelchair, for example, she had learnt to avoid pain by asking her daughter to hold the legs together and moving them as one.

REFERENCES

Adami S, Salvagno G, Guarrera G et al 1985 Dichloromethylene diphosphonate in patients with prostatic carcinoma metastatic to the skeleton. Journal of Urology 134: 1152–1154

Allen K, Johnson T, Hibbs G 1976 Effective bone palliation as related to various treatment regimens. Cancer 37: 984–987

Ashby M 1991 The role of radiotherapy in palliative care. Journal of Pain and Symptom Management 6: 380–388

Baughan C 1991 Treating bony metastases. British Medical Journal 303: 856

Bijvoet O L M 1990 Pamidronate (APD) in cancer therapy: the pharmacological background. In: Rubens R D (ed) Proceedings: The management of bone metastases and hypercalcaemia by osteoclast inhibition. Hogrefe & Huber, Bern

Boonekamp P M, van der Wee-Pals L J A, van Wijk-van Lennep M M L, Thesing C W, Bijvoet O L M 1986 Two modes of action of bisphosphonates on osteoclastic resorption of mineralized matrix. Bone Mineral 1: 27–39

Boop W C, Fischer J A 1981 Methods of pain control. In: Suen J Y, Myers E N (eds) Cancer of the head and neck. Churchill Livingstone, New York, pp 821–838

Carroll D, Rose K 1992 Treatment leads to significant improvement: effect of conservative treatment in pain in lymphoedema. Professional Nurse October: 32–36

Clarke N W, Holbrook I B, McClure J, George N J R 1991 Osteoclast inhibition by pamidronate in metastatic prostatic cancer: a preliminary study. British Journal of Cancer 63: 420–423

Cole D J 1989 A randomized trial of a single treatment versus conventional fractionation in the palliative radiotherapy of painful bone metastases. Clinical Oncology 1: 59–62

Coleman R E, Woll P J, Miles M, Rubens R 1988 3-amino 1, 1 hydroxypropyledine bisphosphonate (ADP) for the treatment of bone metastases from breast cancer. British Journal of Cancer 58: 621–625

Coombes R C, Neville A M, Gazet J C et al 1979 Agents affecting osteolysis in patients with breast cancer. Cancer Chemotherapy and Pharmacology 3: 41–44

Crellin A M, Marks A, Maher E J 1989 Why don't British radiotherapists given single fractions of radiotherapy for bone metastases? Clinical Oncology 1: 63–66

Daley-Yates P T, Dodwell D J, Pongchaidechma M, Coleman R G, Howell A 1991 The clearance and bioavailability of pamidronate in patients with breast cancer and bone metastases. Calcified Tissue International 49: 433–435

Davies J, Trask C, Souhami R L 1979 Effect of mithramycin on widespread painful bone metastases in cancer of the breast. Cancer Treatment Reports 63: 1835–1838

Dodwell D, Bond M, Elwell C et al 1993 Effect of medical audit on prescription of palliative radiotherapy. British Medical Journal 307: 24–25

Editorial 1981 Pathological fractures due to bone metastases. British Medical Journal 283: 748

Elomaa I, Blomqvist C, Porkka L et al 1985 Diphosphonates for osteolytic metastases. Lancet i: 1155–1156

Epstein L, Stewart B, Antunez A et al 1979 Half and total body radiation for carcinoma of the prostate. Journal of Urology 122: 330–332

Fidler M 1973 Prophylactic internal fixation of secondary neoplastic deposits in long bones. British Medical Journal 1: 341–343

Fitzpatrick P J 1981 Wide-field irradiation of bone metasases. In: Weiss L, Gilbert H A (eds) Bone metastasis. G K Hall, Boston, pp 399–427

Fleisch H, Felix R 1979 Diphosphonates. Calcified Tissue International 27: 91–94

Galasko C S B 1974 Pathological fracture secondary to metastatic cancer. Journal of the Royal College of Surgeons of Edinburgh 19: 351–362

Galasko C S B 1988 The role of the orthopaedic surgeon in the treatment of bone pain. In: Hanks G W (ed). Pain and cancer (cancer survey series) vol 7, Oxford University Press, Oxford, pp 103–124

Garmatis C J, Chu F 1978 The effectiveness of radiation therapy in the treatment of bone
    metastases from breast cancer. Radiology 16: 235–237
Garrett I R, Durie B G M, Nedwin G E et al 1987 Production of the bone-resorbing cytokine
    lymphotoxin by cultured myeloma cells. New England Journal of Medicine 317: 526–532
Gilbert H A, Kagan A R, Nussbaum H et al 1977 Evaluation of radiation therapy for bone
    metastases: pain relief and quality of life. American Journal of Roentgenology
    129: 1095–1098
Harinck H I J, Bijvoet O L M, Blanksma J H, Dahlinghaus-Neinhuys P J 1987 Efficacious
    management with APD in Paget's disease of bone. Clinical Orthopaedics 217: 79–88
Hoskin P J 1988 Scientific and clinical aspects of radiotherapy in the relief of bone pain.
    In: Hanks G W (ed) Cancer Surveys, vol 7, no 1. Oxford University Press, Oxford, pp 69–86
Hoskin P J, Ford H T, Harmer C L 1989 Hemibody irradiation for metastatic bone pain in two
    histologically distinct groups of patients. Clinical Oncology 1: 67–69
Kelly C G, Gaze M N, Rodger A 1991 Treating bony metastases. British Medical Journal
    303: 1335
Laing A H, Ackery D M, Bayly R J et al 1991 Strontium-89 chloride for pain palliation in
    prostatic skeletal malignancy. British Journal of Radiology 64: 816–822
Lewington V J, McEwan A J, Ackery D M et al 1991 A prospective, randomized double-blind
    crossover study to examine the efficacy of strontium-89 in pain palliation in patients with
    advanced prostate cancer metastatic to bone. European Journal of Cancer 27: 954–958
Lowik C W G M et al 1988 Migration and phenotypic transformation of osteoclast precursors
    into mature osteoclasts: the effect of a bisphosphonate. Journal of Bone and Mineral
    Research 3: 185–192
Lyss A P 1987 Systemic treatment for prostate cancer. American Journal of Medicine
    83: 1120–1128
Madsen E L 1983 Painful bone metastasis: efficacy of radiotherapy assessed by the patients: a
    randomized trial comparing 4 Gy × 6 versus 10 Gy × 2. International Journal of Radiation
    Oncology, Biology, Physics 9: 1775–1779
Minton M J, Knight R K, Rubens R D, Hayward J L 1981 Corticosteroids for elderly patients
    with breast cancer. Cancer 48: 883–887
Morton A R, Cantrill A R, Pillai G V, McMahon A, Anderson D C, Howell A 1988b Sclerosis
    of lytic bone metastases after disodium aminohydroxypropylidene bisphosphonate (APD) in
    patients with breast carcinoma. British Medical Journal 297: 772–773
Morton A R, Cantrill A R, Craig A E et al 1988b Single dose versus daily intravenous
    aminohydroxypropylidene bisphosphonate (ADP) for the hypercalcaemia of malignancy.
    British Medical Journal 296: 811–814
Nag S, Shah V 1986 Once-a-week lower hemibody irradiation for metastatic cancers.
    International Journal of Radiation Oncology, Biology, Physics 12: 1003–1005
O'Rourke N P, McCloskey E V, Vasikaran S, Eyres K, Fern D, Kanis J A 1993 Effective
    treatment of malignant hypercalcaemia with a single intravenous infusion of clodronate.
    British Journal of Cancer 67: 560–563
Pannuti F, Martoni A, Rossi A P, Piana E 1979 The role of endocrine therapy for relief of pain
    due to advanced cancer. In: Bonica J J, Ventafridda V (eds) Advances in pain research and
    therapy, vol 2. Raven Press, New York, pp 145–165
Parsons V, Dalley V, Brinkley D, Davies C, Vernon A 1974 The effects of calcitonin on the
    metabolic disturbances surrounding widespread bony metastases. Acta Endocrinologica
    76: 286–301
Price P, Hoskin P J, Easton D, Austin D, Palmer S G, Yarnold J R 1986 Prospective
    randomized trial of single and multifraction radiotherapy schedules in the treatment of
    painful bony metastases. Radiotherapy and Oncology 6: 247–255
Qasim M M 1981 Half body irradiation in metastatic carcinoma. Clinical Radiology
    32: 215–219
Ralston S H, Gallacher S J, Patel U et al 1989 Comparison of three intravenous
    bisphosphonates in cancer-associated hypercalcaemia. Lancet ii: 1180–1182
Robinson R G, Preston D F, Spicer J A, Baxter K G 1992 Radionuclide therapy of intractable
    bone pain: emphasis on strontium-89. Seminars in Nuclear Medicine 22: 28–32
Rose K, Taylor H, Twycross R G 1993 Volume reduction of arm lymphoedema. Nursing
    Standard 7: 29–32
Rowland C G, Bullimore J A, Smith P J B, Roberts J B M 1981 Half body irradiation in the
    treatment of metastatic prostatic carcinoma. British Journal of Urology 53: 628–629
Salazar O M, Rubin P, Hendricksen F et al 1986 Single-dose half body irradiation for palliation
    of multiple bone metastases from solid tumours. Cancer 58: 29–36

Siris E S, Hyuman G A, Canfield R E 1983 Effects of dichloromethylene diphosphonate in women with breast carcinoma metastatic to the skeleton. American Journal of Medicine 74: 401–406

Smith J R 1989 Palliation of painful bone metastases from prostate cancer using sodium etidronate: results of a randomized, prospective, double-blind, placebo-controlled study. Journal of Urology 141: 85–87

Smith E I, Macaulay V 1985 Comparison of different endocrine therapies in management of bone metastases from breast carcinoma. Journal of the Royal Society of Medicine 78 (suppl 9): 15–17

Stoll B A 1983 Natural history, prognosis, and staging of bone metastases. In: Stoll B A, Parbhoo S (eds) Bone metastases: monitoring and treatment. Raven Press, New York, pp 1–4

Tannock I, Gospodarowicz M, Meakin W, Panzarella T, Stewart L, Rider W 1989 Treatment of metastatic prostatic cancer with low-dose prednisolone: evaluation of pain and quality of life as pragmatic indices of response. Journal of Clinical Oncology 17: 590–597

Tong D, Gillick L, Hendrickson F 1982 The palliation of symptomatic osseous metastases: final results of the study of the Radiation Therapy Oncology Group. Cancer 50: 893–899

Twycross R G 1977 Care of the terminal patient. In: Stoll B A (ed) Breast cancer management: early and late. Heinemann Medical, London, pp 157–163

Twycross R G, Fairfield S 1982 Pain in far-advanced cancer. Pain 14: 303–310

Watson L 1966 Calcium metabolism and cancer. Australian Annals of Medicine 15: 359–367

Whitehouse J M A 1985 Site-dependent response to chemotherapy for carcinoma of the breast. Journal of the Royal Society of Medicine 78 (suppl 9): 18–22

Wilkins M F, Keen C W 1987 Hemibody radiotherapy in the management of metastatic carcinoma. Clinical Radiology 38: 267–268

Yablon I G, Paul G R 1976 The augmentative use of methyl methacrylate in the management of pathological fractures. Surgery, Gynaecology and Obstetrics 143: 177–183

CHAPTER 25 | Nerve blocks and neurosurgery

NEED FOR NEURODESTRUCTIVE PROCEDURES

The need for neurolytic and neurosurgical procedures has decreased considerably (Fig. 25.1). This relates to the increased use of:

- oral morphine
- secondary analgesics
- spinal analgesia

and better psychosocial support. In places where these are not all available, neurodestructive treatments will be needed more often. Even so, in the UK, it has been said that:

'A localized destructive procedure is better than giving an opioid to the whole

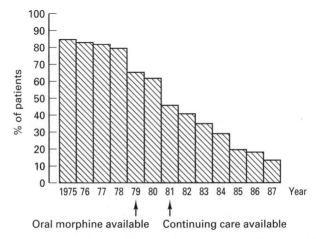

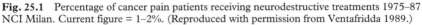

Fig. 25.1 Percentage of cancer pain patients receiving neurodestructive treatments 1975–87 NCI Milan. Current figure = 1–2%. (Reproduced with permission from Ventafridda 1989.)

body just to get some of it into the cerebrospinal fluid. Patients would find it more advantageous if less morphine and more blocks were used because the quality of pain relief when a block works well is much better than that obtained when opioids work well' (Lipton 1989).

'If you are not at least thinking about neurolytic procedures in 10% of your patients, then you are being somewhat blinkered and need to widen your horizons' (Wells 1989).

These comments, however, stem from a Pain Relief Centre where the pain being dealt with will be more resistant to drug therapy than is generally the case. They also predate the more widespread use in the UK of spinal analgesia in patients with advanced cancer. A comment by a neurosurgeon is perhaps apposite:

'We have to admit that patients I will subject to a surgical procedure will be managed by pharmacological, psychological and anaesthesiological techniques in the clinic next door' (Gybels 1992).

Even so, there remains a small group of patients in whom a neurodestructive procedure is crucial.

In the past, lack of data made it difficult to evaluate the long term benefits of neurodestructive treatments. In this respect, one doctor's testimony is noteworthy:

'One of the most vivid images, in my personal experience of 20 years, is of the period when I used to treat pain with neuro-ablative surgery only. I often remember seeing patients, completely relieved of pain after percutaneous cordotomy, kiss my hands the first day, smile at me a week later, and look at me with sadness and even rage after a month. All this because they gradually became aware of the progress of the disease, with its relevant symptoms, and with the consequent deterioration in the quality of life. We must not forget that nausea and vomiting can be worse than the pain itself, and that situations like intestinal occlusion, bedsores, and innumerable other signs of suffering require expert intervention. Control of psychosocial problems represents 50% of the activity to be carried out' (Ventafridda 1987).

Data from the same centre compared two groups of patients, one treated solely by primary and secondary analgesics and the other by a multimodal approach. Patients in the second group had statistically better significant pain relief in weeks 3–5 but not otherwise (Fig. 25.2). The results appear to suggest that, given time, drug measures will achieve equally good pain relief. The two groups of patients, however, were not randomly allocated. Those considered for multimodal management had unilateral pain (possibly because of nerve compression/infiltration). Of 218 patients originally in this group, 118 responded sufficiently well to analgesics to obviate the need to consider proceeding with neurolytic techniques.

Interpretation of the results is further complicated by the inclusion in the multimodal group of 29 patients who had spinal opioids. The other patients underwent:

- coeliac axis plexus block (25)

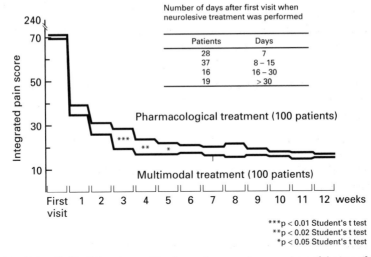

Fig. 25.2   Pain relief in 200 patients with advanced cancer. A comparison of the use of drugs with multimodal management. (Reproduced with permission from Ventafridda et al 1985.)

- percutaneous cordotomy (24)
- chemical rhizotomy (12)
- Gasserian thermocoagulation (7).

A second survey also includes spinal analgesia under 'neural blockade' (Boys et al 1993). Epidural analgesia accounted for 60% of the patients treated (Table 25.1).

LOCAL ANAESTHETIC BLOCKS

Local anaesthetic blocks are of value in:

- diagnosis
- prognosis
- therapy.

A local anaesthetic block can confirm whether a pain is related to a specific nerve, and can act as a predictor of the probable outcome of a neurolytic procedure. The main use of local anaesthetics in a palliative care unit,

Table 25.1   Changes in analgesic medication during 2–6 week follow up after neural blockade

Block	Number	Reduction (%)	Increase (%)	Unchanged (%)
Epidural (single injection)	69	25	6	69
Epidural (infusion)	25	70	8	22
Coeliac plexus	22	44	0	56
Paravertebral	19	22	11	67
Lumbar plexus	16	9	9	82
Intrathecal	4	50	0	50

From Boys et al 1993

however, is therapeutic. Although, theoretically, local anaesthetic blocks are only temporary (Table 25.2), in practice they may provide partial or complete pain relief for an extended period.

Pharmacological considerations

Several local anaesthetic agents are available, more in the USA than in the UK (Bonica 1989). Lignocaine (lidocaine) and bupivacaine are the most widely used (Box 25.A). Lignocaine is short acting (1–2 h), whereas bupivacaine is relatively long acting (8–12 h). Lignocaine but not bupivacaine causes vasodilation and is often used with adrenaline to retard absorption and metabolism.

Giving lignocaine with adrenaline increases the maximum safe dose from 500 mg to about 1 g. Adrenaline should not be used in patients taking a mono-amine oxidase inhibitor or a tricyclic antidepressant, both of which potentiate the pressor effect of sympathomimetic amines. Adverse effects from local anaesthetics are unusual and generally relate to an overdose:

- excitement
  — tremor of lips
  — twitching of corner of mouth
- CNS depression (rare)
- hypotension
  — faintness
  — lightheadedness
- cardiac arrhythmia
  — pallor
  — sweating.

Occasionally, a hypersensitivity reaction may occur manifesting as profound hypotension and tachycardia after only a small dose.

Local anaesthetics have an antimicrobial property. This helps explain why it is relatively safe to leave, for example, an epidural indwelling catheter in place for several days or even weeks.

Indications for use

Therapeutic local anaesthetic blocks should be considered in the following situations:

- myofascial pain
- solitary rib metastasis
- other axial skeletal secondaries
- sacro-iliac pain
- fractured neck of femur (lumbar plexus)
- chest wall pain (paravertebral)
- upper neck and head pain (cervical plexus)
- postherpetic neuralgia.

Table 25.2 Clinical characteristics and doses of local anaesthetics

	Procaine	2-Chloroprocaine	Lignocaine	Mepivacaine	Prilocaine	Tetracaine	Bupivacaine	Etidocaine
Latency (speed of onset)	Moderate	Fast	Fast	Moderate	Moderate	Very slow	Fast	Very fast
Penetration (diffusibility)	Moderate	Marked	Marked	Moderate	Moderate	Poor	Moderate	Moderate
Duration	Short	Very short	Moderate	Moderate	Moderate	Long	Long	Long
Optimal concentrations (%)								
infiltration	0.5	0.5	0.25	0.25	0.25	0.05	0.05	0.1
spinal nerve and plexus block	1.5–2	1–2	0.5–1	0.5–1	0.5–1	0.1–0.2	0.25–0.5	0.5–1
Maximum amount (mg/kg)	12	15	6	6	6	2	2	2

From Bonica 1989

BOX 25.A
LOCAL ANAESTHETIC AGENTS

Esters
Cocaine hydrochloride is a naturally occurring alkaloid used for topical analgesia.

Procaine hydrochloride is the original synthetic local anaesthetic. Unlike cocaine, its surface activity is very poor. Maximum safe dose is about 500 mg. Rapidly absorbed after injection, it is effective for up to an hour if adrenaline is added to counter vasodilatation. Maximum safe dose with adrenaline = 1 g. It is rapidly metabolized by pseudocholinesterase.

Amides
Lignocaine hydrochloride is slightly more toxic than procaine but, because of its greater potency, a smaller dose is necessary. There is little to choose between them in practice. The usual strength for local anaesthesia is 1%. It is more stable in solution than procaine, much more active topically, and causes less vasodilatation. Action lasts 1–2 h. Maximum safe dose in a healthy adult is about 200 mg, or 500 mg with adrenaline.

Bupivacaine hydrochloride is the longest acting of the amide local anaesthetics. It lasts up to 8–12 h, occasionally longer. It produces little if any vasodilatation. It is approximately twice as potent as lignocaine; the standard strength is 0.5%. Maximum safe dose is about 150 mg. It is used therapeutically to break cycles of chronic pain.

Myofascial pain

Stimulation of a myofascial trigger point (TP) by dry needling, intense cold, or injection of physiological saline often produces prolonged pain relief (Melzack 1981). The use of local anaesthetic is probably more reliable. Once a TP has been located by careful palpation, 1–2 ml of 0.5% bupivacaine can be injected into it. If relief is temporary, repeated blocks often relieve the pain for increasingly longer periods.

Solitary rib metastasis

If a patient has pain from a rib metastasis, relief is often obtained with an intralesional injection of bupivacaine and depot methylprednisolone. The technique is described on page 442. Lasting relief is obtained in 70% of patients (Rowell 1988). If benefit is only transient, radiation therapy should be considered.

Other axial skeletal secondaries

It is possible to use the same technique as employed for rib metastases with secondaries involving bony prominences, for example the scapula, iliac crest and pubic symphysis.

At one centre, lignocaine 2% and procaine penicillin are injected directly into bone metastases (Zweig et al 1980). Initially 2–3 ml of 2% lignocaine is injected. Those who obtain relief for 24–72 h are offered a second injection of one part 2% lignocaine and two parts procaine penicillin 6 000 000 units/ml.

The lignocaine is probably adsorbed onto the surface of the poorly soluble procaine penicillin and then slowly released as the procaine penicillin is metabolized. Up to 6 ml is used. Subsequent injections tend to have a longer effect. There is, however, no evidence that this approach is better than bupivacaine and depot methylprednisolone. Both emphasize the value of local anaesthetic injections.

Sacro-iliac pain

Patients with advanced cancer sometimes experience pain in the region of one or both sacro-iliac joints. This may relate to an underlying bone metastasis, notably in breast and prostatic cancer, or to recurrence on the anterior surface of the pelvis from a previously treated intrapelvic cancer, such as rectum, cervix uteri or ovary. If a bone metastasis, it is usually not the only one. The presence of other osteolytic areas on a radiograph indicates the probable cause. With intrapelvic recurrence, there may well be evidence of lumbosacral plexopathy (see p. 89) or an ipsilateral nonfunctioning kidney. Because sacro-iliac pain may be referred pain from the upper lumbar vertebrae, radiographs should include the lumbar spine if there is no local tenderness.

If there is no strong reason for suspecting a metastasis, local injection of bupivacaine and depot methylprednisolone should be considered. Non-malignant sacro-iliac pain is probably more common in patients who have lost weight. The patient should be told:

- sacro-iliac pain is common in patients with cancer
- in this case it appears to be nonmalignant in origin
- an injection of 'local anaesthetic and cortisone' may help considerably
- there will be initial benefit from the local anaesthetic which will wear off 'over the first 8–10 h'
- the maximum benefit will develop over 2 or 3 days as a result of the continuing effect of the 'cortisone'.

Occasionally, patients experience increased pain after the local anaesthetic has worn off, possibly because of a haematoma. This may take several days to settle. The results after the haematoma has resolved are as in other patients:

- some obtain complete relief
- some obtain moderate to good relief
- others obtain minimal or no relief.

Injection of the sacro-iliac joint is done with the patient lying on his side, the painful joint uppermost. Palpation will indicate the site of the sacro-iliac joint. It feels like a ridge of bone in continuity with the posterior part of the iliac crest, lateral to the midline. Bupivacaine 0.5% is used to anaesthetize the skin and SC tissues. With experience, it is often possible to insert the needle into a definite, albeit small, joint space. With the needle still in the joint space, the syringe is changed and the depot methylprednisolone is injected. This may require a modest amount of pressure. If this is the case

1 ml (40 mg) only should be injected into the joint space. Then, after withdrawing the needle a few mm, the rest is injected. The tissues over the joint can then be infiltrated with bupivacaine 4–5 ml.

Fractured neck of femur (lumbar plexus)

This somatic block can be carried out for pain associated with fractures of the femur where surgery is inappropriate. A needle is inserted posteriorly at L3. Its position in the psoas muscle (through which the lumbar nerve roots pass) is confirmed by injecting a water soluble contrast medium. Depot-methylprednisolone 120 mg diluted in 10 ml of 0.5% bupivacaine is injected, followed if necessary by a continuous infusion of 0.5% bupivacaine 1–4 ml/h (Boys et al 1993).

Chest wall pain (paravertebral)

A thoracic paravertebral block can be carried out for pain associated with chest wall involvement (e.g. mesothelioma). Needles are placed in the paravertebral spaces appropriate to the distribution of the pain, monitored by an image intensifier. A mixture of depot methylprednisolone and bupivacaine is injected at each level, up to a total of 120 mg in 20 ml of 0.5% bupivacaine (Boys et al 1993). Continuous infusions of bupivacaine to the paravertebral space can be considered if depot methylprednisolone fails to achieve adequate pain relief. Alternatively, phenol in aqueous glycerine can be injected (see below).

Upper neck and head pain (cervical plexus)

Local anaesthetic nerve blocks of the upper cervical nerves may sometimes be helpful if pain is localized to limited areas supplied by superficial branches of the cervical plexus. The nerves can be injected collectively, as they emerge from under the middle of the posterior border of the sternomastoid muscle.

Postherpetic neuralgia

Pain in postherpetic neuralgia is usually maximal at the proximal and distal ends of the affected dermatome(s). Infiltrating 0.5% bupivacaine 20 ml SC is often helpful. The pain may well be abolished for several *days*, and when it returns, it may not be as intense or as widespread. Although originally considered to be acting locally, the effect may be systemic (Boas et al 1982, Kastrup et al 1986). This means that an injection at any site or IV could be equally effective. To date, however, the technique has not been formally evaluated. Injections can be repeated every 3–6 weeks as necessary.

NEUROLYTIC BLOCKS

'Nothing is more heart warming than the gratitude of a fellow human being who has been relieved of intractable pain by skilful use of a simple nerve block. Nothing can be more guilt provoking than the reproaches of a patient who says he has been harmed. These are the two aspects of a difficult choice that patient and doctor must share when they are considering a chemical nerve lesion' (Wood 1989).

All neurolytic substances are indiscriminate in action and injure large as well as small fibres (Wood 1989). Neurolytic blocks therefore interfere with all aspects of nerve function both sensory and motor. Neuronal membranes are injured, and this opens the way to cross-fibre connections during regeneration. This could lead to inappropriate and possibly painful sensations being triggered by motor activity. This is one explanation for the dysaesthetic pain which frequently occurs several months after a block (Wood 1989).

Clearly, a substance is needed which will leave the neuronal membrane intact but will destroy the neurone itself. The vinca alkaloids and colchicine do this (Csillik et al 1978). It is possible, therefore, that a clinically useful substance will be identified one day.

Neurolytic substances

Phenol

To block peripheral nerves, for example intercostal nerves, 5–7.5% phenol in 50% aqueous glycerine is used. For intrathecal (IT) injection, 5–6% phenol-in-glycerine is used. The glycerine renders the solution hyperbaric and limits the ability of the phenol to mix with CSF.

Chlorocresol

2% chlorocresol-in-glycerine is sometimes used instead of phenol. It is less rapidly fixed to tissues and therefore has a more diffuse effect. This is clearly of benefit in the thoracic spine where there is generally a need to block several adjacent intercostal nerve roots. Chlorocresol and phenol can also be used together (Mehta 1973).

Alcohol

Absolute alcohol is hypobaric and, if used IT, will rise rather than fall in CSF. The use of alcohol, however, is now usually limited to coeliac axis plexus and lumbar sympathetic blocks.

Ammonium sulphate

Ammonium sulphate is more troublesome than phenol in terms of pain on injection and dysaesthesiae (Dam 1965). It is used occasionally for peripheral blocks (Wood 1989).

Thermocoagulation

In thermocoagulation a generator delivers a current to the tip of a special needle which heats up. It is under thermostatic control. Thermocoagulation is used for percutaneous cordotomy (spinothalamic tractotomy) and, in non-cancer patients, for destroying the nerves to the intervertebral facet joints. Needle placement is crucial. If incorrectly placed, either there will be no pain relief or partial relief with dysaesthesiae and allodynia (Wells 1989).

Cryotherapy

A cryoprobe can be used to freeze peripheral nerves (Lloyd et al 1976). Unlike other neurolytic techniques, the nerve membranes remain intact even though the nerve fibres are destroyed. Cryotherapy provides relief for 1–3 months (Anonymous 1982). In some hospitals, cryotherapy is used routinely at thoracotomy and inguinal herniorrhaphy. It has a place in cancer patients with multiple pathological rib fractures.

Coeliac axis plexus block

Coeliac axis plexus block is probably the commonest neurolytic technique still used in the UK. Other blocks which are occasionally used are referred to in Table 25.3.

Coeliac axis plexus block should be considered in patients with intractable epigastric cancer pain, notably pancreatic but also gastric and hepatic. It can be done under local anaesthetic but, in practice, the patient usually has a general anaesthetic. There are no data comparing management of epigastric pain by analgesics and by nerve block. This means that, at present, it is the patients who fail to obtain good relief with opioids who are considered for a coeliac axis plexus block. The block usually does not relieve the back pain if this is caused by malignant infiltration of the posterior abdominal wall.

Coeliac axis plexus block is generally conducted with the patient lying curled up on the more painful side. A 12 cm needle is inserted below the twelfth rib as laterally as possible to avoid puncturing the pleura and lung and passed forward to a point just anterior and adjacent to the first lumbar vertebral body. Monitoring with an image intensifier is essential for the accurate positioning of the tip of the needle. 15–20 ml of 90–95% alcohol on one side is usually sufficient to relieve pain.

This procedure is almost identical to a lumbar sympathetic block, but one vertebra higher. A coincidental lumbar sympathetic block is therefore possible, particularly if large amounts of alcohol are used (40–50 ml). Postural hypotension lasting for several days is common. Rarely it is prolonged and may be incapacitating (Box 25.B). Four cases of paraplegia were noted in a survey of over 2700 cases (Davies 1993, De Conno et al 1993).

Opioid analgesics may still be necessary for one or two days after the block, even when successful. In a group comparison in which 10 patients were treated with analgesics alone and 10 with a coeliac axis plexus block and analgesics, relief was the same in both groups (Mercadante 1993). The opioid requirements in the blocked patients, however, was much less (figures rounded):

- week 1 = 10%

Table 25.3 Nerve blocks for cancer pain

Block	Indications[a]	Method	Results
Trigeminal nerve	Head and neck cancer with trigeminal involvement	Absolute alcohol (<1 ml) → individual branches or → Gasserian ganglion (requires image intensifier[b])	Excellent pain relief. Also numbness but no motor deficit.
Glossopharyngeal nerve	Cancer of mouth and throat	Absolute alcohol injected at jugular foramen (requires image intensifier[c]) *Note* closely related to vagus, accessory and hypoglossal nerves Bilateral block would cause dysphagia	Good relief
Intercostal nerves	Cancer of bronchus and breast, mesothelioma with chest wall involvement	Absolute alcohol or 5% phenol (1 ml) injected subcostally posteriorly. A minimum of three adjacent intercostal blocks should be done. Both alcohol and phenol initially increase the pain; analgesics and sedation needed during procedure	Duration of relief often only days to a few weeks. If block too lateral, lateral cutaneous branch is missed which may reduce relief obtained. Main risk is pneumothorax. Consider radiograph 2 h after blocks.
Sacral nerves	Pelvic metastases causing nerve compression pain	Cryoprobe (or neurolytic substance) inserted through posterior sacral foramina	Good relief for several weeks. Impairment of bladder function unusual with cryoprobe and is reversible.

[a] Assuming that the pain has failed to respond to opioids, NSAIDs and corticosteroids.
[b] Jefferson 1963.
[c] Montgomery & Cousins 1972.

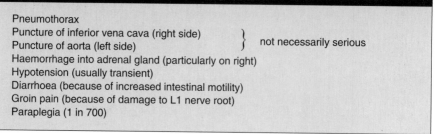

BOX 25.B
UNWANTED EFFECTS ASSOCIATED WITH COELIAC AXIS PLEXUS BLOCK

Pneumothorax
Puncture of inferior vena cava (right side)
Puncture of aorta (left side) } not necessarily serious
Haemorrhage into adrenal gland (particularly on right)
Hypotension (usually transient)
Diarrhoea (because of increased intestinal motility)
Groin pain (because of damage to L1 nerve root)
Paraplegia (1 in 700)

- week 2 = 20%
- weeks 5–7 = 40%.

Adverse drug effects were not significantly different. Three blocked patients had transient orthostatic hypotension (2) or transient diarrhoea (1). Surprisingly, half of the blocked patients had constipation despite lower opioid doses and enhanced intestinal motility (Mercadante 1993).

Lumbar sympathetic block

Lumbar sympathetic blocks are of benefit in patients with pelvic visceral pain, particularly bladder pain or rectal tenesmoid pain. This approach does not usually help peri-anal and perineal pains (Baxter 1984).

Intrathecal neurolysis

As already noted, intrathecal neurolysis may be achieved by use of alcohol (hypobaric), phenol-in-glycerine, or chlorocresol-in-glycerine (both hyperbaric). The most commonly used agent is 5% phenol-in-glycerine. In this concentration there is minimal interference with motor function and with sensations other than pain. Stronger solutions (e.g. 10%) are sometimes used in the treatment of spasticity. Phenol is rapidly fixed to tissues and the amount used (0.3–0.6 ml) generally affects only one or two nerve roots. If the needle or the patient is badly positioned, however, the phenol may drip over the cauda equina. This is likely to result in a more diffuse effect.

2% chlorocresol is not fixed so quickly and is a better agent for the thoracic region where it is necessary to block at least three adjacent intercostal nerves to achieve significant relief. Unlike phenol, it has only a slight early local anaesthetic effect prior to neurolysis. It does not, therefore, cause immediate sensory effects like tingling, numbness or warmth. With phenol these are useful guides to the accuracy of the placement of the neurolytic agent. 5% phenol injures mainly nociceptive fibres. Other fibres may be affected in the following order:

- motor fibres to bladder and rectum

BOX 25.C
COMPLICATIONS OF INTRATHECAL PHENOL

Pain at injection site (phenol)
Headache ± vomiting (post-lumbar puncture)
Meningism
Urinary retention
Faecal incontinence
Paraesthesiae
Sensory loss
Motor weakness

- other sensory fibres
- somatic motor fibres.

With blocks in the lower lumbar region there is a definite risk of producing bladder and anal dysfunction (Box 25.C). Recovery, which is not always complete, takes place in the reverse order.

The duration of pain relief and the incidence of complications following intrathecal neurolytic blockade are difficult to ascertain. Follow up beyond 4 weeks is uncommon and pain rating scales have not been used (Clarke 1984). A survey of 76 major papers on neurolytic blocks published between 1979 and 1983 showed that more than two thirds of papers failed to mention long term complications, and none provided data on physical activity and quality of life (Sbanotto 1984). In one series, the following results were obtained with IT injection of phenol-in-glycerine (Evans & MacKay 1972):

- 50% had pain relief for less than 1 week
- 5% had pain relief exceeding 3 months
- 92% continued to need analgesics after the injection
- 18% had one or more complication
- repeat injections did not improve relief.

A synopsis of results published over a 30 year period is shown in Table 25.4. There is a wide range for each complication. It is not apparent whether the lower figures relate to the skill of the practitioner or to more limited follow up. An incidence of dysaesthesia of nearly 50% is disturbing. The occurrence of this neuropathic complication and the failure of a repeat injection to relieve it is one reason for limiting such blocks to patients with a prognosis of less than 3 months.

Table 25.4 Complications of intrathecal neurolytic blockade (%)[a]

	Weakness	Sphincter disturbance	Sensory loss	Dysaesthesia
Average	11	11	7	10
Range	1–25	0.7–26	1–21	0.3–49

[a] Total number of patients = 832
From Clarke 1984

NEUROSURGERY

It is rare to need neurosurgery to relieve cancer pain. Even pituitary ablation is done much less often than 15 years ago. Anticipated survival time and the location of the pain are important guidelines. When the prognosis is only 1 or 2 months, neurosurgical procedures should *not* be undertaken. Drugs, administered spinally if necessary, and neurolytic procedures should be used instead (Gybels 1992).

For patients with a longer prognosis, there are several options depending on the site of the pain (Table 25.5). In patients likely to survive more than 6 months other alternative procedures may be considered:

- IT opioids with an implanted injection port
- neurostimulation.

Neurostimulation

This is helpful in selected patients with neuropathic pain. The results with dorsal column stimulation and deep brain stimulation (in the region of the posteroventrolateral and posteroventromedial nuclei of the thalamus) are shown in Table 25.6. Dorsal column stimulation, however, is not a simple technique; it is time consuming and expensive (Gybels 1991). Deep brain stimulation is not a routine method; its use is limited to neurosurgeons with a special interest in pain relief. The analgesic effect of deep brain stimulation is reversed by naloxone (Hosobuchi et al 1977).

Percutaneous cordotomy

There are two types of cordotomy (spinothalamic tractotomy):

- percutaneous
- open.

Percutaneous cordotomy means 2 days in a pain relief unit; open cordotomy may mean 2 weeks in a neurosurgical ward.

Percutaneous cordotomy is achieved by inserting a needle in the C1–C2 interspace under image intensification. A thermal lesion is then made in the anterolateral quadrant of the spinal cord using radiofrequency waves. In contrast, surgical cordotomy requires a general anaesthetic and is usually done in the upper thoracic region. The anterolateral quadrant of the cord is cut under direct vision.

Cordotomy is used mainly for intractable *unilateral* pain located in the segments below the midthorax. Bilateral percutaneous high cervical cordotomy is hazardous because of the likelihood of sleep apnoea ('Ondine's Curse') caused by interruption of the motor fibres to the diaphragm. These lie close to the spinothalamic tract and only emerge with the phrenic nerve at the level of C4.

The alleviation of the unilateral pain may unmask a pain on the contralateral side. Further, although the lesion is permanent, the plasticity of the

Table 25.5 Ablative procedures and results

Intervention	Number	Success (%)	Originator	Comment
Open anterolateral cordotomy	542	69	Spiller & Martin 1912	Carried out far less often than formerly.
Percutaneous anterolateral cordotomy	3357	85	Mullan et al 1963	Not easy — requires practice. Good results in unilateral pain.
Selective posterior rhizotomy	80	69	Sindou 1972	Useful in Pancoast syndrome.
Stereotactic mesencephalotomy	270	86	Wycis & Spiegel 1962	Consider in unilateral cephalofacial pain. Percutaneous rhizotomy of the trigeminal, glossopharyngeal and vagus nerves often the initial step. In 7 patients with neuropathic pain, none obtained relief (Bosch 1991).
Commissural myelotomy	235	63	Armour 1927	For bilateral pain in lower half of body. Replaced by spinal morphine and bupivacaine.
Stereotactic C1 central myelotomy	114	71	Hitchcock 1970	
DREZ (dorsal root entry zone) lesion	357	53	Nashold & Ostdahl 1979	

Source: Gybels 1992

Table 25.6   Results of dorsal column and deep brain stimulation in low back, neuropathic and limb ischaemia pain

Pain syndrome	Dorsal column		Deep brain	
	n	Success (%)	n	Success (%)
Low back pain	487	58	254	79
Postcordotomy pain	19	58	20	85
Spinal cord/peripheral nerve	21	38	69	72
Causalgia			26	69
Amputation/phantom limb	103	33	87	67
Postherpetic neuralgia	8	25	47	57
Brachial plexus avulsion	20	20	65	55
Anaesthesia dolorosa			106	42
Paraplegia	21	33	32	34
Poststroke pain			70	27
Severe limb ischaemia	21	71		

From Gybels 1991 (modified)

CNS is such that relief does not generally last for more than 6–18 months. Although this is sufficient for most patients with advanced cancer, for a few it is not.

The results and complications of percutaneous cordotomy are shown in Tables 25.7–25.9. Longitudinal data have been published more recently for patients with cancer of the breast and of the bronchus (Schrottner 1991). Most disturbing is the recurrence of pain resistant to opioids in 40–50% of patients before death (Table 25.10).

PITUITARY ABLATION

Hypophysectomy as a means of inducing a remission in potentially hormone dependent tumours, such as breast and prostate, is not commonly undertaken. The results are not good and the operation is viewed with distaste by

Table 25.7   Pain relief following percutaneous cervical cordotomy

Relief	Success (%)
First cordotomy	
Complete analgesia	80
Rapid disappearance of analgesia	4
Successful long term cordotomies	76
Second cordotomy	
1st cordotomy failures	24
One third refuse 2nd cordotomy	8
Total undergoing 2nd cordotomy	16
Good result obtained in 60%	10
Failures	6
Failures (6) + Refusals (8)	14
Effective	86

From Lipton 1984

Table 25.8 Motor weakness after percutaneous cervical cordotomy

Degree of weakness	Percentage affected
No weakness	10
Slight weakness without disability	40
Obvious weakness without disability	20
Obvious weakness with disability but mobile	20
Immobile but becoming mobile in one month	8
Immobile	2
	100

From Lipton 1984

Table 25.9 Complications of percutaneous cervical cordotomy

Complications	Frequency
Thermo-anaesthesia	All patients
Horner's syndrome	All patients
Headache	Common
C2 neuritis	Occasional
Micturition affected	Rare
Respiration affected	Rare
Ataxia	Very rare
Impotence	Very rare

From Lipton 1984

Table 25.10 Results of percutaneous cordotomy at time of death

	Grade	Lung cancer (n = 46)	Breast cancer (n = 22)
I	Complete relief by invasive procedure	0	0
II	Complete relief with the addition of a nonopioid	7%	14%
III	Complete relief with the addition of an opioid	43%	45%
IV	Incomplete relief despite opioids medication	50%	41%

From Schrottner 1991

most patients and many doctors. On the other hand, hypophysectomy has been used to relieve pain, particularly in patients who have multiple bone pains and in whom it is difficult to achieve complete relief despite the use of analgesics and radiotherapy. Ablation of the pituitary gland may be achieved in one of several ways:

- open surgery
- ^{90}Y implant
- cryosurgery
- alcohol injection.

Although complete destruction of the gland does not always occur with cryosurgery or alcohol injection, the results in terms of pain relief are equally good.

Alcohol is injected through needles inserted by the transnasal transsphenoidal route (Morrica 1968). Up to 2 ml of absolute alcohol is used. Of some 2200 patients treated by Morrica, the originator of the method, 60% experienced complete and immediate relief (Morrica et al 1980). Most of the rest became completely painfree after a second or third injection. In about 4% pain relief remained incomplete, although even in these it was not necessary to continue using strong opioids. Failure to secure complete relief was commonly attributed to psychological factors. 92% of the patients had hormone dependent tumours, mostly breast cancer. Results were equally good, however, in patients with hormone nondependent tumours, for example melanoma and cancers of the bronchus, larynx and bladder. Complications included:

- severe bleeding from the internal carotid
- hyperthermic crises
- hyperphagia
- dehydration.

Most patients experience frontal headache for 2 or 3 days after the injection. This is probably caused by a local chemical meningitis and may be associated with a mild pyrexia. CSF rhinorrhea is occasionally partly responsible for the headache.

Spread of alcohol to involve the optic chiasma and nerves to extraocular muscles may result in visual field defects or ocular palsies. If pupillary dilatation is noted during the injection of the alcohol, the cannula should be withdrawn and the patient turned on his side. Should eye changes occur, hydrocortisone 40–50 mg is injected into the cisterna magna. If this is done, any eye changes disappear within 15 min. At one centre, since implementing this technique, no patient has sustained a visual field defect (Lipton 1981).

Other technical improvements also reduce the overall complication rate of 6–10% and, in one series, a mortality rate of 5% (Editorial 1981). For example, vasoconstrictors can be applied to the nasal mucosa and the sphenoid sinus irrigated with an antibiotic solution. A fibrosing agent, ethyl cyanoacrylate, may be injected before the removal of the cannula to prevent leakage of CSF. After injection, intake of fluids and glucose should be kept high, corticosteroids given, and the polyuria controlled by nasal instillation of the antidiuretic hormone analogue, desmopressin.

Others have not been able to reproduce Morrica's almost total success (Table 25.11). Between 70–80% of patients gain some benefit, although probably no more than 40% obtain complete relief (Franchi 1980). Many patients die of the underlying disease within a few months. Relief persists for more than 4 months in only half of those who survive longer.

It is possible that the discrepancies relate to differences in technique. Morrica commonly used several needles and repeated the procedure until success was achieved. On the other hand, a former colleague disagrees with Morrica's view that pituitary ablation with alcohol is a major step forward in the treatment of diffuse cancer pain. In his opinion, when a patient has

Table 25.11 Results of pituitary injection of alcohol

Reference	Patients	Pituitary injections	Pain relief		
			Good (%)	Partial (%)	None (%)
Lipton et al 1978	106	155	44 (42)	32 (30)	30 (28)
Morrica 1977	822	1906	809 (98)	12 (2)	1
Katz & Levin 1977	13	15	6 (46)	7 (54)	0
Madrid 1979	329		220 (67)	89 (27)	20 (6)

From Lipton 1984

diffuse, poorly relieved pain, the use of radiofrequency percutaneous cervical cordotomy is preferable (Franchi 1980).

Life after hypophysectomy is not always trouble free. Rhinorrhoea often occurs on the first postoperative day, and occasionally lasts longer. Haemorrhage from the nasal mucosa may occur but soon settles. There can be subtle changes postoperatively, such as mild euphoria, but this is uncommon. In one series of 250 patients, there were six deaths associated directly with the technique (Lipton 1984). The deaths were attributed to:

- bacterial meningitis (1)
- hypothalamic injuries (2)
- dehydration (1)
- cerebrovascular accident (1)
- corticosteroid deficiency (1).

Dehydration must be avoided in patients with diabetes insipidus who are often old and very ill. A urinary output of more than 2.5 L warrants the use of nasal desmopressin, particularly at night.

For the first week after a pituitary injection patients are given hydrocortisone replacement therapy. Few require this permanently. Occasionally, a patient develops hypotension for which fludrocortisone needs to be prescribed. Thyroxine is also occasionally required. Patients should have regular endocrinological reviews after pituitary ablation.

How pain relief is produced is not certain. It is known that beta-lipotropin, the precursor of beta-endorphin, is present in large quantities in the intermediate lobe of the pituitary. A massive release of this substance by autolysis may explain the occasional observation of relief within minutes of the injection. Such a mechanism is unlikely, however, to produce a prolonged effect, and an increased endorphin concentration has not been detected in CSF after the injection.

In most cases relief is obtained after 2 or 3 days. A number of other hormonal mechanisms have been postulated (Editorial 1981). For example, prolactin, one of the pituitary hormones, stimulates the production of prostaglandins (PGs). No correlation between suppression of pituitary function and subsequent relief, however, has been demonstrated (Williams et al 1980). Considerable improvement has been seen after minimal changes in hormone levels, whereas one patient who developed panhypopituitarism derived no benefit.

Radiographic studies with a contrast medium have shown that, in about 20% of cases, the contrast is visible in the region of the hypothalamus and the cavity of the third ventricle (Miles 1979). It is possible, therefore, that the alcohol may injure the hypothalamus and its connections.

A better use of analgesics, however, has largely eliminated the need for pituitary ablation. In one paper advocating pituitary ablation for metastatic prostate cancer, a quarter of the patients referred for pituitary ablation were receiving only 'frequent nonopioid analgesics' and two thirds 'frequent oral opioid analgesics' (Fitzpatrick et al 1980). Drug regimens were not discussed and it is not clear whether the analgesics were being given on a regular or 'as needed' basis.

REFERENCES

Anonymous 1982 Cryoanalgesia. Lancet i: 779
Armour D 1927 Surgery of the spinal cord and its membranes. Lancet 1: 691–697
Baxter R 1984 Specialized techniques for the relief of pain. In: Saunders C (ed) The management of terminal malignant disease, 2nd edn. Edward Arnold, London, pp 91–99
Boas R A, Covino B G, Sahnarian A 1982 Analgesic response to IV lignocaine. British Journal of Anaesthesia 54: 501–505
Bonica J J 1989 Local anaesthesia and regional blocks. In: Wall P D, Melzack R (eds) Textbook of pain, 2nd edn. Churchill Livingstone, Edinburgh, pp 724–743
Bosch D A 1991 Stereotactic rostral mesencephalotomy in cancer pain and deafferentation pain. Journal of Neurosurgery 75: 747–751
Boys L, Peat S J, Hanna M H, Burn K 1993 Audit of neural blockade for palliative care patients in an acute unit. Palliative Medicine 7: 205–211
Clarke I M C 1984 Nerve blocks. In: Twycross R G (ed) Clinics in Oncology: Pain relief in cancer, Vol 3: Saunders, London, pp 181–193
Csillik B, Knyihar E, Jojart I, Elshiekh A A, Por I 1978 Perineural microtubule inhibitors induce degenerative atrophy of central nociceptive terminals in the Rolando substance. Research Communications in Chemical Pathology and Pharmacology 21: 467–484
Dam W H 1965 Therapeutic blocks. Acta Chirurgica Scandinavica 343: 89
Davies D D 1993 Incidence of major complications of neurolytic coeliac plexus block. Journal of the Royal Society of Medicine 86: 264–266
De Conno F, Caraceni A, Aldrighetti L et al 1993 Paraplegia following coeliac plexus block. Pain 55: 383–385
Editorial 1981 Pituitary ablation for pain relief 1: 1348–1349
Evans R J, MacKay I M 1972 Subarachnoid phenol nerve blocks for relief of pain in advanced malignancy. Canadian Journal of Surgery 15: 50–53
Fitzpatrick J M, Gardiner R A, Williams J P, Riddle P R, O'Donaghue E P N 1980 Pituitary ablation in the relief of pain in advanced prostatic carcinoma. British Journal of Urology 52: 301–304
Franchi G 1980 Comment of neuroadenolysis. In: Twycross R G, Ventafridda V (eds) Continuing Care of Patients with Terminal Cancer. Pergamon Press, Oxford, p 163
Gybels J M 1991 Indications for the use of neurosurgical techniques on pain control. In: Bond M R, Charlton J E, Woolf C J (eds) Proceedings of the VIth World Congress on Pain. Elsevier, Amsterdam, pp 475–482
Gybels J M 1992 Indications for neurosurgical treatment of chronic pain. Acta Neurochirurgica (Wien) 116: 171–175
Hitchcock E 1970 Stereotactic cervical myelotomy. Journal of Neurology, Neurosurgery and Psychiatry 33: 224–230
Hosobuchi Y, Adams J E, Linchitz R 1977 Pain relief by electrical stimulation of the central gray matter in humans and its reversal by naloxone. Science 197: 183–186
Jefferson A 1963 Trigeminal root and ganglion injections using phenol in glycerine for relief of trigeminal neuralgia. Journal of Neurology, Neurosurgery and Psychiatry 26: 345–352
Kastrup J, Petersen P, Dejgard A, Hilsted J, Angelo H R 1986 Treatment of painful diabetic neuropathy with intravenous lidocaine infusion. British Medical Journal 292: 173

Katz J, Levin A B 1977 Treatment of diffuse metastatic cancer pain by instillation of alcohol into the sella turcica. Anaesthesiology 46: 115–121

Lipton S 1981 Intractable pain: the present position. Annals of the Royal College of Surgeons of England 63: 157–163

Lipton S 1984 Cordotomy and hypophysectomy. In: Twycross R G (ed) Clinics in Oncology: Pain relief in cancer, Vol 3/No. 1. Saunders, London, pp 195–208

Lipton S 1989 Pain relief in active patients with cancer: the early use of nerve blocks improves the quality of life. British Medical Journal 298: 37–38

Lipton S, Miles J B, Williams N, Bark-Jones N 1978 Pituitary injection of alcohol for widespread cancer pain. Pain 5: 73–82

Lloyd J W, Barnard J D W, Glynn C J 1976 Cryoanalgesia: a new approach to pain relief. Lancet ii: 932–934

Madrid J 1979 Chemical hypophysectomy. In: Bonica J, Ventafridda V (eds) Advances in pain research and therapy, vol 2. Raven Press, New York, pp 381–391

Mehta M 1973 Intractable pain. Saunders, London

Melzack R 1981 Myofascial trigger points: relation to acupuncture and mechanisms of pain. Archives of Physical Medicine and Rehabilitation 62: 114–117

Mercadante S 1993 Coeliac plexus block versus analgesics in pancreatic cancer pain. Pain 52: 187–192

Miles J 1979 Chemical hypophysectomy. In: Bonica J J, Ventafridda V (eds) Advances in Pain Research and Therapy, vol 2. Raven Press, New York, pp 373–830

Montgomery W, Cousins M J 1972 Aspects of management of chronic pain illustrated by ninth nerve block. British Journal of Anaesthesia 44: 383–385

Morrica G 1968 The management of cancer pain. In: Progress in Anaesthesiology (Proceedings of IVth World Congress on Anaesthesiology). Excerpta Medica, Amsterdam, pp 266–270

Morrica G 1977 Pituitary neuroadenolysis in the treatment of intractable pain from cancer. In: Lipton S (ed) Persistent pain. Academic Press, London, p 149

Morrica G, Arcuri E, Morricca P 1980 Neuroadenolysis. In: Twycross R G, Ventafridda V (eds) Continuing Care of Patients with Terminal Cancer. Pergamon Press, Oxford, pp 155–163

Mullan S, Harper P V, Hekmatpanah J, Torres H, Dobben H 1963 Percutaneous interruption of spinal-pain tracts by means of a strontium needle. Journal of Neurosurgery 20: 931–939

Nashold B S, Ostdahl R H 1979 Dorsal root entry zone lesions for pain relief. Journal of Neurosurgery 51: 59–69

Rowell N P 1988 Intralesional methylprednisolone for rib metastases: an alternative to radiotherapy? Palliative Medicine 2: 153–155

Sbanotto A 1984 Revisione critica dei risultati antalgici delle tecniche neurolesive. Thesis. University of Milan, Milan

Schrottner O 1991 Results of percutaneous cordotomy in lung and breast cancer: a comparative study with strong support for a multidimensional nature of pain. The Pain Clinic 4: 217–222

Sindou M 1972 Etude de la jonction radiculo-medullaire posterieure. La radicellotomie posterieure selective dans la chirurgie de la douleur. These, Lyon

Spiller W G, Martin E 1912 The treatment of persistent pain of organic origin in the lower part of the body by division of the anterolateral column of the spinal cord. Journal of the American Medical Association 58: 1489–1490

Ventafridda V 1987 Considerations on cancer pain management. Journal of Palliative Care 3 (2): 6–7

Ventafridda V 1989 Continuing care: a major issue in cancer pain management. Pain 36: 137–143

Ventafridda V, Tamburini M, De Conno F 1985 Comprehensive treatment in cancer pain. In: Fields H L, Dubner R, Cervero F (eds) Advances in pain research and therapy, vol 9. Raven Press, New York, pp 617–628

Wells J C D 1989 The use of nerve destruction for relief of pain in cancer: a review. Palliative Medicine 3: 239–247

Williams N E, Miles J B, Lipton S, Hipkin L J, Davis J C 1980 Pituitary function following injection of alcohol into the pituitary fossa. Annals of the Royal College of Surgeons of England 62: 202–207

Wood K M 1989 Peripheral nerve and root chemical lesions. In: Wall P D, Melzack R (eds) Textbook of pain, 2nd edn. Churchill Livingstone, Edinburgh, pp 768–772

Wycis H T, Spiegel E A 1962 Long-range results in the treatment of intractable pain by sterotaxic midbrain surgery. Journal of Neurosurgery 19: 101–107

Zweig J I, Malspies L, Kaus S, Kabakow B 1980 A novel approach to the temporary control of intractable bone pain. Journal of the American Medical Association 244: 245

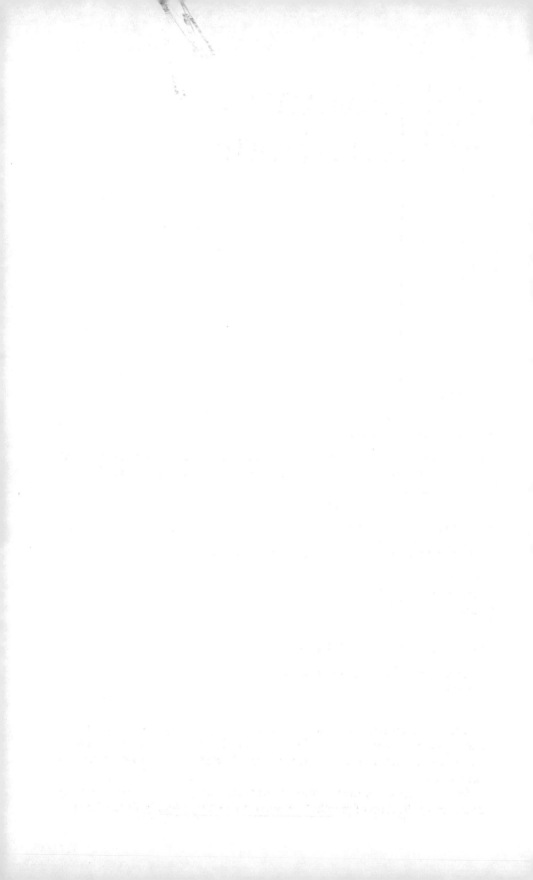

Adjuvant
methods

Various nondrug treatments are discussed in this chapter. They can be grouped under two headings:

- counterirritation
- psychological methods.

Sometimes these methods alone will be adequate. Generally, however, they are used in conjunction with drug and other nondrug treatments. Not all patients, however, find them beneficial.

COUNTERIRRITATION

Counterirritation may be achieved in several ways:

- massage
- chemicals
- cold
- heat.

More sophisticated methods include:

- transcutaneous electrical nerve stimulation (TENS)
- vibration
- acupuncture.

Ointments, ice packs and hot water bottles all help to ease aches and pains in bedfast patients. Relief often outlasts the duration of the counterirritation. If it does not, however, even a short period of relief from a niggling ache is appreciated.

Many analgesic ointments contain menthol, easily detected by its strong odour. An application of menthol ointment to the skin produces a sensation of warmth or cooling which may last several hours. Menthol is often effective in relieving tension headache, muscle spasm and joint pain.

Cold can be applied directly to the painful area with an ice pack, cold damp towels or with a re-usable gel pack. Cold packs can provide relief from headache, muscle spasms, back pain and joint pains caused by immobility. Some people, however, prefer hot packs, heating pads or a hot water bottle, particularly for muscle spasm and back pain. A hot water bottle is also helpful for abdominal colic.

Various theories have been invoked to explain counterirritation. Most are based on the Gate Control Theory of Pain (Melzack 1971) or on the production of endogenous opioids (Anonymous 1976). At home, many patients use some form of counterirritation. It is important, therefore, to make sure that these treatments are available for inpatients. Massage provides both physical and psychological benefits. Human contact reduces the sense of isolation and unworthiness which many terminally ill patients feel; they are no longer 'untouchable'.

Transcutaneous electrical nerve stimulation

Electrical stimulation as a means of modulating pain was used by the Egyptians around 2500 BCE, who used electric fish as current generators (Thompson 1987). It was also used by Hippocrates (400 BCE) and by the Romans. There was a revival of interest in the 18th and 19th centuries when more sophisticated sources of electricity became available. The use of electro-analgesia subsequently waned, because the majority of patients did not benefit from it. More recently, stimulated by the Gate Control Theory of Pain, there has been renewed interest in electrical stimulation.

Transcutaneous electrical nerve stimulation (TENS) is a technique whereby nerves in the skin and subcutaneous tissues are stimulated by surface electrodes connected to a small portable battery powered device (Fig. 26.1). In the past, electrodes were usually made of carbon rubber. Electrical contact with the skin required the use of a special TENS electrode gel or KY jelly. The electrode was then held in place by adhesive plaster. Application to the back, for example, was difficult and sometimes impossible for people living on their own. The advent of self-adhesive electrodes with a life of up to 3 weeks has helped considerably.

With standard high frequency TENS, square wave pulses of frequency 100–150 Hz with a current of 15–35 mA and a pulse width of 200–250 microseconds are used. Although most TENS devices have a variable frequency range, e.g. 2–150 Hz, frequencies of ≥ 100 are generally used for standard TENS (Stamp & Wood 1981, Stamp & Rose 1984).

'Acupuncture-like TENS' is a variant form of TENS in which electrical pulses are delivered in regular bursts, each of which contains a preset number of square wave pulses (Sjolund & Eriksson 1980, Kaada 1982, Kaada 1983). Between the bursts no stimulation takes place. The repetition rate of the bursts is commonly 2 Hz, with the frequency of stimulation in each burst commonly 100 Hz, but may be adjusted to a much slower rate.

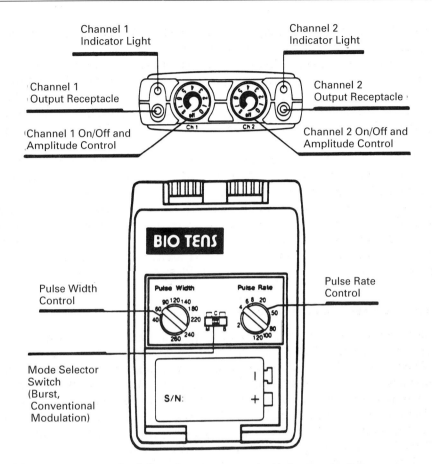

Fig. 26.1   Dual channel transcutaneous electrical nerve stimulator.

TENS is thought to work by stimulating the large A-beta fibres which 'shut the gate' in the substantia gelatinosa of the dorsal horn of the spinal cord (Fig. 26.2). The neurotransmitter most likely to be involved in the production of TENS analgesia is gamma-aminobutyric acid (GABA). In animal experiments, the effect of direct dorsal column stimulation is antagonized by a competitive GABA antagonist (Duggan & Foong 1985).

In order to determine whether opioid mechanisms are also involved, naloxone has been given to subjects after the use of TENS. In two animal studies and in three out of six human studies, naloxone caused either partial or total reversal of stimulation analgesia (Table 26.1). In general, analgesia induced by low frequency stimulation is reversed either partially or totally by naloxone. In contrast, analgesia induced by high frequency stimulation appears to be unaffected by naloxone.

Important factors in the successful use of TENS are the correct positioning of the electrodes and the optimal adjustment of the electrical output. Optimum electrical pulse width, intensity, and rate combinations differ from person to person (Anonymous 1989, Woolf 1989, Johnson et al 1991b). The

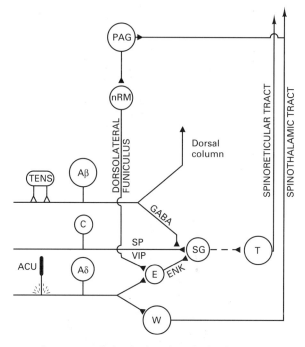

Fig. 26.2 Diagram to show neuronal circuits thought to be involved in TENS and acupuncture (ACU) analgesia. PAG = peri-aqueductal grey; nRM = nucleus raphe magnus; SG = substantia gelatinosa; T = transmission cell; W = Waldeyer cell; GABA = gamma-aminobutyric acid; SP = substance P; VIP = vaso-active intestinal peptide; E = enkephalinergic interneurone; ENK = enkephalin. (Reproduced with permission from Thompson 1988a.)

initial session, including time spent by the patient trying different positions and settings, may well last 2–3 h. Ideally, a suitably trained nurse or physio-therapist should be given responsibility for TENS and the supervision of patients.

The initial session will also identify 'machine phobic' patients and the occasional patient whose pain is made worse by TENS. Patients should use TENS as much as they wish. This varies from 1–2 h/day to the whole day (Johnson et al 1991a). Electrodes must not be placed on ulcerated skin or hyperaesthetic areas.

TENS has been shown to be of benefit in a high proportion of patients suffering from a wide variety of painful conditions, ranging from cramp, colic and arthritis to neuropathic pain from various causes (Woolf 1989). To some extent it is a case of personal response rather than response according to the cause of pain. A myofascial trigger point (TP) is said to be an indication for TENS (Ventafridda et al 1979). Injection of TPs with local anaesthetic is easier, however (see p. 510).

A major problem with TENS is that its efficacy commonly declines with time. The rate of decline varies from trial to trial. Figures of 60–70% initial benefit falling to 10–30% after 1 year are common (Woolf 1989). Loss of effect within 1 or 2 weeks relates to attenuation of the placebo component.

Table 26.1 Effect of naloxone on stimulation analgesia

Subjects	n	Site of stimulation	Frequency	Dose	Effect	Controlled	Reference
Animals							
Rat	41	PAG[a]	Low	1–4 mg/kg	Partial reversal	+	Akil et al 1976
Rat	6	Tail	High	1 mg/kg SC	Partial reversal in both normal and spinal animals	+	Woolf et al 1980
Humans							
Chronic pain patients	6	PAG + PVG[b]	Low	0.2–1 mg IV	Total reversal in 5 patients	–	Hosobuchi et al 1977
Normal volunteers	24	Dental	Low	0.4 mg IV	Partial reversal	+	Chapman & Benedetti 1977
Acute pain patients	6	Intercostal nerves of fractured ribs	?	0.8 mg IV	No reversal	–	Woolf et al 1978
Chronic pain patients	20	Unspecified	Low / High	0.8–1.6 mg IV / 0.8–16 mg IV	Reversal 6/10 / No reversal 10/10	+	Sjolund & Eriksson 1979
Chronic pain patients	12	7 epidural 7 TENS (neck, back and knee)	Low–High	0.4–10 mg IV	No overall change; details of frequency not given	+	Freeman et al 1983
Chronic pain patients	15	TENS (neck, back, shoulders, limbs)	High	0.4–1.2 mg IV	No reversal	+	Abram et al 1981

[a] PAG = peri-aqueductal grey.
[b] PVG = periventricular grey.
From Thompson 1988a

A reduced effect at a later stage probably indicates tolerance (Thompson & Filshie 1993).

In one group of 37 cancer patients only four (11%) experienced a reduction of pain after a month (Ventafridda et al 1979). The best results were seen in 3/13 patients with pain associated with head and neck cancer, 3/6 patients with early phantom limb pain and, to a lesser degree, in 3/8 patients with postherpetic neuralgia.

In practice, the use of TENS is likely to be determined by the presence or absence of a local enthusiast. It is used rarely at Sobell House. In contrast, another centre states:

> 'We utilize TENS in a high proportion of our patients as an adjunct to other more reliably effective modalities. While it rarely relieves pain entirely and there is a significant placebo effect accounting for a decay in efficacy over time, it provides patients with a measure of control that is absent in other aspects of their lives' (Patt 1992).

It is difficult, however, to predict which patients will achieve a lasting response (Bates & Nathan 1980). Even so, a treatment which continues to bring relief to 10–30% of patients is still useful. Personality type, social status, age and gender are not predictive (Johnson et al 1993), but limb pain responds better than trunk pain (Johansson et al 1980). Mental illness, pathological personality traits, and the absence of an obvious physical cause for the pain are all negative factors (Nielzen et al 1982). A significant relationship has been shown between EEG patterns and response to TENS. Poor responders had lower spontaneous and evoked EEG activity across all frequency bands compared with responders (Johnson et al 1993).

Vibration

Percussion analgesia for amputation stump pain was used by veterans of the American Civil War (Editorial 1992). Cutaneous vibration produces an initial increase in pain followed by numbness and analgesia when vibration is continued for a minimum of 30 min. Relief often persists for hours, or even days (Gammon & Starr 1941, Ritchie Russell & Spalding 1950).

One drawback with vibrators is the relative 'user-unfriendliness' of the equipment:

> 'Stationary vibrators, e.g. those incorporated into a chair or bed, are difficult to apply to specific painful areas with enough force to be effective. Moreover, the chairs or beds tend to be extremely expensive and unsuited to patients who are physically active. Hand held vibrators are often bulky and noisy, require a mains power supply, and are obtrusive in use. Small battery operated vibrators may lack the power for long term use and have sexual connotations that can embarrass some patients. However, the small machines are easy to apply, and the high frequencies of some models may be more comfortable and effective than the low frequency vibrators. Even so, vibrators are much more obvious in use than a small transcutaneous nerve stimulator and for this reason patients may reject them even though they are more effective' (Editorial 1992).

Vibration works best if it is applied at around a frequency of 100 Hz near or *distal* to the painful site (Sherer et al 1986), with moderate pressure and maintained for more than 45 min (Lundeberg et al 1984). The area covered in unimportant (Palmesano et al 1989). Benefit is more pronounced in pain arising from nerves or muscles (Lundeberg 1984). Good results with vibration have also been reported in the management of facial pain (McCaffery & Beebe 1989).

Vibration works by stimulation of low threshold large diameter A-beta fibres (McGlone & Marsh 1990); endogenous opioids are not involved (Lundeberg 1985). Vibration is, therefore, more selective than TENS.

Acupuncture

Acupuncture may be performed in several ways, including the manual rotation of pairs of needles and low or high frequency electrical stimulation through them (Man & Ning 1983, Filshie & Redman 1985, Thompson & Filshie 1993). Manual acupuncture is usually carried out with a needle and may be either superficial or deep.

With *superficial acupuncture* the needle is inserted through the skin but no further than the subcutaneous tissues. With *deep acupuncture* the needle passes through skin and subcutaneous tissue into muscle and possibly down to the periosteum. In classical Chinese acupuncture deep needling is used to produce a deep sore aching and numb feeling (called te-chi or dequi) which is considered to be essential if the acupuncture is to be fully effective. Intense pressure (acupressure) may be used, although it is less effective. High intensity stimuli are unpleasant, and activate cutaneous A-delta fibres, or the equivalent Group III fibres in muscle (Bowsher 1976).

In *electro-acupuncture* pairs of needles are connected to an electrical stimulator designed to produce brief square wave pulses (0.2 msec) which are repeated at a slow frequency, e.g. 1–4 Hz. The stimulator is adjusted to deliver high intensity current (30–50 mA). This may cause muscular contraction, a response not always specifically intended by the therapist.

Naloxone reduces or abolishes low frequency electro-acupuncture analgesia in animals and man, but has no effect on analgesia induced by high frequency electro-acupuncture in mice (Editorial 1981). Endogenous opioids are detectable in the cerebrospinal fluid (CSF) during acupuncture (Editorial 1981). The evidence that different forms of acupuncture elicit specific neurohormonal effects gives acupuncture scientific respectability. Despite this, acupuncture is not often offered in palliative care units.

Nearly 200 cancer patients were offered acupuncture at the pain relief clinic of a cancer hospital (Filshie & Redman 1985). Patients who were close to death or who would probably be better treated with a nerve block were excluded. 80% had pain caused by cancer or its treatment, and 20% had pain related to a concurrent disorder, for example postherpetic neuralgia or arthritis. Results are shown in Table 26.2.

Acupuncture was particularly useful for painful muscle spasm and for gynaecological patients. One patient with a fixed flexion deformity of the

Table 26.2   Results of acupuncture treatment in 183 cancer patients

Percentage	Benefit	Comment
18	None	
30	Some	Short duration pain relief; a few hours to 3 days, or increased mobility alone
52	Definite	Multiple treatments often necessary

From Filshie & Redman 1985

left leg following a spinal decompression for metastatic cancer of the lung, could straighten the leg within 5 min of treatment and subsequently began to remobilize.

Bladder spasms were also helped in three patients. Many patients with hyperaesthesia and dysaesthesia were helped. Postherpetic neuralgia and trigeminal neuralgia were often helped. Patients who required multiple treatments exhibited tolerance with time. Tolerance has also been described in an animal model (Han et al 1980).

A comparison of acupuncture and TENS is given in Table 26.3.

PSYCHOLOGICAL METHODS

The somatopsychic nature of pain has already been stressed. A doctor needs to offer skilled companionship (Brewin 1990). He needs to take time not only to listen but also to explain the reason(s) for each symptom, and to encourage the patient in the art of living with cancer. This is important for both the general care of the patient and the relief of pain. Intensity of pain is modulated by the patient's mood and morale, and also by the significance or meaning of the pain for the patient. There is a continuing need to prevent physical isolation which, on occasion, is tantamount to ostracism. The use of TLP ('tender loving physiotherapy') at home or in hospital helps to avoid this (Lichter 1987, Snyder 1992). This should be seen as a specific positive contribution and not as a sop for sagging morale, or worse, as part of a charade to mislead the patient into thinking that he is getting better. To be of maximum benefit, the physiotherapist must be aware of the real intent behind the request for treatment.

Specialized psychological treatments may also be necessary (Box 26.A; Malan 1982, Corsini & Wedding 1989, Brown & Pedder 1991, Tyrer 1992). All members of the caring team must understand the potential benefits of psychological interventions. If not, scepticism on the part of even one person may undermine their impact (Finer 1979).

Distraction

Distraction has been described as a form of 'sensory shielding' (McCaffery 1980). By directing attention to something else, the patient is less aware of noxious stimuli (Broome et al 1992). There are two settings, however, in

Table 26.3 Comparisons of acupuncture and TENS

	Acupuncture	TENS
Stimulation:		
type	Invasive and noxious	Noninvasive and innocuous
afferent neurone	A-delta ± C	A-beta
frequency	Low (1–5 Hz)	High (40–150 Hz)
intensity	High	Low
naloxone reversible	Yes	No[a]
Onset	May be rapid but often slow, e.g. 24 h delay	Usually 15–30 min
Duration of relief	Hours/days/weeks	Minutes/hours
Frequency of treatment	Every 1–2 weeks at increasing intervals	Daily–t.i.d. (more frequent initially)
Number of treatments	10–12; sometimes more	Continued indefinitely
Anatomical effect	Local and distant	Local
Analgesic efficacy:		
most	Headache Musculoskeletal Myofascial	Neuropathic Musculoskeletal Myofascial
less	Visceral Psychological	Visceral Psychological
Success	50–90% helped to varying degrees[b]	25% conventional TENS ⎫ pain reduced 40–50% acupuncture-like[c] ⎭ by 50%
Neurotransmitters/ neuromodulators	Endogenous opioids, Serotonin Noradrenaline ? others	GABA ? others
Advantages	Simple and safe (provided deep anatomy respected by therapist)	Simple and safe (self-treatment usually trouble free)
Disadvantages	Needs special needle and acupuncturist Can be costly Nonresponders Tolerance Infection: bacterial, viral (hepatitis, AIDS)	Needs equipment Patient compliance sometimes poor Can be costly Nonresponders Tolerance
Complications	Increase of pain Broken needle Damage to organs (heart, lung, spinal cord)	Increase of pain Allergy to electrodes, jelly or tape (5%) Skin irritation (30%)[d] Burns (rare)
Contra-indications	Pregnancy (except labour pains) Asthma Mental illnes	Pregnancy (except labour pains) Stimulation of anterior neck Heart pacemaker (unless protected)

[a] Acupuncture-like TENS is reversible.
[b] Richardson & Vincent 1986.
[c] Sjolund & Eriksson 1980
[d] Result of bad technique, i.e. not cleaning old electrode gel (containing sodium chloride) off skin; uncommon with self-adhesive electrodes
Based on Thompson 1988b

BOX 26.A
PSYCHOLOGICAL METHODS AND CANCER PAIN MANAGEMENT

Distraction   Music therapy
Creative activity   Biofeedback
Art therapy   Hypnosis
Imagery   Behavioural therapy
Relaxation   Cognitive therapy

Psychodynamic therapies, e.g.:

- psycho-analysis
- psychodrama
- person-centred therapy
- transactional analysis
- family therapy
- Asian psychotherapies
- multimodal therapy

---

which distraction is hard to provide. One is the busy loneliness of an acute ward (Wilkes 1965). The second is at home where lack of mobility may isolate the patient. Regular attendance at a day hospital is often a powerful corrective for the latter.

A change in approach is required when working with patients who are physically deteriorating:

'Patients who are very weak, or whose cerebration and co-ordination are affected by their disease or medication, will require great sensitivity from the occupational therapist. They will need to be given tasks which are considerably more simple than their previous level of capability. Because this can be both painful and worrying, a skilful therapist will encourage the patient to attempt crafts which he has never tried before. In this way, the comparison with previous standards is not so obvious. Even the simplest item, such as a knitted dish cloth, can give great satisfaction as long as it is something which will be useful. To expect someone to spend their time making something which is neither attractive nor useful is clearly insulting' (Charles-Edwards 1983).

Creative activity

'Poetry seems to be a vehicle for saying a lot in relatively few words. One reacts not just to what is written but to what seems to hover around it unwritten. Though a professional poet can express in very fine verse what it must be like to die, the inexpert poem of a dying person may end up speaking more clearly to the heart' (Frampton 1986).

Creative activity is more than distraction. It speaks to a person's innermost being and enhances self-esteem and hope (Frampton 1986). Palliative care units encourage creativity in various ways. Poetry is a popular art form (Box 26.B).

A major difficulty is that lethargy may make it difficult to get a patient

BOX 26.B
POEMS BY PATIENTS WITH ADVANCED CANCER (Alexander 1991)

Seven types of pain

I get a pain in the back of my neck
that makes me feel as if my head's on wires —
If I turn over too quickly something's gonna snap.

I get a pain in my elbow like shock waves
going down my arm to my fingertip.

I got turned badly the other morning —
the back of my ribs feel as if they're cracking.

I get a pain in the thoracic region,
a sort of clawing —
little crabs sitting in there having a chew.

When I move my legs I get screwdrivers
going through my hip joints.

My knee joints feel as if they've been dislocated.

Then there's the creeping pain.
You think, I'm not doing too badly,
then boom. . .

Other than that we do pretty well.

The long dark tunnel

What will it be like? I ask myself.
A long dark tunnel with a light at the end.
You rise up and look down at your body below
Marvellous!
No pain!
The awful pain of the cancer is gone
The cancer doesn't hurt
Nothing hurts.
Rested, no fear, no pain, at peace. . .
Beautiful
You're not ill any more.

Woodpigeons

Woodpigeons cell in the morning
Making peace with God and the world
The sound is gentle and calming
The sound of coo-ing reminds me
How good it is to be alive
For there are times
When life is too tiring
And it would seem easier to give in
To let it all be over
To not worry friends and relations
To be at peace myself.

But the sun shines
The woodpigeons call
Wonderful is the world!
How can I want to leave
Before my time is here?

to leave the bedside, and there are some who are totally bedfast. It is necessary, therefore, to bring activity to the patient in an attractive and not too demanding way rather than wait for the patient to make the move. An experienced artist can prepare materials and offer support in such a way that, despite limited strength and concentration, something of value is produced.

Art therapy

Creative activity can become a dual experience if overseen by a skilled therapist. This is perhaps most true of art, which can be used as an important means of providing support for psycho-analytical interpretations. Thus, when art is used in combination with psychotherapy the patient is encouraged to interpret what has been drawn or painted (Connell 1992). The impact of art as therapy has been described by a professor of surgery:

'My interest and enthusiasm can be described at two levels. Firstly there is an uncanny thematic similarity running through the works of many of these patients facing life threatening disease. It is as if the experience of cancer stimulates some deeply hidden folk memory to evoke the symbolism of life and death, fear and hope. For example, the tree as an expression of life and hope is a recurring theme in these works of art, which can be traced back through many cultures to the original 'Etz Chaim' (the tree of life) of the Old Testament.

At an individual level, what I found so moving was the obvious cathartic value of using art to express hidden fears and the progression of the imagery from fear to hope as a sign of recovery and sadly in the reverse direction as a sign of deterioration. There is no doubt that art is a powerful medium for self-expression for frightened patients, who don't have the words or the will to express themselves verbally' (Baum 1992).

Imagery

Imagery has been recommended as an adjunct to anticancer treatment. In this, the patient is encouraged to imagine the disease process being successfully attacked by the body's immune system (Simonton et al 1980). In relation to pain relief, however, imagery is a nonphysical form of distraction. A patient may be encouraged to think of a favourite location or activity associated with happy memories (Turk & Rennert 1981). At its best, distraction leads to relaxation. In fact, distraction may well be incorporated into a relaxation training programme.

Relaxation

Relaxation includes a range of techniques (Box 26.C). Muscle tension, emotional arousal and agitation all reduce pain tolerance, and thereby exacerbate pain and distress. In addition, pain may be related to, or exacerbated by, bad posture (Fleming 1988). Anything that reduces arousal and tension, or

BOX 26.C
RELAXATION TECHNIQUES (Fishman 1990)

Passive relaxation
Focuses attention systematically on the sensations of warmth and dissipation of tension in various parts of the body. Verbal suggestions and pleasant imagery are also used.

Progressive muscle relaxation
Focuses attention on the sensations associated with actively tensing and relaxing muscle groups.

Meditation
Mental repetition of a mantra (a word or short sentence) so that attention is removed from distressing feelings and thoughts, and a relaxed state thereby self-induced.

Music therapy
Usually involves a professional therapist who engages the patient in active or passive musical experiences. Music can have both a direct mood altering effect and an indirect relaxing effect through the diversion of attention from pain and stress provoking stimuli.

Biofeedback
Used to train relaxation of specific chronically tense muscles or chronically aroused autonomic functions, thereby aiding general relaxation.

Hypnosis
Enables patients to shift their attention away from pain (dissociation), thereby aiding general relaxation.

improves posture, is likely to ease pain. One of the fundamental messages of relaxation therapy is (Jacobson 1970):

'You can influence your body and your mind, and how they react'.

Meditation develops similar positive attitudes (Magarey 1981). The use of relaxation techniques can be a step towards the re-establishment of self-respect for the patient who feels the helpless victim of circumstances beyond his control: 'At last, there is something I can do!' In relation to pain, the aim is to prevent a vicious spiral of anxiety → muscle tension → muscle pain → more anxiety, and so on.

Published reports evaluating relaxation are summarized elsewhere (Jessup 1989). One study compared relaxation training with either frontal muscle biofeedback or placebo medication (Cox et al 1975). After 4 weeks, both relaxation and biofeedback groups showed a significant decrease in the incidence of headache compared with the placebo group. There was no significant difference between the relaxation and biofeedback groups. Others have reported similar results (Haynes et al 1976). There are a few reports of studies on relaxation and cancer pain (Fleming 1985).

Muscle spasm readily occurs in anxious and frightened cancer patients. Relaxation therapy should be seen as a means of preventing or reducing this. It may also help in more specific pain syndromes (e.g. myofascial and irritable bowel) which are associated with muscle spasm. In cancer pain itself, relaxation therapy will be an adjunct to other treatments.

For maximum benefit, the patient must understand the mechanisms underlying the pain and must comprehend the interaction between anxiety and muscle tone. In fact, the relatively common shoulder girdle pains (supraspinatus, levator scapulae and trapezius muscles) often subside after an explanation as to their cause, without any specific treatment. Simple guidelines about relaxation are available (McCaffery et al 1981), although it is probably expecting too much of most patients to rely on such advice alone. The use of a trained therapist who is prepared also to listen will enhance the use of relaxation. Advice may be re-inforced by the use of taped instructions.

For relief of persistent pain, the patient can be encouraged to practise one or two techniques regularly, such as rhythmic breathing and relaxing with music (Cady 1976). For both, the patient should be in a comfortable position with head supported. He should then close his eyes and listen. For rhythmic breathing, the therapist or tape will repeat the instructions (Box 26.D). For some patients, relaxing with music (or a favourite poem or Bible passage) may be easier (Patel 1981). While listening, the patient may imagine himself drifting or floating with the music. There is evidence that selected music may decrease pain postoperatively (Loscin 1981), possibly by distraction and relaxation.

BOX 26.D
INSTRUCTIONS FOR PATIENTS PRACTISING RHYTHMIC BREATHING
(McCaffery 1980)

Close your eyes.

Breathe in and out slowly and deeply.

Try to breathe from your abdomen.

Every time you breathe out, feel yourself getting more relaxed.

Find out how relaxation feels to you: you may feel light and weightless or you may feel very heavy.

Every time you breathe out, feel yourself getting more and more relaxed.

As you breathe, choose a place which you remember as being peaceful and pleasant. Let your imagination take you there — a beach, a field, a concert . . . Feel the air. Notice the smells. Listen to the sounds.

When you are ready to end your relaxation exercise, count slowly from 1 to 3:

- on 1, move your lower body
- on 2, move your upper body
- on 3, breathe in deeply, open your eyes and as you breathe out slowly, say to yourself: 'I am relaxed and alert'.

Music therapy

One to one music therapy is very profound (Lee 1989, Schroeder-Sheker 1993). It offers a form of expression without words. It requires a trained, skilled and empathic therapist who, in turn, will need psychological supervision and support. Music therapy is available at only a few centres.

Music is also an important aid to relaxation (Munroe 1978, Fagen 1982, Gross & Swartkz 1982, Munroe 1988, Beck 1991). At one palliative care unit, music is used to (Mandel 1991):

- reduce pain perception and anxiety through progressive muscle relaxation exercises with music
- reduce anxiety through the practice of guided imagery with music
- increase distraction from pain by listening to recorded music
- increase interaction with others by playing an instrument or singing with music therapist, family members or friends
- increase verbal or nonverbal expression of thoughts and feelings by creating music or lyrics to music
- increase verbal expression of thoughts and feelings by describing implied meanings and memories associated with selected music.

Biofeedback

Many physiological functions, for example blood pressure and pulse rate, are dependent on the autonomic nervous system. These are traditionally regarded as being beyond self-control. Biofeedback is a technique by which a person is made aware of changes in bodily functions, with the aim of eventually controlling the functions to advantage (Kogeorgos & Scott 1981). Biofeedback is the central component of a wide variety of procedures, all of which have the same principal goal of self-control. It has been used in the management of tension headaches, migraine, low back pain, epilepsy, certain neuromuscular disorders (such as spasmodic torticollis) and anxiety (Editorial 1980).

The basis for the claims of pain relief through biofeedback are several studies of its use in tension headache (Turner & Chapman 1982). In one study, by teaching people how to relax their frontal muscles, headaches were significantly reduced in about two thirds. (Budzynski et al 1973). On the other hand, a study of biofeedback in chronic nonmalignant pain failed to demonstrate significant relief (Melzack & Perry 1975). When used in conjunction with hypnosis, however, over half the patients had a decrease in pain of $\geq 33\%$.

There are no studies of biofeedback with cancer pain (Jessup 1989). When of benefit, biofeedback probably acts by distraction, relaxation, suggestion, and a sense of control over the pain (Melzack 1980). Even in headache, biofeedback is no more effective than relaxation. Relaxation is more straightforward, and is much less costly because it requires no equipment and can be done in groups (Turk et al 1979, Zitman 1981). Accordingly, biofeedback has no real place in the management of cancer pain except as an expensive form of relaxation therapy.

Hypnosis

Hypnosis is a state of alertness characterized by attentive, receptive, focal concentration with diminished peripheral awareness (Debetz 1981). It is a natural ability and has been used for many years as a technique for pain relief and muscle relaxation, and, sometimes, to facilitate healing. It is also a psychotherapeutic tool for alleviating symptoms, uncovering forgotten memories and facilitating behavioural change. Hypnosis does not reduce normal function nor does it affect the patient's mental capacity in a detrimental way. The principal theoretical advantages of hypnosis in cancer pain management are:

- relief of pain without destructive or unpleasant adverse effects
- no reduction of normal functioning or mental capacity
- no development of tolerance to hypnotic effect
- promotion of life enhancing attitudes in patient
- beneficial change in attitudes towards cancer.

Reduction of anxiety by hypnosis will also help (Waxman 1979).

Hypnotic techniques employed for pain relief vary, but generally include some of the following (Barber & Gitelson 1980, Orne 1980):

- directly blocking awareness of pain through the suggestion of anaesthesia or analgesia
- substituting another feeling (such as pressure) for the pain
- moving the perception of the pain to a smaller or less vulnerable area of the body
- altering the meaning of the pain so it becomes less important and less debilitating
- increasing pain tolerance
- in extreme cases, dissociating perception of the body from the patient's awareness.

Hypnosis provides the patient with a tool by which he can exert a measure of control over the effects of cancer. This feeling of personal control reduces the sense of helplessness which many patients experience (Barber 1978). It heightens a person's ability to concentrate on and to live for the moment. This results in a change in the way the cancer is viewed, and thereby promotes life enhancing attitudes.

Autohypnosis, in which the patient hypnotizes himself, is a skill which can be learnt and used to re-inforce therapeutic suggestions (Phelps 1981). The use of tape recorded advice helps to increase the therapeutic effect, and also reduces dependence on the presence of a therapist.

Clinical research of hypnosis in cancer pain is sparse (Table 26.4). A controlled trial comparing hypnosis with cognitive-behavioural therapy in relieving the pain of oral mucositis after marrow transplantation showed a

Table 26.4   Case reports of hypnosis in cancer pain

n	Outcome measures	Follow up	Results	Reference
12	Therapist's judgement	–	All had some relief; unequivocal in 5	Butler 1954
17	Therapist's judgement	–	12 patients had good or excellent improvement	Lea et al 1960
22	Opioid requests	1–20 weeks	13 patients requested less medication	Cangello 1961
8	Therapist's judgement	Not systematic	All showed pain relief	Sacerdote 1962
4	Self-report	–	Pain reduced or eliminated in all cases	Sarcerdote 1970

significant reduction in pain with hypnosis but not with cognitive-behavioural therapy (Syrjala et al 1992). There were two control arms in the trial, namely, 'treatment as usual' and 'therapist contact'.

The main disadvantage of hypnosis is that it requires a degree of concentration which many cancer patients do not have. It is also impossible to predict those who will benefit. Individual patients have been helped considerably by hypnosis (Dempster et al 1976, Zitman 1981, Levitan 1992). Even so, hypnosis has only a limited place in the management of cancer pain. It should be regarded as an adjunct to more traditional forms of treatment.

■ CASE HISTORY

Mark, a 42 year-old drug company representative with testicular cancer, had intense pain in the pelvic area and was fearful of becoming addicted to opioids. He refused to accept that his illness was incurable. He did not comply with instructions and attempted to plan his own treatment. He insisted that there must be a drug to help him and made plans to travel abroad for treatment.

Psychological consultation was requested because of the difficulties the doctors and nurses were experiencing. Hypnosis was suggested as a means of helping Mark. Resistance to this form of intervention was resolved when Mark was taught how to hypnotize the therapist (as a means of increasing his trust). Once he felt he was not being 'used as a guinea pig', he became amenable to hypnotic induction. The hypnotherapy had three aims:

- helping the patient to relax and interact co-operatively with the medical and nursing staff.
- learning self-hypnosis to help relieve pain in the pelvic area.
- working on psychological issues relating to the progress of the disease and the inevitable separation from loved ones.

Relaxation suggestions were given, and Mark became less anxious. He began to re-assess his relationship with his girlfriend and he gradually accepted the physicians' reports about his future. Using a hypnotic technique that allowed him to visually project himself and his girlfriend onto a hallucinated movie screen, he was able to distance himself from his own psychological conflicts about separation. Some resolution was achieved in acknowledging the limitations of the anticancer treatment and the reality that he would die in a few weeks.

Pain relief without opioids was possible until 2 weeks before his death. In order to facilitate self-hypnosis, a 'do not interrupt' notice was fixed to the door of his room during the 20 min periods used for self-hypnosis.

As he became more able to face death, Mark wanted to reconcile family differences. Age regression was employed to help him explore painful childhood memories. Mark asked his parents and brother to visit and to be with him while he was still conscious. He spent the week before his death talking, laughing and crying with his family in a way which would have been impossible before hypnotherapy (Barber & Gitelson 1980).

Cognitive-behavioural therapy

Cognitive therapy is based on a theory which maintains that how one thinks largely determines how one feels and behaves. The therapy is a collaborative process of empirical investigation, reality testing, and problem solving between therapist and patient.

Behavioural therapy emerged in the late 1950s as a systematic approach to the evaluation and treatment of psychological disorders. Behavioural therapy today is marked by a diversity of views and can no longer be defined simply as the clinical application of classical and operant conditioning theory. As behavioural therapy has expanded, the degrees of overlap with other psychotherapeutic approaches has increased.

Cognitive and behavioural approaches have been used effectively in the management of acute and chronic nonmalignant pain (Tan 1982, Turner & Clancy 1986, Jensen et al 1991, Keefe et al 1992). They also have a definite, albeit limited, place in the relief of cancer pain (Turk & Fernandez 1990). Cognitive-behavioural approaches are, however, time consuming and demanding for both patient and practitioner. Some patients may resist intervention of this nature because they feel it implies that their pain is 'all in the head', i.e. imagined and 'not real'.

In situations where cognitive-behavioural therapy is appropriate, however, it is usually possible to overcome this resistance by an explanation of the multidimensional nature of pain and how mind influences matter. The thought of moving from being mastered by pain to exercising mastery over the pain will be attractive to all except the most depressed or despairing patients.

As always, it is important for the practitioner to convey an attitude of 'unconditional positive regard' towards the patient through patience, empathy and sensitivity (Fishman 1990). The following is an example of the rationale which may be given to explain the need for a psychosocial evaluation (Fishman 1990):

'Chronic pain makes people's lives miserable in many ways. It takes the pleasure out of doing things. It makes people generally disinterested. It makes people become upset more quickly. Pain wears down even the strongest person . . . it must be difficult for you too.

It's also hard on family and friends . . . they see you suffering but think they can't help much. That's why it's important for us to find out what your suffering is like and how the pain affects your life. Then we can discuss some new ways of coping which could help you and your family, and reduce the pain.'

Pervasive dysfunctional attitudes such as excessive pessimism, inappropriate (false) guilt, self-blame, catastrophizing and a feeling of lack of control need to be identified. Extensive questioning by the therapist is generally too tiring for a patient with limited strength and concentration. Direct questioning about one's emotional life may also be felt to be intrusive. A lot can be discovered, however, just through conversation and the patient's use of symbols. Gestures and postures also reflect the inner mood of the patient.

Certain assumptions, beliefs and expectations result in excessive distress, helplessness, dependency or unco-operativeness. Examples of pain related dysfunctional attitudes in cancer patients include (Fishman 1990):

'I can't handle pain'
'This pain is driving me crazy'
'This pain is killing me'
'This is my punishment for . . .'
'I can't take drugs — I will become an addict'
'This pain is getting worse all the time — it will never get better'
'I can't enjoy anything if I am in pain'
'I can't do normal things if I have cancer and pain'
'There is nothing I can do about my pain'
'I can't show that I have pain — I am torturing my family'

In most circumstances the goal of cognitive-behavioural therapy is to modify maladaptive thoughts and behaviour. (Maladaptive refers to ideas and behaviours which increase pain and suffering by creating a feeling of personal disintegration and loss of control.) In palliative care, however, it is usually too late to correct the habits of a lifetime. Thus, the goal of cognitive-behavioural therapy in palliative care is not to change but *to support*. This is achieved by using established techniques which help to diminish a patient's frustration, anger and fears. Often, an important first step is to help the patient understand the multidimensional nature of illness, pain and suffering, and the inevitable interaction between mind and body.

Although cognitive and behavioural techniques are divided into the two categories for didactic purposes, specific methods within each category share many common features. In practice they tend to be applied simultaneously in various combinations.

Behavioural techniques focus on coping skills which a patient can acquire (Table 26.5). Cognitive techniques are designed to modify dysfunctional mental processes and to train adaptive coping strategies. They are similar to behavioural techniques except that they are applied to thoughts, images and attitudes. Consequently, they cannot be directly observed.

Cognitive-behavioural therapy is not designed specifically to eliminate a patient's pain, although the intensity of the pain may be reduced as a result

Table 26.5   Behavioural and cognitive techniques[a]

Behavioural	Cognitive
Self-monitoring	Cognitive coping, e.g.
Relaxation	distraction
Systematic desensitization	focusing
Contingency management	Cognitive modification

[a] For details see Fishman 1990.

of increased activity and the acquisition of various cognitive and behavioural coping skills. The therapy is designed to help patients learn to live more satisfying lives despite the presence of discomfort. Other goals include less reliance on the health care system and on analgesics.

The concept of 'pain behaviours' is introduced (Box 26.E). The therapist discusses the important role which spouses or other significant people may play by unwittingly re-inforcing the patient's overt expression of pain and suffering. The patient's spouse is also encouraged to identify examples of the patient's specific pain behaviours, and to complete a diary of the patient's pain behaviours and their responses.

Setting goals is also an integral part of the therapy. As in all aspects of palliative care, the goals must be specific, attainable and measurable. A vague goal of 'to feel better' is inadequate. It must be agreed what will indicate improvement. Goals can be divided into short term, intermediate and long term. They might include:

- medication reduction
- increased activity
- less time lying down
- specific tasks to do at home or at work

BOX 26.E
GLOSSARY OF TERMS FOR DYSFUNCTIONAL PAIN RELATED BEHAVIOURS
(Fishman 1990)

Operant behaviour
A behaviour which occurs in order to avoid pain, e.g. guarding, limping, inactivity, lying down.

Respondent behaviour
A behaviour which occurs in response to pain, e.g. grimacing, groaning, writhing.

Re-inforcer
A behaviour by a second person (spouse, significant other, etc.) which re-inforces operant and respondent behaviours in the patient.

Secondary gain
Being relieved of practical and social responsibilities because of the response by others to displays of pain behaviours.

- recreational activities
- reduced use of the health care system.

Since many chronic pain patients have a sedentary lifestyle which exacerbates their pain, the psychotherapist will enlist the help of a physiotherapist to develop a programme of graded exercises and activity suited to the patient's physical condition, age and gender. The patient should maintain a chart of incremental physical goals from which progress can be measured.

Psychodynamic therapies

Psychodynamic therapies are numerous (Malan 1982, Corsini & Wedding 1989, Brown & Pedder 1991). In this section, it is possible to refer specifically to only a handful.

Psycho-analysis

Psycho-analysis is a system of psychology derived from the work of Sigmund Freud. Originating as a method for treating certain psychoneurotic disorders, psycho-analysis has come to serve as the foundation for a general theory of psychology. By elucidating the influence of unconscious wishes on the physiology of the body, psycho-analysis has made it possible to understand and treat many psychosomatic illnesses.

Freudian psycho-analysis stimulated the evolution of several other psychodynamic therapies, including:

- Jungian
- Adlerian
- logotherapy.

Psychodrama

Psychodrama was developed by Jacob Moreno earlier this century as a method of psychotherapy in which patients are helped to enact situations dramatically in individual, family or group settings. Scenes from the past, present or future, imagined or real, are acted as if they were occurring at the moment. The role playing offers a wealth of diagnostic clues because habitual verbal defenses are circumvented. In the process of working out solutions, patients have an opportunity to discover their capacity for creativity. Psychodrama is a powerful technique which should only be conducted by professionals specifically trained in the method.

Person-centred therapy

Person-centred therapy is an approach to helping individuals and groups in conflict. It was formulated by Carl Rogers, a psychologist, some 50 years ago. In essence, he claimed that a self-directed growth process would occur if relationships are characterized by genuineness, nonjudgmental caring, and empathy. In fact, many palliative care services have intuitively adopted this kind of approach when offering psychological support.

Transactional analysis

Transactional analysis (TA), originated by Eric Berne in the 1950s, is a complete theory of personality. TA is based on the presence of three active, dynamic, and observable ego states labelled the Parent, the Adult, and the Child, each of which exists and operates in any individual. An effective TA therapist facilitates change and growth in clients.

Family therapy

Family therapy attempts to modify relationships within a family to achieve harmony. A family is seen as an open system, created by interlocking triangles, maintained or changed by means of feedback.

Asian psychotherapies

Asian psychologies focus primarily on the existential and transpersonal levels and little on the pathological. They contain detailed maps of states of consciousness, developmental levels, and stages of enlightenment which extend beyond traditional Western psychological maps. Further, they claim to possess techniques for inducing these states and conditions. The two classic families of Asian psychotherapies are *meditation* and *yoga*.

Multimodal psychotherapy

Multimodal psychotherapy is a systematic and comprehensive psychotherapeutic approach developed by Arnold Lazarus, a clinical psychologist. While respecting the assumption that clinical practice should adhere firmly to the principles, procedures and findings of psychology as an experimental science, the multimodal orientation transcends the behavioural tradition by adding unique evaluation procedures and by dealing in great depth and detail with sensory, imagery, cognitive, and interpersonal factors and their interactive effects. A basic premise is that patients are usually troubled by a multitude of specific problems which should be dealt with by a similar multitude of specific treatments.

REFERENCES

Abram S E, Reynolds A C, Cusick J F 1981 Failure of naloxone to reverse analgesia from transcutaneous electrical stimulation in patients with chronic pain. Anesthesia and Analgesia 60: 81–84
Akil H, Mayer D J, Liebeskind J C 1976 Antagonism of stimulation-produced analgesia by naloxone: a narcotic antagonist. Science 191: 961–962
Alexander L 1991 Throwaway lines. Sobell Publications, Oxford
Anonymous 1976 The pain paradox, Lancet i: 945–946

Anonymous 1989 Transcutaneous electrical nerve stimulation to relieve pain. Drug & Therapeutics Bulletin 27: 25–26

Barber J 1978 Hypnosis as a psychological technique in the management of cancer pain. Cancer Nursing Oct: 361–363

Barber J, Gitelson J 1980 Cancer pain: psychological management using hypnosis. CA-A Cancer Journal for Clinicians 30(3): 130–136

Bates J A V, Nathan P W 1980 Transcutaneous electrical nerve stimulation for chronic pain. Anaesthesia 35: 817–822

Baum M 1992 Reflection on the effect of art therapy for patients. Palliative Medicine 6: 24

Beck S L 1991 The therapeutic use of music for cancer-related pain. Oncology Nurses Forum 8: 1327–1337

Bowsher D 1976 Role of the reticular formation in response to noxious stimulation. Pain 2: 361–378

Brewin T B 1990 Not TLC but FPI. Journal of the Royal Society of Medicine 83: 172–175

Broome M E, Lillis P P, McGahee T W, Bates T 1992 The use of distraction and imagery with children during painful procedures. Oncology Nursing Forum 19: 499–502

Brown D, Pedder J 1991 Introduction to psychotherapy, 2nd edn. Routledge, London

Budzynski T H, Stoyva J M, Adler C S, Mullaney D J 1973 EMG biofeedback and tension headaches: a controlled outcome study. Psychosomatic Medicine 35: 484–496

Butler B 1954 The use of hypnosis in the care of the cancer patient. Cancer 7: 1–14

Cady J 1976 Dear pain. American Journal of Nursing 76: 960–961

Cangello V M 1961 The use of hypnotic suggestion for pain relief in malignant disease. International Journal of Clinical and Experimental Hypnosis 9: 17–22

Chapman R A, Benedetti C 1977 Analgesia following transcutaneous electrical stimulation and its partial reversal by a narcotic antagonist. Life Sciences 21: 1645–1648

Charles-Edwards A 1983 The nursing care of the dying patient. Beaconsfield Publishers, Beaconsfield

Connell C 1992 Art therapy as part of a palliative care programme. Palliative Medicine 6: 18–25

Corsini R J, Wedding D 1989 Current psychotherapies, 4th edn. Peacock Publishers, USA

Cox D J, Freundlich A, Meyer R G 1975 Differential effectiveness of electromyographic feedback, verbal relaxation, instructions and placebo medication with tension headaches. Journal of Consultation in Clinical Psychology 43: 892–898

Debetz B 1981 A fresh look at an old phenomenon: hypnosis. Journal of the American Medical Women's Association 36: 109–111

Dempster C R, Balson P, Whalen B T 1976 Supportive hypnotherapy during the radical treatment of malignancies. International Journal of Clinical and Experimental Hypnosis 24: 1–9

Duggan A W, Foong F W 1985 Bicuculline and spinal inhibition produced by dorsal column stimulation in the cat. Pain 22: 249–259

Editorial 1980 Biofeedback and tension headache. Lancet ii: 898–899

Editorial 1981 How does acupuncture work? British Medical Journal 283: 746–748

Editorial 1992 Vibration therapy for pain. Lancet 339: 1513–1514

Fagen E T 1982 Music therapy in the treatment of anxiety and fear in terminal patients. Music Therapy 2: 13–23

Filshie J, Redman D 1985 Acupuncture and malignant pain problems. European Journal of Surgical Oncology 11: 389–394

Finer B 1979 Hypnotherapy in pain and advanced cancer. In: Bonica J J, Ventafridda V (eds) Advances in pain research and therapy, vol 2. Raven Press, New York, pp 223–229

Fishman B 1990 The treatment of suffering in patients with cancer pain. In: Foley K M, Bonica J J, Ventafridda V (eds) Advances in pain research and therapy, vol 16. Raven Press, New York, pp 301–316

Fleming U 1985 Relaxation therapy for far-advanced cancer. The practitioner 229: 471–475

Fleming U 1988 Relaxation as a means of pain control. Journal of Orthopaedic Medicine 1: 21–23

Frampton D R 1986 Restoring creativity to the dying patient. British Medical Journal 293: 1593–1595

Freeman T B, Campbell J N, Long D M 1983 Naloxone does not affect pain relief induced by electrical stimulation in man. Pain 17: 189–195

Gammon D G, Starr J 1941 Studies on the relief of pain by counter-irritation. Journal of Clinical Investigation 20: 13–20

Gross J L, Swartkz R 1982 The effects of music therapy on anxiety in chronically ill patients. Music Therapy 2: 43–52

Han J S, Tang J, Ren M F, Zhou Z F, Fan S G, Qui X C 1980 Central neurotransmitters and acupuncture analgesia. American Journal of Clinical Medicine 8: 31–48

Haynes S, Griffin P, Mooney D, Parise M 1976 Electromyographic feedback and relaxation instructions in the treatment of muscle contraction headaches. Behavioural Therapy 6: 672–678

Hosobuchi Y, Adams J E, Linchitx R 1977 Pain relief by electrical stimulation of the central gray matter in humans and its reversal by naloxone. Science 197: 183–186

Jocobson E 1970 Modern treatment of tense patients. C C Thomas, Springfield: Illinois

Jensen M P, Turner J A, Romano J M, Karoly P 1991 Coping with chronic pain: a critical review of the literature. Pain 47: 249–283

Jessup 1989 Relaxation and biofeedback. In: Wall P D, Melzack R (eds) Textbook of pain, 2nd edn. Churchill Livingstone, Edinburgh, pp 989–1000

Johansson F, Almay B G L, Von Knorring L, Terenius L 1980 Predictors for the outcome of treatment with high frequency transcutaneous electrical nerve stimulation in patients with chronic pain. Pain 9: 55–61

Johnson M I, Ashton C H, Thompson J W 1991a An in-depth study of long-term users of transcutaneous electrical nerve stimulation (TENS): implications for clinical use of TENS. Pain 44: 221–229

Johnson M I, Ashton C H, Thompson J W 1991b The consistency of pulse frequencies and pulse patterns of transcutaneous electrical nerve stimulation (TENS) used by chronic pain patients. Pain 44: 231–234

Johnson M I, Ashton C H, Thompson J W 1993 A prospective investigation into factors related to patient response to transcutaneous electrical nerve stimulation (TENS): the importance of cortical responsivity. European Journal of Pain 14: 1–9

Kaada B 1982 Vasodilation induced by transcutaneous nerve stimulation in peripheral ischaemia (Raynaud's phenomenon and diabetic polyneuropathy). European Heart Journal 3: 303–314

Kaada B 1983 Promoted healing of chronic ulceration by transcutaneous nerve stimulation (TENS) and its vasa. Band 12: heft 3.

Keefe F J, Salley A N, Lefebvre J C 1992 Coping with pain: conceptual concerns and future directions. Pain 51: 131–134

Kogeorgos J, Scott D F 1981 Biofeedback and its clinical applications. British Journal of Hospital Medicine 25: 601–605

Lea P, Ware P, Monroe R 1960 The hypnotic control of intractable pain. American Journal of Clinical Hypnosis 3: 3–8

Lee C A 1989 The efficacy of music therapy for people living with HIV and AIDS. Conference proceedings — new developments in music therapy. British Society for Music Therapy 19–31

Levitan A A 1992 The use of hypnosis with cancer patients. Psychiatry and Medicine 10: 119–131

Lichter I 1987 Communication in Cancer Care. Churchill Livingstone, Edinburgh

Loscin R G 1981 The effect of music on the pain of selected postoperative patients. Journal of Advanced Nursing 6: 19–25

Lundeberg T 1984 Longterm results of vibratory stimulation as a pain relieving measure for chronic pain. Pain 20: 13–23

Lundeberg T 1985 Naloxone does not reverse the pain-reducing effect of vibratory stimulation. Acta Anaesthiologica Scandinavica 29: 212–216

Lundeberg T, Nordemar R, Ottoson D 1984 Pain alleviation by vibratory stimulation. Pain 20: 25–44

McCaffery M 1980 Relieving pain with non-invasive techniques. Nursing 10: 55–57

McCaffery M, Beebe A 1989. Pain: clinical manual for nursing practice. Mosby, St. Louis, pp 142–156

McCaffery M, Morra M E, Gross J, Moritz D A 1981 Dealing with pain. American Cancer Society, Connecticut Division, Yale Comprehensive Cancer Centre, pp 17–22

McGlone F P, Marsh D 1990 Stimulators for treatment of pain. In: Lipton S, Tunks E, Zoppi M (eds) Advances in pain research and therapy, vol 13. Raven Press, New York, pp 79–82

Magarey C 1981 Healing and meditation in medical practice. Medical Journal of Australia 1: 338–341

Malan D 1982 Individual psychotherapy and the science of psychodynamics. Butterworths, London

Man P L, Ning T L 1983 Electroacupuncture and electrostimulation for relief of chronic intractable pain. American Journal of Acupuncture 11: 143–147

Mandel S E 1991 Music therapy in the hospice: 'Musicalive'. Palliative Medicine 5: 155–160

Melzack R 1971 Phantom limb pain: implications for treatment of pathologic pain. Anaesthesiology 35: 409–419

Melzack R 1980 Psychologic aspects of pain. Pain 143–154

Melzack R, Perry C 1975 Self-regulation of pain: the use of alpha-biofeedback and hypnotic training for the control of chronic pain. Experimental Neurology 46: 452–469

Munroe S 1978 Music therapy in palliative care. The Canadian Medical Association Journal 119 (9): 1029–1034

Munroe S 1988 Music therapy in support of cancer patients. In: Senn H J, Glaus A M, Schmid L (eds) Recent results in cancer research, vol 108. Springer, Heidelberg, pp 289–294

Nielzen S , Sjolund B H, Eriksson B E 1982 Psychiatric factors influencing the treatment of pain with peripheral conditioning stimulation. Pain 13: 365–371

Orne M T 1980 Hypnotic control of pain: toward a clarification of the different psychological process involved. Pain 1550–1572

Palmesano T J, Clelland J A, Sherer C, Stullenbarger E, Canan B 1989 Effect of high frequency vibration on experimental pain threshold in young women when applied to areas of different size. Clinical Journal of Pain 5: 337–342

Patel C 1981 Meditation in general practice. British Medical Journal 282: 528–529

Patt R B 1992 Non-pharmacologic measures for controlling oncologic pain. American Journal of Hospice and Palliative Care 9 (6): 41–47

Phelps L A 1981 Suggestion therapy. American Family Physician 23: 145–148

Richardson P H, Vincent C A 1986 Acupuncture for the treatment of pain: a review of evaluative research. Pain 24: 15–40

Ritchie Russell W, Spalding J M K 1950 Treatment of painful amputation stumps. British Medical Journal 2: 68–73

Sacerdote P 1962 The place of hypnosis in the relief of severe protracted pain. American Journal of Clinical Hypnosis 4: 150–157

Sacerdote P 1970 Theory and practice of pain control in malignancy and other protracted or recurring painful illnesses. International Journal of Clinical and Experimental Hypnotherapy 18: 160–180

Schroeder-Sheker T 1993 Music for the dying: a personal account of the new field of music thanatology — history, theories, and clinical narratives. Advances 9: 36–48

Sherer C L, Clelland J A, O'Sullivan P, Doleys D M, Canan B 1986 The effect of two sites of high frequency vibration on cutaneous pain threshold. Pain 25: 133–138

Simonton O C, Matthews-Simonton S, Sparks T F 1980 Psychological intervention in the treatment of cancer. Psychosomatics 21: 226

Sjolund B, Eriksson M 1979 The influence of naloxone on analgesia produced by peripheral conditioning stimulation. Brain Research 173: 295–301

Sjolund B, Eriksson M 1980 Relief of pain by TENS. English translation 1985. John Wiley, Chichester

Snyder R 1992 Physical therapy in terminal illness. Clinical Management 12 (4): 96–100

Stamp J M, Wood D 1981 A comparative evaluation of transcutaneous electrical nerve stimulators (TENS). Sheffield University & Health Authority, Sheffield

Stamp J M, Rose B 1984 A comparative evaluation of transcutaneous electrical nerve stimulators (TENS) Part II. Sheffield University & Health Authority, Sheffield

Syrjala K L, Cummings C, Donaldson G W 1992 Hypnosis or cognitive behavioural training for the reduction of pain and nausea during cancer treatment: a controlled clinical trial. Pain 48: 137–146

Tan S Y 1982 Cognitive and cognitive-behavioural methods for pain control: a selective review. Pain 12: 201–228

Thompson J W 1987 The role of TENS for the control of pain. In: Doyle D (ed) 1986 International Symposium on Pain Control. Royal Society of Medicine, London, pp 27–47

Thompson J W 1988a Pharmacology of transcutaneous electrical nerve stimulation (TENS). Journal of Intractable Pain Society 7 (1): 33–40

Thompson J W 1988b Acupuncture or TENS for pain relief? Bulletin of the Australian Medical Acupuncture Society 7: 8–23

Thompson J W, Filshie J 1993 Transcutaneous Electrical Nerve Stimulation (TENS) and acupuncture. In: Doyle D, Hanks G W, MacDonald N (eds) Oxford Textbook of Palliative Medicine. Oxford University Press, Oxford, pp 229–244

Turk D C, Rennert K 1981 Pain and the terminally ill cancer patient: a cognitive-social learning perspective. In: Sobel H (ed) Behaviour therapy in terminal care, Ballinger, Cambridge, pp 95–123

Turk D C, Fernandez E 1990 On the putative uniqueness of cancer pain: do psychological principles apply? Behaviour Research and Therapy 28: 1–13

Turk D C, Meichenbaum D H, Berman W H 1979 Application of biofeedback for the regulation of pain: a critical review. Psychological Bulletin 86: 1322–1338

Turner J A, Chapman R C 1982 Psychological interventions for chronic pain: a critical review. 1. Relaxation training and biofeedback. Pain 12: 1–21

Turner J A, Clancy S 1986 Strategies for coping with chronic low back pain: relationship to pain and disability. Pain 24: 355–364

Tyrer S 1992 Psychology, psychiatry and chronic pain. Butterworth/Heinemann, London

Ventafridda V, Sganzerla E P, Fochi C, Pozzi G, Gordini G 1979 Transcutaneous nerve stimulation in cancer pain. In Bonica J J, Ventafridda V (eds) Advances in pain research and therapy, vol 2. Raven Press, New York, pp 509–515

Waxman D 1979 Wounds give no pain. Journal of the Royal Society of Medicine 72: 168–171

Wilkes E 1965 Terminal care at home. Lancet ii: 799–801

Woolf C J 1989 Segmental afferent fibre-induced analgesia: transcutaneous electrical nerve stimulation (TENS) and vibration. In: Wall P D, Melzack R (eds) Textbook of pain, 2nd edn. Churchill Livingstone, Edinburgh, pp 884–896

Woolf C J, Mitchell D, Myers R A, Barrett G D 1978 Failure of naloxone to reverse peripheral transcutaneous electro-analgesia in patients suffering from acute trauma. South African Medical Journal 53: 179–180

Woolf C J, Mitchell D, Barrett G D 1980 Antinociceptive effect of peripheral segmental electrical stimulation in the rat. Pain 8: 237–252

Zitman F G 1981 Biofeedback, relaxation training and chronic pain. In: Lipton S, Miles J (eds) Persistent pain, modern methods of treatment, vol 3. Academic Press, London, pp 99–117

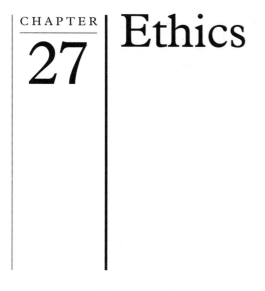

Ethics

The teaching of medical ethics is still patchy, and knowledge of ethics tends to be 'caught' rather than 'taught'. The emphasis in medical training usually results in the newly qualified doctor having a reasonable understanding of acute medical ethics but a poor understanding of chronic and palliative medical ethics.

QUALITY OF LIFE

'The goal of palliative care is achievement of the best possible quality of life for patients and their families' (WHO 1990).

'Quality . . . you know what it is, yet you don't know what it is. But that's self-contradictory. But some things are better than others, that is, they have more quality. But when you try to say what the quality is, apart from the things that have it, it all goes poof! There's nothing to talk about' (Pirsig 1976).

Despite the above comment, it is possible to move towards a definition of quality of life. It relates to subjective satisfaction. Quality of life measures will be flawed, therefore, if they measure only selected objective achievements rather than global satisfaction (van Dam et al 1984, Twycross 1987, Ballatori et al 1993).

Quality of life is influenced by all the dimensions of personhood — physical, psychological, social and spiritual (Cohen & Mount 1992). There is good quality of life when the aspirations of an individual are matched and fulfilled by present experience (Calman 1984). There is poor quality of life when there is a wide divergence between aspirations and present experience. To improve quality of life, it is necessary to narrow the gap between aspirations and what is possible (Fig. 27.1). Thus, a good quality of life in people receiving palliative care is likely to reflect more realism in setting goals as well

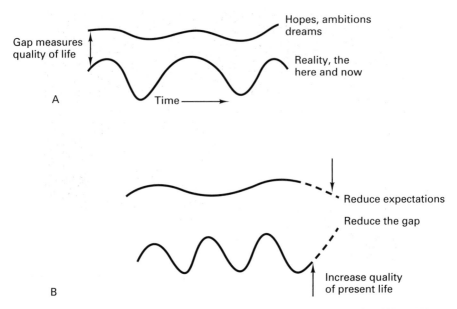

Fig. 27.1   A representation of the gap between reality and hopes, dreams and ambitions (A). Improvement in the quality of life represents either a reduction in expectations or a change in the present mixture of reality (B). (Reproduced with permission from Calman 1984.)

as improved pain and symptom relief. For example, a year after becoming tetraplegic, an ex-gymnastics instructor was able to say (Jonsen et al 1982):

> 'The quality of my life is excellent, though to see me you wouldn't believe it. I've come to terms with my loss and discovered the powers of my mind.'

Similar sentiments were expressed by Andy, a 38 year-old man with congenital neurofibromatosis (Fig. 27.2). He:

- had been paraplegic since the age of 14
- required positive pressure assisted respiration at night and increasingly during the day to maintain adequate oxygenation
- had become progressively less well over the previous year because of a presumed sarcoma of the right thigh
- was temporarily an inpatient at a palliative care unit because of exhaustion brought on by the demands of self-care at home.

He said 2 days before returning home and 4 days before he died:

> 'On a scale of 0–10, my quality of life is 9.5. And when I get over this little blip, it will be back to 10 again.'

The following is an extract from the eulogy given by a friend at Andy's funeral:

> 'It was some years ago, when I was visiting Andy in hospital. He had tubes everywhere, his skin was sore, and every breath seemed to require an effort. I

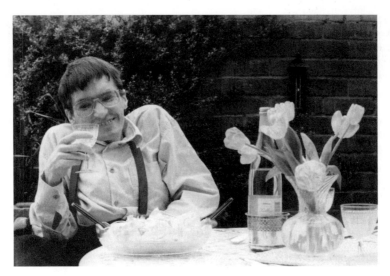

Fig. 27.2   Andy enjoying high quality life despite paraplegia and other physical disabilities.

asked him if he ever felt like giving up, if there were days when the struggle just didn't seem worth the effort. Andy looked rather shocked. "Oh no," he replied "I've had such a wonderful life: I've been so loved." Andy's life was packed full of love and determination and courage, and he went on planning right up to the end.'

MEDICAL OBLIGATIONS AT THE END OF LIFE

The statement of the Council on Ethical and Judicial Affairs of the American Medical Association on 'Withholding or Withdrawing Life-Prolonging Medical Treatment' provides a good summary of the doctor's responsibility to patients at the end of life (Box 27.A). The statement stresses that the ethical standards of professional conduct and responsibility may exceed but are never less than, or contrary to, those required by the law. The following reports are recommended for further reading:

- Hastings Center (1987)
- Appleton Consensus (1989)
- WHO Expert Committee (1990).

ETHICAL PRINCIPLES

The ethical principles governing medical practice have been summarized in four words (Beauchamp & Childress 1983, WHO 1990):

- beneficence
- nonmaleficence
- autonomy
- justice.

BOX 27.A
STATEMENT ON WITHHOLDING OR WITHDRAWING LIFE-PROLONGING MEDICAL TREATMENT (COUNCIL ON ETHICAL AND JUDICIAL AFFAIRS, AMERICAN MEDICAL ASSOCIATION)

The social commitment of the physician is to sustain life and relieve suffering. Where the performance of one duty conflicts with the other, the choice of the patient, or his family or legal representative if the patient is incompetent to act on his own behalf, should prevail. In the absence of the patient's choice or an authorized proxy, the physician must act in the best interest of the patient.

For humane reasons, with informed consent, a physician may do what is medically necessary to alleviate severe pain, or cease or omit treatment to permit a terminally ill patient whose death is imminent to die. However, he should not intentionally cause death. In deciding whether the administration of potentially life-prolonging medical treatment is in the best interest of the patient who is incompetent to act on his own behalf, the physician should determine what the possibility is for extending life under humane and comfortable conditions and what are the prior expressed wishes of the patient and attitudes of the family or those who have responsibility for the custody of the patient.

Even if death is not imminent but a patient's coma is beyond doubt irreversible and there are adequate safeguards to confirm the accuracy of the diagnosis and with the concurrence of those who have responsibility for the care of the patient, it is not unethical to discontinue all means of life-prolonging medical treatment.

Life-prolonging medical treatment includes medication and artificially or technologically supplied respiration, nutrition, or hydration. In treating a terminally ill or irreversibly comatose patient, the physician should determine whether the benefits of treatment outweigh its burdens. At all times, the dignity of the patient should be maintained (Dickey 1986).

Perhaps a better synopsis is one in which medical ethics are portrayed as a series of dichotomies:

- preserve life v. relieve suffering
- do good (beneficence) v. minimize harm (nonmaleficence)
- needs and demands of the individual (autonomy) v. needs and demands of society (justice)

In other words:

- the doctor and the caring team will normally strive to preserve a life of the patient until this is clearly futile
- it is necessary to balance the potential benefits of treatment against potential burdens
- the needs and wishes of an individual are balanced against the needs and wishes of society as a whole

The question of a fair distribution and use of medical resources applies here as elsewhere (WHO 1990, Whedon & Ferrell 1991). In this and other respects, palliative care does not differ in principle from other clinical situations. It affirms life but, at the same time, acknowledges the ultimate inevitability of death. Palliative care, therefore, seeks neither to hasten nor to postpone death (Twycross 1982a). Further, as already noted, palliative care also stresses the importance of regarding the patient and the family as the 'unit of care'.

PARTNERSHIP

Patient autonomy is not an absolute principle (Loewy 1992). For example, a patient cannot force a doctor to act against his professional judgement, or in an unethical or unlawful manner. Likewise, a person cannot force society to accept a course of action which, although considered a benefit by that person, is considered detrimental to the wellbeing of society as a whole. There is, in fact, much to be said for substituting a more broadly based ethic, namely, 'partnership with the patient'. Partnership represents the midpoint on a spectrum between medical paternalism and medical permissiveness (Spreeuwenberg 1989). Partnership necessitates training by a doctor in:

- pain and symptom relief
- psychosocial evaluation
- communication skills
- awareness of how to respond to spiritual issues.

Partnership is creative and profoundly influences the relationship between professional carer and patient (Box 27.B).

Doctors, however, often act as if patients have an obligation to accept all recommended treatment. It is salutary to recall, therefore, that a doctor is laying himself open to legal censure if he forces treatment upon a patient. A doctor has an obligation to discuss treatment options and their implications with his patients, including those who are frail and elderly or terminally ill.

Treatment against a person's wishes is strictly controlled by statute and, ethically, can be justified only on the grounds of necessity. In the UK, patients who are suffering from mental disorder and pose a threat to the health or safety of themselves, or others, may be considered for compulsory detention and/or treatment under the Mental Health Act 1983.

BOX 27.B
PARTNERSHIP WITH THE PATIENT

Avoid an authoritarian manner.

Explain the reason(s) for the pain and/or other symptoms in straightforward language.

Agree on priorities and goals.

Discuss treatment options and care plans, and jointly decide on any necessary action.

Facilitate the continuing care of the patient at home if that is the patient's wish.

Do not withhold the truth about the illness from the patient at the request of a third party.

Respect the patient's wish to decline treatment even if this may result in the patient dying sooner than otherwise might be the case.

APPROPRIATE TREATMENT

In advanced cancer the primary aim of treatment is no longer to prolong life but to make what life remains as comfortable and as meaningful as possible. It is not a question of 'To treat or not to treat?' but 'What is the most appropriate treatment?' given the patient's biological prospects and his personal and social circumstances. Cardiac resuscitation, artificial respiration, IV infusions, nasogastric tubes, and antibiotics are all primarily supportive measures for use in acute or acute on chronic illnesses, to assist a patient through the initial period towards recovery of health (Fig. 27.3). To use such measures in patients close to death and with no hope of a return to health is inappropriate (Fig. 27.4). If inappropriate, it is bad medicine; a doctor has no legal or ethical duty to prescribe a lingering death (Thompson 1984, Dickey 1986). In other words, he does not have a duty to preserve life at all cost. For example, when pneumonia supervenes in terminal cancer,

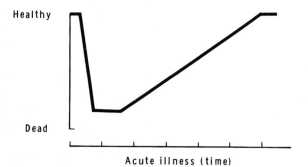

Fig. 27.3 A graphical representation of acute illness. Biological prospects are generally good. Acute resuscitative measures are important and enable the patient to survive the initial crisis. Recovery is aided by the natural forces of healing; rehabilitation is completed by the patient on his own, without continued medical support.

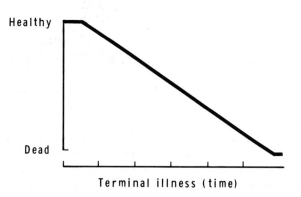

Fig. 27.4 A graphical representation of terminal illness. Biological prospects progressively worsen. Acute and terminal illnesses are therefore distinct pathophysiological entities. Therapeutic interventions that can best be described as prolonging the distress of dying are both futile and inappropriate.

morphine and hyoscine are commonly prescribed to quieten the cough and reduce troublesome secretions; antibiotics are inappropriate in this situation (Twycross 1982b).

Medical care is a continuum, ranging from complete cure at one end to symptom relief at the other. Many types of treatment span the entire spectrum of care, notably radiotherapy. It is important, therefore, to keep the therapeutic aim clearly in mind when ordering investigations and planning treatment. In palliative care, the key points to bear in mind are:

- the patient's general condition and medical prognosis
- the therapeutic aim of each treatment
- the potential benefits of treatment from the patient's point of view
- the adverse effects of treatment
- the need not to prescribe a lingering death.

Treatment remains active however; 'passive care' is a contradiction in terms. Efficient, good quality care is what is called for, not just 'tender loving care' — a term sometimes used to justify neglect (Saunders 1982).

In patients who are close to death it is often appropriate to 'give death a chance'. All patients must die eventually; ultimately nature will take its course. In this respect, the art of medicine is to decide when life sustenance is futile and, therefore, when to allow death to occur without further impediment. For example, although antibiotics are generally appropriate for a patient with advanced cancer who develops a chest infection while still relatively active and independent, pneumonia should still be 'the old man's friend' in those who are close to death. In this circumstance, it is generally appropriate not to prescribe antibiotics.

If it is difficult to make a decision, the 'two days rule' should be invoked, i.e. if after two or three days of symptom relief the patient is holding his own, prescribe an antibiotic but, if the patient is much worse, do not. Not all terminally ill patients who develop a chest infection die from it. A few recover spontaneously, instinctively fighting on. Some progress only to 'grumbling pneumonia' but no further. A continuing wet cough is often distressing and may interrupt sleep. In this circumstance, if the patient is neither better nor worse after several days, an antibiotic is indicated for symptom relief.

LETTING NATURE TAKE ITS COURSE

It is sometimes said that the ethical justification for 'letting nature take its course' relies on the principle of acts and omissions. This states that, in certain situations, a failure to perform an act (e.g. to prescribe an antibiotic for a patient with terminal cancer who develops pneumonia) is less bad than performing a different act (e.g. administering a lethal overdose) which has identical predictable consequences. In other words, it is more reprehensible to kill someone than to allow a person to die. The principle of acts and omissions, however, is rarely relevant in palliative care. In practice, therapeutic recommendations are based on a consideration of the possible advantages and disadvantages which might accrue to the patient.

A doctor is not a technician and there are generally several courses of action which might legitimately be adopted. Arguments in favour of a certain treatment revolve around the question of the anticipated effectiveness of intervention. Linked with this are considerations of the consequences or implications for the patient, his family, and society as a whole. In other words, the doctor seeks, on the basis of the biological and social facts at his disposal, to offer the patient the most appropriate form of care.

■ CASE HISTORY

A 52 year-old man had disseminated small cell cancer of the lung which was resistant to second line chemotherapy. He became lethargic, weak and confused as a result of hypercalcaemia. The patient had had nerve compression pain which was now relieved. He had spoken repeatedly of his fear of developing pain again and had stated that he wanted 'no heroics' to prolong his life. After discussion with his wife and children, his doctor decided that this patient, who was now confused, would not want even this initial hypercalcaemic episode to be reversed. The wife's agreement was documented, and the patient was classified 'do not resuscitate' in accordance with hospital policy. IV fluids were not started. Analgesics and other comfort measures were maintained and he died peacefully 4 days later (Lack 1984).

When a person is within a few days of death, interest in hydration and nutrition often becomes minimal. This is a situation when it is wrong to force a patient to accept fluid and food, if clearly he does not wish to. The disinterest or positive disinclination should be seen as part of the process of 'letting go'. If the distinction between acute and terminal illness is ignored, however, the situation will not be evaluated in terms of what is biologically appropriate (and therefore in the patient's best interest) but will be seen as a question of 'to treat or not to treat?' A failure to resolve what appears to be an ethical dilemma commonly results in unnecessary suffering for the patient as life sustaining measures continue to be used despite their essential futility (Twycross 1982a, 1982b). The following case history describes how inappropriate interventions prolonged a woman's dying and added greatly to her suffering.

■ CASE HISTORY

A 65 year-old woman had extensive head and neck cancer which was resistant to radiation and chemotherapy. She gradually became unable to swallow or speak. Pain relief was a constant problem and she began to self-administer SC morphine q4h. On this she was alert and able to live alone, although not completely painfree. Several attempts at passing an oesophageal tube failed. Prolonged staff discussions took place on whether it was ethical to allow her to 'starve to death'. The patient refused to return to the hospital and wrote that, although weak, she was not hungry and wanted no further surgery. She was found in a coma by the visiting nurse and was admitted to hospital. A gastrostomy was performed and she was transferred to a nursing home where she died a month later. The nursing home was unable to maintain 'round-the-clock' opioid administration and her sister stopped visiting because she could not bear to see her sister in pain (Lack 1984).

PUTTING THEORY INTO PRACTICE

■ CASE HISTORY

In 1992, an experienced rheumatologist in the UK was convicted of manslaughter for killing a terminally ill patient with intravenous potassium chloride. According to reports in the media, the patient suffered from severe rheumatoid arthritis, was bedbound, had a gastric ulcer and bedsores; all agreed that her life expectancy was very short. Some days before, the patient had begged the doctor to end it all — a request which he refused. She in turn refused to continue taking corticosteroids — possibly in the hope that stopping them might speed up her dying. The doctor prescribed diamorphine (exact dose and schedule not known) and diazepam (exact dose and schedule not known). The combination failed to relieve the patient's pain. In desperation the doctor decided to kill the patient in order to kill the pain. Reactions to his conviction varied widely. Some felt that the conviction of a doctor for an act of compassion in a dying woman was abhorrent; others felt that the suspended sentence was inadequate and that, in the words of the judge, the doctor had betrayed the medical profession.

When reflecting on the dilemma facing the doctor, the key question is: is it ever necessary to kill a dying patient in order to kill the pain? It the answer is no, then clearly doctors cannot plead necessity (*force majeure*). In other words, if suffering can be relieved within the law, doctors cannot justify stepping outside it. It is important, however, not to oversimplify the potential dilemma. As already noted, doctors have two general responsibilities, namely, to preserve life and to relieve suffering — and inevitably there will be times when the two are in conflict.

When a terminally ill patient is close to death, preserving life becomes increasingly meaningless and the emphasis on relieving suffering becomes paramount. Even here, however, the doctor is obliged to achieve his objective with minimum risk to the patient's life. This means that treatment to relieve pain and suffering which co-incidentally brings forward the moment of death by a few hours or days is acceptable (the principle of double effect) but administering a drug such as potassium or curare, whose primary action is to cause death, is not acceptable. As Lord Justice Devlin stated in the UK in the late 1950s:

'A doctor who is aiding the dying does not have to calculate in minutes, or even in hours, and perhaps not in days or weeks, the effects upon a patient's life of the medicines he administers or else be in peril of a charge of murder.'

Similar sentiments have been expressed by others:

'A physician cannot be held criminally liable for undertaking or continuing the administration of appropriate palliative care in order to eliminate or reduce the suffering of an individual, only because of the effect that this action might have on the latter's life expectancy' (Law Reform Commission 1983).

'The duty of the physician consists more in striving to relieve pain than in prolonging as long as possible with every available means a life that is no longer fully human and that is naturally coming to its conclusion' (Pope Paul VI, quoted by Colombo 1980).

Giving drugs to relieve pain should not, therefore, be equated with giving a lethal dose deliberately to end life (Roy 1987, Carlson 1990, Hennepin County Medical Society 1990). Sometimes the use of an opioid may marginally shorten the patient's life, but if given for sound medical reasons and in an appropriate dose, the giving of such a drug plays no part in the legal causation of death. Nor is it the moral equivalent of killing the patient deliberately, because the drug is given for the relief of pain. If the patient dies as a result, it is considered from a moral viewpoint to be a secondary effect — foreseeable maybe, but not directly intended (Roy 1988).

In practice, however, and contrary to popular belief, the appropriate use of morphine in the relief of cancer pain carries less risk than the use of aspirin or other NSAID. Morphine given regularly, particularly by mouth, is a very safe drug. If the patient is dying from exhaustion, however, as a result of weeks or months of intolerable pain associated with insomnia and poor nutrition, any drug with a sedative effect is likely to tip the scales in the direction of death. Generally, the correct use of morphine *prolongs* a patient's life rather than shortens it because he is more rested and painfree.

So in this case, what more could the doctor have done to ease his patient's pain and suffering? The answer is: quite a lot. What he *should* have done, however, depends on the diagnosis:

- was he giving doses of diamorphine which were too small?
- was he endeavouring to relieve pain which was poorly responsive to opioids with diamorphine alone?
- was he dealing with a case of morphine induced pain?
- was he dealing with 'terminal anguish' and relying on diazepam alone to relieve this?

It is possible that the doctor simply failed to increase the dose of diamorphine high enough and fast enough. On the other hand, to rely on diamorphine alone to relieve pain related to movement, particularly in someone with arthritis, is a fundamental mistake — but one still made. In this circumstance, a NSAID and a strong opioid should be prescribed concurrently. Ideally therefore, the patient should have been persuaded to continue any long term arthritic analgesic medication.

She had a gastric ulcer: did that mean she had stopped taking a NSAID? With the various gastroprotective agents on the market, a gastric ulcer is not an absolute contra-indication to the continued use of a NSAID (Roth et al 1989, Lancaster-Smith et al 1991, Fenn & Robinson 1991). Further, several NSAIDs can be given by suppository or SC infusion in patients who are too ill to swallow. Thus, my advice would have been to give diamorphine by continuous SC infusion using a portable syringe driver, together with a NSAID by either suppository or SC infusion.

The question of morphine induced pain is clearly important (see p. 257). As noted elsewhere, reports of this rare condition link it with high doses of *intrathecal* morphine and diamorphine and with *multigramme* IV doses, i.e. doses much greater than those used in this case. But supposing it *was* morphine induced pain, what could the doctor have done? After taking advice from a palliative medicine or pain relief clinic colleague he could have changed to fentanyl or methadone — both of which are readily available in parenteral forms. And if those colleagues were unaware of morphine induced pain, he would undoubtedly have been advised to render the patient unconscious until her imminent death ensued.

What about distress in the dying? As with other symptoms, careful evaluation is important (Back 1992). A full bladder or rectum may be the cause. However, assuming there is no readily correctible cause, an anxiolytic-sedative should be given — as happened in this case. But, although diazepam may sometimes be a good drug in this situation, it is not always so. Many patients need a neuroleptic such as haloperidol or chlorpromazine. Indeed, a combination of a benzodiazepine and a neuroleptic is often needed.

In a few patients, however, sedation serves only to make matters worse as the patient panics in response to drug induced drowsiness. This condition, usually associated with a confusional state, has been called 'terminal anguish' (Twycross & Lichter 1993). Possibly, this is what the doctor was faced with here. It is distressing for all concerned and may respond only to heavy sedation with a benzodiazepine (diazepam or midazolam) *and* a neuroleptic (haloperidol, chlorpromazine or methotrimeprazine). Alternatively, some centres recommend chlormethiazole or a barbiturate (phenobarbitone, amylobarbitone or thiopentone).

The dose of benzodiazepine and neuroleptic is arbitrary; it depends on what has previously been used and failed (i.e. even higher doses). The dose of IV chlormethiazole is that recommended in the British National Formulary for use in status epilepticus. The dose of SC phenobarbitone also varies: 100–200 mg stat and 600–1200 mg/24 h by SC infusion. Guidelines for IV amylobarbitone and IV thiopentone are available (Greene & Davis 1991). The aim with all of these manoeuvres is to relieve the patient's distress. Usually, this necessitates the patient being kept unconscious until death.

What is the difference between this and what the rheumatologist did? After all, both result in the patient's death. One difference is that the use of heavy sedation in this circumstance is both ethical and legal, whereas what the rheumatologist did is not. If a doctor can achieve his goal within the law, he cannot claim necessity as a reason for breaking the law. So should the law be changed? After all, IV potassium is quicker, easier and cheaper than the cocktails referred to above. In my opinion the answer to that is an emphatic 'no'. Deliberate death acceleration (euthanasia) would take the medical profession and society over a dividing line which, however thin it may become on rare occasions, they cross at their peril (Gaylin et al 1988, Twycross 1990). The experience in the Netherlands shows beyond reasonable doubt that abuse follows use of euthanasia as an instrument to relieve terminal pain and distress (van de Maas et al 1991, Gunning 1991, Ferguson et al 1991, Keown 1992, van de Wal et al 1992).

The dividing line is based on intent. With one path of action, the primary intent is to relieve suffering while respecting an ultimate prohibition on the taking of life. With the other, the primary intent is to take life in order to relieve suffering. And, as stressed in a Report from the World Health Organization:

> 'Now that a practicable alternative to death in pain exists, there should be concentrated efforts to implement programmes of palliative care, rather than a yielding to pressure for legal euthanasia' (WHO 1990).

In this connection, it is salutary to note that patients tend to be sedated when the carers have reached the limit of their resources and are no longer able to stand the patient's problems without anxiety, impatience, guilt, anger or despair (Main 1957). A sedative will alter the situation and produce a patient who, if not dead, is at least quiet.

> 'Perhaps many of the desperate treatments in medicine can be justified by expediency, but history has an awkward habit of judging some as fashions, more helpful to the therapist than to the patient' (Main 1957).

AT THE END OF THE DAY

Palliative care developed as a reaction to the attitude, spoken or unspoken, that ' there is nothing more that we can do for you' with the inevitable consequence for the patient and family of a sense of abandonment, hopelessness and despair. It was stressed that this was never true — there is always something that can be done. Yet, while this is generally so, there are times when a nurse or doctor has nothing specific to do for a patient and, in consequence, feels that she/he has nothing to offer. In such a situation, we are thrown back on who we are as individuals.

> 'Slowly, I learn about the importance of powerlessness. I experience it in my own life and I live with it in my work. The secret is not to be afraid of it — not to run away. The dying know we are not God . . . All they ask is that we do not desert them' (Cassidy 1988).

There are circumstances, therefore, in which it is necessary to relinquish the 'Dr Fix-it' and 'Nurse Fix-it' attitudes imbued during training. When there is nothing to offer except ourselves, a belief that life has meaning and purpose helps to sustain the carer. However, to speak glibly of this to a patient who is in despair serves only to distance the carer from the patient. At such a time companionship is crucial, and actions (i.e. the continuing attention of the doctor) are better than words. By what we *do*, we seek to convey the essential message:

> 'You matter because you are you.
> You matter to the last moment of your life,

and we will do all we can

not only to help you die peacefully,

but to live until you die' (Cicely Saunders).

REFERENCES

Appleton Consensus 1989 Suggested international guidelines for decisions to forego medical treatment. Journal of Medical Ethics 15: 129–136

Appleton Consensus 1989 Suggested international guidelines for decisions to forego medical treatment. Ugeskr Laeger 151: 700–706

Back I N 1992 Terminal restlessness in patients with advanced malignant disease. Palliative Medicine 6: 293–298

Ballatori E, Roila F, Basurto C et al 1993 Reliability and validity of a quality of life questionnaire in cancer patients. European Journal of Cancer 29a (suppl 1): S63–S69

Beauchamp T L, Childress J F 1983 Principles of biomedical ethics, 2nd edn. Oxford University Press, Oxford

Calman K C 1984 Quality of life in cancer patients an hypothesis. Journal of Medical Ethics 10: 124–127

Carlson P J 1990 Response to the joint guidelines of the Hennepin Country Attorney and the Hennepin County Medical Examiner. Minnesota Medicine 73: 35–36

Cassidy S 1988 Sharing the darkness. Darton, Longman & Todd, London, pp 61–64

Cohen S R, Mount B M 1992 Quality of life in terminal illness: defining and measuring subjective well-being in the dying. Journal of Palliative Care 8(3): 40–45

Colombo G (quoting Pope Paul VI) 1980 In: Twycross R G, Ventafridda V (eds) The continuing care of terminal patients. Pergamon Press, Oxford, p. xix

Dickey N W 1986 Withholding or withdrawing life-prolonging medical treatment. Journal of the American Medical Association 256: 471

Fenn G C, Robinson C G 1991 Misoprostol: a logical therapeutic approach to gastroduodenal mucosal injury induced by nonsteroidal anti-inflammatory drugs. Journal of Clinical Pharmacy and Therapeutics 16: 385–409

Fergusson A, George R, Norris P, Twycross R, Winter R 1991 Euthanasia. Lancet 338: 1010–1011

Gaylin W, Kass L R Pellegrino E D, Siegler M 1988 Doctors must not kill. Journal of the American Medical Association 259: 2139–2140

Greene W R, Davis W H 1991 Titrated intravenous barbiturates in the control of symptoms in patients with terminal cancer. Southern Medical Journal 84: 332–337

Gunning K F 1991 Euthanasia. Lancet 338: 1010

Hastings Center Report 1987 Guidelines on the Termination of Life-Sustaining Treatment and the Care of the Dying. Indiana University Press, Bloomington

Hennepin County Medical Society 1990 Position paper on management of pain and suffering in the dying patient. Minnesota Medicine 73: 36–37

Jonsen A R, Siegler M, Winslade W J 1992 Clinical ethics. A practical approach to ethical decisions in clinical medicine. Bailliere Tindall, London

Keown I J 1991 The law and practice of euthanasia in the Netherlands. The Law Quarterly Review 108: 51–78

Lack S A 1984 Non-invasive measures. In: Twycross R G (ed) Clinics in oncology. Pain relief in cancer, vol 3, number 1. W B Saunders, London, pp 167–180

Lancaster-Smith M J, Jaderberg M E, Jackson D A 1991 Ranitidine in the treatment of nonsteroidal anti-inflammatory drug associated gastric and duodenal ulcers. Gut 32: 252–255

Law Reform Commission 1983 Euthanasia, aiding suicide and cessation of treatment. Law Reform Commission of Canada, Ottawa, p. 32

Loewy E H 1992 Advance directives and surrogate laws. Achieve of Internal Medicine 152: 1973–1976

Main T F 1957 The ailment. British Journal of Medical Psychology 30: 129–145

Pirsig R M 1976 Zen and the art of motorcycle maintenance. Transworld, Buffalo

Roth S, Agrawal N, Mahowald M et al 1989 Misoprostol heals gastroduodenal injury in patients with rheumatoid arthritis receiving aspirin. Rheumatoid Archives of Internal Medicine 149: 775–779

Roy D J 1987 Ethics in palliative care. Journal of Palliative Care 3: 3–5

Roy D J 1988 Decisions and dying: questions of clinical ethics. In: Bolaria B, Dickinson H D (eds) Sociology of health care in Canada. Harcourt Brace Jovanovich, Toronto, pp 527–536

Saunders C 1982 Principles of symptom control in terminal care. In: Reidenberg M M (ed) The Medical clinics of North America. Volume 66/Number 5. Clinical Pharmacology of Symptom Control. W B Saunders, Philadelphia, pp 1169–1183

Spreeuwenberg C 1989 Terminale thuiszorg: sterven in Nederland. Medisch Contact 44: 179–181

Thompson I 1984 Ethical issues in palliative care. In: Doyle D (ed) Palliative care. The management of far-advanced illness. Croom Helm, London, pp 461–485

Twycross R G 1982a Euthanasia: a physician's viewpoint. Journal of Medical Ethics 8: 86–95

Twycross R G 1982b Ethical and clinical aspects of pain treatment in cancer patients. Acta Anaesthesiologica Scandinavica 74: 83–90

Twycross R G 1987 Quality before quantity. A note of caution. Palliative Medicine 1: 65–72

Twycross R G 1990 Assisted death: a reply. Lancet 336: 796–798

Twycross R G, Lichter I 1993 The terminal phase. In: Doyle D, Hanks G W, MacDonald N (eds) The Oxford textbook of palliative medicine. Oxford University Press, Oxford, pp 649–661

Van Dam F S A M, Linssen C A G, Couzijn A L 1984 Evaluating quality of life in cancer clinical trials. In: Buyse M E, Staquet M J, Sylvester R J (eds) Cancer clinical trials: methods and practice. Oxford University Press, Oxford, pp 26–43

Van der Maas P J, van Delden J J M, Pijnenborg L, Looman C W N 1991 Euthanasia and other medical decisions concerning the end of life. The Lancet 338: 669–674

Van del Wal G, Leenen H J J, Spreeuwenberg C 1992 Reported cases of euthanasia: More often reported, less frequently prosecuted (in Dutch). Medisch Contact 47: 1023–1028

Whedon M, Ferrell B R 1991 Professional and ethical considerations in the use of high-tech pain management. Oncology Nursing Forum 18: 1135–1143

WHO Expert Committee Report 1990 Cancer Pain Relief and Palliative Care. Technical Report Series No. 804. World Health Organization, Geneva

Index